Surgical Treatment of Rheumatoid Arthritis

Surgical Treatment of Rheumatoid Arthritis

THOMAS P. SCULCO, M.D.

Clinical Professor of Orthopaedic Surgery
Cornell University Medical College
Associate Director of Orthopaedic Surgery
Co-Director, Surgical Arthritis Service
Hospital for Special Surgery
Consultant, Memorial Sloan Kettering Cancer Center
New York, New York

Forewords by
Lee Ramsay Straub, M.D.
Graham R.V. Hughes, M.D., F.R.C.P.

Mosby Year Book

St. Louis Baltimore Boston Chicago London Philadelphia Sydney Toronto

Mosby Year Book
Dedicated to Publishing Excellence

Sponsoring Editors: James D. Ryan, Jr./Joyce-Rachel John
Assistant Director, Manuscript Services: Frances M. Perveiler
Production Manager: Nancy C. Baker
Proofroom Manager: Barbara Kelly

Mosby-Year Book, Inc.
11830 Westline Industrial Drive
St. Louis, MO 63146

1 2 3 4 5 6 7 8 9 0 CL/MV 96 95 94 93 92

Library of Congress Cataloging-in-Publication Data

Surgical treatment of rheumatoid arthritis / [edited by] Thomas P. Sculco.
p. cm.
Includes bibliographical references and index.
ISBN 0-8016-6279-6
1. Rheumatoid arthritis—Surgery. I. Sculco, Thomas P.
[DNLM: 1. Arthritis, Rheumatoid—surgery. WE 346 S9613]
RD686.S874 1992
617.4'72059—dc20
DNLM/DLC 91-46178
for Library of Congress CIP

This text is dedicated to the many patients I have cared for afflicted with rheumatoid arthritis. From their courage and perseverance we as physicians gain strength to strive continually to solve and unravel the mysteries of this disabling disease.

Contributors

Michael M. Alexiades, M.D.
Assistant Professor of Orthopaedic Surgery
Cornell University Medical College
Assistant Orthopaedic Attending
Hospital for Special Surgery
New York, New York

David A. Behrman, D.M.D.
Assistant Professor of Surgery, Oral and Maxillofacial Surgery
Cornell University Medical College
Associate Attending Surgeon, Oral and Maxillofacial Surgery
The New York Hospital
New York, New York

Roberta Brockman, M.D.
Assistant Professor of Surgery (Orthopaedics)
Cornell University Medical College
Assistant Attending Orthopaedic Surgeon
Hospital for Special Surgery
New York, New York

Charles L. Christian, M.D.
Professor of Medicine
Cornell University Medical College
Physician-in-Chief
Hospital for Special Surgery
New York, New York

Edward F. DiCarlo, M.D.
Assistant Professor of Pathology
Cornell University Medical College
Assistant Pathologist
The Hospital for Special Surgery
New York, New York

Mark P. Figgie, M.D.
Instructor in Surgery
Cornell University Medical College
Assistant Attending Orthopaedic Surgeon
Hospital for Special Surgery
New York, New York

William F. Flynn, Jr., M.D.
Fellow in Orthopaedic Surgery
Cornell University Medical College
Junior Attending Orthopaedic Surgeon
Hospital for Special Surgery
New York, New York

Sandy B. Ganz, M.S., P.T.
Adjunct Instructor
Hunter College
Clinical Supervisor/Physical Therapy
Department of Rehabilitation
The Hospital for Special Surgery
New York, New York

Mark J. Geppert, M.D.
Fellow, Foot and Ankle Service
The Hospital for Special Surgery
New York, New York

Michelle Gerwin, M.D.
Senior Clinical Associate in Surgery
Cornell University Medical College
Senior Resident, Orthopeadic Surgery
The Hospital for Special Surgery
New York, New York

Bernard Ghelman, M.D.
Associate Professor of Radiology
Cornell University Medical College
Attending Radiologist
The Hospital for Special Surgery
New York, New York

Toni I. Golin, O.T.R.
Adjunct Instructor
Hunter College
Chief Occupational Therapist
Department of Rehabilitation
The Hospital for Special Surgery
New York, New York

Louis L. Harris, M.S., P.T.
Associate Professor
Hunter College School of Physical Therapy
Director, Department of Rehabilitation
The Hospital for Special Surgery
New York, New York

Allan E. Inglis, M.D.
Clinical Professor of Cell Biology and Human Anatomy
Professor of Clinical Surgery
Cornell University Medical Center
Director, Reconstructive and Surgical Arthritis Center
Beth Israel North
Hospital for Special Surgery
New York, New York

Norman A. Johanson, M.D.
Associate Professor of Orthopaedic Surgery
Temple University Medical School
Associate Attending Orthopaedic Surgeon
Temple University Hospital
Philadelphia, Pennsylvania

Matthew J. Kraay, M.S., M.D.
Clinical Instructor in Orthopaedics
Case Western Reserve University
Attending Orthopaedic Surgeon
University Hospitals of Cleveland
Cleveland, Ohio

Thomas J. A. Lehman, M.D., F.A.A.P., A.C.R.
Associate Professor of Pediatrics
Cornell University Medical Center
Chief, Division of Pediatric Rheumatology
Hospital for Special Surgery
New York, New York

Barry M. Libin, D.D.S., M.S.D.
Clinical Instructor in Surgery, Dentistry
Cornell University Medical College
Assistant Attending Dentist
The New York Hospital
New York, New York

Jay D. Mabrey, M.D.
Fellow in Biomechanics
Department of Biomechanics
The Hospital for Special Surgery
New York, New York

Michael J. Maynard, M.D.
Fellow in Orthopaedic Surgery
Cornell University Medical College
Junior Attending Orthopaedic Surgeon
Hospital for Special Surgery
New York, New York

Nancy Nichols, O.T.R.
Adjunct Instructor
Hunter College
Senior Occupational Therapist
The Hospital for Special Surgery
New York, New York

James C. Otis, Ph.D.
Associate Professor of Biomechanical Engineering in Surgery (Orthopaedics)
Cornell University Medical College
Senior Scientist
Department of Biomechanics
The Hospital for Special Surgery
New York, New York

Hollis G. Potter, M.D.
Assistant Professor of Radiology
Cornell University Medical College
Assistant Attending Radiologist
The Hospital for Special Surgery
New York, New York

Chitranjan S. Ranawat, M.D.
Professor of Orthopaedic Surgery
Cornell University Medical College
Attending Surgeon
Hospital for Special Surgery
New York, New York

Kevin V. Sanborn, M.D.
Clinical Associate Professor of Anesthesiology
Cornell University Medical College
Associate Attending Anesthesiologist
Hospital for Special Surgery
New York, New York

Thomas P. Sculco, M.D.
Clinical Professor of Orthopaedic Surgery
Cornell University Medical College
Associate Director of Orthopaedic Surgery
Co-Director, Surgical Arthritis Service
Hospital for Special Surgery
Consultant, Memorial Sloan Kettering Cancer Center
New York, New York

Mark Sobel, M.D.
Senior Resident Orthopaedic Surgery
The Hospital for Special Surgery
New York, New York

Foreword

Rheumatoid arthritis is a complex disease of many presentations. It may truly be the "Great Imitator" in our collection of painful inflammatory chronic diseases. Painful swollen joints, one or many, acute or chronic, may be tuberculous or gout or even luetic. These conditions may look alike clinically. These and other diseases, as well as trauma and stress, may be borne in mind when considering a differential diagnosis. Rheumatoid arthritis is a disastrous disease both personally and nationally in economic loss.

The course of disease in rheumatoid arthritis is unpredictable. It may remain at low levels for many years, or may progress rapidly in spite of therapy. Thirty years ago we followed a patient who suffered from severe juvenile rheumatoid arthritis. She had complete ankylosis of both elbows and serious limitation of motion in both knees. She had not been outside her apartment for about 10 years, spoke no English, and knew no trade. In a prolonged hospital stay, a carefully planned program included arthroplasties with her own fascia lata to both elbows and osteotomies to straighten both knees. During each operative period, the patient received intensive physical therapy for strength and walking (the first time she had walked). During her entire hospital stay, this intelligent young woman received occupational therapy, learning to be a seamstress of children's clothes and doll dresses. During this year she also learned to read, write, and converse in English. After leaving the hospital, she provided partial self-support doing work at home with her sewing. She was able to leave her apartment with assistance and lives now with limited family support. I tell this patient's story to illustrate the importance of treating the rheumatoid patient in a comprehensive manner. There is truth to the statement, "Surgery alone will not cure rheumatoid arthritis." This patient had a comfortable, though limited, lifestyle for about 7 years. She then noticed a gradual recurrence of her disease; pain and swelling of knees and elbows leading to dislocation, and further reconstructive surgery and intensive medical treatment allowed improved function again.

Dr. Richard Freyberg came from the University of Michigan to the Hospital for Special Surgery in 1944 as Chief of Rheumatic Diseases. He brought a great stimulus to both clinical and laboratory research. For years there had been a medically-oriented "Arthritis" clinic, as Dr. James Knight, who founded the Hospital for the Relief of Ruptured and Crippled (The R & C; changed to Hospital for Special Surgery in 1940), was an internist and was opposed to surgery.

Dr. Freyberg arrived at a very crowded HSS and was forced to share private offices and examination rooms with me. This proved to be most enjoyable, for proximity led to ready consultation and better evaluation and care. Our discussions led eventually to the formation of a special consultative arthritis clinic and conference staffed by internists, orthopaedic surgeons, rheumatologists, nurses, physical therapists, occupational therapists, medical students, and interested staff. This was named the "Comprehensive Arthritis Program" [C.A.P.], covering a separate clinic, scheduled operative time and case presentation conference. The regular arthritis clinics and conferences now continue manned by the same research-clinician group. A review of the chapter titles in this book shows the study areas in this program. It can hardly cover the value of the tissues made available to research. Nor can the value of the numerous informal personal ideas and discussions stimulated by this combined program be recorded. It is hoped that careful evaluation of all therapeutic techniques, medical and surgical, will lead to great improvement in the treatment of this miserable disease.

Lee Ramsay Straub, M.D.
Professor Emeritus
Department of Orthopaedic Surgery
The Hospital for Special Surgery
Professor of Orthopaedic Surgery
Cornell University Medical College
New York, New York

Foreword

In 1969 to 1970, together with a number of other rheumatology research fellows, I followed my chief, Dr Charles Christian from Presbyterian Hospital in New York City, to the Hospital for Special Surgery where he assumed the role of Physician-in-Chief. The immediate impression of this hospital was one of enormous team spirit—at every level and in every department. It was an impression which my colleagues shared and which has remained with me.

At a clinical level, this spirit produced results which have been admired and emulated worldwide. It is almost universally accepted that a combined approach to patients with long-term and complex diseases such as rheumatoid arthritis pays dividends. In practice, however, this combined approach frequently falters. Orthopaedic surgeons are, and must always be, pragmatists. Rheumatologists, dealing with less-than-perfect treatments, with chronic pain, and with small successes, are doubters. On the face of it, the two specialties sit together uncomfortably.

In practice, the combination of these specialties has, in certain groups of patients, resulted in real improvements in patient care.

That combined—even multidisciplinary—clinics are now accepted worldwide is, in large part, due to the pioneering work of a small number of centers, one of which was, and is, the Hospital for Special Surgery.

In this volume, Dr. Tom Sculco has brought in many colleagues from HSS's well-known Comprehensive Arthritis Program to provide a uniquely experienced overview of the surgical management of rheumatoid arthritis.

Graham R.V., Hughes, M.D. F.R.C.P.
Head, Lupus Arthritis Research Unit
The Rayne Institute
St. Thomas' Hospital
London, England

Preface

Rheumatoid arthritis remains an unsolved disease. Despite extensive and continued research its etiology remains unclear. The disease itself manifests a varied spectrum of clinical presentation from a transient oligoarticular disease pattern to a rapidly devastating polyarthritis with severely impaired upper and lower extremity function. The clinician must also be aware of the severe extraskeletal components of the disease which can lead to cardiopulmonary, renal, and ocular complications. In fact, rheumatoid arthritis may be a generic name for a wide spectrum of diseases with varying presentations which are all labelled under the general umbrella of rheumatoid arthritis.

The disease has its predilection for children and adults in their early years. Because of its skewed incidence in young women, it may be particularly disruptive to a young family. The economic impact of the disease is considerable both because of the chronic need for medical and surgical care and the lost income by the affected patients during their most productive years. Children afflicted with the disease require the most complex medical care and familial support, and may never be able to function in society in a successful manner.

The severity of the disease and its multifaceted character require that these patients be cared for in a comprehensive fashion. Comprehensive implies a multidisciplinary approach to the clinical, social, and psychologic aspects of the disease, and that solutions are developed in a collaborative manner. Clinical input is important from rheumatologist, nurse, physical and occupational therapist, social worker, orthopaedic surgeon, and at times psychiatrist. At the Hospital for Special Surgery this is carried out in a combined service, the Surgical Arthritis Service (formerly the Comprehensive Arthritis Program). Patients with rheumatoid arthritis are presented in a combined forum with input from all subspecialties. A treatment plan is then developed and effected with the same clinical team following the patient as they become in-patients. When in-patient care is completed patients are returned to the outpatient setting and cared for by the same health team. This not only ensures a complete evaluation and treatment plan to the patients but continuity of care is possible because the same clinical team follows the patient in the ambulatory and in-patient setting.

This text emphasizes this comprehensive, collaborative approach to rheumatoid arthritis. The first part of the book concentrates on the medical treatment of the disease with its pathologic and radiologic features. The latter part of the text addresses the nonsurgical and surgical treatment by anatomic area. A thorough rehabilitation section is also provided to detail the modalities available for the rheumatoid patient in the outpatient setting and as part of the recovery process after reconstructive surgery.

A text which encompasses this broad topic cannot be completed without the help of many individuals. Firstly, my gratitude to my co-authors and colleagues who labored so hard to meet deadlines and put up with many harassing calls and messages. Hopefully a current and much needed text on rheumatoid arthritis makes the task well worth it. Joyce-Rachel John at Mosby–Year Book, Inc. deserves particular recognition for keeping the book moving in a prodding but pleasant way. Also much thanks to Jim Ryan, also of Mosby–Year Book, Inc., who was there when the final push was needed. My family saw less of me during the past year and I especially owe a debt of gratitude to them. And finally (so this does not sound like an Oscar acceptance speech), to Joel Herring, the illustrator who kept a close schedule and was always available, especially down the home stretch.

Thomas P. Sculco, M.D.

Contents

Foreword by Lee Ramsay Straub ix

Foreword by Graham R.V. Hughes xi

Preface xiii

PART I: GENERAL CONSIDERATIONS 1

1 / Medical Concepts and Treatment in Rheumatoid Arthritis 3
by Charles L. Christian and Thomas J.A. Lehman

1A / Adult Rheumatoid Arthritis 5
by Charles L. Christian

1B / Juvenile Rheumatoid Arthritis 11
by Thomas J.A. Lehman

2 / Radiographic Evaluation 23
by Hollis G. Potter and Bernard Ghelman

3 / Pathology 45
by Edward F. DiCarlo

PART II: SURGICAL CONSIDERATIONS 55

4 / Introduction to the Rheumatoid Patient Undergoing Surgical Treatment 57
by Thomas P. Sculco

5 / Anesthesia 69
by Kevin V. Sanborn

Special Section on the Temporomandibular Joint 76
by Barry M. Libin

6 / The Temporomandibular Joint 83
by Barry M. Libin and David A. Behrman

7 / The Cervical Spine 103
by Thomas P. Sculco and Michael M. Alexiades

8 / The Shoulder 127
by Matthew J. Kraay and Mark P. Figgie

9 / The Elbow 147
by Allan E. Inglis

10 / The Wrist 161
by Michelle Gerwin, Chitranjan S. Ranawat, and Roberta Brockman

11 / The Hand 189
by Allan E. Inglis

12 / The Hip 211
by Michael J. Maynard, Chitranjan S. Ranawat, and William F. Flynn, Jr.

13 / The Knee 237
by Thomas P. Sculco

14 / Bilateral Hip and Knee Replacement 265
by Thomas P. Sculco

15 / The Hindfoot 273
by Mark P. Figgie, Mark Sobel, and Mark J. Geppert

16 / The Forefoot 315
by Thomas P. Sculco, Mark J. Geppert, and Mark Sobel

17 / Lower Extremity Function 343
by Jay D. Mabrey and James C. Otis

18 / Soft Tissue 353
by Michael M. Alexiades

19 / Surgery in Juvenile Rheumatoid Arthritis *361*
by Norman A. Johanson

PART III: REHABILITATION *377*

20 / Rehabilitation in Rheumatoid Arthritis *379*
by Sandy B. Ganz, Louis L. Harris, Toni I. Golin, and Nancy Nichols

20A / Physical Therapy *381*
by Sandy B. Ganz and Louis L. Harris

20B / Occupational Therapy *397*
by Toni I. Golin and Nancy Nichols

Index *409*

PART I

General Considerations

CHAPTER 1

Medical Concepts and Treatment in Rheumatoid Arthritis

Charles L. Christian, M.D.

Thomas J. A. Lehman, M.D.

CHAPTER 1A

Adult Rheumatoid Arthritis

Charles L. Christian, M.D.

INTRODUCTION

The term *rheumatoid arthritis* (RA) first appeared in an 1859 communication by Alfred Baring Garrod; from his experience he described a syndrome that seemed to him distinct from gout and rheumatism (acute rheumatic fever). Except for inclusion of inflammatory Heberden's nodes, his description, by and large, fits modern concepts of RA. The syndrome is more complex than clinical synovitis, in most patients systemic manifestations are prominent, and in some subjects morbidity relates more to extraarticular involvement than to joint disease. For a comprehensive and reasonably contemporary review of RA, readers are referred to a textbook.[12]

Rheumatoid arthritis is relatively common—the incidence in most populations is in the range of 1% to 2%,—it affects all ages, and is more common in women than men (epidemiologic studies suggest that the incidence of RA may be decreasing[6]). There are genetic markers that identify persons with higher than normal risk for development of RA. Concordance for disease is observed in 50% or more of monozygotic twin pairs. Pathologic changes reflect the full range of multiple cellular and humoral factors mediating inflammation. Etiologic stimuli have not been identified but immunologic mechanisms are clearly implicated in pathogenesis.

Rheumatoid arthritis as currently defined is a strikingly diverse syndrome; some of the variables that characterize subsets are summarized in Table 1A–1. Classifications have taken into consideration: the presence or absence of rheumatoid factor (seropositive vs. seronegative RA); major histocompatibility complex (MHC) class I and II markers (HLA-B27, HLA-DR4, etc.), anatomic variations (polyarticular vs. pauciarticular, ankylosing vs. subluxing patterns, symmetric vs. asymmetric); the presence or absence of nodules, vasculitis, and other extraarticular manifestations; and the synovial histologic findings (presence or absence of lymphoid features). The clinical heterogeneity may reflect multiple etiologies or, alternatively, varied host responses to a single or restricted range of etiologies.

PATHOLOGY

Lesions of articular cartilage, bones, and periarticular tissues in RA are related to the generation of a hyperplastic synovium (pannus) which, via collagenase and other hydrolytic enzymes, can degrade these tissues. In addition, there is a wide range of humoral events that may mediate injury of connective tissue substrates. They include: (1) release of vasoactive amines; (2) generation of enzymes from plasma substrates or from cells that affect tone and permeability of blood vessels, and promote blood coagulation or fibrinolysis; (3) activation of complement, yielding chemotactic, anaphylactic, and cytotoxic principles; (4) production of prostaglandins and leukotrienes via the action of enzymes on arachidonic acid; (5) formation of oxygen-derived products; (6) release of lysosomal enzymes from inflammatory cells; and (7) the synthesis and release of numerous cytokines (e.g., interleukins, growth factors, tumor necrosis factor).

Granulocytes predominate in RA synovial fluid but the cellular composition of hyperplastic synovial tissues is complex and varied. It includes fibroblastic cells, macrophages, endothelial cells, lymphocytes, plasmacytes, and mast cells. Aggregates of T lym-

TABLE 1A–1.
Rheumatoid Arthritis: Subset Variations

Feature	Variations
Serologic (rheumatoid factor)	Seropositive vs. seronegative
HLA antigens	HLA-DR4–positive vs. –negative
	HLA-B27–positive vs. –negative
Number of joints	Polyarticular vs. pauciarticular
Anatomic patterns	Symmetric vs. asymmetric
	Ankylosing vs. subluxing
	Erosive vs. nonerosive
Histology	Lymphoid vs. nonlymphoid
Extraarticular features	Prominent vs. not prominent
Course	Sustained vs. remittive

phocytes are present in some RA synovial specimens; the cells express the helper/inducer phenotype (CD4) and markers of activation (increased class II MHC products, LFA-1, and other adhesion molecules).

The chronic inflammatory lesions noted above are present in rheumatoid nodules and, in patients with severe systemic disease, they can be found in other extraarticular tissues, e.g., heart, lungs, eye, peripheral nerves, often in association with manifestations of systemic vasculitis.

EXPERIMENTAL MODELS OF CHRONIC SYNOVITIS

There are several animal models of synovitis that mimic features of RA; most are induced by infectious agents or products of microorganisms. The microbial species involved include bacteria, mycoplasma, chlamydia, and viruses. Adjuvant arthritis results from the injection of mycobacterial antigen into Lewis strain rats. (Special interest in this model relates to the hypothesis that the mechanism for induction involves cross-reactivity between a 65-kilodalton mycobacterial heat shock protein and a protein present in cartilage proteoglycan and that analogous molecular mimicry might underlie the development of RA[4]). Variable patterns of acute and chronic synovitis are inducible in some strains of rats with bacterial cell wall preparations,[5] and in another model that resembles RA, by immunization with type II collagen.[11] Spontaneous synovitis resembling RA occurs in a murine strain (MRL/lpr) that is characterized by expression of multiple autoimmune specificities, including rheumatoid factors.[3]

ETIOLOGY

According to current concepts, the pathogenesis of RA involves: (1) the interaction of one or more environmental (etiologic) stimuli with (2) host regulatory variables (genetic, immunologic, etc.) which initiate (3) cellular and humoral processes mediating tissue injury.[7] The best characterized of these three phases is the last, i.e., the pathophysiology of inflammation. Consideration of etiologic events is in the realm of hypothesis but there is an impressive body of information focusing attention on infection. Supporting evidence includes: (1) extrapolation from animal models (reviewed above), (2) characterization of Lyme borreliosis (its manifestations may include acute and chronic synovitis[10]), (3) elucidation of the role of multiple bacterial species in the development of Reiter's syndrome and other postinfectious arthropathies, and (4) association of acute arthritis with viral infection in human subjects, i.e., rubella, parvorvirus B19, etc. (reviewed in reference 9).

DIAGNOSIS

Paramount in the diagnosis of RA is the exclusion of many other syndromes, some with defined etiologies, that can be associated with synovitis. Approximately three fourths of patients with RA, as currently defined, are seropositive for rheumatoid factor but the presence of this autoantibody is not diagnostic of RA. It is observed as well in other connective tissue syndromes, chronic infectious diseases, and (in low frequency) in healthy subjects.

The American Rheumatism Association (now the American College of Rheumatology) has developed criteria for classifying RA.[1] The criteria are: (1) morning stiffness in and around joints lasting at least 1 hour before maximal improvement; (2) soft tissue swelling (arthritis) of three more joint areas observed by a physician; (3) swelling (arthritis) of the proximal interphalangeal, and metacarpophalangeal, or wrist joints; (4) symmetric swelling (arthritis); (5) rheumatoid nodules; (6) the presence of rheumatoid factor; and (7) radiographic erosions or periarticular osteopenia in the hand or wrist joint(s). Criteria (1) through (4) must have been present for at least 6 weeks. Rheumatoid arthritis is defined by the presence of four or more criteria, and no further qualifications (classic, definite, or probable) or list of exclusions are required. In addition, a "classification tree" schema is presented which performs equally as well as the traditional (four of seven) format. The criteria demonstrated 91% to 94% sensitivity and 89% specificity for RA when compared with non-RA rheumatic disease control subjects.

The most critical aspect of the differential diagnosis of arthritis is the early recognition of syndromes other than RA for which more specific, sometimes curative, therapies are indicated, i.e., infection, crystal arthropathies, mechanical derangements.

CLINICAL COURSE AND NATURAL HISTORY

In the majority of subjects, RA (as currently defined) is a chronic illness characterized by alternating periods of improvement and exacerbation. Complete remissions are observed in the range of 10% to 15% of patients who meet the criteria for classification of RA; in some of these patients the remission is permanent. (Future studies may demonstrate that the etiologies of acute remittent, chronic intermittent, and chronic sustained patterns of RA are different.)

MANAGEMENT AND TREATMENT

Basic Management

The basic management relevant to all patients with RA includes: (1) education, realistic reassurance regarding prognosis, review of the overall treatment strategy, and emphasis on the patient's role in management; (2) use of aspirin or an equivalent nonsteroidal anti-inflammatory drug (NSAID), and (3) a physical medicine program tailored to the pattern of disease and disability.[8]

Physical Medicine Measures

The goals of physical therapy are (1) to combat or reverse muscle weakness, (2) to preserve, to the extent possible, normal alignment of joints, and (3) to maintain joint motion. Achievement of these objectives rests with the institution of an exercise program that the patient can maintain; adjuvant measures are heat (hot packs, hydrotherapy, diathermy, or ultrasound), rest, and splints. Physical therapy programs need to be individualized. If synovitis is very acute, nothing more than rest, isometric exercises, and gentle passive motion may be appropriate. Rest (avoidance of loaded or weightbearing exercises) for patients with active synovitis is not inconsistent with the goals of maintaining muscle power and motion.

Nonsteroidal Anti-inflammatory Drugs

For nearly all forms of synovitis, sustained or intermittent use of an NSAID is appropriate. Included in this class of drugs are salicylate preparations, indomethacin, phenylbutazone, and several newer agents, which are listed along with recommended dosages in Table 1A–2. (The dose range for each NSAID indicates the requirement for anti-inflammatory action as opposed to the lower requirements for analgesia.) All these compounds inhibit prostaglandin biosynthesis, but there are other actions that may mediate, in part, anti-inflammatory effects. Newer drugs have levels of anti-inflammatory activity not far removed from that of aspirin, but relative to aspirin some appear to have lower levels of gastrointestinal toxicity. Benefits from NSAID therapy require sustained and systematic use. A common error is to conclude that a given medication brought

TABLE 1A–2.
Nonsteroidal Anti-inflammatory Drugs

Generic Name	Proprietary Name	Dose Range (mg)	
Aspirin		600–1,200	q.i.d.
Choline magnesium trisalicylate	Trilisate	600–900	q.i.d.
Diclofenac sodium	Voltaren	50–75	b.i.d.
Flurbiprofen	Ansaid	50–100	t.i.d.
Ibuprofen	Motrin,Rufen	300–800	t.i.d.
Indomethacin	Indocin	25–50	t.i.d.
Ketoprofen	Orudis	50–100	t.i.d.
Meclofenamate sodium	Meclomen	50–100	q.i.d.
Naproxen	Naprosyn	250–500	b.i.d.
Phenylbutazone	Butazolidin	100–200	t.i.d.
Piroxican	Feldene	20	q.d.
Salsalate	Disalcid	600–900	q.i.d.
Sulindac	Clinoril	150–200	b.i.d.
Tolmetin sodium	Tolectin	400	t.i.d.

no benefit, when in fact such therapy was not given an adequate trial. Salicylate preparations have two important advantages relative to other NSAIDs: (1) low cost, and (2) questions of absorption or toxicity can be easily checked by obtaining salicylate levels.

Disease-Modifying Drugs

Table 1A–3 lists medications applicable to the treatment of RA that are generally reserved for patients who have not responded to the basic regimen described above.[2] These agents, collectively called "disease-modifying antirheumatic drugs" (DMARDs), share three features: (1) their modes of action are unknown but seem to be independent of direct anti-inflammatory effect, (2) they are slower-acting (i.e., require several weeks or more of therapy before improvement ensues), and (3) efficacy in an individual patient is not predictable. Of the therapeutic agents listed in Table 1A–3, gold compounds have had the widest and longest application, and are still the first choice of many rheumatologists, but methotrexate

TABLE 1A–3.
Disease-Modifying Antirheumatic Drugs Used in the Treatment of Rheumatoid Arthritis

Generic Name	Proprietary Name	Initial Dose	Maintenance Dose	Toxicity
Gold compounds				
Auranofin	Ridaura	3 mg/day po	6–9 mg/day (po)	Skin rash
Aurothioglucose	Solgonal	Weekly injections (IM) beginning 10 mg increasing to 50 mg until total dose 1,000 mg or remission	50 mg at 2–4 wk intervals	Myelosuppression
Gold sodium thiomalate	Myochrysine			Renal disease
Antimalarial drugs				
Hydroxychloroquine sulfate	Plaquenil	200 mg/day	200–400 mg/day	Skin rash Corneal deposits Retinitis (careful ophthalmologic examination recommended at 3–6 month intervals) Gastrointestinal (GI) intolerance
Penicillamine	Cuprimine Depen	125–250 mg/day increasing by 125–250 mg increments every 2–3 months until remission ensues or toxicity develops (maximum daily dose 1,000 mg)	Maintain level of therapy associated with remission, gradually decreasing dose if remission continues	Skin rash Myelosuppression Nephritis Loss of taste
Methotrexate	Rheumatrex	5.0–7.5 mg (po or IM) *weekly*	7.5–15 mg (po to 15 mg) *weekly*	GI intolerance Myelosuppression Stomatitis Pneumonitis
Sulfasalazine	Azulfidine	1–2 g/day (divided doses)	3–4 g/day (divided doses)	GI intolerance Allergic reactions
Other cytotoxic drugs				
Cyclophosphamide Azathioprine	Cytoxan Imuran	100–200 mg/day in single A.M. dose	Maintain level of therapy associated with remission, gradually decreasing dose if remission continues	Myelosuppression (additional toxicity associated with cyclophosphamide includes hair loss, gonadal failure, hemorrhagic cystitis, and bladder tumors; large volume of water ingestion and frequent emptying of bladder recommended

has gained acceptance; relative to the other DMARDs, it has an earlier onset of action and a higher incidence of efficacy. With the exception of methotrexate, cytotoxic drugs are generally reserved for patients with high risk patterns of disease that are not responsive to other modes of therapy.

Adrenocortical Steroid Therapy

Corticosteroid drugs are the most potent of the anti-inflammatory agents, but the incidence of toxicity associated with systemic administration limits their use in patients with RA. Patients with very high levels of disability that do not respond to more conservative regimens may be candidates for systemic corticosteroid therapy; in such cases, accepting the risk of drug toxicity may be preferable to that of chronic invalidism. Maintenance therapy should be restricted to low dose levels, preferably 10 mg of prednisone or less daily.

There is a pattern of relatively mild seronegative arthropathy in elderly subjects for which low-dose prednisone (5–10 mg/day) is sometimes more effective and better tolerated than NSAID therapy.

When major levels of disability are attributable to one or few joints, intraarticular administration of steroid preparations such as methylprednisolone acetate (20–40 mg) may induce periods of improvement that last for several weeks or more. Injections in individual joints should not be repeated more frequently than every 2 or 3 months because of the risk of accelerated cartilage destruction.

Surgical Rehabilitation

Discussions elsewhere in this book consider in detail the indications and techniques for various surgical procedures that have revolutionized the management of chronic RA. Improvements in the techniques of total joint replacement over the past decade have made this the treatment of choice for patients with major joint destruction. Because of the availability of these salvage procedures, early (prophylactic) synovectomy is performed less frequently, but it is still an appropriate consideration for patients with sustained synovitis who are exhibiting early signs of bone or cartilage erosion.

REFERENCES

1. Arnett FC, Edworthy SM, Block DA, et al: The American Rheumatism Association 1987 Revised Criteria for the Classification of Rheumatoid Arthritis. *Arthritis Rheum* 1988; 31:315.
2. Felson DT, Anderson JJ, Meenan RF: The comparative efficacy and toxicity of second-line drugs in rheumatoid arthritis: Results of two metanalyses. *Arthritis Rheum* 1980; 33:1449.
3. Hang L, Theofilopoulos AN: A spontaneous rheumatoid arthritis-like disease in MRL/l mice. *J Exp Med* 1982; 155:1690.
4. Holoshitz J, Drucker I, Yaretzky A, et al: T lymphocytes of rheumatoid arthritis patients show augmented reactivity to a fraction of mycobacteria cross-reactive with cartilage. *Lancet* 1986; *i*:305.
5. Lehman TJA, Allen JB, Plutz PH, et al: Polyarthritis in rats following the systemic injection of *Lactobacillus casei* cell walls in aqueous suspension. *Arthritis Rheum* 1983; 26:1259.
6. Linos A, Worthington JW, O'Fallen WM, et al: The epidemiology of rheumatoid arthritis in Rochester, Minnesota: A study of incidence, prevalence, and mortality. *Am J Epidemiol* 1980; 111:87.
7. Lutz M, Vaughan JH: Rheumatoid arthritis, in Samter M (ed): *Immunological Diseases,* ed 4. Boston, Little, Brown & Co, 1988, pp 1365–1416.
8. Pinals RS. Rheumatoid arthritis: A pharmacologic overview. *Am Fam Physician* 1988; 37:145.
9. Saag MS, Bennett JC: *Semin Arthritis Rheum* 1987; 17:1.
10. Steere AC. Lyme disease, in Kelley WN, Harris ED Jr, Ruddy S, et al (eds): *Textbook of Rheumatology,* ed 3. Philadelphia, WB Saunders Co, 1989, p 1602.
11. Trentham DE: Collagen arthritis as a relevant model for rheumatoid arthritis. *Arthritis Rheum* 1982; 25:911.
12. Utsinger PD, Zvaifler NJ, Ehrlich GE: *Rheumatoid Arthritis, Etiology, Diagnosis, and Management.* Philadelphia, JB Lippincott Co, 1985.

CHAPTER 1B

Juvenile Rheumatoid Arthritis

Thomas J. A. Lehman M.D.

INTRODUCTION

Juvenile rheumatoid arthritis (JRA) is the most common form of chronic arthritis in childhood. It is a protracted inflammatory synovitis with varying presentations and prognoses. Children may present as acutely ill, with fever, rash, and an elevated sedimentation rate suggesting an acute infectious episode, or with the insidious onset of painless joint contracture. To care for children with JRA properly it is necessary to understand JRA's varied presentations and their impact on prognosis and therapy.

Juvenile rheumatoid arthritis is defined by the onset before age 16 years of arthritis of at least 6 weeks' duration in two or more joints (see box). If only a single joint is involved, the arthritis must be present for at least 3 months before the diagnosis is considered "definite." Infections, tumors, and other forms of chronic childhood arthritis which may mimic JRA must be excluded.[1, 3] By definition, the presence of arthritis requires at least two characteristic signs of inflammation, including pain, swelling, limitation of motion, or redness. Pain alone is inadequate.

Definition of "Definite" JRA

Chronic arthritis of two or more joints for at least 6 weeks or a single joint for more than 3 months *for which other causes have been excluded*

When reviewing the literature it is important to distinguish the terms *juvenile arthritis* (JA), *juvenile chronic arthritis* (JCA), and *juvenile chronic polyarthritis* (JCP) from JRA (see box). These terms arose because it is often difficult to exclude early manifestations of other forms of chronic childhood arthritis when diagnosing JRA. The intent was to prompt recognition that not all children with arthritis have JRA. However, these terms are often used to group children with diverse arthritides without distinction. The natural history, prognosis, and optimal therapy of these diverse diseases differ, making proper interpretation of such series uncertain. Spondyloarthropathies and "psoriaform" arthritis are two forms of chronic childhood arthritis that are often confused with JRA. They are included in this chapter because they are often referred for care with a diagnosis of JRA.

Juvenile Arthritis

Juvenile arthritis (JA)
Juvenile chronic arthritis (JCA)
Juvenile chronic polyarthritis (JCP)
These terms refer to any of the many different forms of arthritis which occur in childhood, not just JRA.

EPIDEMIOLOGY

Short-lived joint pains in childhood are extremely common. As many as 350,000 children in the United States experience an episode of arthritis sufficient to prompt medical consultation in any given year.[2] Most are children with infectious or reactive arthritis associated with viral or bacterial infection. The prevalence of definite JRA in the United States is unclear, but is estimated to be 100,000 cases in any given year.[11] The frequency of chronic forms of childhood arthritis such as spondyloarthropathies and psoriaform arthritis has not been determined.

ETIOLOGY AND GENETICS

The etiology of JRA is unknown. The histopathologic picture is a nonspecific chronic synovitis without differentiating factors. No common infectious agent or pathologic event is recognized. Although certain histocompatibility antigens are more common among children with specific subtypes of JRA, there is no consistent pattern across the subtypes.[5, 7, 10] This suggests that even the diagnosis of definite JRA takes in a heterogeneous population encompassing different disorders.

NATURAL HISTORY

Because of its various manifestations the prognosis and therapy of JRA are closely linked to the three characteristic onset subtypes.[4] These subtypes are pauciarticular onset (involving four or fewer joints during the first 6 months), polyarticular onset (involving more than four joints), or systemic onset (presentation with high spiking fevers and rash) (see box). The onset subtypes are defined not by the number of joints involved initially, but by the number involved during the first 6 months of disease.

Subtypes of JRA

- Pauciarticular onset
  - Young children (typically less than 5 years of age)
  - Four or fewer large joints affected
  - Increased risk of eye disease (greatest if ANA-positive)
  - Girls affected more than boys
  - Should be rheumatoid factor–negative
  - Most do well
- Polyarticular onset
  - More than four joints affected
  - Girls affected more than boys
  - Variable prognosis
  - Young children are usually rheumatoid factor–negative
  - Older rheumatoid factor–positive children may do poorly
- Systemic onset
  - Onset with high spiking fevers and rash
  - May be very ill with systemic manifestations
  - High frequency of pericarditis
  - Boys affected as often as girls
  - Should be rheumatoid factor–negative

Thus a child who presents with a swollen knee for 3 weeks, but develops swelling of multiple joints over the next 3 months has polyarticular-onset disease.

Each subtype of JRA has its own clinical picture, etiologic hypotheses, serologic findings, complications, diseases with which it may be confused, and guidelines for medical therapy. The specific medications used in treating children with JRA are discussed at the end of this chapter. Patient and family education, physical and occupational therapy, and broad-based psychosocial support of the children and their families are important components of the therapy of every type of JRA.

PAUCIARTICULAR-ONSET JRA

This onset type accounts for nearly 50% of children with JRA. It typically begins between 1 and 5 years of age with the gradual onset of joint swelling and morning stiffness. Most often it involves a single knee, but it may involve elbows, wrists, or ankles and may spread to as many as four joints. Small joints of the hands and feet are typically spared. These children often do not complain of pain, but are limping or noted to have a swollen joint when a parent is dressing them. Significant constitutional symptoms, including fever, are normally absent.

This form of JRA more often involves girls than boys, but either sex may be affected. Genetic studies have shown a high incidence of specific HLA-DR antigens in this subgroup.[7] It occurs with a greater than expected frequency in blond-haired blue-eyed girls, and is less often encountered in blacks and orientals.[4] These children typically have only mildly elevated erythrocyte sedimentation rates. Mild anemia and a mild elevation of the platelet count may be present. Marked anemia (hemoglobin <9 g), thrombocytopenia, or Westergren erythrocyte sedimentation rates greater than 50 mm/hr should prompt careful reconsideration of the diagnosis. IgA deficiency and mild panhypogammaglobulinemia also occur more often than expected in these children.

These children are almost never rheumatoid factor–positive. Antinuclear antibodies (ANAs) are frequently present and should be sought in every child because chronic ocular involvement (iridocyclitis) occurs predominantly among ANA-positive children with pauciarticular onset. Eye involvement is painless, but may lead to permanent visual impairment without warning. ANA-positive children require ophthalmologic evaluation every 4 months at least until 10 years of age, and every 6 months after that.

There is no correlation between the presence or severity of eye disease and the severity or activity of the arthritis. Children have developed visual impairment years after the arthritis resolved. Although it is hypothesized that the ciliary body of the anterior chamber of the eye functions in a filtering capacity and so may become inflamed by the presence of immune complexes much like the synovium of joints, the explanation for the concordance of pauciarticular-onset JRA and iridocyclitis is unknown.

Children with pauciarticular-onset JRA often recover completely, but some will experience relapses. Relapses may be separated by asymptomatic periods of years throughout childhood and even into adulthood. The subset of these children who develop polyarticular arthritis later in the course of their disease often do poorly.

The major orthopaedic complications for children with pauciarticular JRA are leg length discrepancies, and contractures. Because of the hyperemia associated with inflammation of the joint during a period of rapid growth, the affected limb is often longer than the unaffected limb although contractures may cause it to appear shorter.

Exclusions

HLA-B27-positive boys with asymmetric large joint arthritis (e.g., knees, hips) in the preadolescent and adolescent age groups (roughly 8 years of age and older) are described by some as a subgroup of pauciarticular JRA.[9] Their prognosis, natural history, and response to therapy are entirely unrelated to pauciarticular JRA of early childhood. They are better considered separately under the category of spondyloarthropathy.

Hip involvement is an important exclusion in the evaluation of pauciarticular JRA. Although JRA frequently spreads to involve the hip, early hip involvement is rare (excluding older children with spondyloarthropathies). Isolated hip involvement in a young girl should prompt extensive search for an alternative diagnosis such as infection, osteoid osteoma, transient osteoporosis, or chondrolysis.

Some children with pauciarticular JRA present with involvement of four or fewer joints but have dactylitis of either fingers or toes. These children represent another subgroup with a differing natural history. They tend to have greater anemia and more significantly elevated erythrocyte sedimentation rates. Although they do not have psoriasis they often have a first-degree relative who does (see psoriaform arthritis below). Their prognosis is guarded. Their disease more often evolves into severe polyarticular disease than is the case with other children with pauciarticular onset and they may prove resistant to normal therapy.

Three additional diseases which may present with involvement of four or fewer joints should be familiar to anyone caring for children with pauciarticular JRA. Tuberculous arthritis in childhood may present as a smoldering subacute monarticular arthritis. Whenever monarticular arthritis is present in a child with a socioeconomic background that places him or her at risk, or fails to respond to therapy as expected, tuberculin testing should be performed. If tuberculin testing is positive the joint should be aspirated for appropriate cultures.

Lyme disease is an endemic problem in New England and other parts of the United States. Children with Lyme arthritis may mimic pauciarticular JRA with recurrent arthritis that rapidly resolves even without therapy. Joint fluid aspirates are usually benign. Often the child is thought to have benign reactive arthritis, which draws attention only because it is recurrent. Appropriate Lyme disease testing should be performed in these children. In nonendemic areas it is important to seek a history of travel to endemic areas (see box).

Diseases to Be Excluded From Pauciarticular JRA

Lyme disease
Osteomyelitis
Septic arthritis (including tuberculous arthritis)
Plant thorn synovitis
Spondyloarthropathies
Psoriaform arthritis
Neoplastic diseases

Plant thorn synovitis is another frequently unrecognized cause of monarticular arthritis. It often occurs in young children who fall on a palm frond or similar plant material while playing and suffer a puncture wound penetrating the knee joint. The wound initially heals without difficulty and is forgotten when the knee becomes extremely inflamed 6 to 8 weeks later. Although cultures are negative, the arthritis is extremely aggressive and unresponsive to medical therapy. The diagnosis is established by polarized light microscopy of a synovial biopsy specimen demonstrating starchlike material of herbaceous origin within the inflamed synovium. Synovectomy is the treatment of choice.

Medical Treatment

Pauciarticular-onset JRA is usually responsive to nonsteroidal anti-inflammatory drugs such as acetylsalicylic acid, naproxen, ibuprofen, or tolmetin sodium (Tolectin). Children whose disease proves resistant to these agents may benefit from the prudent use of intraarticular corticosteroids, but recurrent injections are unwise. Occasional children who have not responded to other nonsteroidal anti-inflammatory agents respond well to indomethacin but this drug must be used with caution.

Intramuscular gold salts are an effective therapy for children whose pauciarticular JRA has not responded to nonsteroidal agents. Only a rare child with pauciarticular-onset JRA will require methotrexate or other immunosuppressive agents in the absence of polyarticular disease. Hydroxychloroquine and sulfasalazine (Azulfidine) may be beneficial for children with arthritis that did not respond to nonsteroidal anti-inflammatory drugs alone, but was not of sufficient severity to warrant immunosuppressive therapy. Corticosteroids have no role in the treatment of pauciarticular JRA except for ocular complications or intraarticular injection.

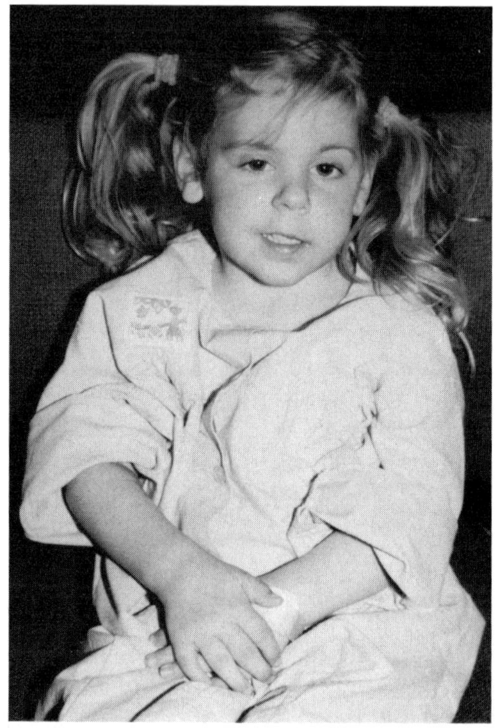

FIG 1B–1.
Seven-year-old child with polyarticular JRA.

POLYARTICULAR JRA

This onset subtype accounts for about 40% of children with JRA (Fig 1B–1). Like pauciarticular-onset JRA it is more frequent in girls than boys. Blacks and orientals are likewise infrequently affected. In young children polyarticular-onset JRA often has a slowly progressive onset similar to that of pauciarticular-onset JRA. The child may be brought to the physician complaining of knee or wrist pain, but within the first few months of disease symmetric involvement of the small joints of the hands becomes evident. In others involvement of more than four large joints is evident.

The extent of the arthritis may not be recognized by the family at presentation. These children often present with a complaint of stiffness or limping much like a typical pauciarticular JRA. The prognosis for younger children (under age 6 years) with rapidly progressive polyarticular disease is guarded. Many recover and do well, but those with continuing active disease despite therapy are at risk of significant functional impairment.

Early adolescent and teenage girls with rheumatoid factor–positive polyarticular JRA represent a distinct subgroup. This group shares the HLA-DR4 preponderance seen in adult rheumatoid arthritis.[11] The onset of rheumatoid factor–positive polyarthritis in this age group is often rapidly aggressive and severe. Rheumatoid nodules and other extraarticular manifestations identical to those seen in adults with rheumatoid arthritis are common.

Anemia and significantly elevated erythrocyte sedimentation rates are common in children with both types of polyarticular JRA. Although rheumatoid factor remains rare in children under the age of 10 years, it becomes progressively more common with increasing age. ANAs may be found in both age groups. The risk of ocular involvement is less than that seen in children with pauciarticular JRA, but ophthalmologic examinations every 6 months remain necessary.

Progressive joint destruction with aggressive erosive disease is characteristic of both subsets of polyarticular JRA. Without aggressive therapy permanent joint deformity and loss of function are common. The hips, knees, and wrists are particularly susceptible target organs.

In younger patients diffuse joint involvement at a time of rapid growth may produce permanent disfigurement. Growth impairment and micrognathia occur even without corticosteroid therapy. Because of the markedly altered appearance and functional abilities of these children, extensive psychosocial support is critical to attaining the best possible long-term outcome.

Exclusions

Infectious entities that produce polyarthritis need to be excluded in this group but should be evident before 6 weeks of illness. Gonococcal arthritis in the girl who denies sexual exposure is of particular concern in this regard. Other forms of chronic collagen-vascular disease may be confused with polyarticular JRA. One must be particularly careful not to overlook systemic lupus erythematosus or mixed connective tissue disease (see box).

Diseases to Be Excluded From Systemic-Onset or Polyarticular JRA

Infectious arthritis (gonococcal arthritis, hepatitis, etc.)
Rheumatic fever
Other collagen-vascular diseases (e.g., spondyloarthropathies, systemic lupus erythematosus)
Neoplastic diseases

Children with mixed connective tissue disease often have both rheumatoid factor and ANAs prompting referral for JRA. Mixed connective tissue disease may be distinguished from polyarticular JRA by the presence of a very strongly positive ANA (characteristically with a "speckled" pattern), rheumatoid factor, and marked elevation of the total protein with a normal or low albumin suggesting hypergammaglobulinemia. Elevation of creatinine phosphokinase (CPK) is also suggestive since this does not normally occur in children with JRA. On special testing these children can be shown to have antibodies to ribonucleoprotein (RNP) but not Sm. These children normally require corticosteroid therapy.

Psoriatic arthritis, arthritis associated with inflammatory bowel disease, and other spondyloarthropathies may be differentiated from polyarticular JRA by the presence of enthesopathic symptoms or recognition of the underlying condition. A few children have presented with typical polyarticular JRA only to develop manifestations of systemic lupus erythematosus years later. These children are considered to have had both diseases and illustrate overlapping disease predisposition.[8]

Leukemia and lymphoma also may present with arthritis. While these children commonly manifest pain at the long bone metaphyses and not arthritis, children with leukemia may present with true synovial effusions. Thrombocytopenia in a child with apparent JRA should always prompt examination of the bone marrow. Still, an occasional child will be followed with "typical polyarticular JRA" only to suddenly develop obvious acute lymphatic leukemia.

Medical Therapy

Polyarticular JRA may be a permanently deforming disease. Children with this onset subtype (or who develop polyarticular disease after either pauciarticular or systemic onset) require aggressive intervention. Many children respond to therapy with nonsteroidal anti-inflammatory drugs alone. Acetylsalicylic acid, naproxen, tolmetin sodium, and ibuprofen are the nonsteroidal anti-inflammatory drugs of choice. Indomethacin is a useful second-line agent. For children with rapidly progressive disease unresponsive to nonsteroidal anti-inflammatory drugs, the decision to advance to a "disease-modifying agent" such as gold sodium thiomalate (Myochrysine) should be made rapidly (within 3–6 months of disease onset), before significant joint destruction has accumulated. Too often, aggressive efforts to modify the course of polyarticular JRA are deferred until after significant joint destruction has become widespread.

Methotrexate is a useful immunosuppressive agent for children with polyarticular JRA unresponsive to gold sodium thiomalate therapy. Other immunosuppressive agents may prove useful if the child does not respond to methotrexate. All immunosuppressive agents have worrisome and potentially life-threatening toxicities. But, with proper monitoring the risks can be minimized and are clearly justified in view of the permanent psychological damage and functional impairment which may result from uncontrolled polyarticular disease.

The use of corticosteroids in these patients is controversial. Although high-dose alternate-day corticosteroids are advocated by some, they are associated with a significant risk of osteoporosis and avascular necrosis. Corticosteroids also contribute to short stature and the many undesirable effects associated with Cushing's syndrome.

Large doses of intravenous "pulse" methylprednisolone (30 mg/kg up to 1,000 mg) given daily for 3 days may be a useful stopgap measure in children with uncontrolled disease. Alternatively, low-dose corticosteroids (0.25 mg/kg/day of prednisone or its equivalent) may provide short-term relief for the child unable to carry out the necessary activities of daily living. Optimally, introduction of corticosteroids is coupled with institution of a disease-modifying agent so that the corticosteroids may be gradually withdrawn as the disease-modifying agent takes effect.

SYSTEMIC-ONSET JRA

Systemic-onset JRA is characterized by the occurrence of high spiking fevers, a fleeting, recurrent salmon-pink maculopapular rash, and varying degrees of arthritis. Unlike the other forms of JRA it occurs with almost equal frequency in both sexes, and occurs with a more uniform distribution throughout childhood. It is hypothesized that this disease may be a viral infection unrelated to the other forms of JRA. Approximately 10% of children with JRA have this onset subtype.

The diagnosis of systemic-onset JRA cannot be considered definite in the absence of arthritis. However, once arthritis is present the total number of joints involved is irrelevant to the diagnosis. The onset of systemic-onset JRA is often acute. Many children appear acutely ill and have been hospitalized for an extensive diagnostic evaluation prior to consideration of systemic-onset JRA. Unlike the other subtypes of JRA, systemic-onset disease may have immediate life-threatening complications.

The diagnosis of systemic-onset JRA is strongly suggested by daily fever spikes in excess of 38.5° C with the fever falling to normal at least once every day. Patients frequently present with fevers in the late afternoon and late evening. The rash is usually fleeting, but apparent when the fever is present. These children are often distinguished from those with tumors or infections by their improved affect during afebrile periods.

The prognosis of children with systemic-onset JRA is highly variable. Many children with minimal joint involvement will recover without residual joint damage, but others may succumb to the systemic manifestations of the disease. Pericarditis is common and may be severe. Pneumonitis occurs, but is rarely clinically significant. Lymphadenopathy and hepatosplenomegaly are common. Liver involvement may be exacerbated by drug therapy. Occasional patients will develop a picture of diffuse intravascular coagulation that may be life-threatening. The severity of the articular and extraarticular involvement determines the long-term prognosis.

The articular involvement of systemic-onset JRA is often minimal at first, but may become progressively more severe. Some children evolve directly from the systemic phase of the disease to diffuse articular involvement. Others may have recurrences of systemic disease over a period of months or years with only mild arthritis followed by the sudden development of severe polyarthritis without systemic manifestations. Polyarticular arthritis in children with systemic onset is often very aggressive and permanently disabling.

Laboratory evaluation of the child with systemic-onset JRA should show anemia, a markedly elevated erythrocyte sedimentation rate, leukocytosis, thrombocytosis, and hypergammaglobulinemia, often with a low albumin. The thrombocytosis is an important finding since platelets are an acute phase reactant. Thrombocytopenia should prompt immediate reevaluation and bone marrow aspiration to exclude the possibility of neuroblastoma, leukemia, or lymphoma. Patients with these malignancies referred for treatment of systemic-onset JRA are common in every pediatric rheumatology program. ANA and rheumatoid factor are absent in most patients with systemic-onset JRA. Ocular involvement is infrequent. Still, children with systemic-onset disease should receive ophthalmologic examinations every six months.

Exclusions

Infection is the major diagnostic exclusion when evaluating a child with possible systemic-onset JRA. Malaria should be suspected in the child with an appropriate travel history. Fevers which do not return to normal each day are sufficiently infrequent to prompt exhaustive investigation of other possible explanations before accepting the diagnosis of systemic-onset JRA. Bacterial endocarditis, neuroblastoma, leukemia, and lymphoma all may present with fever, anemia, leukocytosis, and "bone pain."

Other collagen-vascular diseases may present with fever, rash, and arthritis. Systemic lupus erythematosus, dermatomyositis, acute rheumatic fever, and Kawasaki disease all may present with findings suggesting systemic-onset JRA.

Medical Therapy

Initial medical therapy of systemic-onset JRA is similar to therapy for other forms of JRA, but it must be tempered by a heightened sensitivity to drug toxicity. Diffuse intravascular coagulation may occur shortly after the initiation of salicylate or gold sodium thiomalate therapy in children with systemic-onset JRA. The etiology of this complication and its association with drug therapy is not well understood. Many children with systemic-onset JRA are unresponsive to naproxen, tolmetin sodium, or ibuprofen, but respond well to indomethacin. Gold sodium thiomalate is an effective agent, but like other drugs must be used with increased attention to the possibility of toxicity in children with systemic-onset JRA. Children who do not respond to the gold compound may require methotrexate or other immunosuppressive agents.

Systemic-onset JRA can be controlled in most children by a combination of nonsteroidal anti-inflammatory drugs and immunosuppressive agents without corticosteroids. However, prednisone or its equivalent (1–2 mg/kg/day) may be the only suitable therapy for acutely ill children with severe systemic-onset JRA. Intravenous pulse methylprednisolone may be necessary for acute control of severe disease. Large doses of alternate-day corticosteroids are used in some centers, but are associated with significant toxicity.

SPONDYLOARTHROPATHIES

The recognition of spondyloarthropathies in childhood came about following widespread HLA-B27 antigen testing. Ankylosing spondylitis is rare in childhood because the erosive sacroiliac joint changes required for diagnosis rarely develop before adulthood. When HLA-B27 testing became widely available, many boys with asymmetric large joint arthritis involving the hips or knees, and limited reversal of their lumbar curve on anterior forward flexion (positive Schober test) were recognized. Enthesopathic symptoms (tendon insertion inflammation) were also common in these children. Many had heel spurs, plantar fasciitis, Achilles tendon insertion pain, and other periarticular manifestations (see box).

Hallmarks of Spondyloarthropathy

- Onset in late childhood or early adolescence
- Asymmetric joint involvement
- Frequent involvement of the hips, low back
- Enthesopathic symptoms (tendon insertion pain, especially heel and ankle)

These children initially were thought to represent the early onset of ankylosing spondylitis. However, with further investigation it became apparent that many children with this constellation of findings are not HLA-B27–positive and few develop ankylosing spondylitis over time. The syndrome is now recognized as "spondyloarthropathy" or seronegative enthesopathy arthropathy (SEA syndrome). Affected children are usually adolescents. They may be male or female.

The principal characteristic of spondyloarthropathies is the presence of enthesopathic inflammation, tenderness of the sacroiliac joints, and limited anterior forward flexion. Not all findings are always present. Spondyloarthopathy is the most common cause of arthritis in adolescent males. The prognosis for these children is unclear. Few go on to develop full-fledged ankylosing spondylitis, but many have recurrent low back pain and arthritis. The spectrum of disease varies, from children with severe limitation of their lumbar spine and active synovitis of large joints to children with only mild heel pain and limited anterior forward flexion. The arthritis that complicates inflammatory bowel disease is a spondyloarthropathy and special attention should be paid to excluding bowel disease in these patients.

Laboratory evaluation is typically unrewarding, with HLA-B27 testing being a useful confirmation if positive, but of little significance if negative since only 60% of patients with this entity are HLA-B27-positive. Although children with active synovitis may have anemia and elevated erythrocyte sedimentation rates during periods of active disease, many with mild disease have entirely normal laboratory results.

Medical Therapy

It is important to differentiate this syndrome from pauciarticular JRA because of its different natural history and its different therapy. Spondyloarthropathies typically respond well to tolmetin sodium or indomethacin. Gold sodium thiomalate is not recommended. In severe cases sulfasalazine or methotrexate may provide relief. Corticosteroids and immunosuppressive drugs are rarely appropriate for these children.

PSORIAFORM ARTHRITIS

This is a recently described entity whose characterization is still in progress. Some authors refer to these children as having psoriatic arthritis in the absence of psoriasis,[3] but the resulting confusion is undesirable. Tentatively established criteria for the diagnosis of psoriaform arthritis are arthritis plus any three of the following four criteria: dactylitis, nail pitting, psoriasis-like rash, or a family history of psoriasis in a first- or second-degree relative.[3, 12] A child with arthritis and any two of the criteria may be classified as having probable psoriaform arthritis (see box).

Psoriaform Arthritis

Arthritis plus at least two of the following:
- Dactylitis or asymmetric large joint arthritis
- Nail pitting
- Psoriasis-like rash
- Family history of psoriasis

The importance of this subset lies in the recognition of its more severe prognosis and differing therapy. Psoriatic arthritis is a spondyloarthropathy, but psoriaform arthritis may be recognized in a young girl with only dactylitis of one or two fingers and a positive family history of psoriasis. This child would otherwise be labeled as having pauciarticular JRA. However, children with psoriaform arthritis are more likely to have chronic recurrent disease with anemia and an elevated sedimentation rate. Whether they will all ultimately develop psoriasis (as suggested[3]) remains unknown. Medical therapy for these children is the same as for the other spondyloarthropathies.

DRUG THERAPY

Nonsteroidal anti-inflammatory drugs are the first-line agents in the treatment of chronic synovitis in childhood. Although acetylsalicylic acid remains effective and inexpensive, public fears of Reye's syndrome, the need for dosing every 6 hours to maintain levels, and the need to monitor carefully for hepatic toxicity have reduced its acceptance. Although many other nonsteroidal anti-inflammatory drugs are available, naproxen, tolmetin sodium, and ibuprofen are the three most often used in childhood. Naproxen and ibuprofen have the advantage of liquid preparations for small children, and naproxen has the advantage of dosing twice a day. Tolmetin sodium is often more effective for children who appear to have a spondyloarthropathy, but is also a more common source of gastrointestinal discomfort.

Indomethacin is an extremely effective nonsteroidal anti-inflammatory drug, but should be used only after the other nonsteroidal anti-inflammatory drugs have failed to provide adequate relief. Headaches, dizziness, behavior changes, and gastrointestinal irritation are all more frequent with indomethacin. Apparent hepatic toxicity and death in children with JRA who were receiving indomethacin has occurred.[6]

Some physicians criticize nonsteroidal anti-inflammatory drugs because they are not disease-modifying agents. This is an inaccurate characterization. The nonsteroidal anti-inflammatory drugs decrease pain and inflammation. In so doing they allow the child to maintain strength, function, and endurance and continue a more nearly normal program of activities of daily living. Maintaining the child's functional abilities is an important goal which directly impacts on the long-term outcome. Inasmuch as nonsteroidal anti-inflammatory drugs contribute to this goal they directly alter the outcome and are clearly disease-modifying agents despite the absence of a documented effect on the radiographic progression of disease.

Aurothioglucose (Solganal) and gold sodium thiomalate are injectable gold salts commonly used in childhood by pediatric rheumatologists. Because these agents have potentially fatal toxicities they should not be prescribed by physicians who are unfamiliar with appropriate monitoring. However, these agents clearly offer the best hope of inducing disease remission in children with active JRA that has proved unresponsive to nonsteroidal anti-inflammatory drugs. Auranofin is an oral gold preparation that has similar toxicity to the injectable gold salts without comparable efficacy.[3]

Methotrexate, azathioprine, chlorambucil, and cyclosporine are immunosuppressive drugs that may be of benefit in the treatment of children with severe progressive JRA. Methotrexate is currently receiving widespread use. It is generally effective, but the disease tends to become exacerbated when the drug is withdrawn. Toxic side effects of methotrexate have not been troubling to date, but the long-term experience with this drug in children with arthritis is not yet substantial. Azathioprine, chlorambucil, and cyclosporine are generally reserved for use by experienced pediatric rheumatologists in children with severe destructive arthritis unresponsive to other agents. Although there are serious toxicities associated with each of these agents, their use is justified if they can restore normal or near-normal function to a child who is otherwise disabled or dependent on chronic corticosteroid therapy.

Corticosteroids are useful agents for promptly suppressing JRA when all other therapies have failed. However, they have profound effects on growth that frequently result in undesirably short stature in children with severe JRA. In addition, the profoundly altered appearance of Cushing's syndrome has dramatic effects on the psychological development of children and adolescents. These difficulties, combined with the predisposition of patients on large doses of corticosteroids to develop osteoporosis and avascular necrosis, highlight the need to avoid chronic corticosteroid therapy. Except for systemic-onset JRA, chronic corticosteroid therapy is rarely indicated. When necessary, corticosteroids should be used in the lowest possible dose for the briefest possible period. The exception is the use of pulse intravenous methylprednisolone (30 mg/kg/dose up to a maximum of 1 g given once or daily for up to 3 days). This therapy may provide dramatic relief in a child with otherwise uncontrolled polyarticular or systemic-onset JRA. Although it has had profound and long-lasting effects in some patients, it should be regarded as a temporary measure to provide relief while other therapies take effect.

Two additional agents that may be used in the therapy of JRA are hydroxychloroquine and sulfasalazine. Hydroxychloroquine is a slow-acting agent that is effective in chronic JRA. It has a potential for retinal toxicity, but this is extremely rare when appropriate dosage guidelines are followed. Sulfasalazine has limited success in the treatment of JRA but is a useful adjunct in the treatment of spondyloarthropathies (Table 1B–1).

ANCILLARY THERAPIES

Physical and occupational therapy is a major adjunct to the treatment of children with JRA. No matter the onset type, the major goal of the treating team must be the maintenance of strength and range of motion. Physical and occupational therapy plays an invaluable role in accomplishing these goals. When medical therapy is failing, hospitalization to allow 2 and even 3 hours per day of physical and occupational therapy with heat, icing, and passive range-of-motion exercises may serve to preserve function that would otherwise be lost. Splinting and, in particular wrist splints to prevent flexion contractures and

TABLE 1B–1.

Recommended Dosages for Antirheumatic Agents in Childhood*

Agent	Dosage
Nonsteroidal anti-inflammatory drugs	
Acetylsalicylic acid (aspirin)	80 mg/kg/day divided q. 6 h. (maintain a blood level of 10–20 mg/100 mL)
Naproxen	10–20 mg/kg/day divided q. 12 h.
Ibuprofen	20–40 mg/kg/day divided q. 6 h.
Tolmetin sodium	20–40 mg/kg/day divided q. 6 h.†
Indomethacin	1–3 mg/kg/day divided q. 12 h.
Gold salts	
Aurothioglucose	1 mg/kg/wk up to 50 mg IM‡
Gold sodium thiomalate	1 mg/kg/wk up to 50 mg IM‡
Immunosuppressive agents	
Methotrexate	5–10 mg/m^2/wk§
Other agents	
Hydroxychloroquine	7 mg/kg/day up to 200 mg
Sulfasalazine	30–50 mg/kg/day up to 3 g

*The dosages recommended here are commonly accepted by the community of pediatric rheumatologists, but do not necessarily reflect the recommendations of the manufacturer or the Food and Drug Administration. The reader is directed to the *Physicians Desk Reference* for up-to-date prescribing information.

†Tolmetin sodium may be given effectively divided every 8 or 12 hours, but this schedule is not endorsed by the manufacturer.

‡These medications are given weekly intramuscularly with careful monitoring for hematologic or nephrologic toxicity and only after successful completion of a series of test doses.

§This medication is given weekly with careful monitoring for hematologic or hepatic toxicity and only after successful completion of a series of test doses. Higher doses have been utilized by some centers.

"night resting splints" to retard or prevent the development of knee flexion contractures, are valuable aids in the long-term management of children with severe JRA.

Every effort must be made to avoid wheelchair dependence. In our own program the need for a wheelchair is viewed as an acute medical and surgical emergency prompting immediate hospitalization. The use of a wheelchair clearly provides improved mobility for the child with arthritis, but the probability that a child who has been wheelchair-dependent for more than a few weeks will ever resume ambulation is low. Every effort must be made to avoid the child's or family's acceptance of this level of function. With aggressive use of physical therapy, medications, and surgical intervention (including total joint replacement) wheelchair dependancy can usually be avoided.

It is extremely difficult to restore ambulation to children who have become wheelchair-dependent. Selected highly motivated children confined to a wheelchair may be restored to ambulation with an intensive program of medical and surgical intervention combined with excellent physical and occupational therapy. The multidisciplinary team and facilities necessary to accomplish this goal are often found only in large institutions with extensive experience in the management of severe JRA. The child, the family, and the multidisciplinary team must be committed to the goal and prepared for repeated long hospitalizations over a 6- to 12-month period. However, the improved self-esteem and prognosis of an ambulatory patient justify such intervention when possible.

The successful multidisciplinary team for the care of children with JRA also will include a nurse-educator (clinical nurse specialist), a social worker, and a psychologist. Often patient-family compliance is a greater determinant of long-term outcome than the medical or surgical resources available to the treating physicians. Too often families leave the physician's office confused not only about what to expect but about what is expected of them as well. Nurse-educators provide a vital role by educating the family regarding the normal developments to be expected in the course of the child's JRA and the importance of medications, laboratory evaluations, when to contact the physician emergently, and appropriate follow-up visits. Families will frequently provide information to a friendly nonphysician that they are afraid to discuss directly with the physician. An experienced nurse-educator also may facilitate school referrals and coordinate activities for patients throughout the medical establishment.

The social worker is valuable in helping families deal with both insurance companies and the myriad government agencies charged with assisting children with chronic handicapping conditions. In addition, the social worker can provide limited psychological counseling to patients and their families in times of emotional stress and provide appropriate referral to the team psychologist when necessary. Chronic disease is a major stress upon the afflicted child, and his or her parents and siblings. Divorce is a frequent complication of JRA. Families have divergent coping patterns in dealing with the increased needs of the child with JRA. In some families parental guilt or other factors drive the parents to pour all their resources into the care of the afflicted child. When the needs of the other children in the family are ignored they may act out against the parents or the afflicted child. This produces a feeling of guilt in the child with JRA which further exacerbates the situation. Suicide is an ever-present risk in children with severe polyarticular JRA. Every effort should be made to provide the family with a comprehensive system of supports that reaches every member to provide the optimum outcome.

CONCLUSION

JRA is a complex group of diseases with a varying prognosis. While many children have mild disease requiring only a brief period of nonsteroidal anti-inflammatory drug therapy, others will have chronic and potentially debilitating disease. With aggressive medical and surgical management and appropriate provision of supporting services by an experienced multidisciplinary team, the chance of a successful outcome for children with JRA can be maximized. For all but the most severely affected children, normal or near-normal function can be restored. Even for severely affected children, optimal management may result in a well-adjusted individual who will make the most of his or her abilities, both vocationally and intellectually, with a satisfactory long-term outcome.

REFERENCES

1. Cassidy JT, Levinson JE, Bass JC, et al: A study of classification criteria for a diagnosis of juvenile rheumatoid arthritis. *Arthritis Rheum* 1986; 29:274.
2. Cassidy JT, Nelson AM: The frequency of juvenile arthritis. *J Rheumatol* 1988; 16:535.
3. Cassidy JT, Petty RE (eds): *Textbook of Pediatric Rheu-*

matology, ed 2. New York, Churchill Livingstone Inc, 1990.

4. Hanson V, Kornreich HK, Bernstein B, et al: Three subtypes of juvenile rheumatoid arthritis (correlations of age at onset, sex, and serologic factors). *Arthritis Rheum* 1977; 20:184.
5. Howard JF, Sigsbee A, Glass DN: HLA genetics and inherited predisposition to JRA. *J Rheumatol* 1985; 12:7.
6. Jacobs JC: Sudden death in arthritic children receiving large doses of indomethacin. *JAMA* 1967; 199:932.
7. Maksymowych WP, Glass DN: Population genetics and molecular biology of the childhood chronic arthropathies. *Clin Rheumatol* 1988; 2:649.
8. Ragsdale CG, Petty RE, Cassidy JT, et al: The clinical progression of apparent juvenile rheumatoid arthritis to systemic lupus erythematosus. *J Rheumatol* 1980; 7:50.
9. Schaller JG, Ochs HD, Thomas ED, et al: Histocompatibility antigens in childhood onset arthritis. *J Pediatr* 1976; 88:926.
10. Sher MR, Schultz JS, Ragsdale CG, et al: HLA-DR and MT associations with the clinical and serologic manifestations of pauciarticular onset juvenile rheumatoid arthritis. *J Rheumatol* 1985; 12:114.
11. Singsen BH: Epidemiology of Rheumatic Disease—Rheumatic diseases of childhood. *Rheum Dis Clin North Am* 1990; 16:581.
12. Southwood TR, Delgado E, Wood B, et al: Psoriatic arthritis in childhood. *Arthritis Rheum* 1988; 31(suppl):119.

CHAPTER 2

Radiographic Evaluation

Hollis G. Potter, M.D.

Bernard Ghelman, M.D.

INTRODUCTION

The role of the radiologist in the management of patients with rheumatoid arthritis is multifold, and encompasses diverse imaging techniques, ranging from plain film radiography to magnetic resonance imaging (MRI). The initial assessment of a patient presenting with ill-defined "joint pains" may prove a diagnostic dilemma for the clinician. The detection of specific radiographic signs narrows the clinician's differential considerations and aids in the assessment of both the extent and severity of disease. Clearly, radiographic criteria are but one of several diagnostic clues. Detailed patient history, serologic testing, and a thorough physical examination all provide additional information which enable an accurate diagnostic outcome.

IMAGING OF THE APPENDICULAR SKELETON

Plain Film Analysis

Plain film radiography is the imaging mainstay for the initial evaluation and ongoing assessment of arthritic conditions. A high-resolution, slow-speed film–screen system is needed to provide the necessary anatomic detail. The affected joint is examined in at least two (and often more) projections.

Since inflammatory arthritides commonly affect the small joints of the hands, the plain film is often the initial examination requested by the clinician. Posteroanterior (PA), lateral, and oblique (approximately 45-degree supination from the PA) views are recommended. The lateral film provides invaluable information concerning alignment of the carpus. The Norgaard, or anteroposterior (AP) oblique view (Fig 2–1), has been said to reveal the earliest changes of an inflammatory arthritis. Further, since this position is passively achieved by the patient, and not rigidly fixed by the technologist, reversible subluxations may become more apparent.[5] The advantage of the Norgaard over conventional views is controversial,[25] however, and it is therefore not routinely performed in many radiology departments.

Early radiographic findings of rheumatoid arthritis include periarticular soft tissue swelling, osteoporosis, loss of the subchondral bony plate, and minimal, symmetric joint space narrowing (Fig 2–2). With progressive proliferation of inflamed synovium, marginal erosions appear at the "bare" bony regions unprotected by articular cartilage at the site of ligament insertion.[21] (Fig 2–3).

Later radiographic findings in rheumatoid hands include diffuse osteoporosis, reflective of the regional hyperemia due to persistent synovial inflammation. Diffuse osteoporosis is characteristic of advanced rheumatoid arthritis, and helps to distinguish it from the seronegative spondyloarthritides. Erosions occurring primarily at the radial aspect of the metacarpal heads, in combination with inflammation of the adjacent ligaments and tendons and

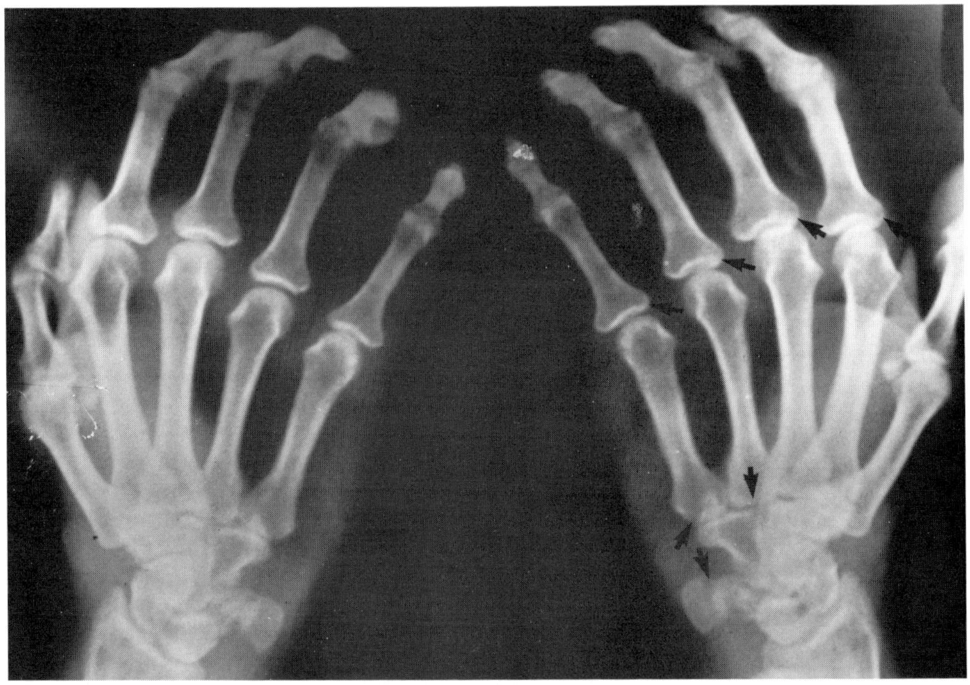

FIG 2–1.
Norgaard view of the hands in a normal patient. *Arrows* mark the areas where erosions may become apparent before their appearance on conventional views.

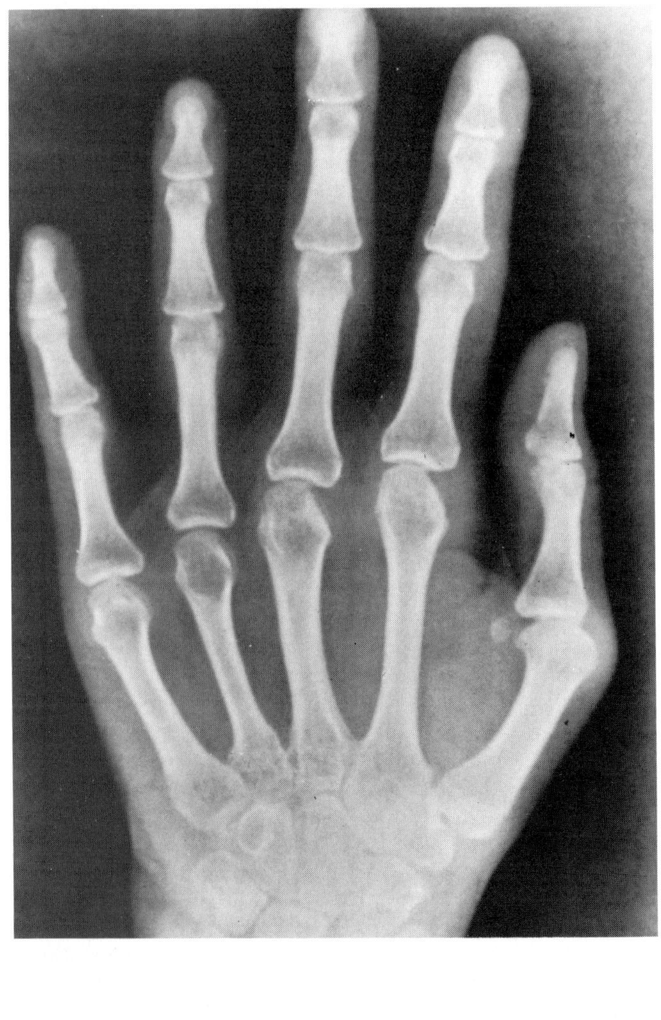

FIG 2–2.
PA view of the hand in a female patient with early seropositive rheumatoid arthritis. Subtle periarticular osteoporosis of the metacarpophalangeal and proximal interphalangeal joints is evident.

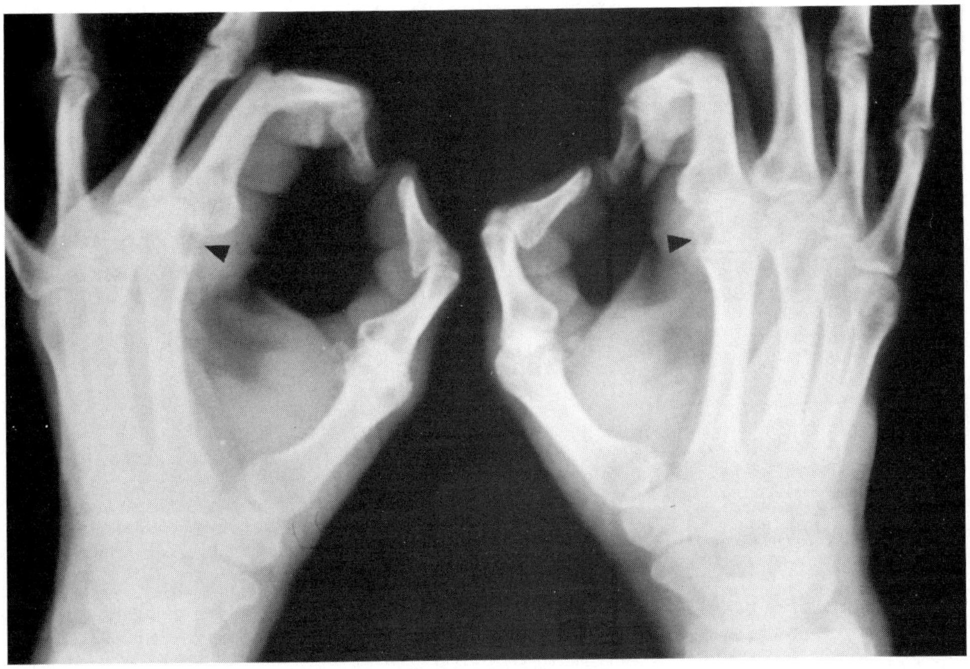

FIG 2–3.
Oblique view of the hands demonstrating symmetric erosions at the radial aspect of the metacarpophalangeal joints *(arrowheads).*

further joint destruction leads to ulnar subluxation and progressive deformity[15] (Fig 2–4). The characteristic erosion of the ulna styloid process reflects its proximity to the prestyloid recess of the radiocarpal joint compartment, as well as the extensor carpi ulnaris tendon. Late compressive-type erosions occur due to muscular action upon osteoporotic bone, and may be seen in both the hands and in the hips (Fig 2–5).

Joint ankylosis may occur following joint space obliteration. Although fibrous ankylosis may occur in any affected joint, noniatrogenic osseous ankylosis distal to the carpus is unusual in rheumatoid arthritis, and should suggest a rheumatoid variant[5] (Fig 2–6,A and B). In the rare instances that bony ankylosis of the metacarpophalangeal or interphalangeal joints is noted in a patient with established rheumatoid arthritis, it should suggest longstand-

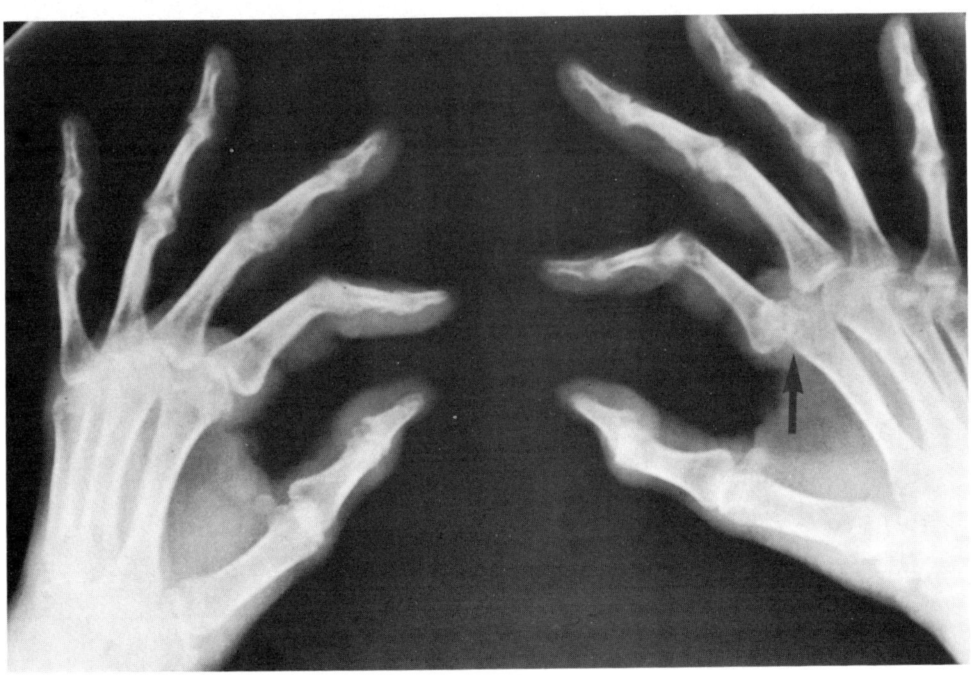

FIG 2–4.
Oblique view of the hands showing marginal erosions with resultant ulnar subluxation *(arrow).*

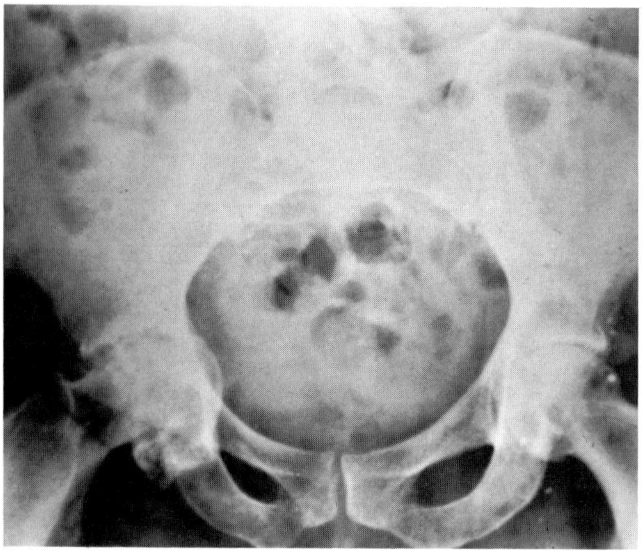

FIG 2–5.
AP view of the pelvis demonstrating a protrusio deformity of the right hip due to severe axial joint space narrowing and late, compressive-type erosions. Mild axial joint space narrowing is evident on the left side.

ing, more severe disease.[17] Quantitative scoring methods, based on plain film analysis of hand films, have been devised and applied to statistically significant measures of clinical status.[18] These methods entail a detailed assessment of bony changes, including the degree of erosion, joint space narrowing, and malalignment. Radiographs of advanced rheumatoid arthritis reflect the sequelae of ongoing synovial inflammation, destruction, and deformity (Fig 2–7).

Despite these characteristic findings, the clinician may be presented with conflicting clinical and radiographic findings. Cystic change occurring in bone with a relative lack of osteoporosis and clinical disability has been described in physically active patients,[7] and is known as rheumatoid arthritis of the robust reaction type.[10] The cystic changes are thought to be the result of increased articular pressure forcing synovial fluid or granulation tissue into the bone,[7] a process which may become accelerated with a greater degree of physical activity[19] (Fig 2–8).

Bone proliferation, either related to enthesopathy, or to osteophyte production, is atypical of rheumatoid arthritis, and should suggest alternative diagnoses (Fig 2–9). It is important to remember, however, that older patients with longstanding rheumatoid arthritis may present a mixed radiographic picture of an inflammatory arthritis with superimposed degenerative joint disease.

Soft tissue involvement with synovial inflammation of bursae leads to osseous erosion[6] and spontaneous tendon rupture[37] noted on both plain films (Fig 2–10,A) and arthrography (Fig 2–10,B).

FIG 2–6.
A, PA view of the wrist in a patient with rheumatoid arthritis, demonstrating bony ankylosis of the radioscaphoid and radiolunate joints. The extension of the radiocarpal joint to the prestyloid recess accounts, in part, for the erosion of the ulna styloid process. **B,** PA view of the hand in a patient with psoriatic arthritis showing more severe involvement of the distal interphalangeal joints, with partial osseous ankylosis of the fifth ray *(arrow)*. The distribution of both erosions and ankylosis would be highly atypical of rheumatoid arthritis.

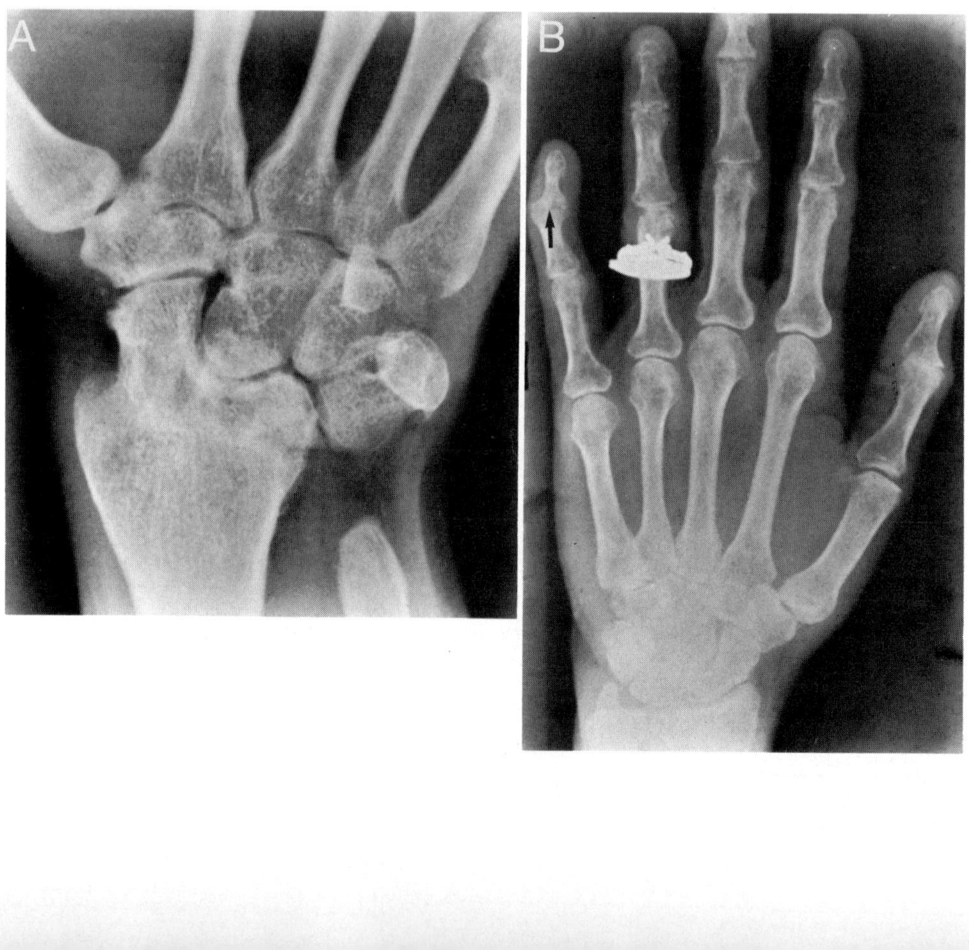

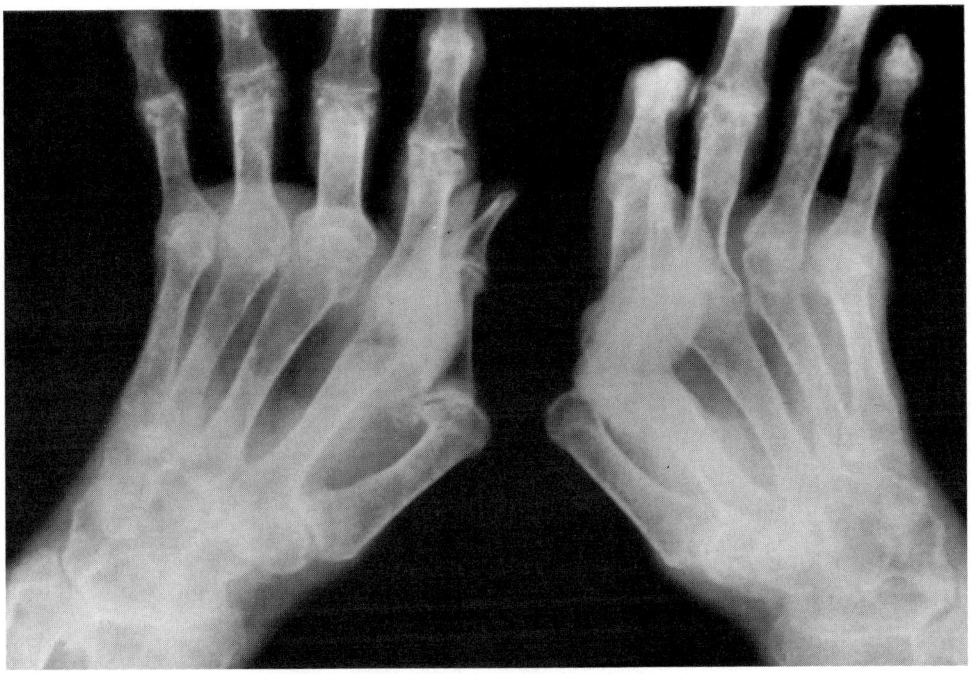

FIG 2–7.
Advanced rheumatoid arthritis. Diffuse, symmetric joint space narrowing and osteoporosis, as well as severe ulnar subluxation of the metacarpophalangeal joints, lead to the characteristic clinical deformity.

Arthrography

Single and double contrast athrography provides an effective means to evaluate the synovial inflammation and complications of rheumatoid arthritis (see Fig 2–10,B). Irregularity of the capsule, early lymphatic filling, and diminished joint capacity reflect capsulitis (Fig 2–11,A and B). Arthrography may also be of use following surgical intervention (Fig 2–12,A and B), when the presence of metallic prostheses may interfere with more sophisticated modalities owing to image artifacts.

Ultrasound

Attempts have been made to search for diagnostic modalities that will provide information with less invasive techniques. Ultrasound has been used to evaluate popliteal cysts,[14] and rotator cuff tears,[16, 35]

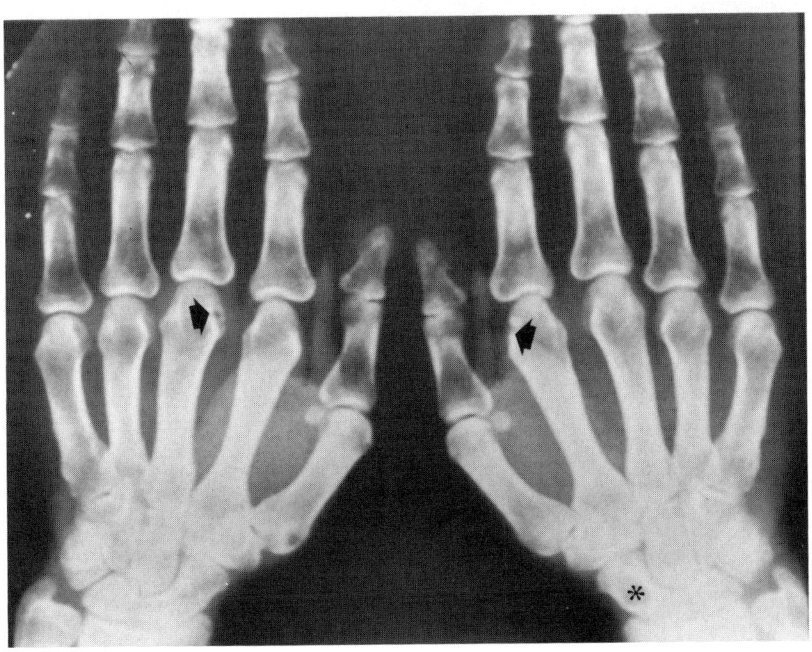

FIG 2–8.
PA view of the hands in a manual laborer with rheumatoid arthritis. Cystic changes in the carpus *(asterisk)* and marginal erosions of the metacarpophalangeal joints *(arrows)* are evident. Bone mineralization is relatively normal.

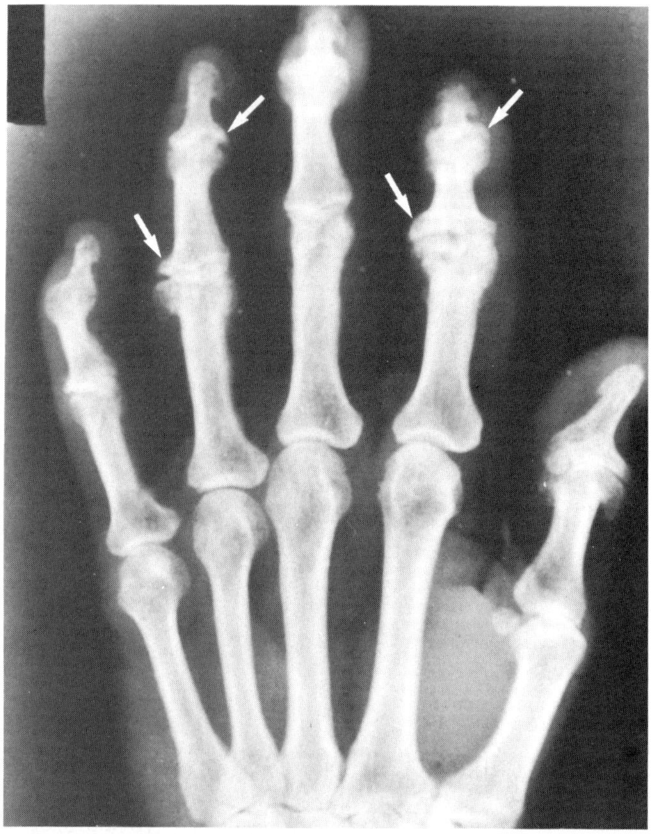

FIG 2–9.
PA view of the hands in an older patient with erosive osteoarthritis. Typical radiographic changes include an interphalangeal joint distribution, with relative sparing of the metacarpophalangeal region, and exuberant osteophyte formation *(arrows).*

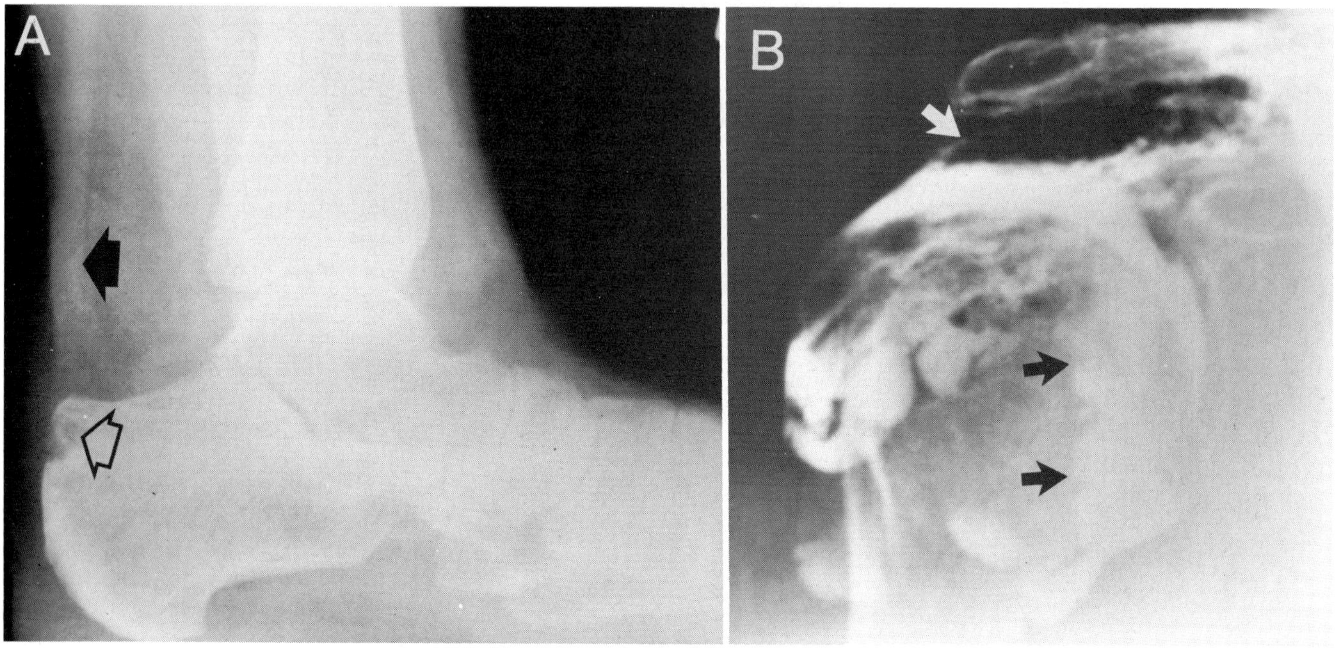

FIG 2–10.
A, lateral view of the calcaneus in a rheumatoid patient. The erosion at the superior aspect of the calcaneus *(open arrow)* reflects the inflammation of the retrocalcaneal bursa and the adjacent Achilles tendon *(closed arrow).* **B,** double contrast shoulder arthrogram demonstrating air in the subacromial-subdeltoid bursa *(white arrow),* indicative of a full-thickness rotator cuff tendon tear. Irregularity of the axillary recess *(black arrows)* reflects the underlying synovial inflammation in this rheumatoid patient.

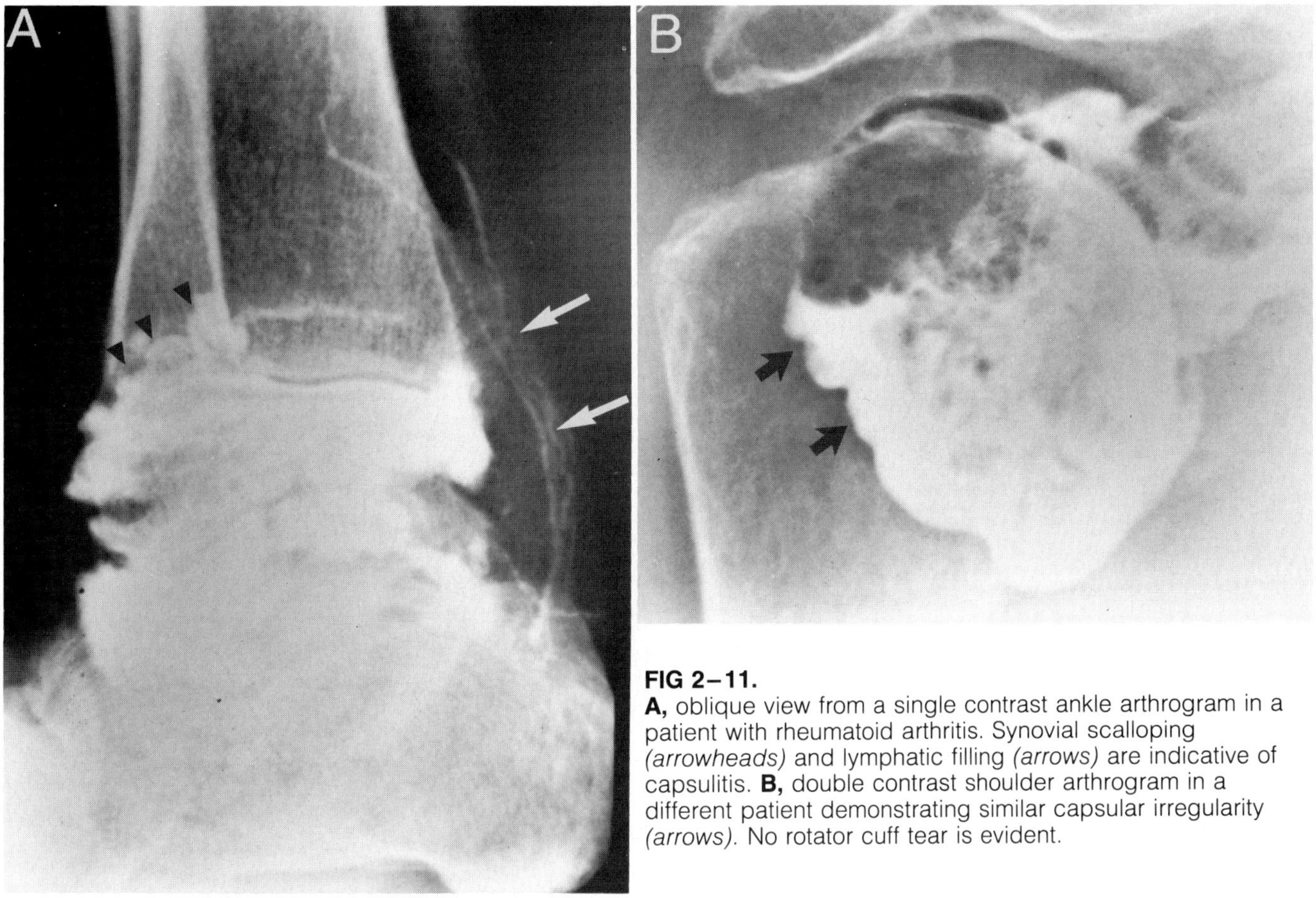

FIG 2–11.
A, oblique view from a single contrast ankle arthrogram in a patient with rheumatoid arthritis. Synovial scalloping *(arrowheads)* and lymphatic filling *(arrows)* are indicative of capsulitis. **B,** double contrast shoulder arthrogram in a different patient demonstrating similar capsular irregularity *(arrows)*. No rotator cuff tear is evident.

with reported specificities as high as 75%.[16] The reproducibility of such results, however, has proved difficult due to conflicting sonographic critieria[4] and extremely subjective operator dependency.

Scintigraphy

Bone scintigraphy provides an assessment of both disease distribution and activity. The use of bone scanning agents in the evaluation of the painful prosthesis is discussed later in this chapter. Scintigraphic abnormalities may precede conventional radiographic findings.[38] The most commonly used agent is technetium 99m methylene diphosphonate (^{99m}Tc MDP), which is injected intravenously, and is distributed to the bone based on several factors, including regional blood supply and bone turnover. The hyperemia and reactive bone turnover associated with inflammatory arthritis results in areas of increased activity detected by the gamma camera. The diphosphonate compounds are preferred because of their relatively high target-nontarget ratio within 2 to 3 hours following injection.[24] Rapid sequential images obtained following injection provide regional flow information, which may aid in assessing both disease activity and pathologic fracture (Fig 2–13).

COMPUTED TOMOGRAPHY

The use of more sophisticated imaging techniques provides increased sensitivity in the detection of disease severity, and may help to plan for the surgical management of the patient. High-resolution computed tomography (CT) of affected joints shows with greater detail the degree of joint involvement (Fig 2–14). The data obtained from these studies may be used for the design and manufacture of a joint prosthesis.

Computed tomography has also been used to improve the detection of rheumatoid involvement of the soft tissues. Rheumatoid lung disease encompasses a wide range of pathologic changes, from the more common pleuritis and pleural effusion, to mul-

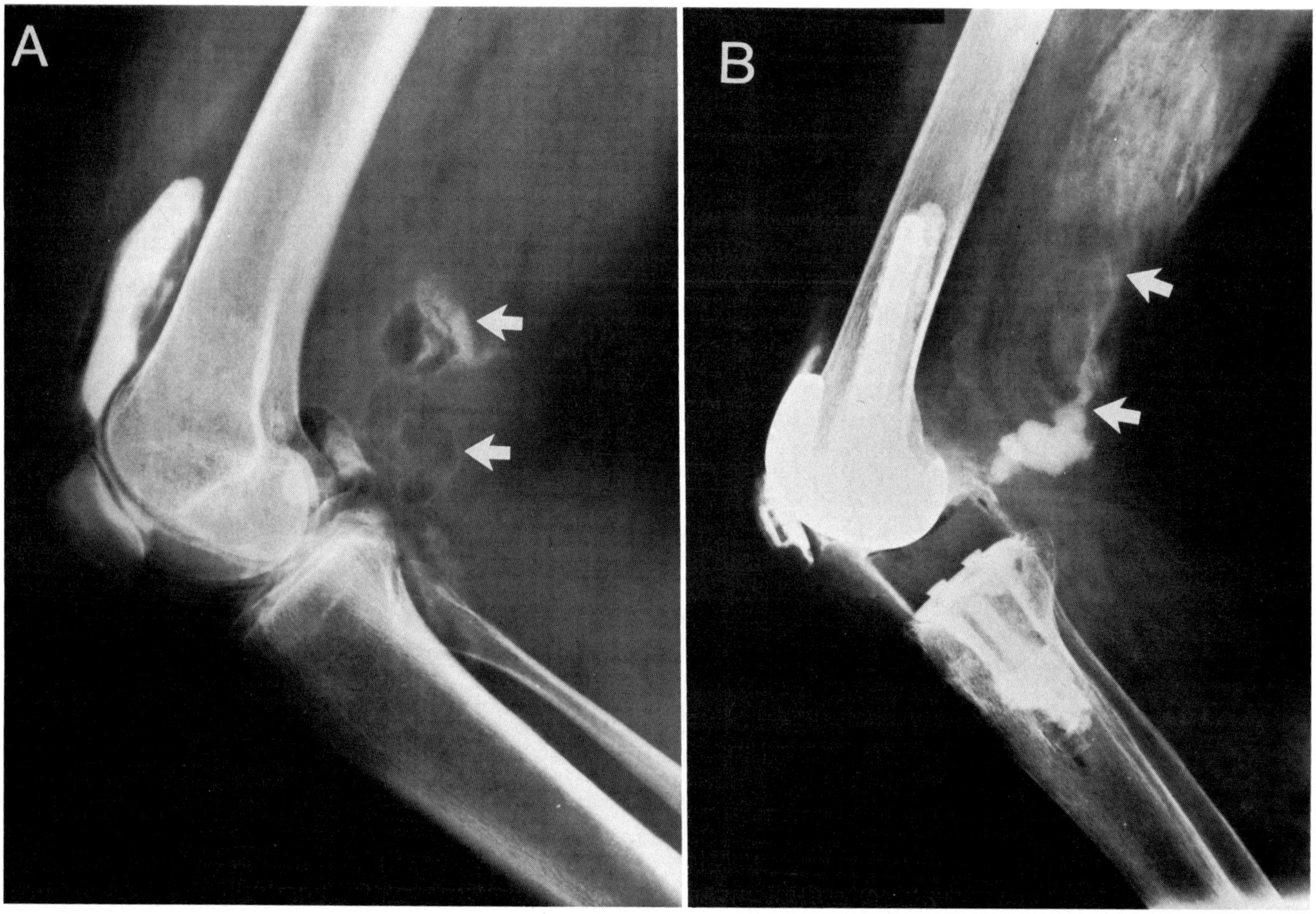

FIG 2–12.
A, preoperative knee arthrogram in a patient with rheumatoid arthritis showing a large, ascending popliteal cyst *(arrows)*. **B,** postoperative arthrogram, obtained following total joint replacement, demonstrating rupture of the popliteal cyst *(arrows)*. (From Pavlov H, Steinbach L, Fried SH: *Clin Orthop* 1983; 179:204. Used by permission.)

tiple parenchymal "necrobiotic" nodules.[33] These nodules are typically found in the periphery of the lung, and often cavitate, forming thick walls with smooth inner linings.[28] Lung disease is not a presenting sign in rheumatoid patients, as it typically arises in association with longstanding arthritis with multiple subcutaneous nodules.[33] While plain film radiography may serve as a cost-effective means in the interval assessment of disease, high-resolution chest CT demonstrates the pathologic changes to better advantage (Fig 2–15,A and B).

MAGNETIC RESONANCE IMAGING

Unlike CT, MRI provides multiplanar imaging capabilities without loss of anatomic detail. MRI entails the placement of the patient in an external magnetic field, which causes the alignment of a vector quantity of the patient's protons with the axis of the external field. Subsequently, a radiofrequency (RF) pulse is applied, which will disturb the mobile protons out of the axis of the external field (longitudinal magnetization), to the plane of transverse magnetization. As thermal equilibrium is regained, electromagnetic energy is released, which will induce a current in the imaging coil, and generate an MR signal.

The T1-weighted images, which provide the better anatomic detail, rely on differential speeds of recovery of longitudinal magnetization, following the RF pulse. Fat has a short T1 relaxation time, yielding a bright signal, while water remains dark (low signal intensity) due to its long T1 relaxation time. Conversely, T2-weighted images maximize tissue contrast, based on decay or loss of transverse magneti-

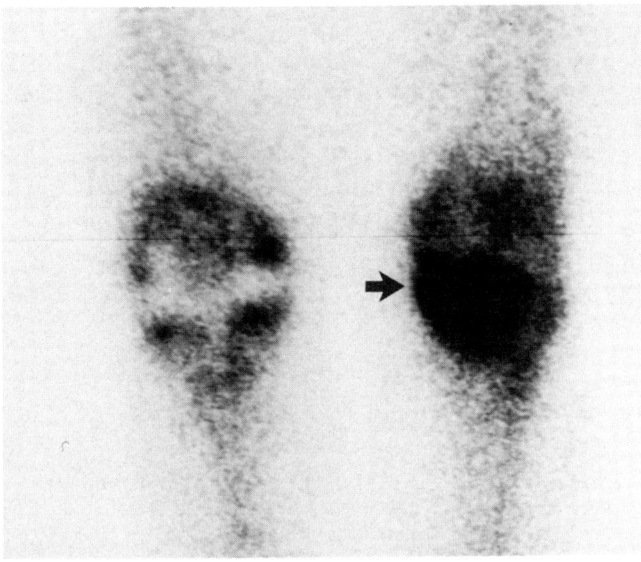

FIG 2–13.
Third (bone) phase from a three-phase ^{99m}Tc MDP bone scan in a rheumatoid arthritis patient with left knee pain. A region of intense radiotracer localization in the left tibia was noted on all three phases *(arrow)*, and reflects an insufficiency-type stress fracture. The photopenic region in the right knee is due to the presence of a total joint prosthesis. Plain films obtained at the time were normal.

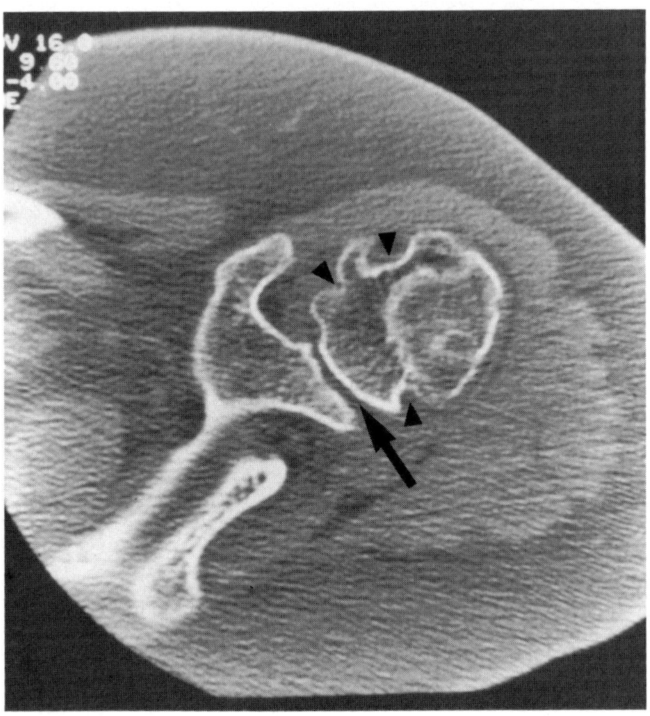

FIG 2–14.
Transaxial CT image through the shoulder of a patient with rheumatoid arthritis, demonstrating glenohumeral joint space narrowing *(arrow)* and adjacent marginal erosions *(arrowheads)*. The examination was performed to aid in the development of a custom joint prosthesis.

zation. Water maintains its signal coherence in the transverse plane longer than fat, allowing for the brighter (or "whiter") signal from water on the T2-weighted images.

Given the superior tissue contrast of MRI over plain film radiography, it has become popular in the evaluation of all musculoskeletal disease. In patients with rheumatoid arthritis, marginal erosions are better demonstrated, probably in part due to the tomographic nature of the technique[3, 11] (Fig 2–16). Furthermore, MRI enables detection of both cartilage destruction[41] (Fig 2–17) and secondary soft tissue abnormalities occurring as a result of longstanding synovial inflammation (Fig 2–18).

Pannus, representing inflammation of the synovium with a resultant increase in synovial water content, is usually an intermediate signal intensity on T1-weighted images, with a corresponding increased signal on T2-weighted images.[36, 41] Areas of synovial proliferation that maintain a relatively low signal intensity on all pulse sequences may represent more fibrotic, inactive pannus formation.[41] In addition, areas of low signal intensity on T2-weighted images may reflect hemosiderin deposition within the hypertrophied synovium.[3]

In most cases of active disease, pannus will show relative increased signal intensity on T2-weighted images, making it difficult to distinguish from the bright signal intensity of joint effusion. The intravenous use of the MR contrast agent gadolinium diethylenetriamine pentaacetic acid (DTPA) (Gd DTPA;0.1 mmol/kg body weight), which primarily acts to shorten T1 relaxation times, may help in this regard. Synovial proliferations will typically exhibit a marked increase in signal intensity following contrast administration, as opposed to minimal enhancement of the synovial effusion[30] (Fig 2–19,A–C). It is attractive to speculate that Gd DTPA might be used to assess the activity of disease; however, no definite correlation between the signal intensity and the clinical estimate of disease activity has yet been found.[30]

IMAGING OF THE SPINE

The frequency of radiographic and clinical involvement of the cervical spine has been reported to be as high as 88%.[9] Discovertebral instability, synovial inflammation, and ligamentous laxity lead to subluxations with resultant neurologic injury. Early involvement of the cervical spine is manifested by

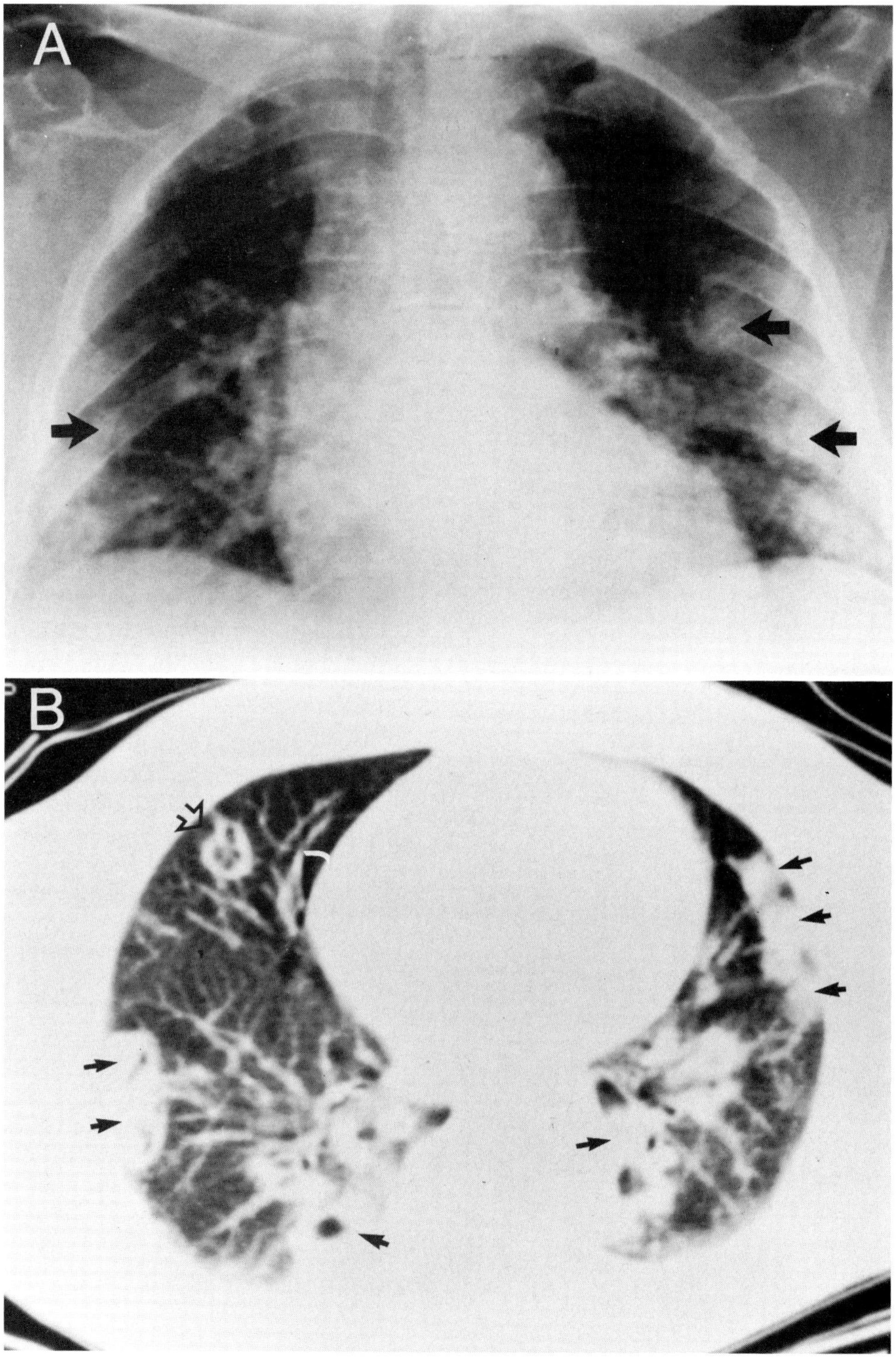

FIG 2–15.
A, conventional chest radiograph in a patient with rheumatoid lung disease. Ill-defined nodules are apparent in the lower lobes *(arrows).* **B,** transaxial CT image in the same patient demonstrates the numerous necrobiotic nodules *(arrows),* with cavitation *(open arrow)* that is not apparent on the routine chest film.

erosion of the odontoid; apophyseal joint erosion or sclerosis, or both; and subaxial subluxation, usually in an anterior direction.[39]

Conventional radiography should be the initial imaging method employed in evaluation of the spine. Standing lateral films, taken in neutral position, as well as *passive* flexion and extension, will demonstrate the degree of dynamic instability (Fig 2–20,A and B). Water-soluble contrast myelography affords visualization of thecal sac and nerve root

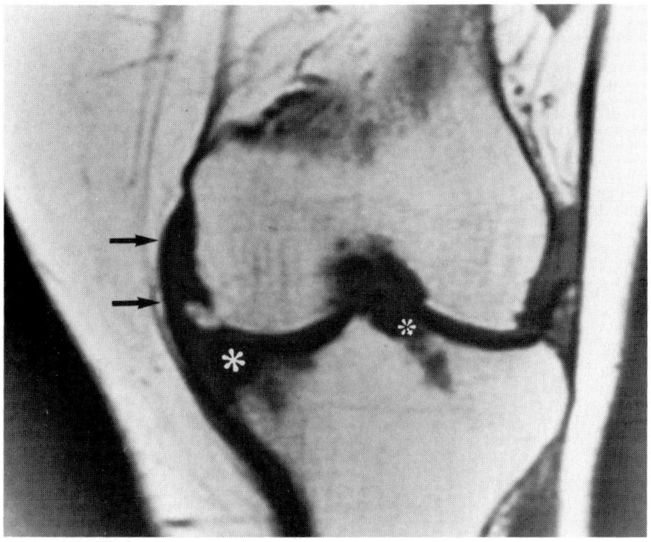

FIG 2–16.
Coronal T1-weighted (TR = 500 ms, TE = 12 ms) MR image demonstrates marginal erosions *(asterisks)*. The superficial fibers of the medial collateral ligament are bowed by both joint effusion and fluid in the adjacent bursa *(arrows)*.

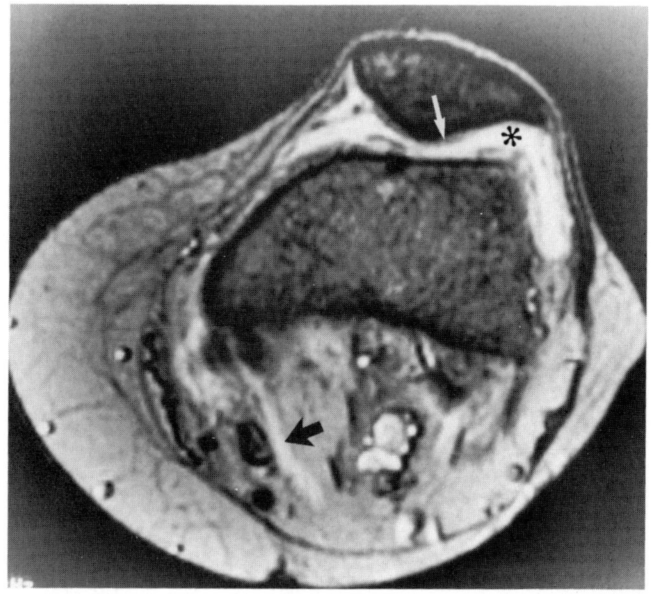

FIG 2–17.
Transaxial gradient echo MR image (TR = 350 ms, TE = 18 ms; flip angle 30 degrees) of the knee in the same patient as in Figure 2–16. Almost complete erosion of the patella cartilage is evident, with a small amount remaining at the patella apex (gray or intermediate signal, *white arrow*). The high signal intensity *(asterisk)* is joint fluid. A partially collapsed popliteal cyst is noted posteromedially *(black arrow)*.

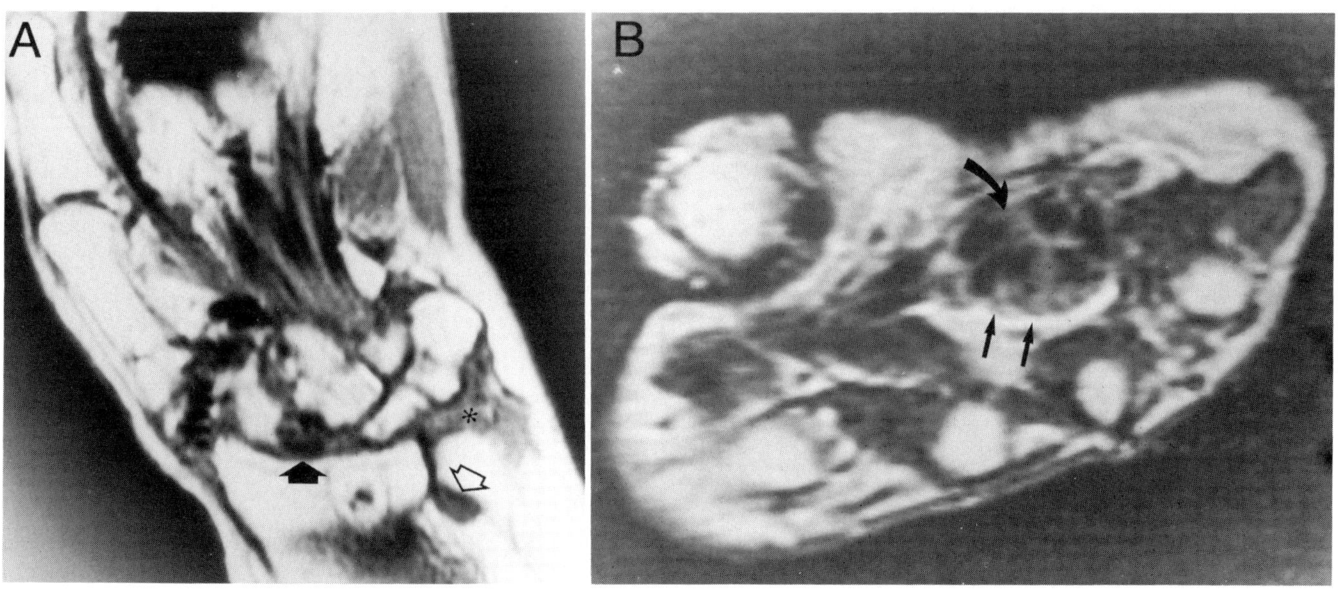

FIG 2–18.
A, coronal MR image (TR = 2,000 ms, TE = 16 ms) through the wrist in a patient with rheumatoid arthritis and suspected carpal tunnel syndrome. (The thumb is to the viewer's left.) Erosions at the radioscaphoid joint are apparent *(closed arrow)*. Also noted is fluid in the distal radioulnar joint *(open arrow)*, and pannus in the triangular fibrocartilage complex *(asterisk)*. **B,** transaxial T2-weighted (TR = 2,000 ms, TE = 80 ms) MR image in the same patient slightly distal to the osseous carpal tunnel. High signal intensity fluid *(straight black arrows)* is noted in the ulna bursa, surrounding the deep flexor tendons. Disruption of the normal flexor tendon configuration is noted, and the adjacent median nerve *(curved black arrow)* is compressed.

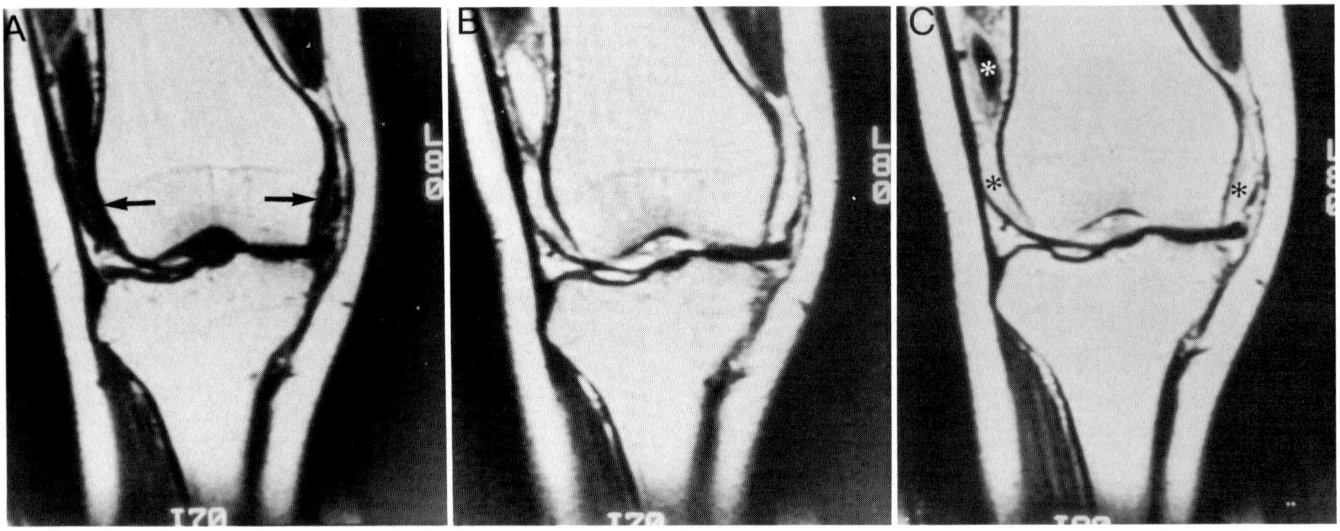

FIG 2–19.
A, coronal T1-weighted MR image demonstrates areas of low signal intensity at both aspects of the joint line *(arrows)*. **B,** T2-weighted MR image obtained at the same level shows corresponding increased signal intensity in the same areas. One cannot distinguish synovial fluid from inflammatory pannus. **C,** T1-weighted MR image, obtained following Gd DTPA contrast administration, distinguishes the marked enhancement of the pannus *(black asterisks)* from the poorly enhancing effusion *(white asterisk)*.(Courtesy of Sevil Kursunoglu-Brahme, M.D., San Diego.)

compression due to the osseous instability (Fig 2–21,A). Most institutions routinely follow the cervical myelogram with thin-section transaxial CT examination, which will disclose the degree of cervical cord compression at a specific level (Fig 2–21,B). Sagittal reformations from the CT-acquired data enable visualization of the pathologic changes in additional planes, albeit with slightly diminished resolution.

The multiplanar capabilities of MRI make its ap-

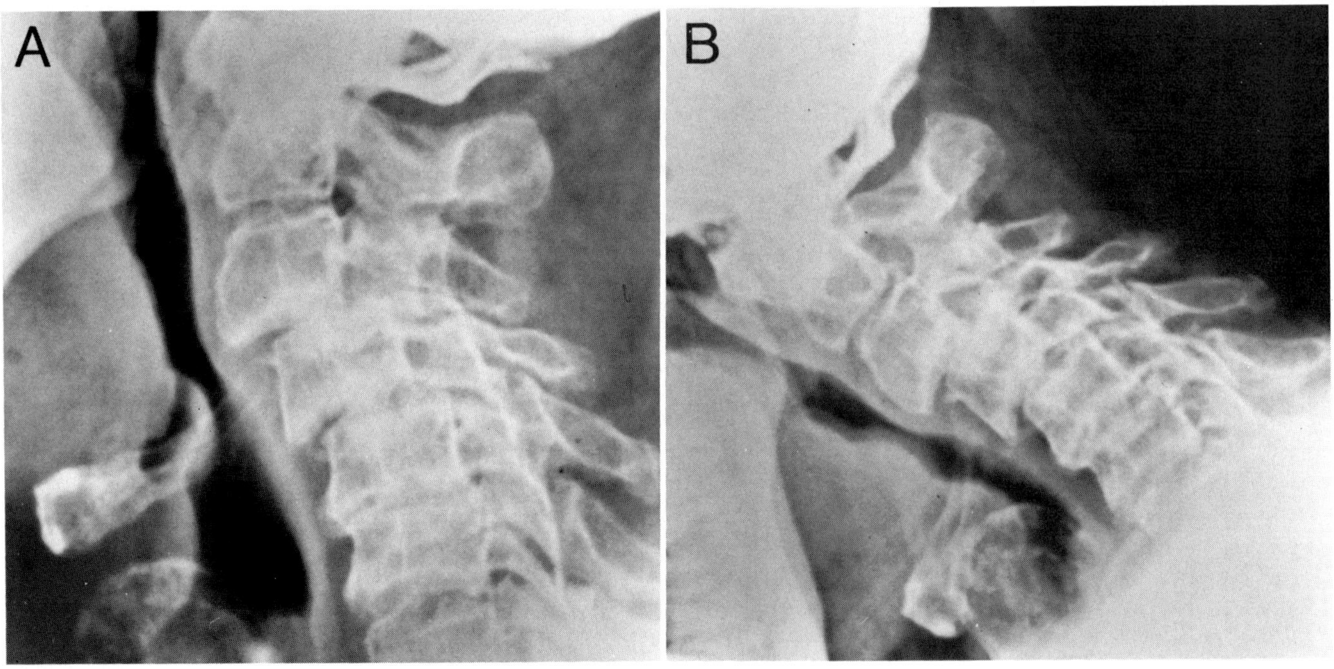

FIG 2–20.
Standing lateral view of the cervical spine in a rheumatoid patient, taken in neutral **(A)** and passive flexion **(B)** positions. Extensive subluxation of C3 on C4, and C4 on C5 is noted.

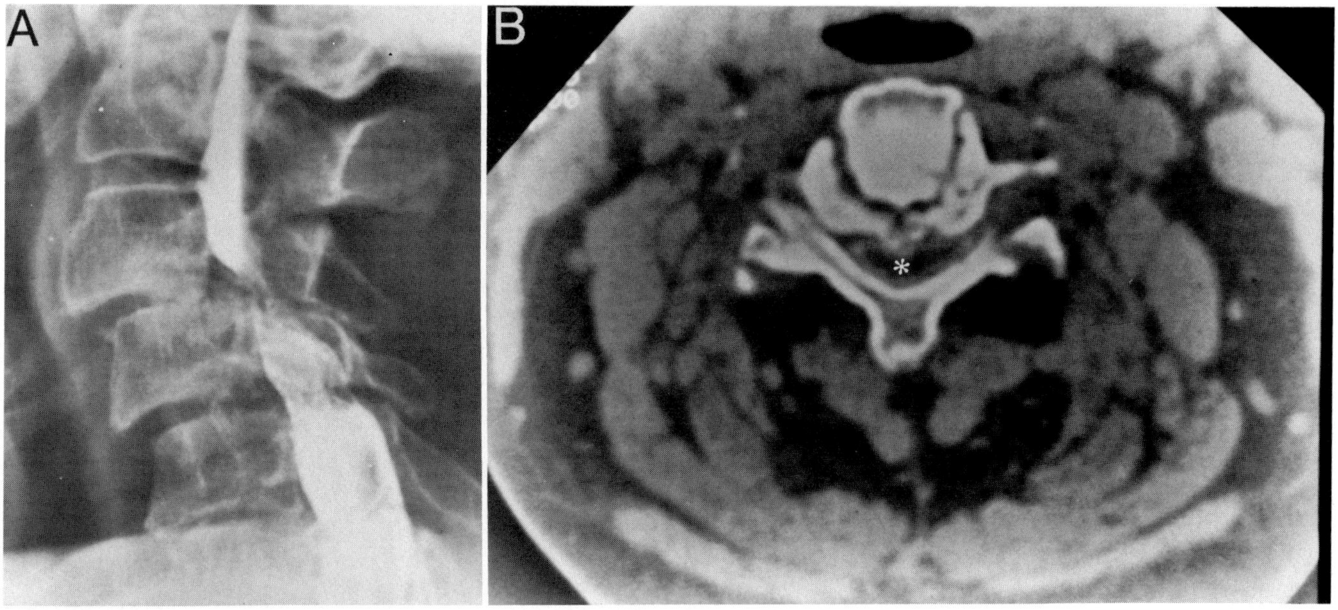

FIG 2–21.
A, same patient as in Figure 2–20. Marked constriction of the thecal sac at the C3–4 level is noted on this water-soluble myelogram. **B,** transaxial CT image at the C3–4 level demonstrates the osseous subluxation as well as the degree of cervical cord *(asterisk)* compression.

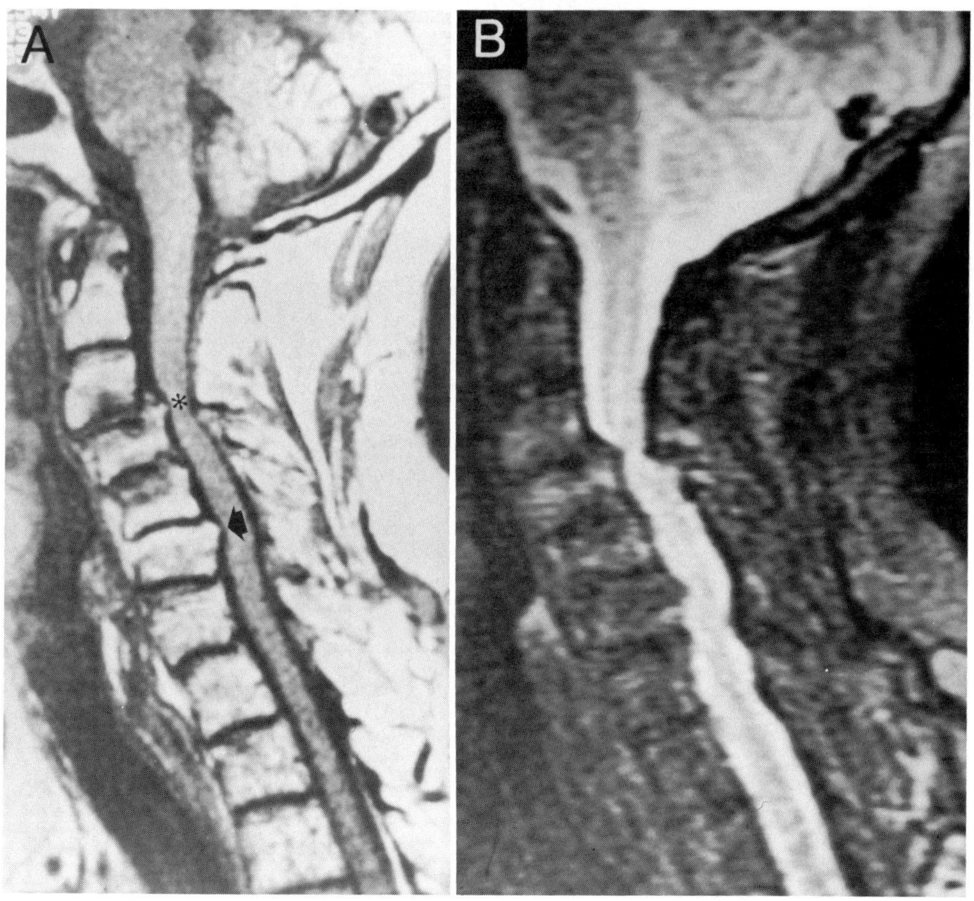

FIG 2–22.
A, Sagittal T1-weighted (TR = 600 ms, TE = 20 ms) MR image in the same patient discloses the degree of cervical cord compression at C3–4 *(asterisk).* Also apparent is slight cord compression at C6 *(arrow),* which is only seen upon retrospective review of the myelogram (see Fig 2–21,A). **B,** T2-weighted (TR = 2,000 ms, TE = 80 ms) MR image provides a myelographic effect.

plication to spine imaging self-evident. The use of a dedicated cervical spine surface coil, as well as sagittal and axial planar imaging, will disclose any cord compression (Fig 2–22,A). If available, volumetric thin-section examination (1.5 mm with no interslice gap) enables improved visualization of associated cervical disc disease. The T2-weighted sequences will provide a "myelographic" effect due to the high signal intensity of the cerebrospinal fluid, and will thus further demonstrate any cord compression or edema caused by vertebral compression (Fig 2–22,B).

Abnormalities of the upper cervical region deserve special mention, as they are common pathologic features of the rheumatoid spine.[1, 39] Atlantoaxial distance is generally measured on plain films between the posterior aspect of the anterior arch of C1, and the anterior aspect of the odontoid. This distance should not exceed 3 mm in adults, or 5 mm in children.

Plain film analysis of "cranial settling," or basilar invagination, usually relies on a series of measurements obtained by lines drawn on a lateral view of the cervical spine. Perhaps the two most commonly used are McGregor's and Chamberlain's lines, being lines drawn from the posterior margin of the hard palate to either the posterior aspect of the foramen magnum (Chamberlain's[8]), or the most caudal point on the occipital curve (McGregor's[22]) (Fig 2–23). In normal cases, the odontoid process should not project above Chamberlain's line, and any case in which the odontoid is 6.6 mm (2 SD) above this level, or 4.5 mm above McGregor's line, would be indicative of basilar invagination.

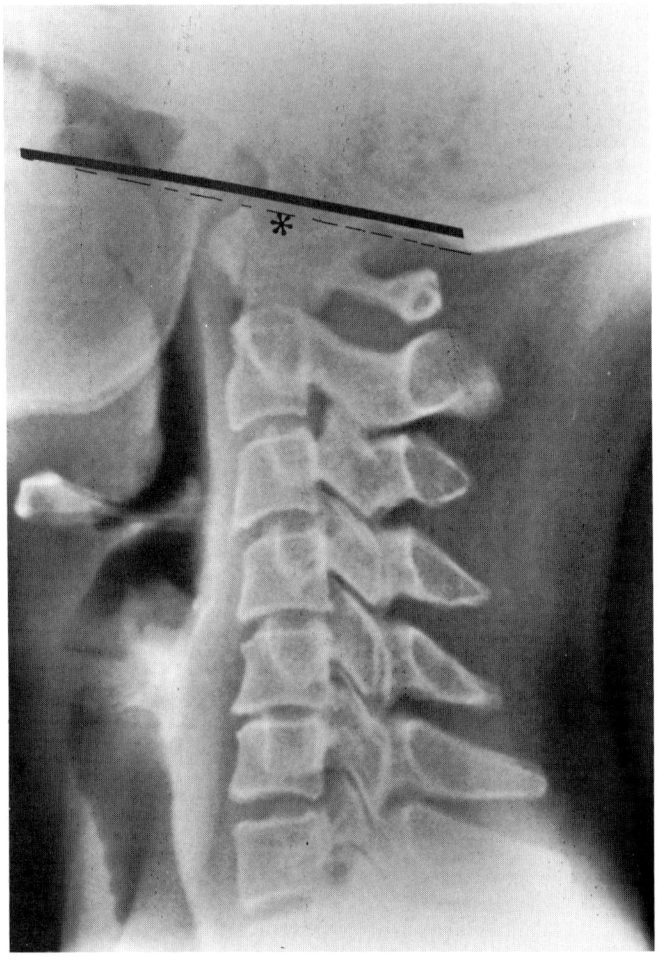

FIG 2–23.
Lateral view of the cervical spine in a normal patient, showing the normal relationship of the odontoid *(asterisk)* to Chamberlain's *(solid line)* and McGregor's *(dotted line)* lines.

Practical considerations limit the use of these lines, however, owing to limited visualization of the distal tip of the odontoid when erosions are present. Sagittal reformations of transaxial CT sections may provide improved resolution (Fig 2–24,A). MRI affords improved visualization of the odontoid owing to the contrast between the fatty marrow of the odontoid anteriorly (bright or "white" on T1-weighted images), and the cerebrospinal fluid posteriorly (low signal or "black" on T1-weighted images) (Fig 2–24,B). Areas of hypertrophic synovium may be seen also around the odontoid.

MRI in flexion and extension provide more dynamic information regarding spine stability, and more fully demonstrate the degree of cord or medullary compression (Fig 2–25,A and B). This process, however, lengthens the time of the examination, and may require special neck coils to allow for an adequate signal-to-noise ratio in the different positions.

It bears mention that in a patient with coexistent atlantoaxial and subaxial subluxation, and presenting with long tract signs, the neurologic compromise is most likely due to the more caudal level of abnormality. Owing to the increasing diameter of the spinal canal as it approaches the foramen magnum, atlantoaxial subluxation may exist without significant neurologic deterioration.

Once surgical reduction of the subluxation is achieved, the presence of posterior wire fixation may limit the use of CT or MRI owing to streak artifact or localized disturbance in the magnetic field, respectively. At that time, plain films and complex-motion tomography may be used to assess any subsequent instability.

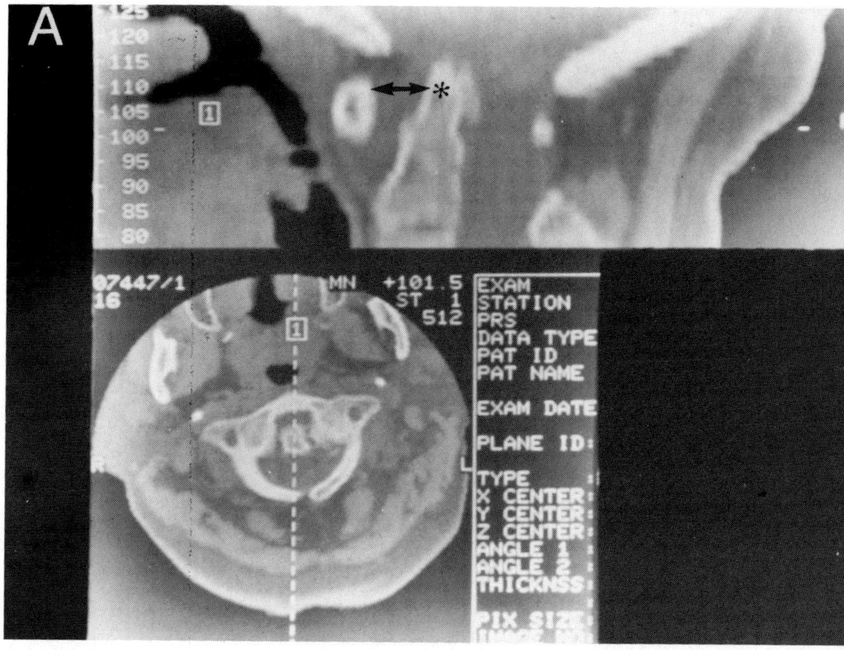

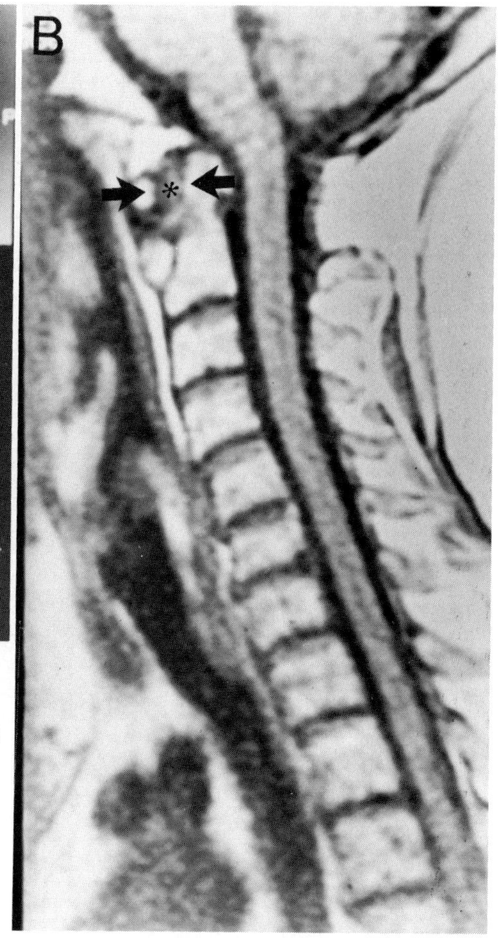

FIG 2–24.
A, sagittal CT re-formation from data acquired in the axial plane. The improved resolution of CT over plain films allows for better visualization of the odontoid erosion *(asterisk).* The atlantoaxial distance is widened in neutral position *(arrows).* **B,** T1-weighted MR image in the same patient shows the intermediate signal pannus *(asterisk)* between the anterior arch of C1 and the odontoid *(arrows).*

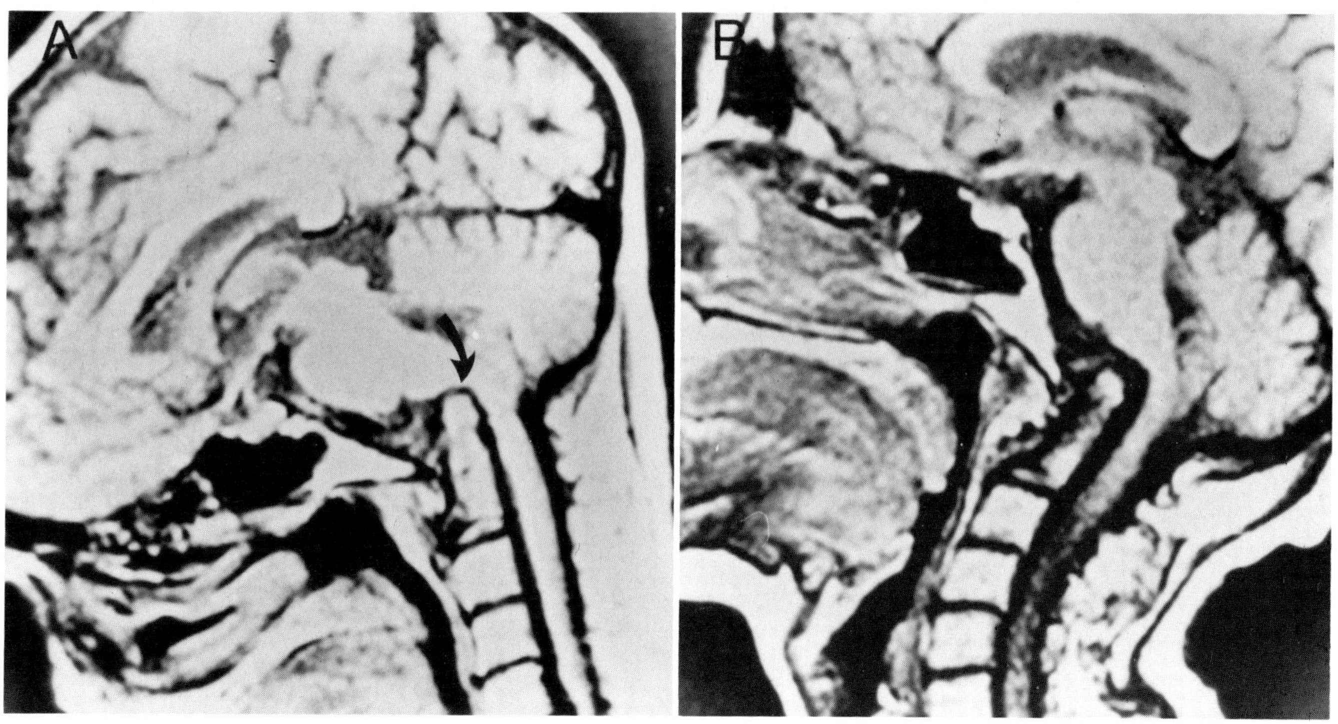

FIG 2–25.
T1-weighted MR images, taken in flexion **(A)** and extension **(B),** in a patient with basilar invagination and rheumatoid arthritis. The medullary compression is maximized in flexion *(curved arrow).*

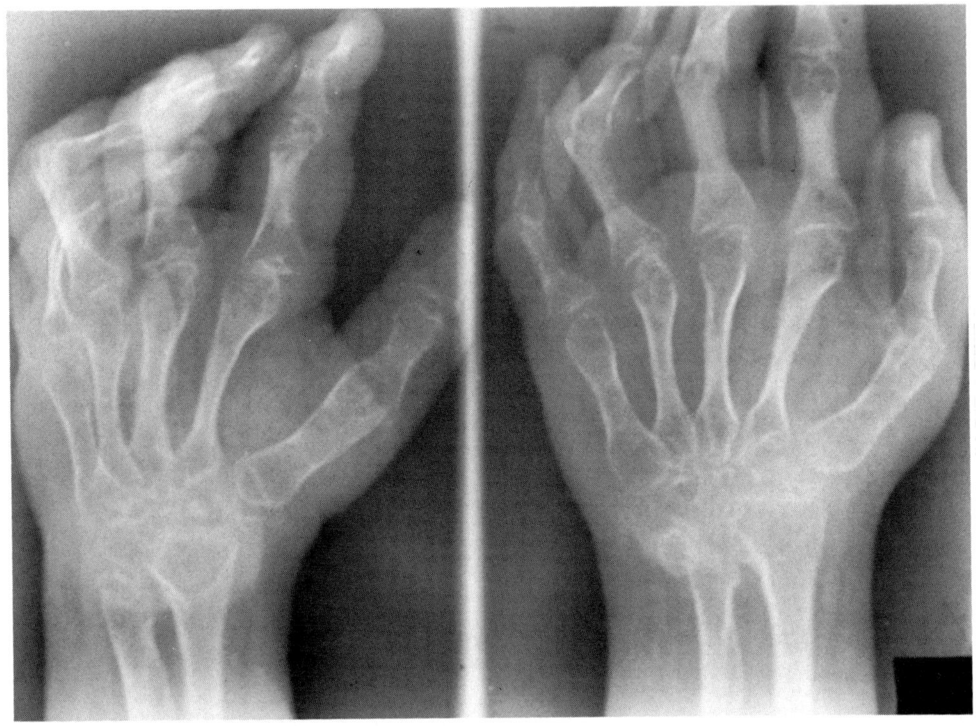

FIG 2–26.
PA and oblique views of the hands in a patient with juvenile chronic arthritis. Advanced skeletal maturation has led to premature epiphyseal fusion, with resultant brachydactyly.

IMAGING OF THE JUVENILE RHEUMATOID PATIENT

Owing to its lack of ionizing radiation, MRI has been used to evaluate patients with juvenile rheumatoid arthritis.[41] Sedation may be required, however, depending on both the age and degree of cooperation of the child, because of image susceptibility to motion degradation. Radiographic imaging of children requires great attention to radiation dose, as these patients will require serial examinations over many years. Plain film analysis demands particular attention to adequate gonadal shielding and x-ray beam collimation.

The spectrum of juvenile chronic arthritis includes many distinct disease entities, including juvenile-onset ankylosing spondylitis, psoriatic and other seronegative spondyloarthritides, adult-type (seropositive) rheumatoid arthritis, and Still's disease, which accounts for approximately 70% of all juvenile chronic arthritis.[5]

Typically assuming a pauci- or monarticular pattern,[31] the classic radiographic features of Still's disease include periarticular soft tissue swelling, periostitis, osteoporosis, and advanced skeletal maturation, with premature epiphyseal fusion. Early physeal closure leads to decreased bone length (Fig 2–26). The regional hyperemia promotes epiphyseal enlargement, with a resultant "balloon" deformity

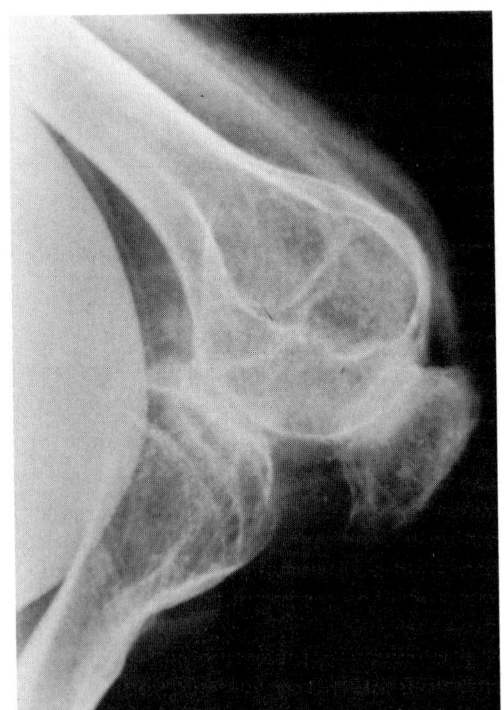

FIG 2–27.
Lateral view of the knee in a patient with Still's disease. Typical epiphyseal expansion, as well as osteoporosis, is noted.

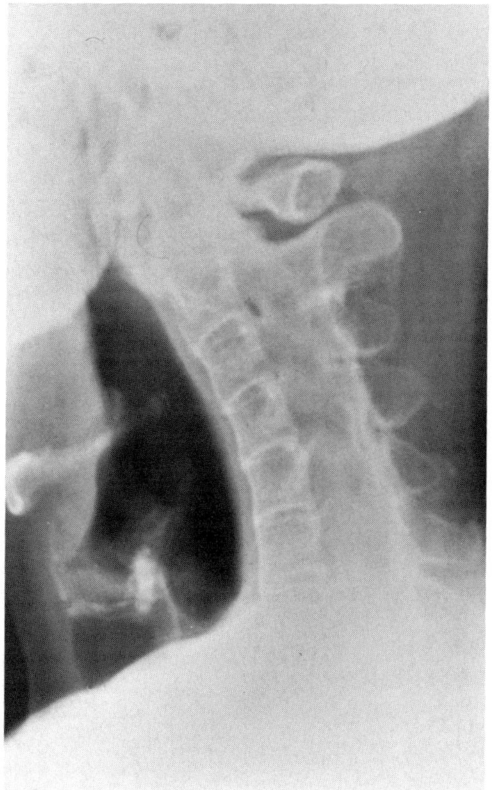

FIG 2–28.
Cervical spine involvement in juvenile rheumatoid arthritis. Diffuse ankylosis of the apophyseal joints is noted.

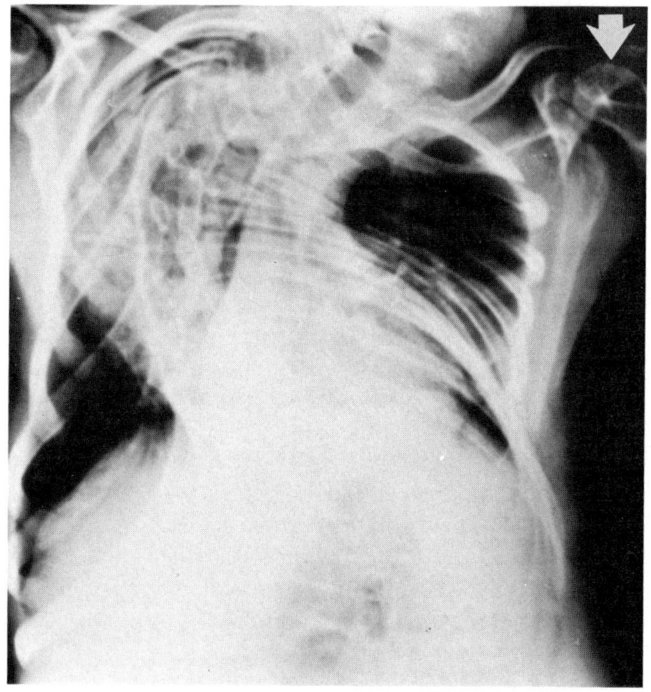

FIG 2–29.
AP view of the thoracic spine in a juvenile rheumatoid arthritis patient with severe scoliosis. Characteristic epiphyseal expansion of the proximal humerus is noted *(arrow).*

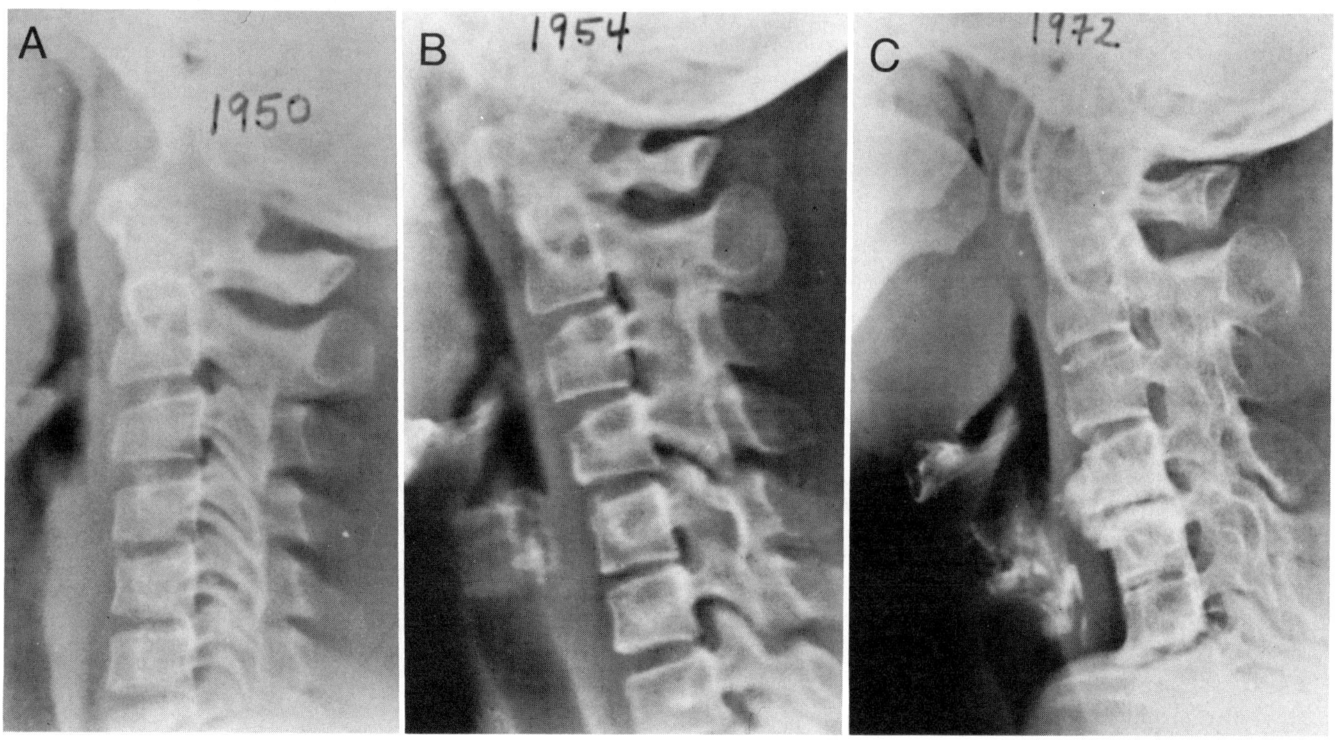

FIG 2–30.
A–C, serial lateral radiographs of the cervical spine demonstrate progressive apophyseal joint ankylosis, with development of a pseudarthrosis at C4–5.

(Fig 2–27). Growth deformity, rather than erosions and joint space narrowing, dominates the radiographic picture.[5] It should be noted that monarticular involvement may be simulated by both intraarticular osteoid osteoma and septic arthritis. A careful history may help to distinguish these entities. If infection is still a diagnostic consideration, aspiration in combination with arthrography is recommended.

Spine involvement is characterized by apophyseal joint ankylosis (Fig 2–28), with the predominant effect on the upper cervical region.[5] Thoracolumbar involvement is relatively rare; when present, scoliosis may occur, possibly due to both apophyseal joint arthritis and muscle imbalance[31] (Fig 2–29). Interval radiographic assessment is crucial in these children, as complications of joint ankylosis may become manifest radiographically prior to development of clinical exacerbations (Fig 2–30,A–C).

IMAGING OF THE POSTOPERATIVE PATIENT

Complications of both disease progression and surgical intervention may first become apparent on the radiographic image. Both contrast venography and duplex Doppler ultrasonography[32] have been used to diagnose deep venous thrombosis in the postoperative patient (Fig 2–31).

Skeletal scintigraphy may be used in the detection of both loosening and infection of painful joint replacements (Fig 2–32,A and B). If there is a high clinical index of suspicion for infection, joint aspiration-arthrography is recommended,[13] as both gallium and technetium agents may nonspecifically show increased uptake in either loosening or infection.[2]

Areas surrounding joint replacements may show reactive uptake of radiotracer for a variable amount of time in the immediate postoperative period. A useful general rule is that a cemented prosthesis should not demonstrate increased uptake at 1 year following surgery. Factors affecting uptake include stress reactions with resultant cortical thickening, and the amount of preexisting bone deformity.

Conversely, in porous-coated arthroplasty, ingrowth of bone and fibrous tissue occurs onto the prosthesis, with corresponding areas of increased radionuclide uptake.[27] Uptake of ^{99m}Tc MDP, occurring as a result of continued bone remodeling, may be seen in the *absence* of loosening or infection for up to 24 months of postoperative study, particularly at the distal and lateral prosthetic tip segments.[27] Furthermore, the activity noted in these regions may increase over time. Oswald et al.[27] suggest that uptake occurring at areas not covered by porous coating may reflect micromotion at the metal-bone interface.

Indium 111–labeled white blood cell (In WBC) scintigraphy will disclose areas of inflammation sur-

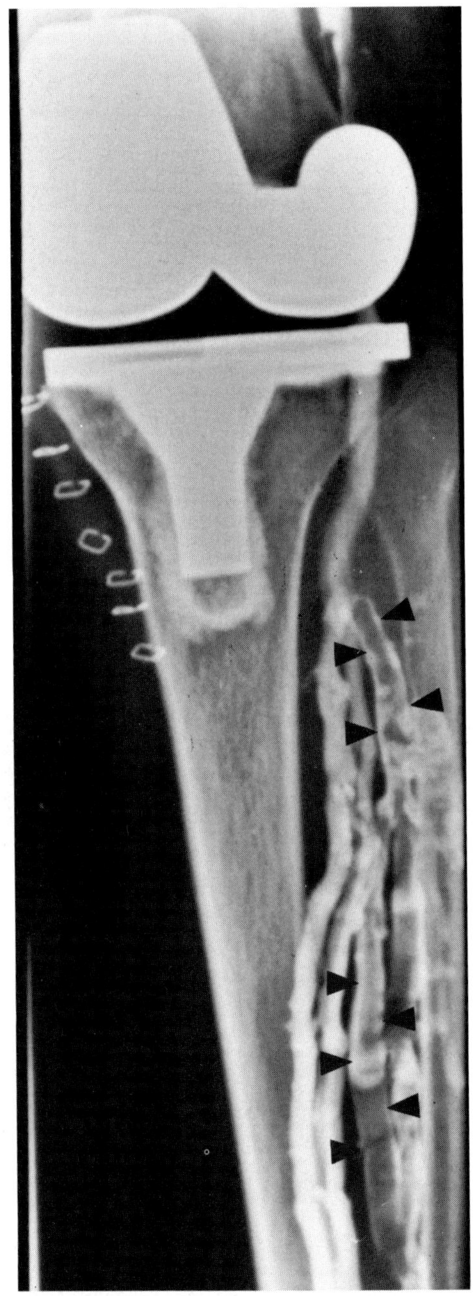

FIG 2–31.
AP view of the leg obtained during contrast venography. Multiple deep venous thrombi cause filling defects, creating a characteristic "tram-track" appearance *(arrowheads)*.

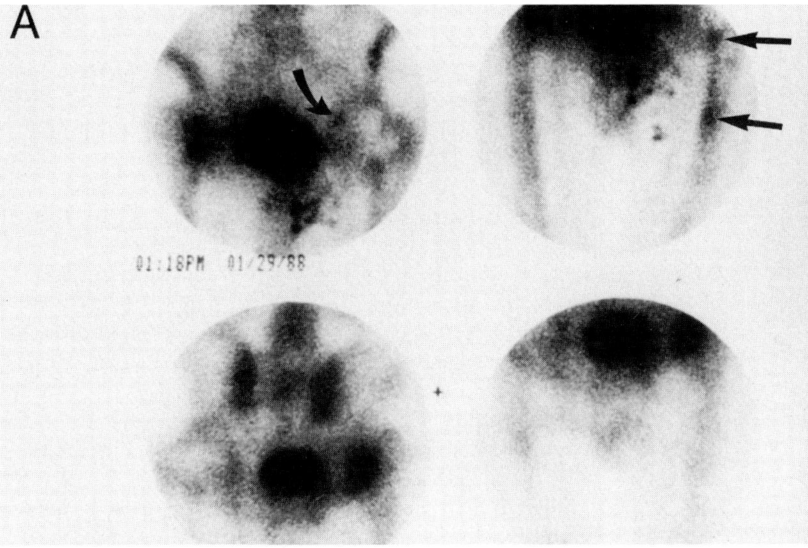

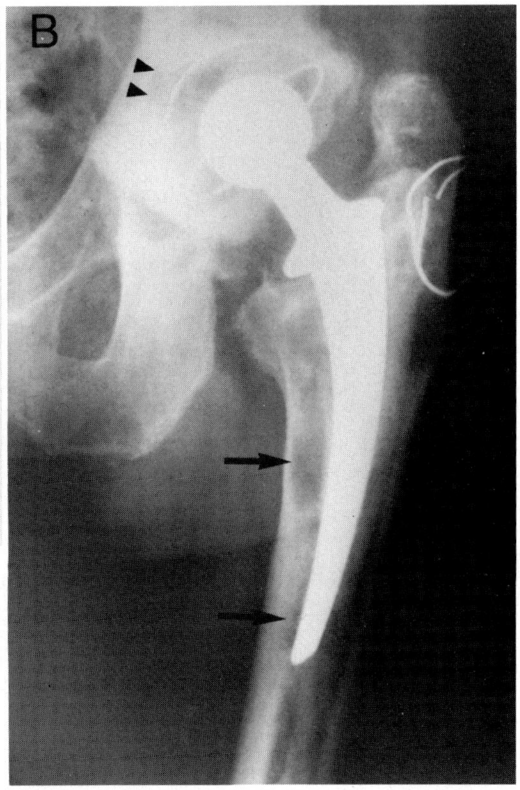

FIG 2–32.
A, images obtained from a ^{99m}Tc MDP bone scan in a patient with a painful left hip prosthesis. Foci of increased activity at the neck and stem of the prosthesis *(straight arrows)* suggest loosening of the femoral component. Slightly increased activity at the medial aspect of the acetabular component *(curved arrow)* reflects an additional site of abnormality. **B,** corresponding plain film in the same patient. The prominent lucency at the superomedial aspect of the acetabular component *(arrowheads)* proved to be focal loosening at surgery. Extensive osteolysis due to histiocytic resorption at the bone-cement interface of the femoral component is noted *(arrows).*

rounding painful joint prostheses, with a higher accuracy in the detection of infection than sequential technetium-gallium scanning.[23] False-positive indium scans, however, have been noted in the presence of prosthetic loosening, particularly in the knee, when joint effusion may contain inflammatory cells in the absence of infection.[29]

In addition, porous-coated hip prostheses may show focal In WBC uptake in the absence of infection. Such uptake may be seen both at the femoral tip and acetabular regions of hip prostheses for up to 2 years post surgery.[26, 27] The possibility of infection should be raised, however, when (1) serial In WBC scans show an increase in abnormal activity after the initial 6-month postoperative period; (2) the In WBC scan is more intense than the ^{99m}Tc MDP uptake; (3) the increased flow or nondiffuse blood pool activity is noted after 3 months post arthroplasty; or (4) the increased In WBC activity is at any time greater than the ipsilateral iliac crest (a useful reference point).[26, 27]

It is clear from these data that there is no one specific, noninvasive test which is 100% specific for prosthesis infection. It is further apparent that the type of prosthesis will greatly affect the diagnostic interpretation of the test. The importance of plain film correlation, as well as a knowledge of the location of the porous coating, cannot be overstated.

Small joint replacements and bone implants made of silicone polymers may cause a reactive synovitis with focal bone destruction[12, 34, 40] and foreign body granuloma formation.[20] Radiographic findings include implant deformity, intramedullary lucencies, and erosion of the adjacent bone (Fig 2–33). Although this phenomenon has been described in both carpal bone implants and small joint replacements, it appears more commonly in association with the bone implants, possibly owing to the increased compressive loading forces.[34]

CONCLUSIONS

The radiologist plays an integral role in the diagnosis and ongoing assessment of the patient with rheumatoid arthritis. The multiplanar capabilities of MRI, as well as its superior tissue contrast, has made it an

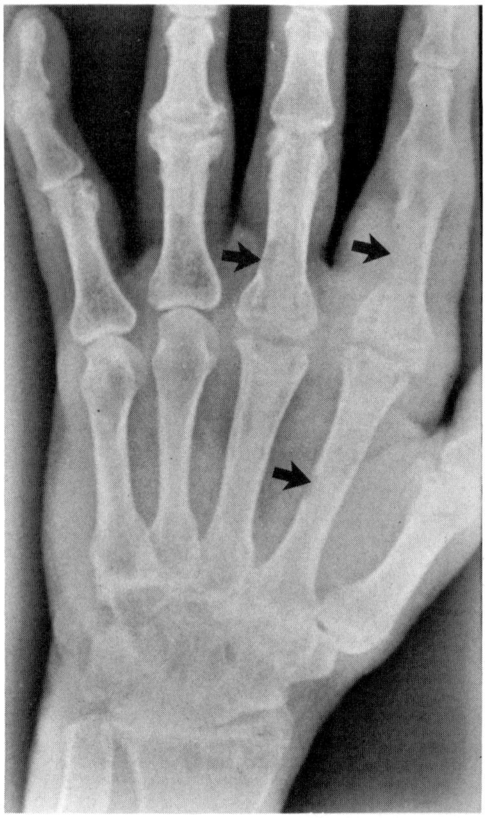

FIG 2–33.
PA view of the hand in a patient with advanced rheumatoid arthritis who has undergone silicone joint replacement of the second and third metacarpophalangeal and fourth proximal interphalangeal joints. Focal resorption and osteolysis surrounding the prosthesis suggest silicone synovitis *(arrows).*

important diagnostic tool in the evaluation of joint disease. Despite the increasing availability of more sophisticated techniques, however, it must be emphasized that plain film radiography remains the imaging mainstay of articular pathologic study.

REFERENCES

1. Aisen AM, Martel W, Ellis JH, et al: Cervical spine involvement in rheumatoid arthritis: MR imaging. *Radiology* 1987; 165:159–163.
2. Aliabadi P, Tumeh SS, Weissman BN, et al: Cemented total hip prosthesis: Radiographic and scintigraphic evaluation. *Radiology* 1989; 173:203–206.
3. Beltran J, Caudill JL, Herman LA, et al: Rheumatoid arthritis: MR imaging manifestations. *Radiology* 1987; 165:153–157.
4. Brandt TD, Cardone BW, Grant TH, et al: Rotator cuff sonography: A reassessment, *Radiology* 1989; 173:323–327.
5. Brower AC: *Arthritis in Black and White.* Philadelphia, WB Saunders Co, 1988.
6. Bywaters EGL: Heel lesions of rheumatoid arthritis. *Ann Rheum Dis* 1954; 13:42–51.
7. Castillo BA, El Sallab RA, Scott JT: Physical activity, cystic erosions, and osteoporosis in rheumatoid arthritis. *Ann Rheum Dis* 1965; 24:522–527.
8. Chamberlain WE: Basilar impression (platybasva). *Yale J Biol Med* 1939; 11:487.
9. Conlon PW, Isdale IC, Rose BS: Rheumatoid arthritis of the cervical spine: An analysis of 333 cases. *Ann Rheum Dis* 1966; 25:120–126.
10. De Haas WH, De Boer W, Griffioen F, et al: Rheumatoid arthritis of the robust reaction type. *Ann Rheum Dis* 1974; 33:81–85.
11. Gilkeson G, Polisson R, Sinclair H, et al: Early detection of carpal erosions in patients with rheumatoid arthritis: A pilot study of magnetic resonance imaging. *J Rheum* 1988; 15:1361–1366.
12. Gordon M, Bullough PG: Synovial and osseous inflammation in failed silicone-rubber prostheses. *J Bone Joint Surg [Am]* 1982; 64:574–580.
13. Gould ES, Potter HG, Bober SE: Role of routine percutaneous hip aspirations prior to prosthesis revision. *Skeletal Radiol* 1990; 19:427–430.
14. Grant EG, Ear NJ, Richardson JD, et al: High-resolution real-time sonography: The study of superficial body parts. *Med Clin North Am* 1984; 68:1609.
15. Hakstian RW: Ulnar deviation of the fingers: The role of joint structure and function. *J Bone Joint Surg [Am]* 1967; 49:299–316.
16. Hodler J, Fretz CJ, Terrier F, et al: Rotator cuff tears: Correlation of sonographic and surgical findings. *Radiology* 1988; 169:791–794.
17. Kaye JJ, Callahan LF, Nance EP Jr, et al: Bony ankylosis in rheumatoid arthritis: Associations with longer duration and greater severity of disease. *Invest Radiol* 1987; 22:303–309.
18. Kaye JJ, Callahan LF, Nance EP Jr, et al: Rheumatoid arthritis: Explanatory power of specific radiographic findings for patient clinical status. *Radiology* 1987; 165:753–758.
19. Magyar E, Talerman A, Fehér M, et al: The pathogenesis of the subchondral pseudocysts in rheumatoid arthritis. *Clin Orthop Res* 1974; 100:341–344.
20. Manes HR: Foreign body granuloma of bone secondary to silicone prosthesis. *Clin Orthop* 1985; 199:239–241.
21. Martel W, Hayes JT, Duff IF: The pattern of bone erosion in the hand and wrist in rheumatoid arthritis. *Radiology* 1965; 84:204.
22. McGregor M: The significance of certain measurements of the skull in the diagnosis of basilar impression. *Br J Radiol* 1948; 21:171–181.
23. Merkel KD, Brown ML, Dewanjee MK, et al: Com-

parison of indium-labeled-leukocyte imaging with sequential technetium-gallium scanning in the diagnosis of low-grade musculoskeletal sepsis. *J Bone Joint Surg [Am]* 1985; 67:465–476.
24. Mettler FA, Guiberteau MJ: *Essentials of Nuclear Medicine Imaging,* ed 2. New York, Grune & Stratton, Inc, 1986.
25. Mewa, AA, Pui M, Cockshott WP, et al: Observer differences in detecting erosions in radiographs of rheumatoid arthritis. A comparison of posteroanterior, Nøgaard and Brewerton views. *J Rheum* 1983; 10:216–221.
26. Oswald SG, Van Nostrand D, Savory CG, et al: The acetabulum: A prospective study of three-phase bone and indium white blood cell scintigraphy following porous-coated hip arthroplasty. *J Nucl Med* 1990; 31:274–280.
27. Oswald SG, Van Nostrand D, Savory CG, et al: Three-phase bone scan and idium white blood cell scintigraphy following porous coated hip arthroplasty: A prospective study of the prosthetic tip. *J Nucl Med* 1989; 30:1321–1331.
28. Pare JA, Fraser RG: *Synopsis of diseases of the Chest.* Philadelphia, WB Saunders Co, 1983.
29. Pring DJ, Henderson RG, Rivett AG, et al: Autologous granulocyte scanning of painful prosthetic joints. *J Bone Joint Surg [Br]* 1986; 68:647–652.
30. Reiser MF, Bongartz GP, Erlemann R, et al: Gadolinium-DTPA in rheumatoid arthritis and related diseases: First results with dynamic magnetic resonance imaging. *Skeletal Radiol* 1989; 18:591–597.
31. Resnick D, Niwayama G: *Diagnosis of Bone and Joint Disorders,* ed 2, Philadelphia, WB Saunders Co, 1988.
32. Rose SC, Zwiebel WJ, Nelson BD, et al: Symptomatic lower extremity deep venous thrombosis: Accuracy, limitations, and role of color duplex flow imaging in diagnosis. *Radiology* 1990; 175:639–644.
33. Rubin EH: Pulmonary lesions in "rheumatoid disease" with remarks on diffuse interstitial pulmonary fibrosis. *Am J Med* 1955; 19:569.
34. Smith RJ, Atkinson, RE, Jupiter JB: Silicone synovitis of the wrist. *J Hand Surg [Am]* 1985; 10:47–60.
35. Soble MG, Kaye AD, Guay RC: Rotator cuff tear: Clinical experience with sonographic detection. *Radiology* 1989; 173:319–321.
36. Terrier F, Hricak H, Revel D, et al: Magnetic resonance imaging and spectroscopy of the periarticular inflammatory soft-tissue changes in experimental arthritis of the rat. *Invest Radiol* 1985; 20:813–823.
37. Weiss JJ, Thompson GR, Doust V, et al: Rotator cuff tears in rheumatoid arthritis. *Arch Intern Med* 1975; 135:521–525.
38. Weissberg DL, Resnick D, Taylor A, et al: Rheumatoid arthritis and its variants: Analysis of scintiphotographic, radiographic, and clinical examinations. *AJR* 1978; 131:665–673.
39. Wolfe BK, O'Keeffe D, Mitchell DM, et al: Rheumatoid arthritis of the cervical spine: Early and progressive radiographic features. *Radiology* 1987; 165:145–148.
40. Worsing RA, Engber WD, Lange TA: Reactive synovitis from particulate silastic. *J Bone Joint Surg [Am]* 1982; 64:581–585.
41. Yulish BS, Lieberman JM, Strandjord SE, et al: Juvenile rheumatoid arthritis: Assessment with MR imaging. *Radiology* 1987; 165:149–152.

CHAPTER 3

Pathology

Edward F. DiCarlo, M.D.

INTRODUCTION

The pathologic features of the tissues in rheumatoid arthritis (RA) are characteristic but not diagnostic, which explains in part why the diagnosis of RA is clinical and not histologic.[2–4] Pathologic examination, however, may provide useful information regarding the diagnosis and pathogenesis of the disease. Histologic examination will often confirm the clinical impression or it may provide the last piece of information necessary to yield a diagnosis of probable or definite RA in a clinically problematic patient.

The lack of pathognomonic features, however, does complicate pathologic diagnosis. Consequently, in all but very rare cases, a definitive diagnosis of RA cannot be made by a surgical pathologist from histologic examination of synovial or joint tissue. In the Laboratory of Orthopaedic Pathology at The Hospital for Special Surgery (New York City), the reported diagnosis usually reads: "Destructive joint disease with chronic, proliferative and exudative synovitis *consistent with* rheumatoid arthritis." On the other hand, if the findings also include rheumatoid nodules in the accompanying soft tissue or in the synovium itself, current practice would generally provide a diagnosis of RA.

Regardless of other considerations, the manifestations of RA are due to its inflammatory nature, the consequences of which are destruction of connective tissue and articular cartilage. Orthopaedists are involved in the care of rheumatoid patients primarily because of joint disease, but RA is a systemic disorder. In addition to the joints, the skeleton as a whole, both near and away from the joints, the soft tissues, and the lymph nodes may also show pathologic changes.

SYNOVIUM

The synovium, whether lining a diarthrodial joint or a tendon sheath, is the primary tissue manifesting the inflammatory changes of RA. Depending on the degree of activity or chronicity of the disease, the synovium may have a wide range of abnormalities. In early or low-grade disease, the synovium may show no apparent abnormalities. However, in most cases requiring surgery, the disease is usually well established in its clinical course and its tissue manifestations are not usually subtle.

The normal synovial lining is smooth and glistening and somewhat transparent; blood vessels are usually visible through the superficial layers. Microscopically, the superficial lining layer is normally thin and not well defined and contains flat or only slightly plump cells (synoviocytes). The synovium in RA, however, is cloudy and somewhat granular and in early or low-grade disease the lining layer of synovium is also thickened due to an increase in the number and size of the synoviocytes. The sublining tissues may have a slight chronic inflammatory infiltrate that is most often perivascular, as it is in osteoarthritis. This inflammatory infiltrate, however, is characterized by the presence of a large proportion of plasma cells. Plasma cell inflammation is a hall-

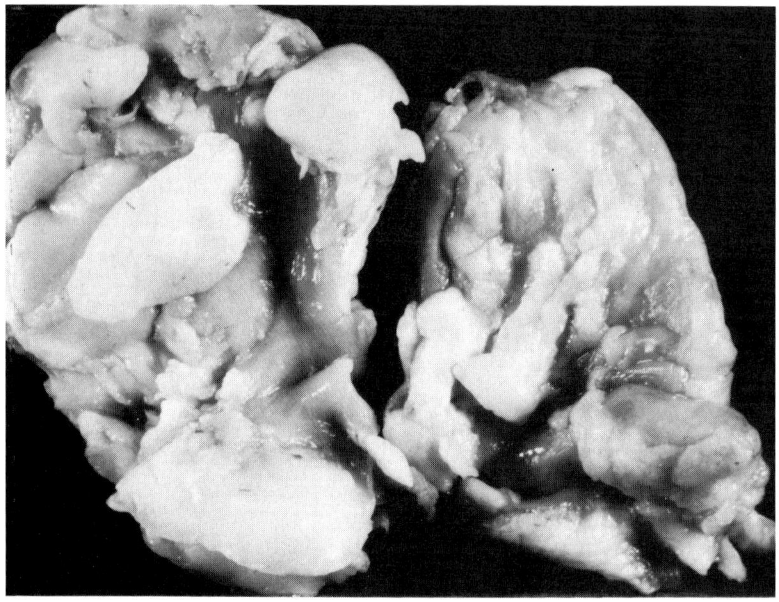

FIG 3–1.
This gross photograph of the synovium of a knee shows the thickened, coarsely nodular, and papillate synovium with adherent masses of congealed fibrin that are characteristic of RA.

mark of rheumatoid synovitis and is not a significant feature of the inflammation in osteoarthritis, which is usually more lymphocytic.

In the florid case, the synovium has a coarsely nodular and papillate, "heaped-up" appearance. The nodules and papillae are plump and soft. The tissue is usually pale tan and variably reddish-brown owing to local interstitial hemorrhage. It is opaque or only slightly translucent; subsynovial features, such as blood vessels, are not usually visible. The surfaces may be glistening but are more frequently granular and partially covered by waxy, yellow-tan, fibrinous material (Fig 3–1). This material may be congealed into clumps that adhere to the synovial surface and may cause the hypertrophic papillae to be matted together. When the clumps of fibrinous material float freely in the synovial fluid within the joint they produce what are called rice bodies (Fig 3–2).

The cut surfaces of the rheumatoid synovium are usually tan or slightly gray. Areas of frank hemorrhage or necrosis are not usually apparent. The synovium of older, more chronic disease is usually not as hypertrophic, but is generally tougher, more fibrous, and dryer.

The microscopic appearance of florid rheumatoid synovitis is characterized by hypertrophy of the synovium due to hyperplasia of the synovial lining

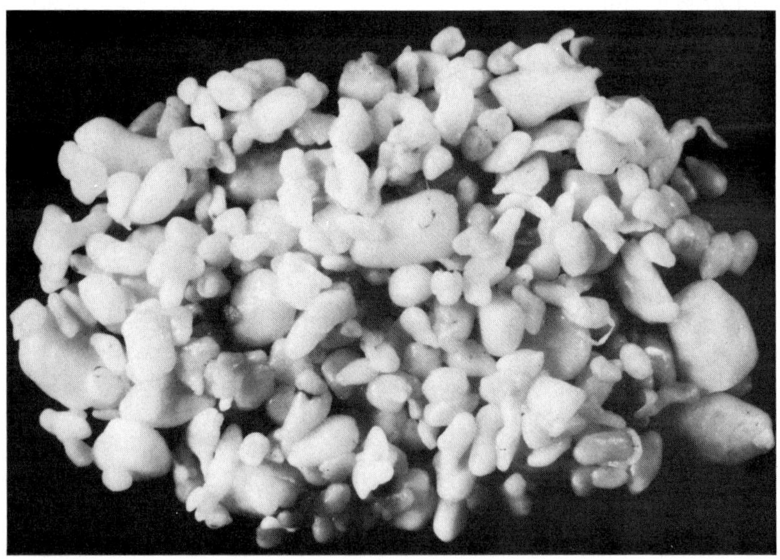

FIG 3–2.
This gross photograph shows the characteristic appearance of rice bodies which are usually numerous.

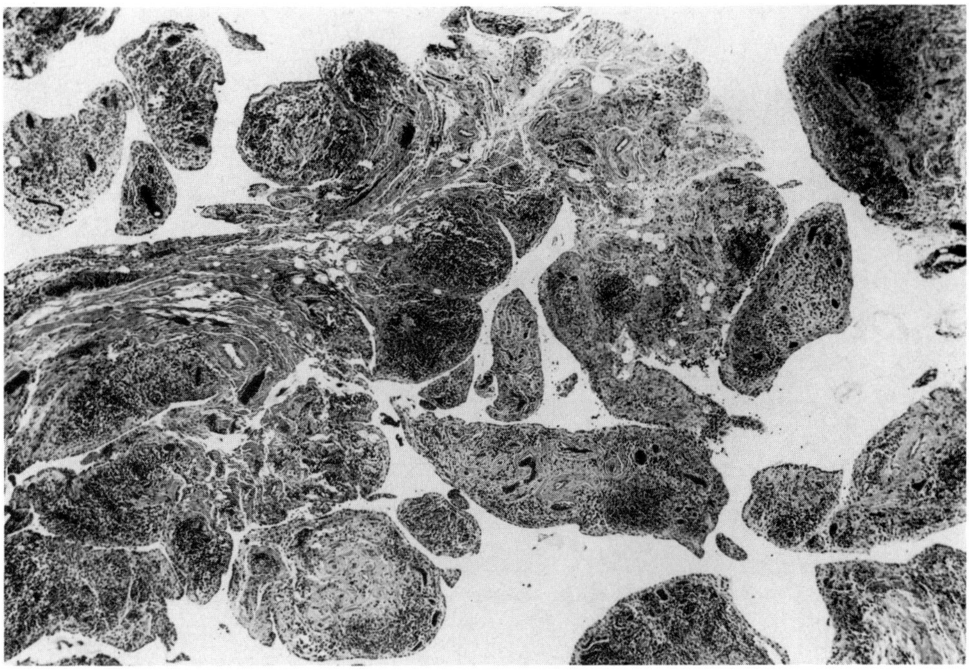

FIG 3–3.
This low-power photomicrograph of rheumatoid synovium shows the thickening of the synovial papillae with dense infiltrates of cells that, on higher power, prove to be lymphocytes and plasma cells (hematoxylin-eosin, X2.5).

layer and infiltration of the sublining layers by chronic inflammatory cells. Low-power magnification shows the thickened folds of the synovium with aggregates of densely packed lymphoid tissue (Fig 3–3).

The lining layer of synoviocytes is generally thickened, and contains cells that are plump and crowded (Fig 3–4). The thickness of the superficial layer, however, is not uniform throughout the synovium and in some areas may be thin and delicate as in normal synovium. Although there is no absolute correlation, the thickest linings are likely to be present in the most active cases. In these active cases, it is not uncommon to find binucleate or even multinucleate cells in or just below the lining layer.

The synovium is variably infiltrated by chronic inflammatory cells consisting of lymphocytes and plasma cells. In contrast to the inflammation that

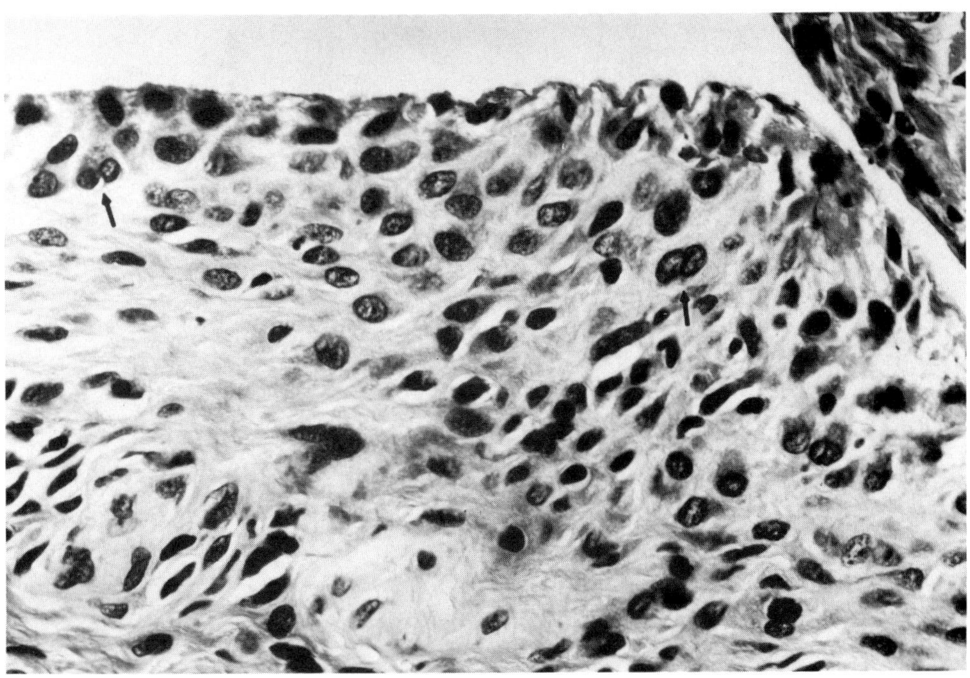

FIG 3–4.
This high-power photomicrograph shows the ill-defined thickened synovial lining layer containing plump synoviocytes. Cells marked with *arrows* are binucleate (hematoxylin-eosin, X40).

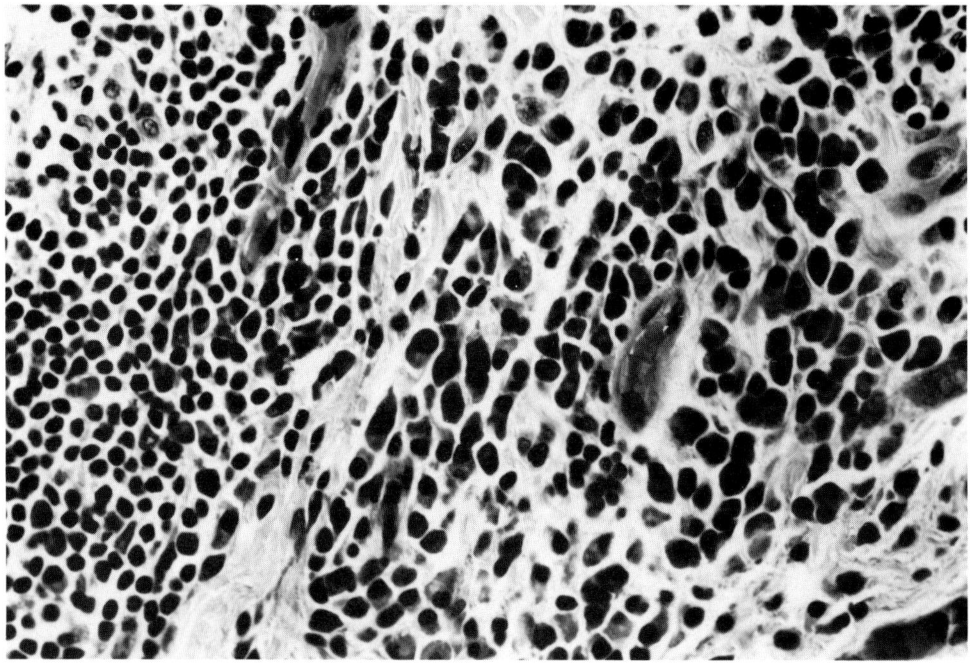

FIG 3–5.
This high-power photomicrograph shows the dense lymphoplasmacytic inflammatory infiltrate with a high proportion of plasma cells as seen in the center and to the right of the photograph (hematoxylin-eosin, X40).

might be present in osteoarthritis, inflammation in active RA is not limited to a perivascular location but is more frequently diffusely spread beneath the sublining layer. The most important feature of the inflammation of RA that distinguishes it from that of osteoarthritis is the large proportion of plasma cells, some of which may be large and binucleate (Fig 3–5). In many cases, Russell bodies, aggregates of immunoglobulin, may be present within the plasma cells or free within the tissue (Fig 3–6). Rarely, the intensity of the inflammation may be so great as to produce structures resembling the follicles and germinal centers of lymph nodes and other lymphoid tissues (Fig 3–7). These germinal center–like structures have been called Allison-Ghormley bodies.

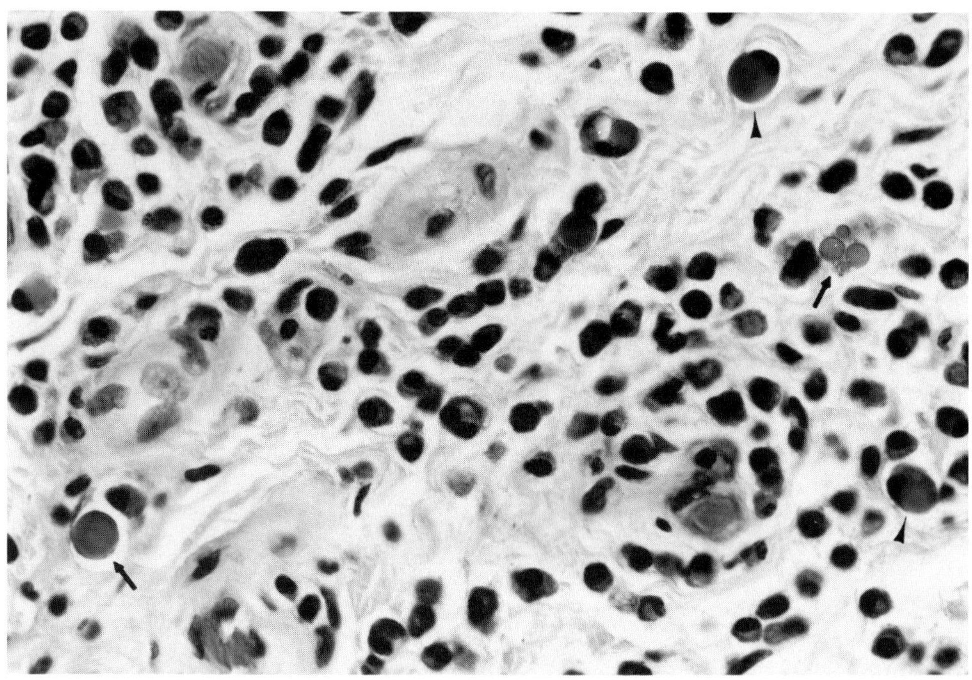

FIG 3–6.
This high-power photomicrograph shows an area of plasma cell infiltration with numerous round Russell bodies free *(arrows)* and within enlarged plasma cells *(arrowheads)*. A binucleate plasma cell is also present (hematoxylin-eosin, X40).

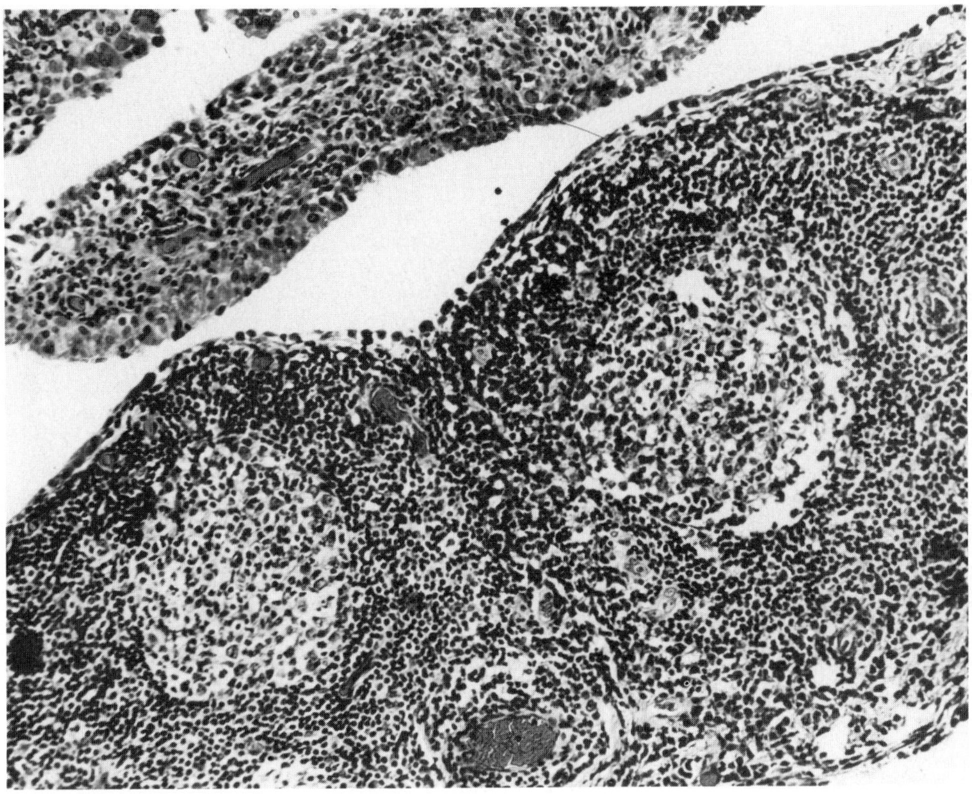

FIG 3–7.
This intermediate-power photomicrograph shows two germinal centers in an intensely inflamed papilla of synovium. This is an uncommon finding (hematoxylin-eosin, X12).

DIARTHRODIAL JOINTS

The synovium is attached to the most peripheral part of the articular cartilage and does not normally cover it. When a joint is affected by RA the early changes are therefore found at the periphery of the articular surfaces, in contrast to those in osteoarthritis, which develop more centrally. As the inflammatory synovium becomes hyperplastic and thickened, it extends into the joint space and contacts the surfaces of the articular cartilage and other intraarticular structures such as menisci. The inflamed synovial tissue then becomes adherent and covers the exposed surfaces, and when it does, it is referred to as a *pannus* (Fig 3–8).

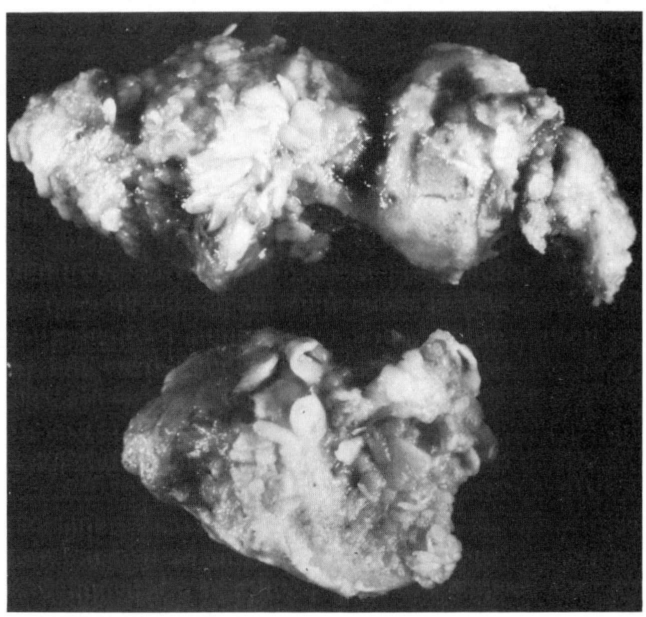

FIG 3–8.
This gross photograph of elbow joint components shows a pannus of papillate rheumatoid synovium covering most of the articular surfaces.

Articular Cartilage

In early RA, the periphery of the articular surface is covered by the adherent pannus and has an irregular margin due to erosion of the articular cartilage. In joints such as the knee, the pannus also causes erosion and distortion of menisci. As the disease continues, progressively more of the joint surface is destroyed, leaving pitted, raw, and hemorrhagic surfaces (Fig 3–9). Over time, the bone, devoid of

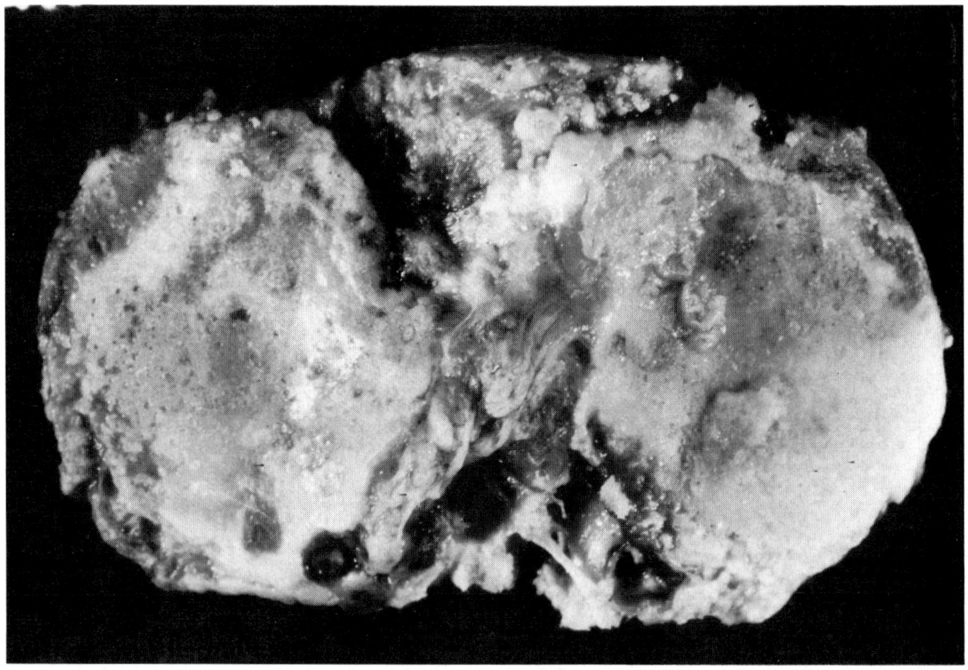

FIG 3–9.
This gross photograph of a tibial plateau shows erosion and pitting at the joint margins and loss of most of the articular cartilage. The surfaces at the intercondylar regions are slightly eburnated in this case of late RA.

cartilage, may become sclerotic and resemble an osteoarthritic joint, but this is not usually seen until late in the so-called burned-out state. Osteophytes are not seen in active disease, but may develop late and not to the degree usually seen in osteoarthritis.

Microscopically, the pannus overlying the articular surface is composed of fibrous tissue with inflammatory cells including predominantly lymphocytes and plasma cells with fewer neutrophils and mast cells. The destructive processes resulting from the inflammatory infiltrate in the pannus cause erosion of the articular cartilage beginning at the periphery. The cartilage underlying the pannus often has a porous appearance; the "pores" are called Weichselbaum lacunae and result from the destruction of chondrocytes with subsequent invasion of the chon-

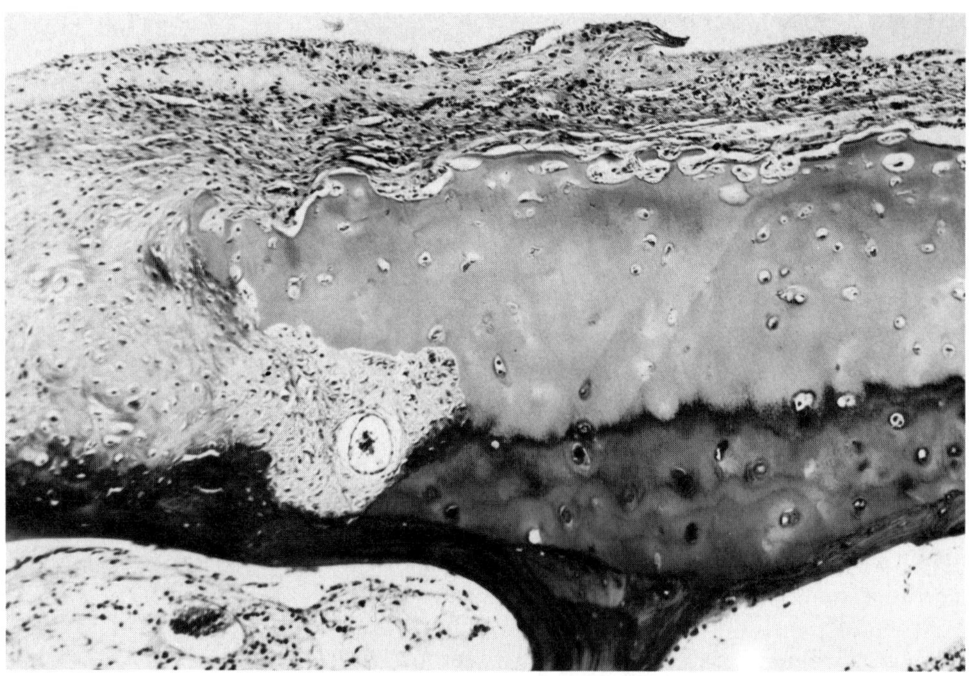

FIG 3–10.
This low-power photomicrograph of the articular surface in a rheumatoid joint shows the pannus overlying the cartilage, erosion of the edge of the cartilage, and Weichselbaum lacunae at the surface of the cartilage just below the pannus (hematoxylin-eosin, X8).

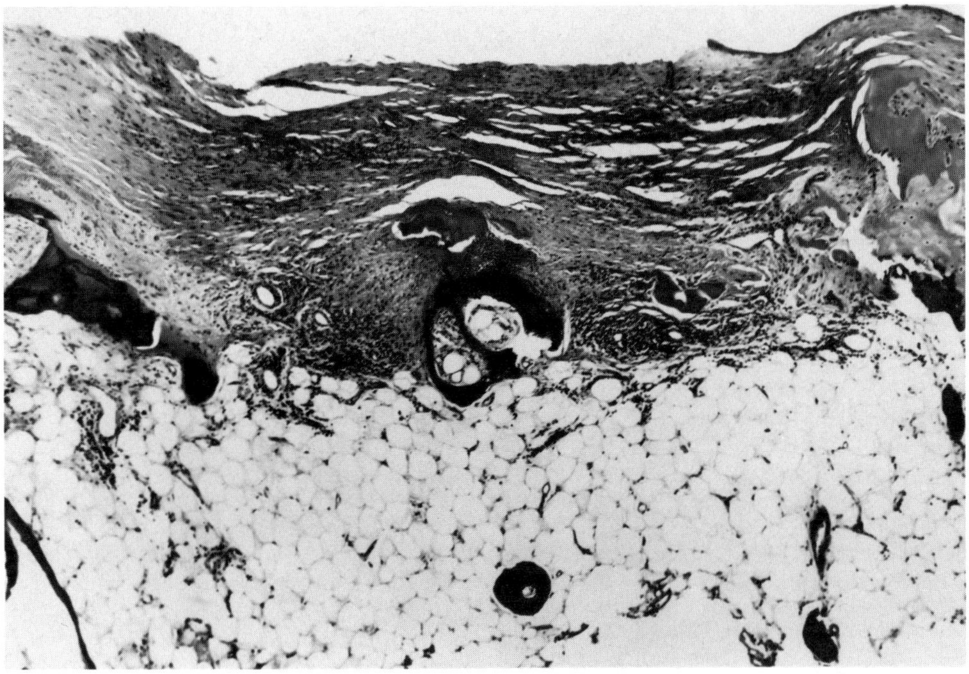

FIG 3–11.
This low-power photomicrograph of an articular surface in late RA shows the inflamed fibrous pannus with only minimal residual bony end plate. The superficial bone marrow is chronically inflamed and the bony trabeculae are decreased in size and number, indicating osteoporosis (hematoxylin-Eosin, X8).

drocytic lacunae by fibrous, vascular, and inflammatory tissue (Fig 3–10).

Bone

The bone beneath the articular cartilage is also altered by the inflammatory process. The marrow space immediately beneath the subchondral bony end plate is hypervascular and contains a variably intense inflammatory infiltrate of lymphocytes and plasma cells. Rarely, germinal center–like structures may also be present. The bony end plate itself is eroded by osteoclasts and where it is absent, only an ill-defined layer of inflammatory fibrous tissue may remain (Fig 3–11). The trabeculae of the cancellous bone are thin and delicate and are the tissue evidence of the osteoporosis that occurs in the bones around involved joints. In the later stages of the disease, especially when there is no remaining articular cartilage, the marrow inflammation decreases and sclerosis of the cancellous bone may develop.

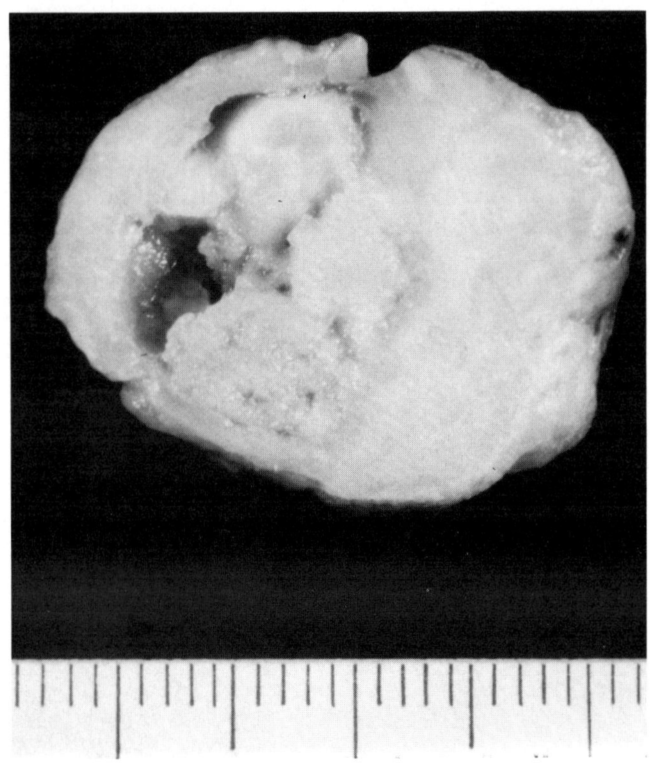

FIG 3–12.
This gross photograph of a rheumatoid nodule shows fragmentation of the central necrotic zone which is surrounded by a serpiginous margin. The necrotic zone is yellow and the surrounding tissue is gray or tan.

SOFT TISSUE

Rheumatoid arthritis manifests itself in the extraskeletal soft tissues predominantly as rheumatoid nodules[5] and, less commonly, as lymphadenopathy.[1]

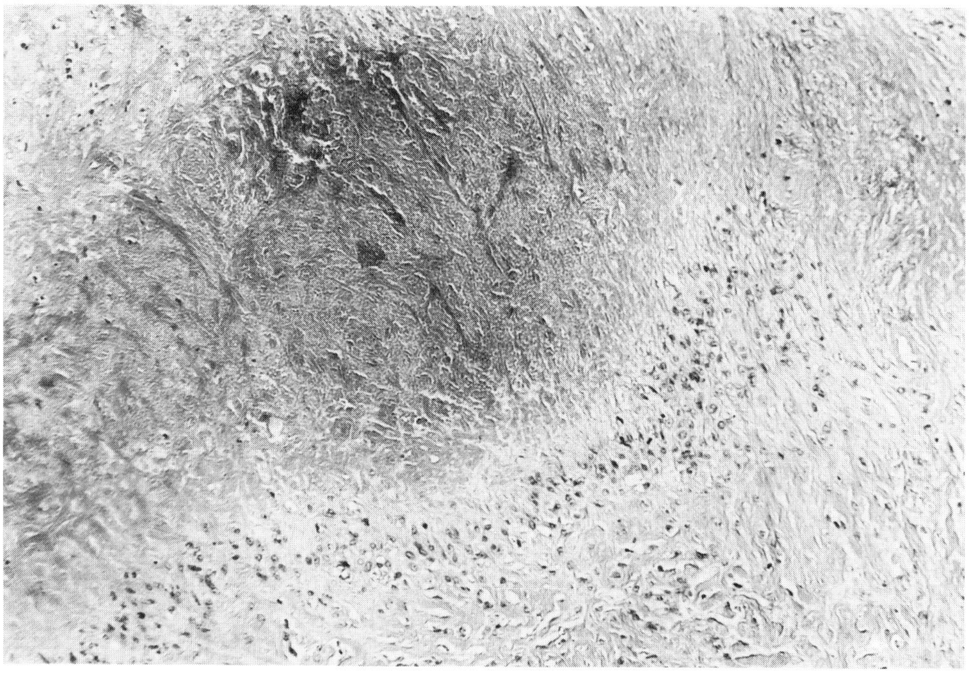

FIG 3–13.
This intermediate-power photomicrograph of a rheumatoid nodule shows the irregular boundary of palisaded histiocytes separating the necrotic tissue in the *upper left* from the viable fibrous tissue in the *lower right* (hematoxylin-eosin, X10).

Rheumatoid Nodules

Rheumatoid nodules are rubbery, well-defined nodules in the subcutaneous tissues, most frequently on the extensor surface of the forearms. However, they may also be present in the fingers and toes, especially around actively arthritic joints. On cut section rheumatoid nodules have geographic yellow regions that represent necrosis of the collagenous connective tissues (Fig 3–12). The microscopic features of rheumatoid nodules are characteristic. The nodule is composed mostly of fibrous tissue without significant inflammation in most cases. The central regions contain necrotic, denatured collagen. The boundary between the central necrotic region and the viable fibrous tissue consists of an irregular line of plump cells (histiocytes) arranged in a palisade with the long axes of the cells pointing into the necrotic zone (Fig 3–13).

FIG 3–14.
This low-power photomicrograph of a rheumatoid lymph node shows the abnormally shaped and enlarged germinal centers (hematoxylin-eosin, X10).

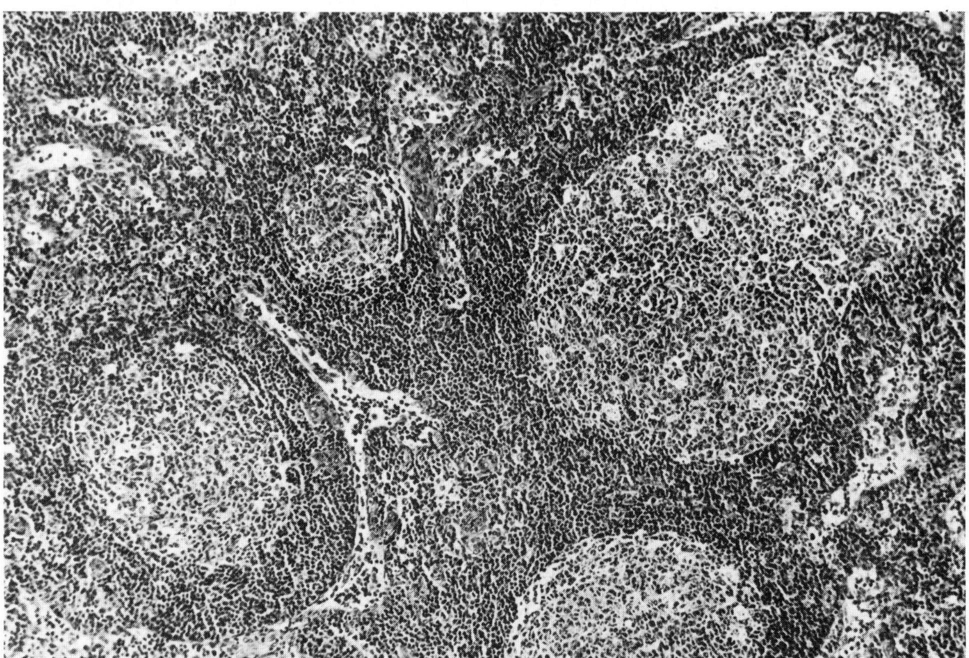

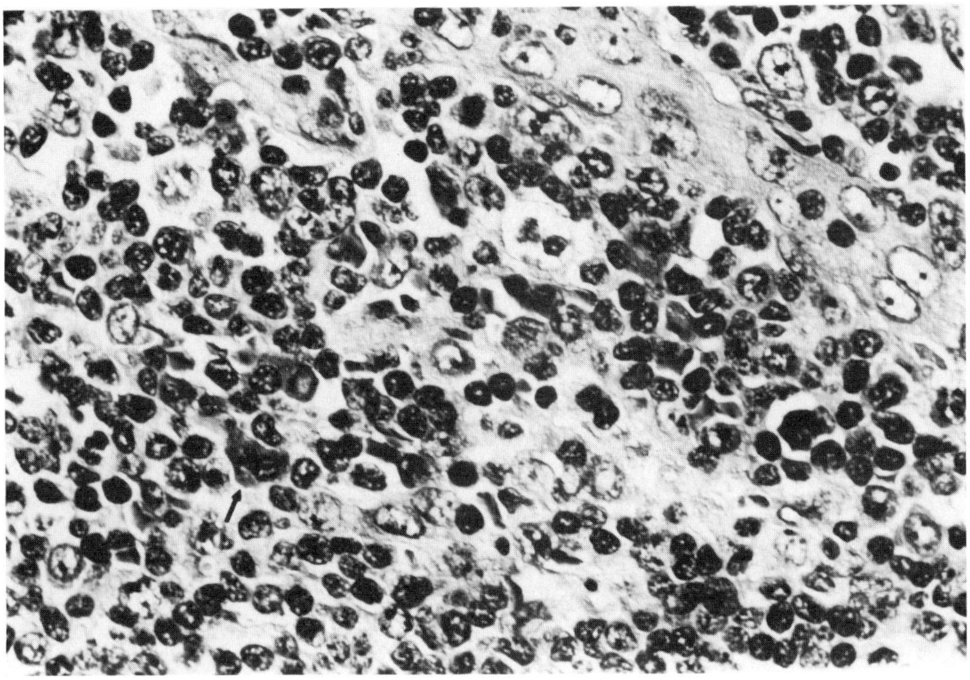

FIG 3–15.
This high-power photomicrograph of a rheumatoid lymph node shows increased numbers of plasma cells, one of which is binucleate *(arrow)* (hematoxylin-Eosin, X40).

In rare cases, rheumatoid nodules may be found within the synovial tissues themselves. This is perhaps the only finding that would permit a histologic diagnosis of RA based on joint material.

Lymph Nodes

Systemic or localized lymphadenopathy in RA is not uncommon, but rarely, a rheumatoid patient develops a severe condition requiring a biopsy to exclude the possibility of lymphoma. The lymph nodes are large, nontender, and mobile and do not necessarily drain affected joints. On sectioning, the nodes are soft and fleshy and pale gray; they may be focally yellow due to necrosis. A nodular appearance is discernible on the cut surface in both the cortical and medullary zones.

Microscopically, the nodules are hyperplastic, irregularly shaped follicles with actively proliferating germinal centers that contain the usual complement of follicular center cells with numerous mitotic figures (Fig 3–14). The sinuses in the medullary region are filled with hypertrophic endothelial cells and the perifollicular and medullary zones usually have an increase in the number of plasma cells. Russell bodies may also be present (Fig 3–15). Necrosis in the germinal centers is evidenced by the presence of macrophages filled with nuclear debris, deposits of hyaline pink material, and scattered clusters of neutrophils.

CONCLUSION

The pathologic features of joint and synovial disease in RA are not specific and, apart from the presence of rheumatoid nodules, cannot by themselves provide a definitive diagnosis. Similar features may be encountered in any of the primary inflammatory arthropathies including juvenile RA, systemic lupus erythematosus, and psoriatic arthritis. The diagnosis of RA is therefore not histologic. The pathologic features present in the joints and synovium of rheumatoid patients must ultimately be interpreted in the light of the clinical situation.

REFERENCES

1. Ioachim HL: *Lymph Node Biopsy,* Philadelphia, JB Lippincott Co, 1982, pp 114–117.
2. Rodnan GP, Schumacher HR (eds): *Primer on the Rheumatic Diseases,* ed 8., Atlanta, Arthritis Foundation, 1983, pp 38–48.
3. Short CL, Bauer W, Reynolds WS: *Rheumatoid Arthritis.* Cambridge, Harvard University Press, 1957.
4. Silberberg R: Disease of joints, in Kissane JM (ed): *Anderson's Pathology,* ed 8. St Louis, Mosby–Year Book, Inc, 1985, pp 1828–1836.
5. Williams HJ, Biddulph EC, Coleman SS, et al: Isolated subcutaneous nodules (pseudorheumatoid). *J Bone Joint Surg [Am]* 1977; 59:73.

PART II

Surgical Considerations

CHAPTER 4

Introduction to the Rheumatoid Patient Undergoing Surgical Treatment

Thomas P. Sculco, M.D.

INTRODUCTION

In the context of musculoskeletal patient care there exists no more complex clinical setting than the patient afflicted with polyarticular rheumatoid arthritis.[6, 12] These patients manifest not only the destructive signs and symptoms of their bone and joint disease but also a spectrum of associated problems that demand comprehensive and thorough evaluation and treatment. The operating surgeon, able to reconstruct a ravaged joint, must also be aware of the diversity of the patient's associated illnesses which will impact on the success of the surgical treatment. The patient with profound joint involvement will commonly be taking a myriad of medications including immunosuppressive drugs that may have an adverse effect on wound healing and the ability to ward off infection. The patient with rheumatoid arthritis may have psychosocial needs[15] that must be addressed if an optional functional response is to be achieved with surgical treatment. To insure a successful surgical intervention in these patients the surgeon must (1) carefully evaluate the patient preoperatively, (2) plan the intraoperative management, (3) develop a perioperative rehabilitative program, and (4) identify and aggressively manage the long-term complications which may occur in these patients. This process forms the basis for the comprehensive management required by the rheumatoid patient undergoing surgical treatment.

PREOPERATIVE EVALUATION

A thorough preoperative evaluation is necessary in patients with rheumatoid arthritis undergoing reconstructive surgery. This must include knowledge of the associated medical conditions in rheumatoid arthritis (e.g., pericarditis, pulmonary fibrosis, vasculitis). The rheumatoid patient additionally will have medical problems not related to his or her disease and which may negatively influence surgical treatment. The fundamental understanding of the patient's disease process and its natural history are best provided by the rheumatologist. The surgeon must be in close contact with the patient's rheumatologist who is most often best acquainted with the patient and thus aware of the patient's various medical conditions, their treatment, and their severity. The rheumatologist can provide invaluable information regarding the duration and severity of the disease process itself and a close collaborative relationship with the rheumatologist before and during the patient's hospital stay is requisite for uncomplicated medical and arthritic management. The rheumatoid patient has usually been on a series of anti-inflammatory medications and may forget the sequence and rationale for discontinuing various medications. If the rheumatologist is not closely monitoring the patient with the surgeon, the current medications may be confused by the patient and this may lead to an exacerbation of the arthritis postoperatively. At the time of the surgical consultation the patient may not recall a recent course of corticosteroid medication and this can lead to acute adrenal insufficiency postoperatively with severe febrile illness. The surgeon may mistake this response as an operative complication and needless consternation and ineffective treatment may ensue. The rheumatologist has been the primary physician to the patient preoperatively, will continue as such after discharge from the hospital, and it is strongly advocated that he or she consult on the patient and follow the patient's care during surgical admission. This allows for better management of the patient's medical, arthritic, and drug-related complications should they occur.

The preoperative evaluation by the surgeon and the close working relationship with the rheumatologist is but one part in the comprehensive multidisciplinary approach to the care of the patient with rheumatoid arthritis. Because of the complexity of the disease process and its ramifications, which extend beyond the musculoskeletal involvement, the preoperative evaluation should include nursing, occupational and physical therapy, and social work staff as well as rheumatologist and surgeon[4] (Fig 4–1). It has been demonstrated that this comprehensive approach improves the patient's mental and physical well-being.[1]

The Comprehensive Arthritis Program (CAP) was established at The Hospital for Special Surgery (New York City) in 1967 to provide multidisciplinary care to the patient with rheumatoid arthritis. The service is composed of physical and occupational therapists, nurses, social workers, rheumatologists, orthopaedic surgeons with a special interest in arthritis surgery, and an administrative secretary (see Fig 4–1). All clinic patients who are under consideration for surgical treatment are presented in a joint forum with input encouraged from all health care members. In this way, all facets of the disease process, including its psychological and socioeconomic impact, are weighed in planning the optimal approach to the care of the patient whether or not surgery is ultimately performed. The cross-fertilization of information and ideas from varied perspectives is educational for all members of the team and provides a holistic appraisal of the patient.

The team also includes orthopaedic residents and postgraduate fellows from orthopaedic surgery and rheumatology who spend 6-week to 1-year rotations on this service. Because many of these patients undergo multiple medical and surgical admissions over the course of many years of disease, the attending staff rheumatologists and orthopaedic surgeons provide the long-term perspective and treatment plan for these patients. Additionally, to prevent fragmentation in the care of these complex polyarticular patients, the service's orthopaedic team of surgeons have the expertise to manage any area of musculoskeletal involvement, from cervical spine to forefoot. This care prevents patients from being referred to specialty clinics for surgical treatment of a particular joint affliction, thereby preserving the service's comprehensive overview of the patient. The same CAP team follows and cares for patients when they move to an inpatient setting. Postoperatively, the patient returns to the CAP outpatient clinic and is followed in this clinic by the entire CAP team.

Even in a setting where a comprehensive arthritis program does not exist, a thorough preoperative evaluation is recommended. The level of functional disability tends to be widespread and it is beneficial if the physical and occupational therapists can examine and interview the patient preoperatively. Their input is often invaluable in preparing the patient for postoperative rehabilitation and the interaction allows the patient to ask questions and be reassured. Additionally, they will frequently advise ways to

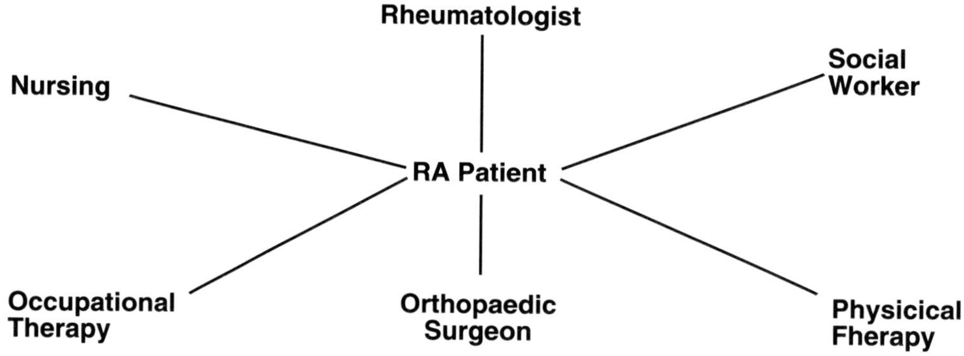

FIG 4–1.
Schematic representation of the interrelationship between the clinical team and the rheumatoid patient.

hasten the patient's recovery. When lower extremity surgery is contemplated these therapists can be helpful in recognizing difficulties the patient may have with crutches or canes. Modification of these assistive devices implemented preoperatively can improve the postoperative rehabilitation in these patients. Recommendations from therapists has also led to the fabrication of other assistive devices for improvement in both upper and lower extremity function. Careful evaluation of muscle function and joint range of motion throughout the musculoskeletal system by occupational and physical therapy can provide in-depth information of underlying joint function and disability.

In a similar fashion, the nursing staff can provide insights into the patient's recovery process which may be overlooked by the surgeon. They view the patient from a different perspective and can recommend measures to enhance nutrition, skin care, and bowel and bladder function. Questions concerning medications, particularly analgesics, can be addressed at the preoperative interview by the floor nursing staff. The day-to-day care plan of the patient is supervised by the nursing staff and can be reviewed with the patient. The patient with rheumatoid arthritis is often fearful of admission to the hospital and the loss of his or her independent functioning at home. Support systems are usually in place in the home environment and these patients have developed a mechanism to cope with the dependent needs provoked by their disease. There may be family, friends, or home medical personnel who assist the patient with his or her daily activities. In the hospital setting, patients enter alien surroundings and are often apprehensive of whether assistance will be necessary should they require it and are unable to provide for themselves. Nursing is pivotal to allaying these anxieties and providing a smooth transition into a hospital setting and monitoring the patient's progress as postoperative recovery unfolds.

Because patients with severe rheumatoid arthritis have such a multitude of needs when they return to their outpatient setting, the social worker should also be involved, preferably in the preoperative period. The surgeon should not expect other health team members to assume complete responsibility for postoperative discharge planning, but should be conversant with the patient's home situation and possible options at discharge. The concerns that support services (e.g., visiting nursing care, physical therapy, home health care services) will not be available when the patient has recovered sufficiently to leave the hospital will increase the fear and anxiety already produced by the operative procedure. De-

TABLE 4–1.

Roles and Responsibilities of Members of the Comprehensive Arthritis Team

- Orthopaedic surgeon
  - Develops a surgical plan for musculoskeletal area involved
  - Coordinates perioperative care with rheumatologist, physical and occupational therapists, social worker, nursing staff
  - Effects surgical reconstruction with improved function
- Social worker
  - Aware of home setting, advises and implements home support systems
  - Assists with long term inpatient rehabilitation if needed
  - Provides psychological support and reassurance to patient
- Nursing staff
  - Preoperatively evaluate and counsel patient and develop appropriate care plan
  - Postoperatively implement care plan
    - Nutrition
    - Skin care
    - Bowel and bladder function
    - Medications
    - Active coordination with physical and occupational therapists
    - Medical recovery
- Rheumatologist
  - Ongoing care of arthritis
  - Conversant with patient's medications, their effectiveness, side effects
  - Aware of patient's medical history and provides general medical care
- Physical therapist, occupational therapist
  - Preoperatively evaluate, counsel patient, and suggest alterations necessary in recovery rehabilitation
  - Postoperatively provide musculoskeletal, pulmonary, and associated rehabilitation

pression may result and this may greatly impede postoperative recovery. If the patient is reassured by the social service that the medical staff is aware of his or her special needs and discharge planning is under way as soon as the patient enters the hospital, the hospital stay will be less traumatic and more beneficial.

From the inception of operative planning and care for the rheumatoid patient the concept of a comprehensive approach must be emphasized (Table 4–1). More than any other patient undergoing orthopaedic surgery the patient with rheumatoid arthritis will require this multidisciplinary approach.[7, 15] This is best done in the preoperative period whenever possible to allow all suggestions for the care of these patients to be effected or at least planned prior to admission to the hospital. A concerted evaluation will improve the care, and produce a less complicated perioperative course and better surgical result.

INTRAOPERATIVE PLANNING

The patient with rheumatoid arthritis presents a singular subset of problems that must be recognized and addressed prior to surgical reconstruction. These include the systemic and musculoskeletal components of the disease which may make anesthetic management difficult. The rheumatoid patient may have compromised pulmonary function from parenchymal fibrosis, cervical spine instability, or a compromised mandibular excursion, all of which greatly complicate anesthetic management. Although regional anesthesia solves some of the problems outlined and is strongly recommended, these patients tend to be quite frail and are uncomfortable in a given position for long periods owing to the diffuse nature of their disease. Thus regional anesthesia may not be completely without drawbacks. Preoperative anesthetic consultation is strongly advised if special airway or medical conditions are present.

Local tissue deficiencies must be considered in operative planning. Osteopenia is present in almost all patients with rheumatoid arthritis and is probably due to several factors. Disuse of a painful limb will produce localized osteopenia which will aggravate the osteopenia that may be a component of the disease process itself (Fig 4–2). Corticosteroids produce mineral loss in bone and vertebral compression and long bone fractures are common. The surgeon must be careful not to cause an intraoperative fracture by injudicious use of force during limb manipulation at

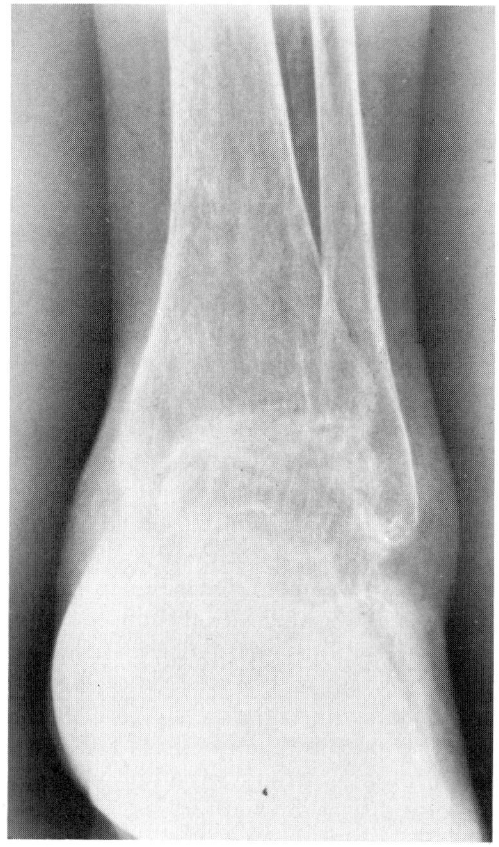

FIG 4–2.
Severe periarticular osteopenia and ankle joint destruction in a patient with rheumatoid arthritis.

surgery. Levering on bony surfaces with surgical instruments may crush bone and compromise the substrate needed for support of implants during arthroplasty. Oscillating-power cutting tools should be used rather than bone chisels and osteotomes, whenever possible. The underlying bone is soft and is crushed rather than cut by these hand instruments. Large cavitary deficits and smaller cysts may be present within bone as a result of erosion and infiltration of synovium. The surgeon must be prepared to graft these areas with autogenous bone or, allografts (Fig 4–3,A and B).

Along with bony deficiency, soft tissue coverage of affected joints may be poor. Soft tissue handling must be careful and atraumatic. During exposure of a joint for reconstruction, large skin flaps should be avoided. These flaps, if extensive, denude subcutaneous fat from skin and can lead to delayed wound healing and sloughing. If deformities are severe, wound closure may be complex; ample, soft tissue coverage without tension is necessary for proper wound healing. Previous incisions should be uti-

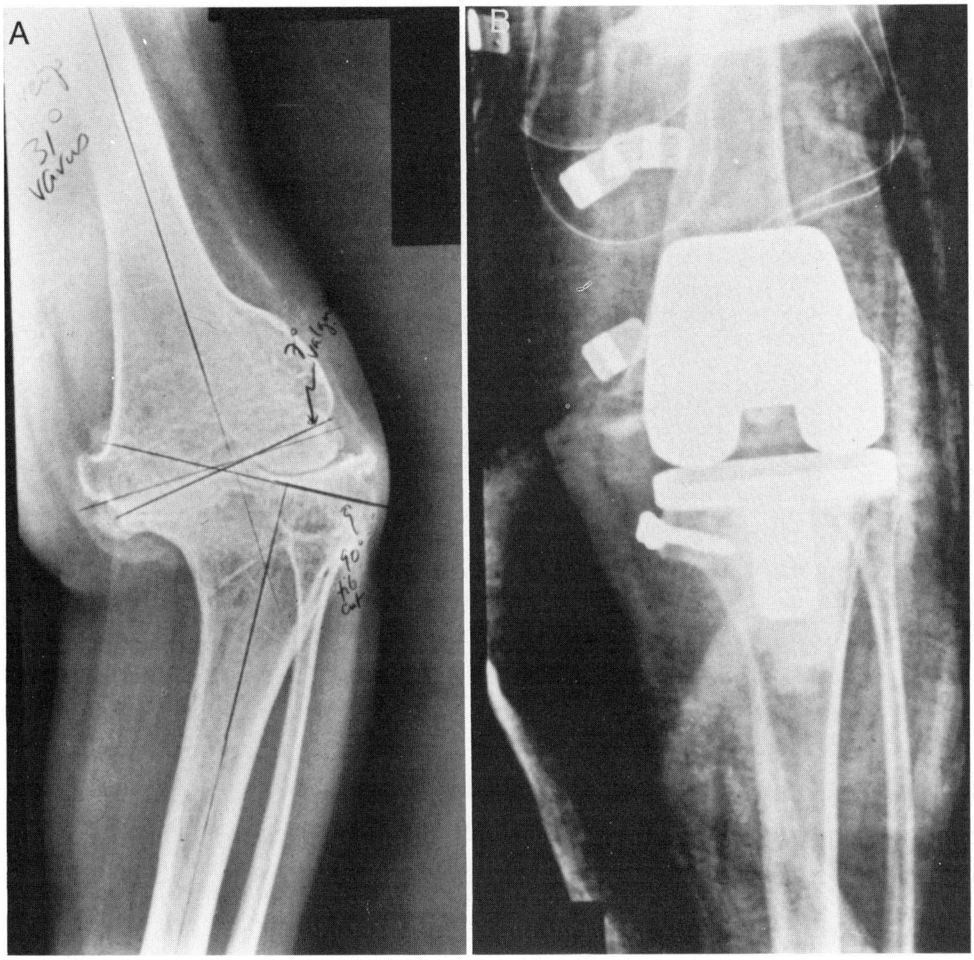

FIG 4–3.
A, severe deformity of the knee joint with bone loss in a patient with juvenile rheumatoid arthritis. **B,** total knee replacement in the same patient with autogenous bone grafting for tibial deficiency.

lized whenever possible and adjacent parallel incisions that leave a devascularized zone should not be used.

Many patients with rheumatoid arthritis, especially those with juvenile rheumatoid arthritis, are small (Fig 4–4) and care must be given in selection of size and type of prosthetic implant. The availability of all potentially needed implants must be insured before embarking upon the operative procedure. Radiographic measurements and computed tomography (CT) imaging, if necessary, should be performed on all patients in whom the size of the implant may be a problem. In those patients in whom conventional devices are not applicable, the surgeon should arrange for fabrication of a custom implant.

An integral part of operative planning in patients with rheumatoid arthritis is the avoidance of postoperative infection. Many studies have documented the increased risk of infection in these patients due to local factors, immunosuppressive medications, and poor host resistance.[2, 5, 6, 8, 13, 14] Vasculitic ulcerations are a common source of infection of prosthetic joints. Localized areas of infection related to nodules, skin breakdown over areas of deformity, poor dentition, chronic urinary tract infection, and so forth should also be treated before proceeding with surgical treatment. Perioperative antibiotics, atraumatic handling of soft tissues at surgery, and individualized rehabilitation depending upon the wound progress will reduce wound problems and infection. Should evidence of wound breakdown or infection be noted, the surgeon must be prepared to act rapidly and aggressively to convert a potential catastrophic complication to a healthy wound.

Perioperative blood replacement is another important consideration. Most patients prefer to deposit autologous blood preoperatively when there is a question of need at surgery or postoperatively. This practice should be encouraged in the rheumatoid patient although anemia may preclude this. Designated donors may be used for blood replace-

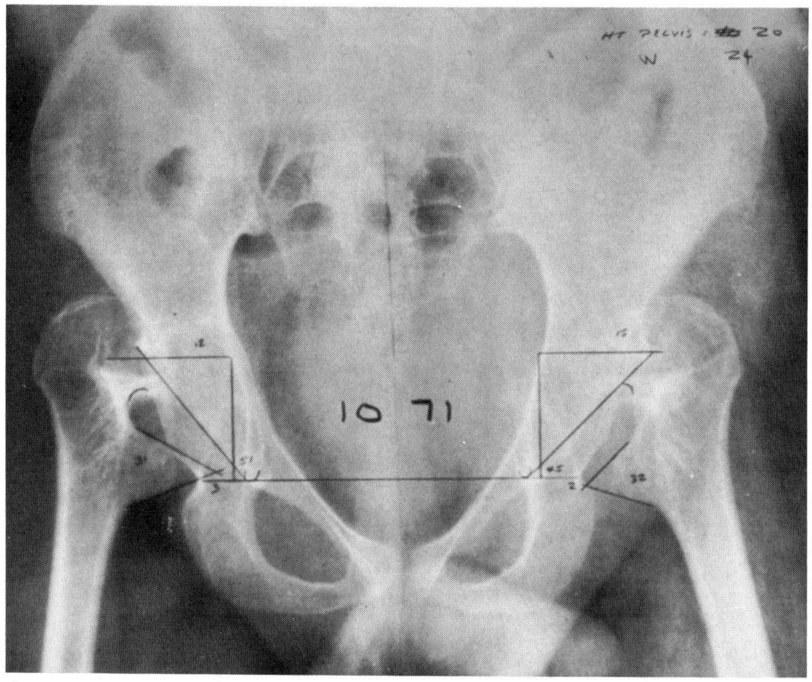

FIG 4–4.
Severe destruction of bilateral hip joints and marked dysplasia of proximal femur and acetabula.

ment in these patients. The role of erythropoietin as a bone marrow stimulant is currently being explored in patients who are unable to predeposit their own blood because of a low hemoglobin.[10] Blood may also be salvaged intraoperatively by use of a cell saver. This is particularly useful in procedures where intraoperative blood loss is greater than 1,000 mL. About 60% of blood shed intraoperatively can be retrieved and the surgeon should plan to have a cell saver available in revision hip replacement and bilateral hip procedures. Postoperative retrieval of blood by suction drainage may also be considered in patients in whom postoperative sanguineous drainage is expected to be greater than 400 to 500 mL. Knee and hip replacement surgery, especially bilateral procedures, and revision joint replacement entail significant blood loss postoperatively and patients should be considered for reinfusion of blood from drainage collection systems. It is strongly recommended that cells be washed prior to reinfusion in a cell washer as hypotensive events have been reported[3] in unwashed red cell infusions.

Careful and thorough intraoperative planning facilitates surgical treatment in the rheumatoid patient. It is important to the ultimate success of the surgical treatment that the surgeon spend time reviewing the intraoperative problems that may be encountered and be prepared to deal with them when they occur. Preoperative planning is best done when the decision to proceed with surgery has been made by patient and surgeon. The next consideration for surgery in rheumatoid arthritis is the postoperative rehabilitation.

POSTOPERATIVE REHABILITATION

Consideration of rehabilitative care after surgical reconstruction has to begin preoperatively. This must include consultation with occupational and physical therapists. The social worker also plays a role in assisting with appropriate home care rehabilitative services. In the severely disabled patient an inpatient intensive rehabilitation program may be necessary. The surgeon should set functional outcome goals prior to surgical treatment and thoroughly review these with the patient. This basic interaction with the patient prevents unreasonable expectations by the patient and allows the surgeon and the patient to approach the surgical procedure with similiar projected end points.

There are parameters that will guide the clinical team regarding the functional outcome after surgery.[11] If these preoperative functional indicators are present singly or in combination the difficulty of postoperative rehabilitation will be greatly compounded. In the lower extremity, painless ambulation is the goal of any surgical procedure. Polyarticular involvement of more than one lower extremity

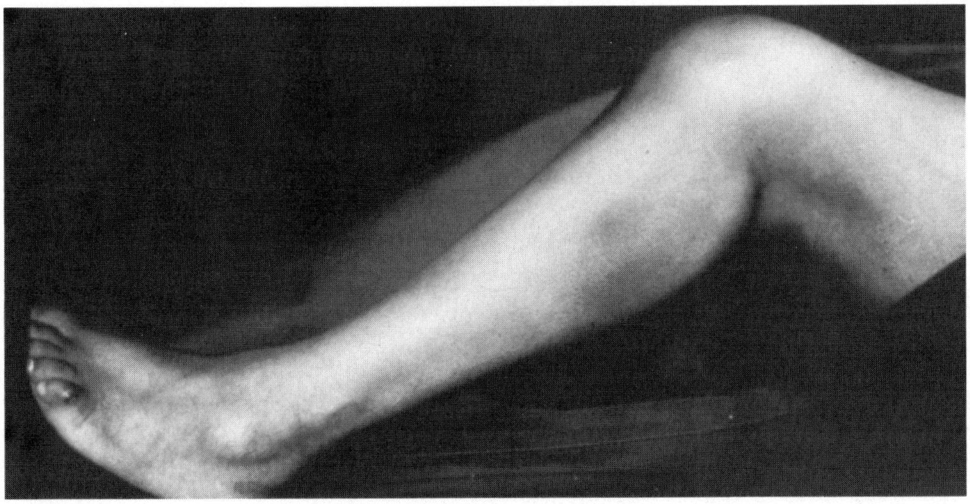

FIG 4–5.
Marked flexion contracture of the knee joint in a patient with longstanding rheumatoid arthritis.

joint will hinder rehabilitation if the limiting joints and involved musculoskeletal areas are not corrected. If ambulation is prevented because of hip and knee joint destruction, these areas must be addressed to insure maximum potential benefit from lower extremity surgery. The surgeon should be prepared preoperatively to deal with disabling lower extremity joints. Bilateral knee and hip procedures may be necessary during the hospital stay to promote postoperative rehabilitation and ambulation. Hindfoot or forefoot surgery may also need staging in the same polyoperative planning. Poorly planned and incomplete treatment of the polyarticular rheumatoid patient will significantly jeopardize the functional result of surgical treatment.

A second indicator that may be used preoperatively to determine postoperative rehabilitative goals is the period of time that the patient has been nonambulatory. The greater the duration of nonambulatory status, the greater the difficulty in establishing an ambulatory patient postoperatively. In a review of patients undergoing four lower extremity joint replacements (bilateral hip and knee replacement), return to ambulation was uncommon in patients who were chairbound for greater than 6 months.[9] Joint contractures (Fig 4–5) muscle atrophy, and osteopenia contribute to failure to ambulate. An advanced degree of deformity and concomitant poor muscle function will slow recovery from reconstructive surgery. The surgeon must broach this subject with the nonambulatory patient preoperatively when discussing the postoperative functional status and degree of physical therapy required after surgery. A period of inpatient rehabilitation should be planned postoperatively after the acute phase of surgical recovery.

A third factor that plays a role in the plan of rehabilitation after lower extremity surgery is the degree of disease severity in the upper extremities. If the ability to grip assistive ambulatory aids is limited by hand deformity, the surgeon must plan for platform- or forearm-supported devices. Weak or arthritic upper extremities will make arising from a seated position and stair climbing more difficult. Physical and occupational therapists can provide invaluable assistance in the design and fabrication of these assistive devices.

A fourth component in planning postoperative rehabilitation is the rheumatoid patient's motivation to participate in the recovery program. Depression or other psychological impediments to recovery should be identified and treated prior to surgery. Personality traits that may pose problems for the postoperative therapy program must be addressed. The surgeon must be frank in his or her discussion with the patient and family members concerning the importance of full compliance in the program. An excellent surgical result as judged radiographically will become a poor functional result if the patient fails to actively assist the therapist after surgery (Table 4–2).

The surgeon must also consider the patient's general medical status. In rheumatoid patients with multiple and complex medical problems, particularly

TABLE 4–2.
Poor Rehabilitative Indicators in Rheumatoid Arthritis

Severe polyarticular upper and lower extremity disease
Prolonged nonambulatory status
Associated cervical myelopathy, myositis, or myopathy
Poor motivation
Significant medical disease

cardiopulmonary problems, their general well-being may be poor and therefore complicated rehabilitative programs may be too onerous and fatiguing. Emphasis should be on recognizing these factors preoperatively and considering their role in the rapidity of the patient's recovery. A frail patient with multiple disabling medical problems will advance far more slowly and this should be anticipated and planned for. Long-range physical therapy at a rehabilitation facility is generally beneficial to these patients and should be reviewed and arrangements established early in the recovery period.

Cervical spine disease may produce a myelopathy that can retard recovery after lower extremity surgery and interfere with ambulatory ability (Fig 4–6). A careful neurologic examination should be performed on all patients undergoing reconstructive surgery. Cervical spine films in flexion and extension are recommended routinely in patients undergoing major reconstructive surgery. If evidence of spinal cord compression and myelopathy is present, a neurologic evaluation should be obtained and surgical treatment directed to the cervical spine first.

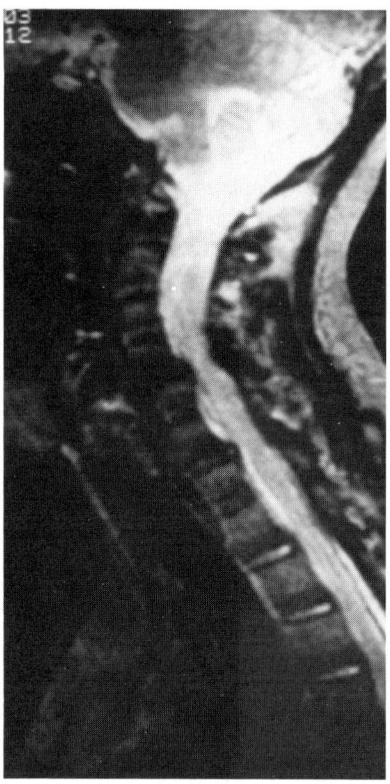

FIG 4–6.
Subaxial subluxation in a 32-year-old woman with rheumatoid arthritis, spinal cord compression, and cervical myelopathy.

This is especially true if neurologic function is deteriorating. If myelopathy is present and undetected, postoperative rehabilitation will be greatly hindered and the functional outcome will be compromised. Myositis or myopathy as an associated condition in rheumatoid arthritis will retard the rehabilitative progress. Identification of this problem and appropriate treatment should begin prior to surgery. Surgical reconstruction is best delayed if active or progressive myositis is present.

In planning for rehabilitation in the upper extremity the goals of surgical reconstruction must be to relieve pain, promote improved joint stability, and increase range of motion and thereby facilitate activities of daily living. In planning postoperative rehabilitation, many of the same factors as previously outlined for lower extremity surgery should be considered prior to surgery. Whereas upper extremity function plays a key role in lower extremity recovery and ambulation, the converse is not true. Rehabilitation of the upper extremity can occur even in the wheelchairbound patient.

In the upper extremity, splinting is often necessary. Rehabilitation of the upper extremity requires close communication between surgeon and occupational therapist to insure that proper precautions are observed for soft tissue reconstruction and goals are clear to patient and therapist. The splint must be comfortable and easily applied and removed. Compliance with splinting is often central to the surgical result in upper extremity surgery and the patient must be fully aware of why it is worn and how it should be maintained. The surgeon must be cognizant of the patient's willingness to work with the therapist prior to recommending surgical intervention.

In the upper extremity, joint disease in contiguous joints will interfere with return of function. If shoulder replacement is performed rehabilitation will be slow and functional improvement of the upper extremity more limited if elbow flexion is poor or hand function impaired. Therapy should be planned to treat all upper extremity joints, with emphasis on the joint(s) operated on (Fig 4–7,A and B).

Muscle dysfunction in upper extremity joints must be documented before surgery. If weakness is profound, intensive rehabilitation will be needed. Absent rotator cuff function preoperatively will greatly alter recovery from total shoulder arthroplasty. The cause or source of the weakness must be clearly defined. Cervical myelopathy will lead to both upper and lower extremity weakness. This is often subtle and manifested by alterations in upper

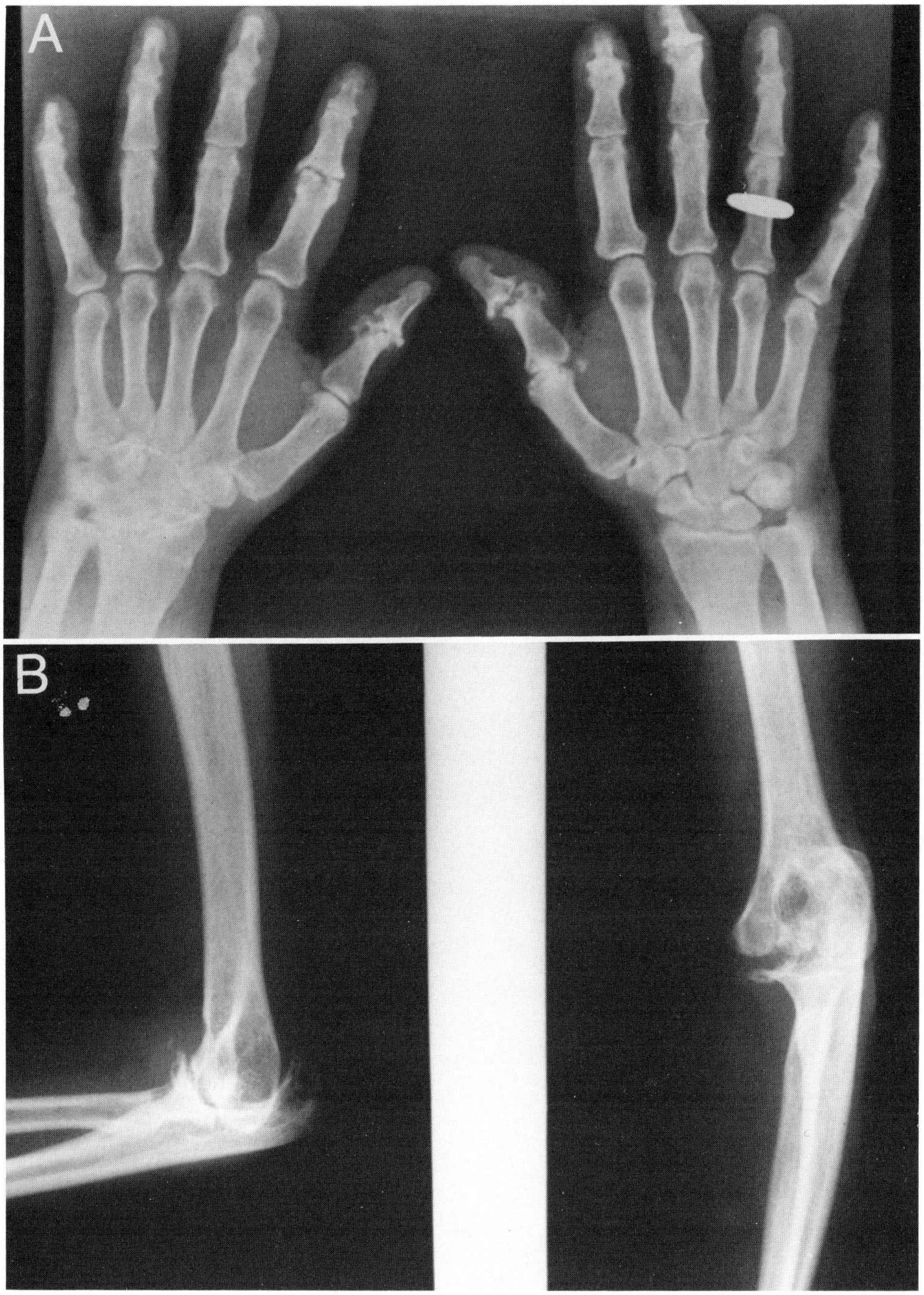

FIG 4–7.
A,B, multiple upper extremity joint involvement—hand, wrist, and elbow—in a 53-year-old patient with rheumatoid arthritis.

extremity function and fine coordination, and increased difficulty with other activities of daily living. Muscle weakness, be it of central or peripheral origin, should be measured prior to surgery and at intervals postoperatively. This is important in documenting progress or improvement. Occupational therapists must instruct the patient with poor muscle power in strengthening programs for the entire upper extremity.

AWARENESS OF POSTOPERATIVE COMPLICATIONS

As the surgeon approaches surgical treatment in the rheumatoid patient he or she must be aware of the increased risk of complications in these patients. The surgeon must communicate these concerns to the patient in a frank and comprehensive discussion

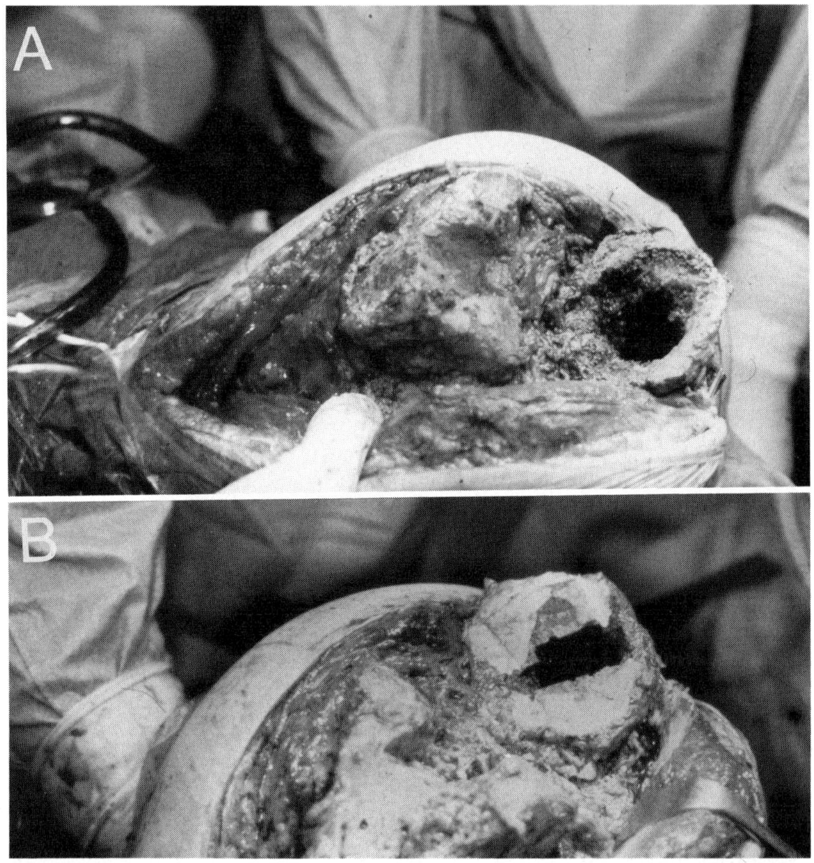

FIG 4–8.
A, bone loss in revision knee replacement in a 60-year-old woman with rheumatoid arthritis. **B,** same patient treated by allograft to the proximal tibia.

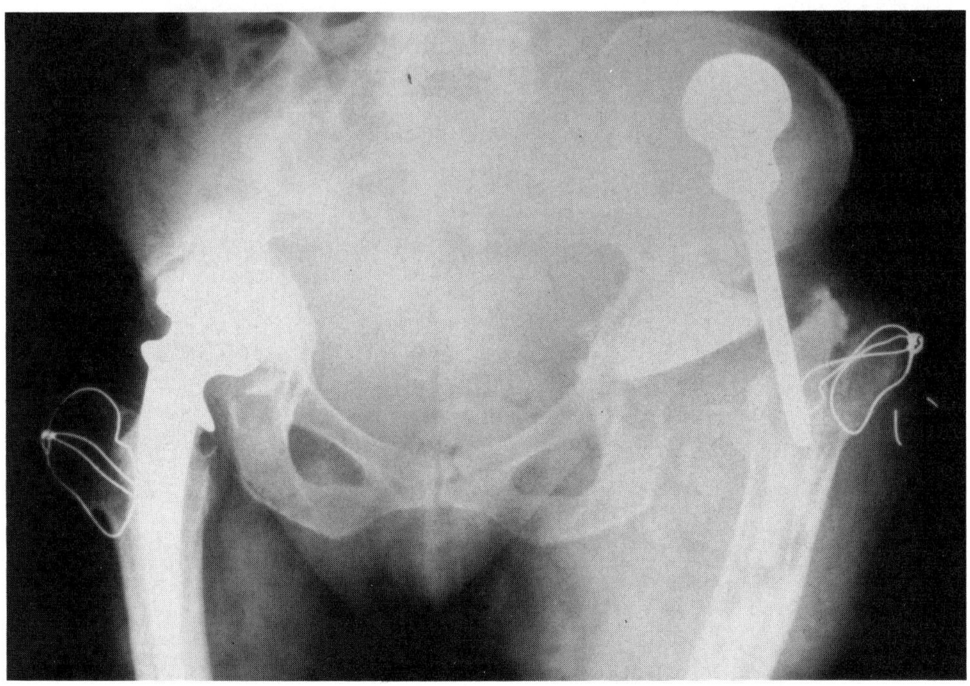

FIG 4–9.
Loosening with dislocation of total hip replacement in a patient with severe osteopenia and rheumatoid arthritis.

preoperatively. It is important to answer the patient's questions and concerns without increasing the fear and anxiety already present in these patients.

Complications may be local or systemic. Wound problems are the most common local problem after surgery. Delayed wound healing and skin sloughing may occur if tissues are not handled with care. The patient must be aware that should a wound healing problem occur, delay in rehabilitation and further surgical treatment may be necessary. Superficial wound infection and deep periprosthetic infection are often catastrophic and must be treated expediently if the implant is to be salvaged. The patient should be aware that deep infection will usually require implant removal, prolonged parenteral antibiotics, and reimplantation (see Chapter 13).

Because of the osteopenia, fractures may complicate hip or knee replacement either during surgery or afterward (Figs 4–8,A and B, and 4–9). Poor bone quality may also be responsible for mechanical loosening (see Fig 4–9), and osteopenic bone may be a contraindication to use of a porous prosthesis in these patients. Localized pressure areas may lead to ulceration and possible secondary infection. Those areas most commonly affected—elbow, heel, sacrum—must be protected and the patient counseled to avoid undue pressure locally. Pads and protective lamb's wool–type devices should be used to prevent pressure sores.

Systemically, the rheumatoid patient is at a greater risk to develop pulmonary problems if interstitial fibrosis is present. It is common for rheumatoid patients to be anemic and this may require that an increased number of blood units be transfused postoperatively. Patients may develop adrenal insufficiency if the cortisone supplement is inadequate. A flare of the patient's rheumatoid disease may also be seen after surgery and this must be treated aggressively with the assistance of the rheumatologist.

CONCLUSIONS

In the approach to the patient with rheumatoid arthritis the most important message is that open communications between surgeon and patient is vital to surgical success. Surgical goals, concerns regarding rehabilitation after surgery, and a review of complications and their treatment should be discussed in great detail with the patient. The other key to successful surgical results is the involvement of the clinical team in the care of these patients. The nurse, social worker, physical and occupational therapist, surgeon, and rheumatologist must all be actively involved. The team approach insures that all aspects of the patient's hospital stay and discharge plan are in place and the appropriate referrals made.

REFERENCES

1. Ahlmen M, Sullivan M, Bjelle A: Team versus non-team outpatient care in rheumatoid arthritis. *Arthritis Rheum* 1988;31:471–479.
2. Baum J: Infection in rheumatoid arthritis. Rheum. 14:135–137.
3. Clements D, Sculco TP, Levine DB, et al: Reinfusion of postoperative sanguinous drainage, washed versus unwashed cells. Presented at the American Academy of Orthopaedic Surgeons Meeting, Anaheim, Calif, February 1991.
4. Duff IF, Carpenter JO, Neukom JE: Comprehensive management of patients with rheumatoid arthritis: Some results of the regional control program in Michigan. *Arthritis Rheum* 1974;17:635–645.
5. Goldenberg DL: Infectious arthritis complicating rheumatoid arthritis and other chronic rheumatic disorders. *Arthritis Rheum* 1987;32:496–502.
6. Harris ED: Rheumatoid arthritis, pathophysiology and implications for therapy. *N Engl J Med* 1990;322:1277–1289.
7. Katz S, Vignos PJ Jr, Moskowitz, RW, et al: Comprehensive outpatient care in rheumatoid arthritis: A controlled study. *JAMA* 1968;206:1249–1254.
8. Perhala RS, Wilke WS, Clough JD, et al: Local infectious complications following large joint replacement in rheumatoid arthritis patients treated with methotrexate versus those not treated with methotrexate. *Arthritis Rheum* 1991;34:146–152.
9. Sculco TP, Adams W, Fried S, et al: Four joint replacement in rheumatoid arthritis, long term follow-up, Presented at the American Academy of Orthopaedic Surgeons, Atlanta, February 1984.
10. Sculco TP: Randomized trial of HuEpo in patients undergoing joint replacement surgery and unable to give autologous blood. Clinical trials in progress.
11. Spiegel JS, Spiegel TM, Ward NB, et al: Rehabilitation for rheumatoid arthritis patients: A controlled trial, *Arthritis Rheum* 1986;29:628–637.
12. Tillman K: Recent advances in the surgical treatment of rheumatoid arthritis. *Clin Orthop* 1990;258: 62–72.

13. Turner RA, Schumacher HR, Myers AR: Phagocytic function of polymorphonuclear leukocytes in rheumatic diseases. *J Clin Invest* 1973;52:1632–1635.
14. Van Albada-Kuipers GA, Linthorst J, Peeters EAJ, et al: Frequency of infection among patients with rheumatoid arthritis versus patients with osteoarthritis or soft tissue rheumatism, *Arthritis Rheum* 1988;31:667–671.
15. Vignos PJ Jr, Thompson HM, Katz S, et al: Comprehensive care and psychosocial factors in rehabilitation in rheumatoid arthritis, a controlled study. *J Chronic Dis* 1972;25:457–567.

CHAPTER 5

Anesthesia

Kevin V. Sanborn, M.D.

With a Special Section on the Temporomandibular Joint

Barry M. Libin, D.D.S, M.S.D.

INTRODUCTION

The patient with rheumatoid arthritis (RA) poses many challenges in anesthetic management. Because of the diffuse nature of the disease, which is both systemic and musculoskeletal, these patients require thorough preoperative, intraoperative, and postoperative monitoring. In addition to the medical problems they present, emotional lability and depression may further complicate their anesthetic management. The anesthesiologist must be knowledgeable about the spectrum of systemic manifestations of the disease and interact closely with the rheumatologist and orthopaedic surgeon to facilitate an uncomplicated perioperative course.

GENERAL CONSIDERATIONS FOR PREOPERATIVE EVALUATION

Metabolic Rate

During active inflammatory disease, there is a hypermetabolic state.[39] This increase in metabolic rate, estimated at about 30% for the average patient with active RA, results in increased oxygen transport requirements and may account for otherwise unexplained sinus tachycardia frequently seen in the perioperative period.

Effects of Steroids

Steroid therapy, either current or past, may adversely affect the response to stress, as in the induction of anesthesia or surgery. A patient who has received exogenous steroids within 1 year of surgery may develop sudden hypotension during stress.[24] The mechanism of circulatory collapse is based upon suppression of adrenocorticotropic hormone (ACTH) secretion by negative feedback. The normal adrenocortical axis is able to increase the output of hydrocortisone when the body is exposed to stress, but a patient treated chronically with steroids may be unable to do this. Chronic steroid therapy may be associated with adrenocortical atrophy and adrenal insufficiency.[15] The perioperative doses of glucocorticoids that are currently recommended for patients with adrenal insufficiency are *supra*physiologic and are rationalized on the grounds of preventing hemodynamic instability, cardiovascular collapse, and death. However, recent studies in monkeys have failed to show any benefit of such high doses over physiologic doses.[36, 41]

Treatment

Patients with adrenocortical insufficiency who require surgery should have measurements of blood sugar and electrolytes and an assessment of hypovolemia, and any abnormalities should be corrected. Assuming 70 kg body weight, methylprednisolone

40 mg may be given intramuscularly (IM) on the night before surgery and hydrocortisone 100 mg should be given intravenously (IV) prior to anesthesia and surgery. Intravenous fluid therapy should address the potential for hypoglycemia, hyponatremia, and hypokalemia that exists in patients with adrenocortical insufficiency perioperatively.[28]

Increased Risk of Infection

Owing to immunologic defects in both humoral and cellular mechanisms of host defense, patients with RA have an increased susceptibility to infection. Therefore, it is imperative that the anesthesiologist take extraordinary precautions concerning sterility in the performance of invasive procedures. In addition, antibiotics should be used in patients with RA who are monitored invasively.

Anemia of Chronic Disease

Patients with RA may suffer from anemia of chronic disease and therefore can be expected to have a lower hematocrit than what is normally required for elective surgery. Since these patients may be taking nonsteroidal anti-inflammatory drugs (NSAIDs) and steroids, anemia secondary to gastrointestinal bleeding should be excluded. There is no evidence that preoperative transfusion is beneficial to the patient suffering from chronic anemia.[6] The anemia of chronic disease can be managed in much the same way that the anemia associated with chronic renal failure is managed. In the absence of significant congestive heart failure, patients maintain normal oxygen transport down to a hematocrit of 24%, by simply increasing cardiac output (Fig 5–1). In patients who are chronically adapted to anemia, other mechanisms are at work to enhance oxygen transport, including a rightward shift of the oxyhemoglobin dissociation curve.

Cardiovascular Disease Associated With Rheumatoid Arthritis

The subject of heart disease associated with RA has been thoroughly reviewed by Pizzarello and Goldberg.[23]

Pericarditis

Children with juvenile rheumatoid arthritis (JRA) are at risk for the development of pericarditis. Pericarditis has been reported to occur in 7% to 10% of children with JRA.[3] Symptoms include chest pain, palpitation, tachypnea, dyspnea, weakness, anxiety due to hypoxia, pallor, and clammy sweaty skin. Physical findings include tachycardia, muffled heart sounds, distended neck veins, or hepatomegaly due to chronic passive congestion.[3] In addition to pericarditis, patients with JRA have also been shown by electrocardiogram (ECG) and echocardiogram studies to have myocardial dysfunction during episodes of systemic JRA.[17] In adults with RA, pericarditis has been detected in 30% at autopsy but the fre-

FIG 5–1.
Graph showing that patients with anemia can maintain normal oxygen transport if they are able to increase their cardiac output and have normal arterial oxygen saturation (Sat). Hgb = hemoglobin in PaO_2 = partial pressure of arterial oxygen.

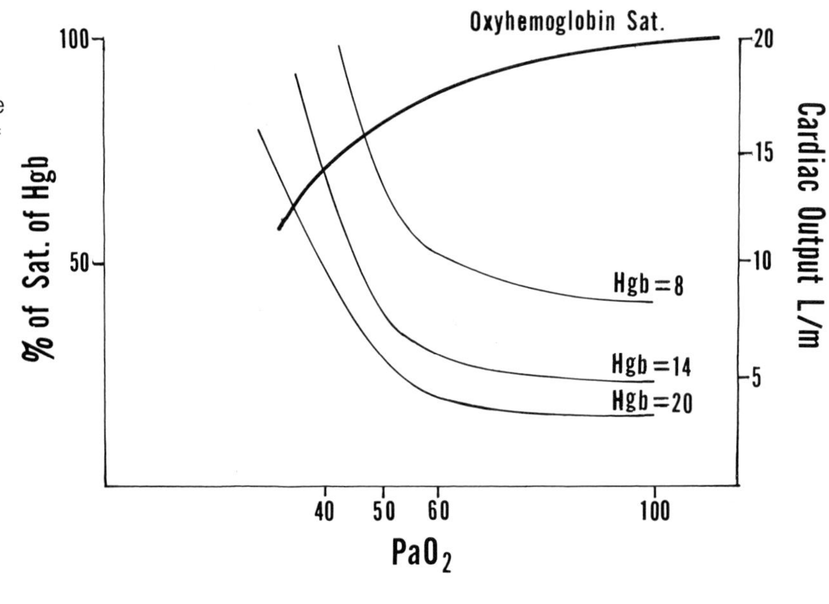

quency of clinically evident pericarditis varies from 2% to 10%.[18]

Myocardial Disease

Nonspecific or granulomatous inflammatory reaction in the myocardium is found in 4% to 30% of necropsy patients with RA. This condition is usually clinically silent or benign. When it becomes severe, congestive heart failure, arrhythmias, and conduction delays may occur. ECG abnormalities will include ST-T changes, conduction abnormalities, and disturbances of rate and rhythm.[1]

Conduction Abnormalities

Conduction abnormalities occur in about 8% to 10% of patients with RA, and are believed to be due to inflammatory disease or arteritis of the conducting tissue. Complete heart block is rare.

Coronary Artery Disease

Cathcart and Spodick found an increased prevalence of coronary artery disease, but other studies failed to show that association.[7] Pizzarello and Goldberg[23] report a 15% to 20% incidence of coronary *arteritis* at necropsy and state that these lesions rarely express themselves clinically. Thrombosis is rarely present. When anginal chest pain does occur, the cause is almost always atherosclerotic coronary artery disease, not inflammatory coronary arteritis. Rare exceptions are in patients with severe systemic vasculitis or in young people without associated cardiac risk factors. When inflammatory coronary arteritis is suspected, then steroids should be considered in addition to regular antianginal therapy. The incidence of atherosclerotic coronary artery disease in patients with RA is about equal to age-matched controls.

Valvular Disease

The incidence of valvular heart disease at necropsy in patients with RA varies from 6% to 62%, although the average is about 30% to 40%. Any of the valves may be involved, either alone or in combination. Mitral insufficiency of varying severity is the most common lesion. Mitral stenosis is unreported. Atrial arrhythmias may occur, and patients may require treatment with digitalis and diuretics. Aortitis with associated aortic insufficiency is a well-known extraarticular manifestation of ankylosing spondylitis and other HLA-B27–associated spondyloarthropathies in adults. One study reported a 12.5% incidence of aortic insufficiency in patients with ankylosing spondylitis.[35]

Pulmonary Disease Associated With Rheumatoid Arthritis

Pulmonary Fibrosis

Approximately 30% to 40% of patients with RA demonstrate either radiographic or pulmonary function abnormalities indicative of interstitial fibrosis or restrictive lung disease. The severity of pulmonary fibrosis is not associated with rheumatologic symptoms or the duration of the associated RA, nor is there any clear relation to the extraarticular features of RA or serologic findings. Survival rates in patients with coexisting RA and pulmonary fibrosis are similar to those of patients with idiopathic pulmonary fibrosis. Some patients have a slowly progressive course for 10 years whereas others may have a rapidly deteriorating course resulting in death within 4 months of the onset of pulmonary symptoms. In a study of 39 patients with RA and pulmonary fibrosis, 56% died within 5 years of detection of pulmonary involvement.[30, 40]

Pleural Effusion

The reported incidence of pleural effusion in patients with RA varies from 3.0% to 12.5%. Pleural effusion most commonly appears in the sixth decade and is unusual below the age of 40 years. It may be transient, chronic, relapsing, or complicated by the development of empyema or hydropneumothorax. The effusions are characteristically small, may be unilateral or bilateral, and are frequently asymptomatic. However, pleuritic pain can occur and large effusions may produce dyspnea.[21]

Pulmonary Nodules

Pulmonary necrobiotic nodules, a rare pulmonary complication of RA, are round pulmonary lesions histologically identical to subcutaneous rheumatoid nodules. Although usually asymptomatic, they may rupture into a bronchus, causing cough and hemoptysis.

Other Respiratory Abnormalities

Patients with RA have increased susceptibility to pulmonary infection. Recently, it was shown that among 15 patients with RA who had normal chest films, 9 patients had decreased inspiratory muscle strength. The authors suggested steroid myopathy and rheumatoid myositis as possible etiologies.[12] A study by Hyland et al. *failed* to demonstrate a higher incidence of obstructive lung disease in a group of 155 patients with RA compared with 95 control subjects.[13] Pulmonary hypertension is a rare but serious complication of RA. In 19 reported cases, 11 patients died within 12 months of the diagnosis. The reported causes of pulmonary hypertension in RA include interstitial fibrosis, pulmonary vasculitis, serum hyperviscosity, and idiopathic pulmonary hypertension.[43]

Personality Disorders Associated With Rheumatoid Arthritis

Neurotic symptoms are common in RA and have generally been regarded as a consequence of the disabling physical illness. The view that RA is a psychosomatic disease with a psychogenic origin in personality conflicts has *not* been supported despite much suggestive evidence. Patients with RA have shown consistently abnormal patterns on the Minnesota Multiphasic Personality Inventory (MMPI), especially elevations in the hysteria, hypochondriasis, and depression subscales.[25, 29] Other personality scales such as the Eysenck Personality Inventory have also revealed "neurotic" patterns in RA patients, more in those who were seronegative, and more in patients with chronic as opposed to new-onset disease. Some of these abnormal patterns may be the result of long-term adaptation to the illness.[8, 19] Unlike systemic lupus erythematosus (SLE), RA rarely affects the central nervous system (CNS), so that an organic brain syndrome based on RA is extremely unlikely.

Patients with RA may suffer from the neuropsychiatric side effects of therapeutic agents used to treat the disease. The corticosteroids may produce psychiatric side effects. Studies have shown that 3% to 5% of patients who are started on significant doses of prednisone develop severe psychiatric syndromes. Psychosis, mania, and hypomania were the most common patterns with depression being a small component. Depression has also been associated with ibuprofen, fenoprofen, and naproxen. Cognitive dysfunction associated with naproxen and ibuprofen has been reported in the elderly.[29] These neuropsychiatric disturbances can create difficulties for the anesthesiologist during the clinical management of patients with RA in the operating room and intensive care unit. During regional anesthesia, additional sedation and reassurance may be required. Such patients may be subject to emotional outbursts normally associated with a more juvenile level of maturity.

PERIOPERATIVE MONITORING

Arterial Lines

An arterial line is strongly recommended for perioperative monitoring of the rheumatoid patient undergoing major reconstructive surgery. Placement of a radial arterial line may be difficult in patients with advanced RA owing to:

1. Positioning: distortion of the wrist joint may require a steep angle of approach and painful, rigid wrist and elbow joints may limit ideal positioning.
2. Arteritis: narrowed lumen and tendency to spasm when instrumented. Targeting a more proximal portion of the radial artery and using a 22-gauge catheter may be helpful.

Intravenous Access

Intravenous access is frequently difficult in patients with advanced disease. Peripheral veins tend to be small and fragile or absent altogether. Access to the internal jugular vein may require a reassessment of the superficial neck anatomy, which may be distorted. Using the so-called central approach to the internal jugular, the vein may be found in a more medial relation to the triangle formed by the sternocleidomastoid muscle and the clavicle than is found in normal subjects (Fig 5–2).

Skin

Special care must be exercised when using adhesives to secure IV, epidural, or monitoring catheters. Patients on steroid therapy for extended periods of time may have very friable skin which can be avulsed merely by removing adhesive tape applied to dressings or lines, or by rough handling of the skin.

CHOICE OF ANESTHESIA

Choice of anesthesia should be based on a consideration of the patient's safety and comfort, the surgeon's needs, and the skills of the anesthesiologist. In our opinion, regional anesthesia should be

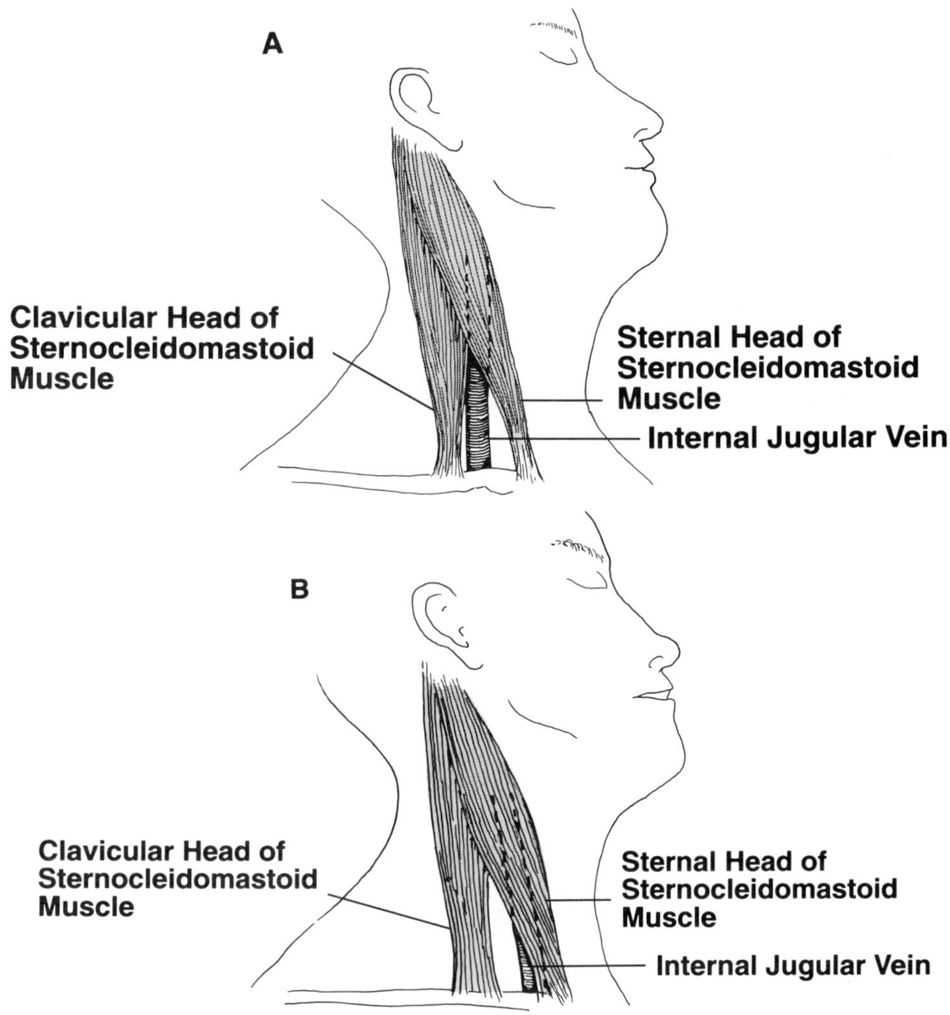

FIG 5–2.
A, normal location of the internal jugular vein. **B,** location of the internal jugular vein in some patients with advanced RA.

strongly emphasized for patients with RA except when the regional technique required is not included among the anesthesiologist's skills. This opinion is based upon the difficulty in achieving control of the airway in patients with RA as well as the fact that patients with RA frequently require orthopaedic surgery on their extremities and such surgery can be nicely facilitated with regional anesthesia techniques.

Regional Anesthesia

The performance of regional anesthesia in patients with RA can be complicated by: (1) increased sedation requirements based upon personality disorders and increased metabolic rate; and (2) positioning difficulties based upon decreased range of motion of joints and chronic pain in joints not involved in the regional technique.

Epidural or *spinal* anesthesia is recommended for procedures on the hip, knee, and ankle joints. Spinal anesthesia has the disadvantage that it may result in dural puncture headache in younger patients. The performance of spinal or epidural anesthesia in patients with RA may be difficult due to lordosis of the lumbar spine. The use of a paramedian approach overcomes that difficulty in all but the most extreme cases. Patients with ankylosing spondylitis usually have fused lumbar interspaces, making spinal or epidural anesthesia extremely difficult or impossible, although caudal anesthesia may be easily accomplished.

Potential Benefits of Epidural Anesthesia

There are several potential benefits of epidural anesthesia in the patient with RA. During total hip replacement, epidural anesthesia can be used to provide a remarkably dry field for the surgeon and a significant reduction in blood loss for the patient.[33, 38, 42] These benefits result from the smooth pattern of intraoperative hemodynamics that is characteristic of epidural anesthesia, assuming that the relative hypotension produced is not overcorrected with vasopressors.[34] Pain relief following total hip or total knee replacement can be enhanced by using epidural analgesia. Low concentrations of local anesthetics, usually bupivacaine, with or without narcotics, may be infused via epidural catheters for 2 to 3 days after surgery. This type of analgesia has the advantages of obtunding the stress response to surgery and minimizing respiratory depression and dysphoric responses to conventional analgesics. However, postoperative epidural analgesia has not yet been shown to improve survival, enhance rehabilitation, or lower the rate of cardiopulmonary complications.

Axillary block is recommended for procedures on the hand, wrist, and elbow. Contrary to previous reports, axillary block provides excellent anesthesia for elbow surgery, including total elbow replacement.[32] If frequent movement of a painful shoulder joint during surgery is anticipated, then it is very helpful to perform an "analgesic" interscalene brachial plexus block, using about 10 mL of local anesthesia just after performing the axillary block. Some patients with RA have such severe disease in the shoulder joint that it may be difficult or impossible to access the axilla. In such cases, it may be necessary to perform an interscalene brachial plexus block instead of the axillary block. However, interscalene brachial plexus block often fails to produce adequate anesthesia of the T1 and C8 nerve roots, requiring that local anesthesia or sedatives be used to supplement the block when operating on the hand or wrist.

Interscalene brachial plexus block is recommended for procedures on the shoulder, including total shoulder replacement. It can also be used for procedures on the elbow, especially when immobility of the shoulder makes the positioning for axillary block difficult or impossible.

Ankle block is recommended for surgery of the forefoot and toes. The use of 0.75% bupivacaine *without* epinephrine provides prolonged analgesia, reducing the need for narcotic analgesics postoperatively.

General Anesthesia

When general anesthesia is unavoidable, the main focus is on control of the airway. The authors advise against attempts at blind nasal or oral laryngoscopy whenever the preoperative evaluation reveals that the airway is compromised in a patient with RA. Such attempts may lead to swelling and bleeding from damaged fragile mucous membranes. Instead, we recommend that the fiberoptic intubating bronchoscope (e.g., the Olympus LF-1) be used to intubate the trachea on an elective basis. In our practice, this is accomplished using minimal sedation, topical local anesthesia, and nasal oxygen. A lubricated 6.0-mm armored endotracheal tube is loaded onto the intubating bronchoscope and passed over the scope after the scope has been introduced through the nose into the trachea. Balanced anesthesia is then induced and the patient is extubated in the operating room fully awake. There is a significant danger of upper airway obstruction postoperatively if emergence from general anesthesia is not complete before extubation. Using this approach, it has not yet been necessary to perform preoperative elective tracheos-

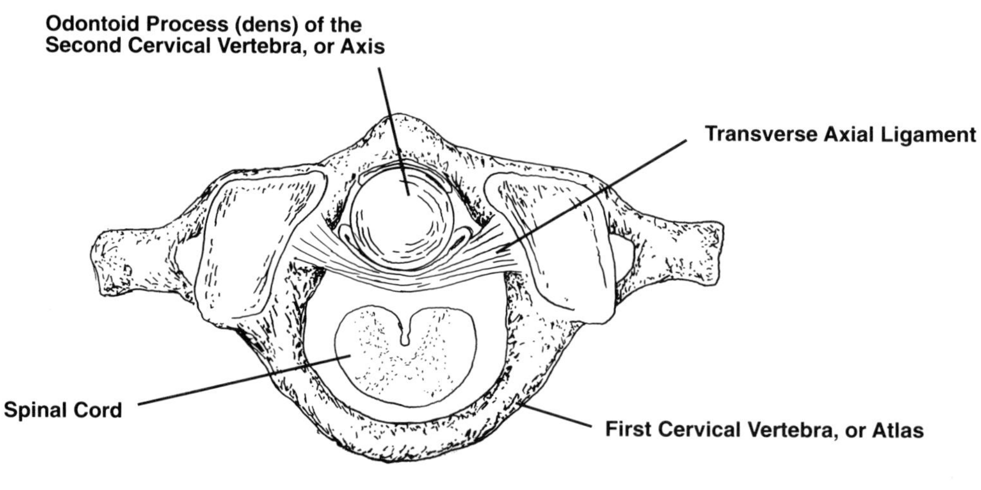

FIG 5–3.
The dens, or odontoid process of the axis, is held in place against the anterior arch of the C1 vertebra by the transverse axial ligament.

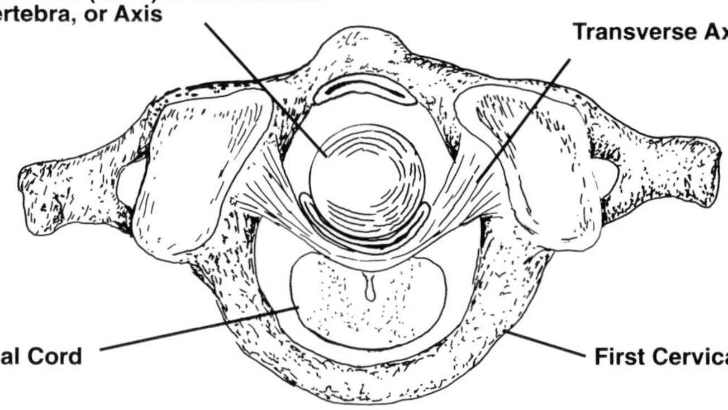

FIG 5–4.
Laxity or disruption of the transverse axial ligament by disease process leads to mobility of the odontoid within the spinal canal. Then, in flexion, the odontoid may remain in its position while the arch of C1 and the spinal cord move anteriorly.

tomy, nor has it been necessary to perform an emergency tracheostomy perioperatively.

AIRWAY ABNORMALITIES

Cervical Spine

The incidence of clinically evident involvement of the cervical spine in RA is stated to be 25% to 90%, depending on the study.[22] Atlantoaxial subluxation occurred in 61% and subaxial subluxation in 31% of 163 patients with RA who had complaints about the cervical spine.[22] The dens, or odontoid process of the axis, is held in place against the anterior arch of the C1 vertebra by the transverse axial ligament. (Fig 5–3) Laxity or disruption of this ligament by disease process leads to mobility of the odontoid within the spinal canal. Then, in flexion, the odontoid may remain in its position while the arch of C1 and the spinal cord move anteriorly.[2] (Figs 5–4 and 5–5) This can endanger the spine, so patients with atlantoaxial subluxation must be maintained in slight extension because excessive flexion may result in neurologic injury. Neurologic injury may include compression of the C2 nerve root, posterior column dysfunction, and ultimately quadriparesis or quadriplegia. Con-

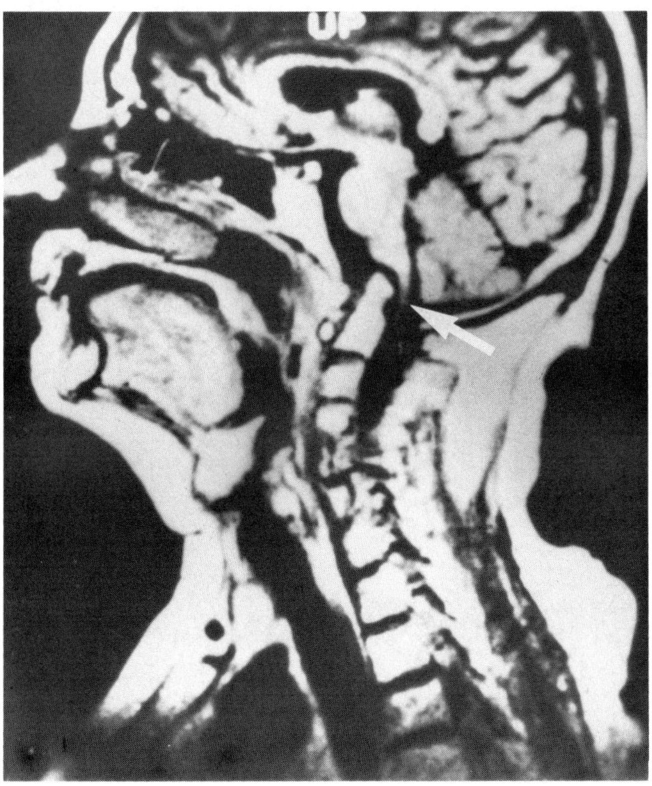

FIG 5–5.
Magnetic resonance image of the cervical spine of a patient with severe RA. The axis or odontoid process of C2 is impinging on the brainstem and spinal cord *(arrow).*

versely, it is frequently impossible for such patients to achieve the degree of cervical spine *extension* required for oral intubation.

Because there is poor correlation between symptoms and pathologic findings, it is advised to obtain cervical spine radiographs before undertaking *general* anesthesia on any patient with RA of more than 5 years' duration.[5, 22]

The Temporomandibular Joint

Barry M. Libin, D.D.S, M.S.D.

Fifty percent to 75% of patients with RA have pathologic changes in the temporomandibular joint (TMJ).[37] The symptoms and severity of TMJ involvement vary, but the major symptoms are intermittent pain, swelling, and limitation of movement. Radiographic changes in the TMJ occur eventually in the majority of cases, but may not be apparent until the later stages of the disease (Fig 5–6,A and B). There are two problems that concern the anesthesiologist: (1) limitation of the mandibular opening that will prevent endotracheal intubation; and (2) the loss of upper pharyngeal airway space, which can result in complete airway obstruction with sedation or anesthesia.

Limitation of Mandibular Opening

Anterior displacement of articular discs and osseous resorption resulting in disfigurement of the mandibular condyle or temporal bone may make mandibular opening difficult, if not impossible, especially in the supine position. In a study of 123 patients with RA, almost 50% had some restriction in mouth opening, although no patient had such severe restriction (less than 10 mm) to suggest ankylosis.[37] Indeed, the literature suggests that complete restriction of joint movement as a result of osseous fusion is a rare and late finding in RA. Limitation of mandibular opening may be due to abnormality of the joint itself or from malfunction of the muscles that power jaw opening. Following inflammatory disease of the TMJ, the repair process may result in fibrous adhesions between the articular disc and the temporal bone. Such adhesions may prevent the disc from moving easily backward and forward with the mandibular condyle. It may also result in the loss of the normal anatomic disc–condyle relationship, producing a locking of the joint as the condyle is unable to negotiate past an anteriorly displaced disc (Fig 5–7). Restriction of the opening may also be due to severe mandibular muscle contraction, a common finding in patients with RA. In this situation, the muscles are either "guarding" the injured joint, preventing motion, or are fatigued from overuse, as may result from tooth clenching or occlusal dysfunction.

Upper Airway Obstruction

Destruction of the TMJ may result in a supraglottic obstruction of the airway that has been related to apnea and dysphagia.[10] This is especially significant in patients with severe reduction of ramal height or micrognathia, as occurs in JRA. In such cases, there is considerable distal movement of the body of the mandible, one of whose sequelae is tongue retraction, often into the pharyngeal space (Fig 5–8). Redlund-Johnell studied 400 patients with RA, 76 of whom had destruction of the TMJ. Thirty patients (39%) had upper airway obstruction, especially in the supine position, and 53 patients (70%) had episodes of airway obstruction. Many of these patients had airway obstruction or apnea perioperatively under sedation or after general anesthesia.[27]

Preanesthesia Examination of the TMJ

History

The history should include the following questions:

Is there a history of symptoms related to the TMJ? Has the patient had difficulty in opening the mouth? Has the patient experienced clicking of the joints or locking of the jaws upon jaw opening or closing?

Physical Examination

The physical examination is carried out as follows:

1. Evaluate jaw opening with the patient supine.

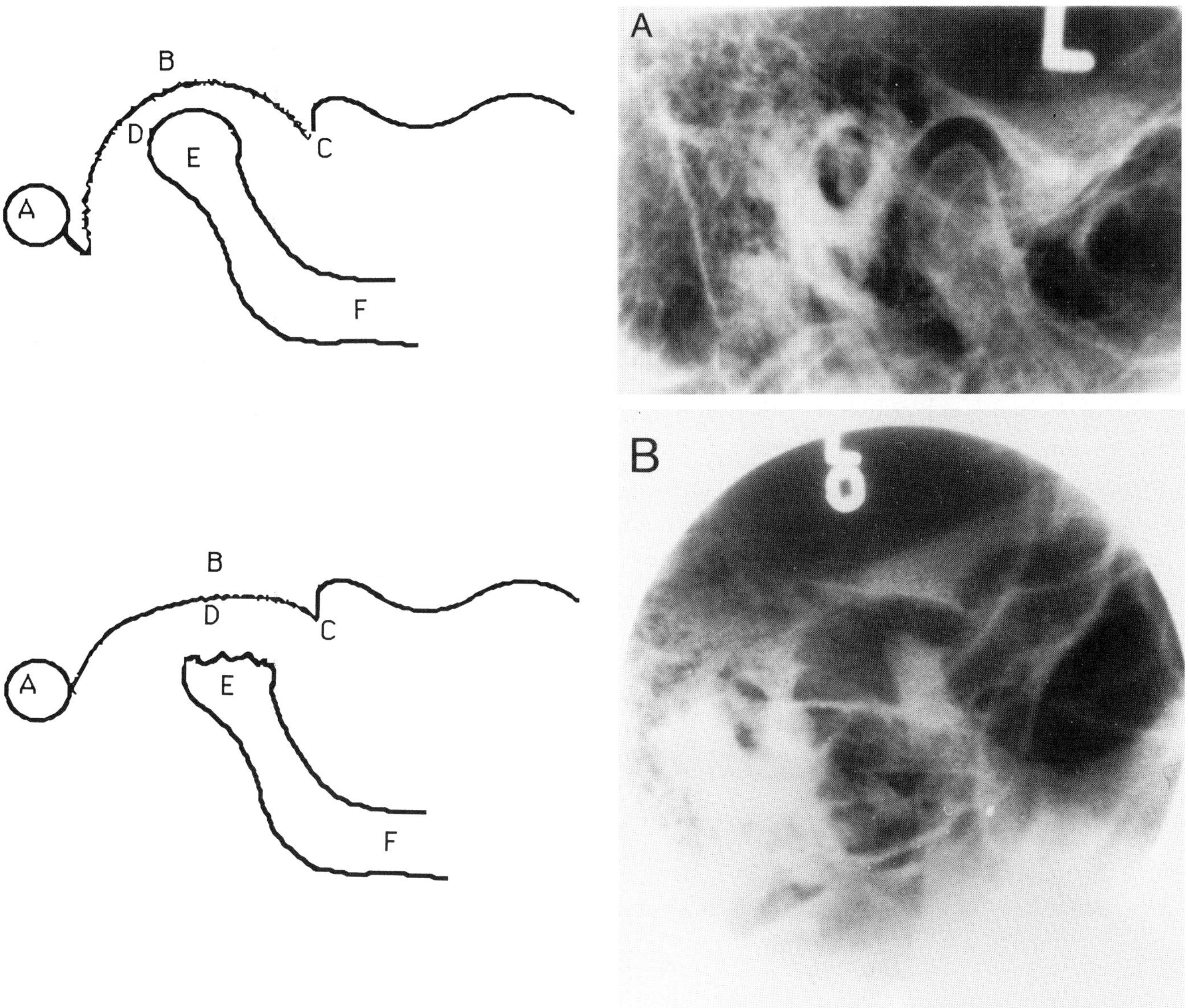

FIG 5–6.
Two x-ray studies of the temporomandibular joint, showing the normal appearance **(A),** and a patient with advanced RA **(B).** *A* = external auditory meatus; *B* = temporal bone; *C* = articular eminence of temporal bone; *D* = temporal fossa; *E* = head of the mandibular condyle—note flattening and resorption resulting from RA; *F* = body of the mandible.

2. Listen with the stethoscope for clicking and crepitus. Clicking is associated with a displaced disc and crepitus is associated with radiographic evidence of erosion.

3. The normal amount of mouth opening allows three of the patient's fingers to be placed vertically between the maxillary and mandibular teeth. If the mouth opening is limited to two fingers or less, then a problem may result during oral endotracheal intubation.

4. Try to manipulate the mandible to full opening. If the articular disc is dislocated ahead of the condyle, it may be possible to place your thumb on the molar tooth on the side of the lock and move the mandible inferiorly to clear the thickness of the disc and then forward to bring the mandibular condyle back under the disc (Fig 5–9). It is important for the anesthesiologist to realize that the joint may not lock all the time, but may lock most often upon awakening if the patient was clenching the night before.

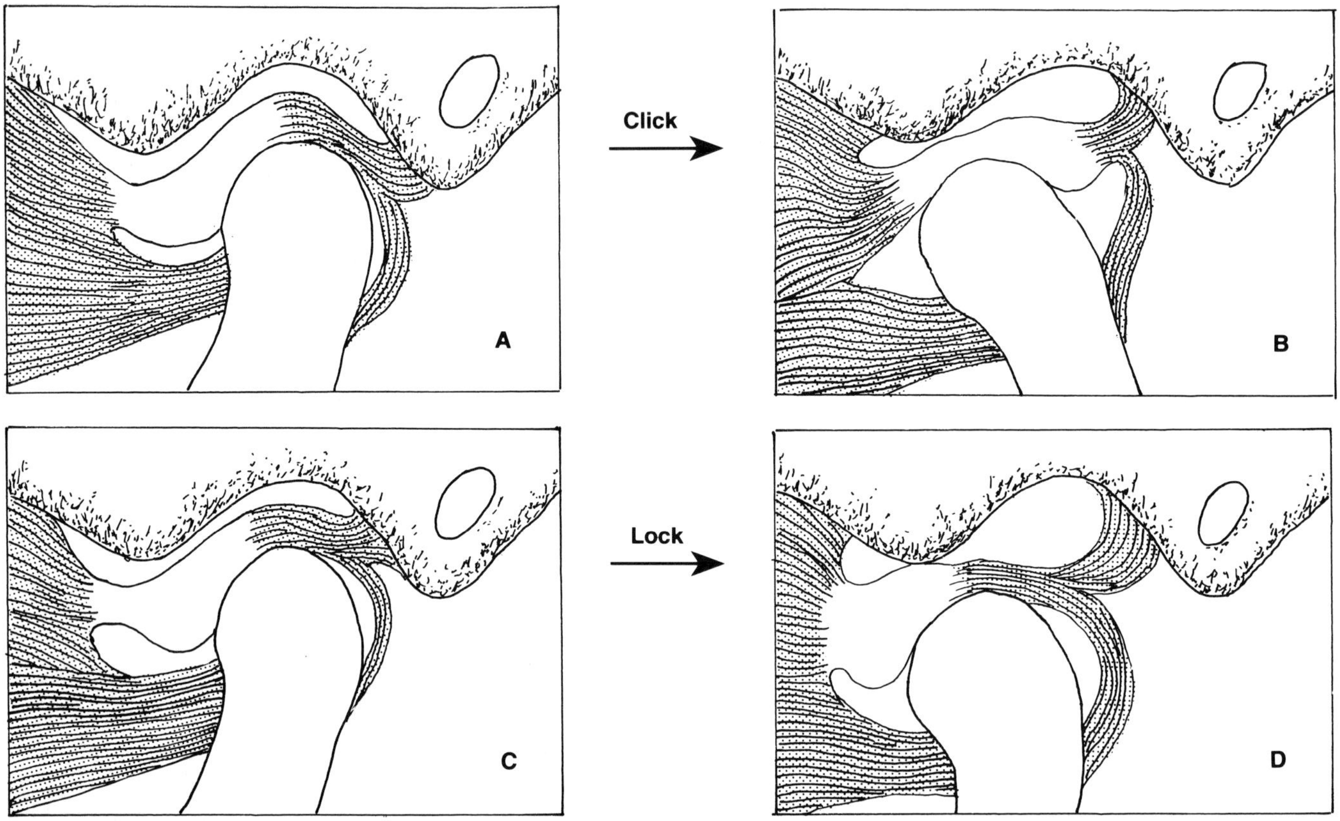

FIG 5–7.
Anterior displacement of the articular disc of the temporomandibular joint.

FIG 5–8.
Airway obstruction: condylar bone loss may result in posterior shifting of the mandible and the attached soft tissue on the floor of the mouth, including the tongue. This may result in impingement and obstruction of the airway.

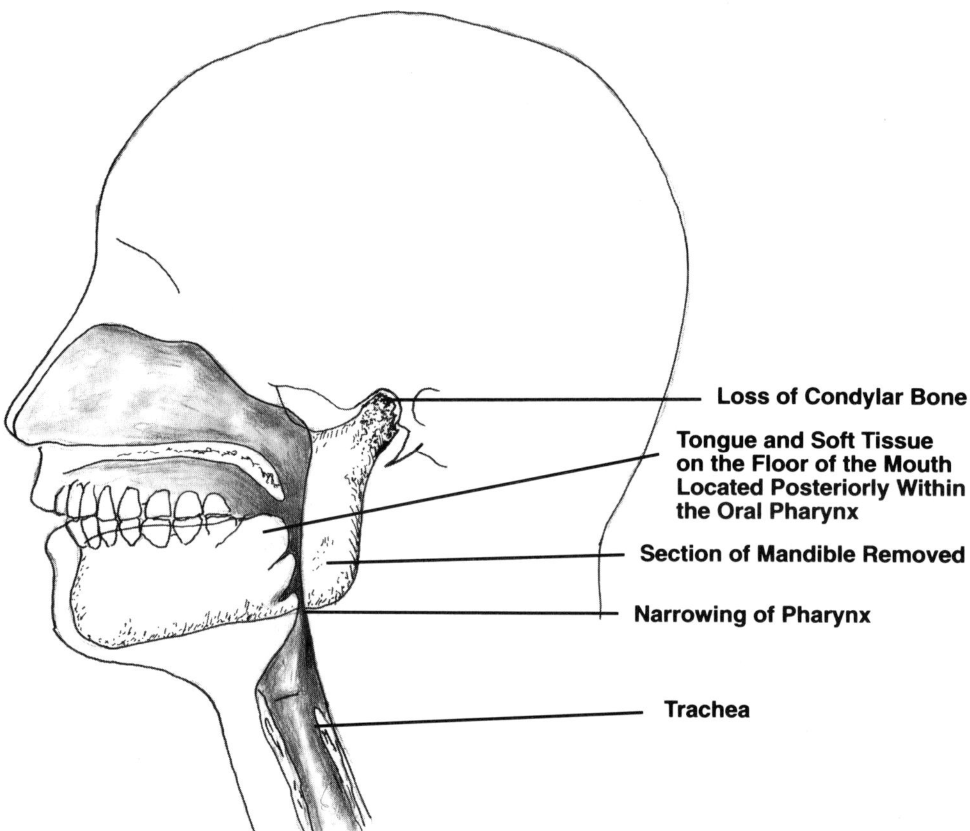

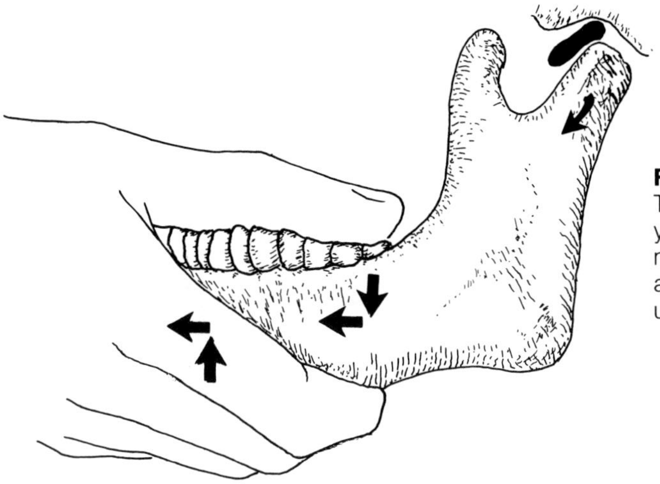

FIG 5–9.
Technique for reduction of dislocated articular disc: place your thumb on the molar tooth on the side of the lock and move the mandible inferiorly to clear the thickness of the disc and then forward to bring the mandibular condyle back under the disc.

Radiography

Radiographic changes in the TMJ are present in 50% to 65% of all patients with RA, and there is a correlation between severity of subjective and clinical dysfunction and radiographic findings.[20]

Larynx

Arthritis of the cricoarytenoid joints is found in at least 26% of patients with RA.[4, 14, 16] Arthritic involvement of the cricoarytenoid joints produces progressive narrowing and fixation of the vocal cords in adduction, thus compromising the airway (Fig 5–10). For this reason, *a narrow internal diameter should be chosen when selecting an endotracheal tube.* When the inflammation of the cricoarytenoid joints is acute, there may be redness and swelling of the false and true cords and the aryepiglottic fold. Palpation of the larynx during the preoperative evaluation may elicit tenderness. In addition, the patient may give a history of stridor, wheezing, hoarseness, or dysphagia. Occasionally, a patient may have satisfactory compensation of airway obstruction at the level of the larynx while awake, but this compensation may disappear when the patient is sedated or anesthetized owing to relaxation of the upper airway joints and muscles, resulting in complete airway obstruction. Following a long procedure with endotracheal intubation, extubation must be performed with great caution, since swelling of an already compromised airway may result in complete airway obstruction in a patient who cannot easily be reintubated.[11]

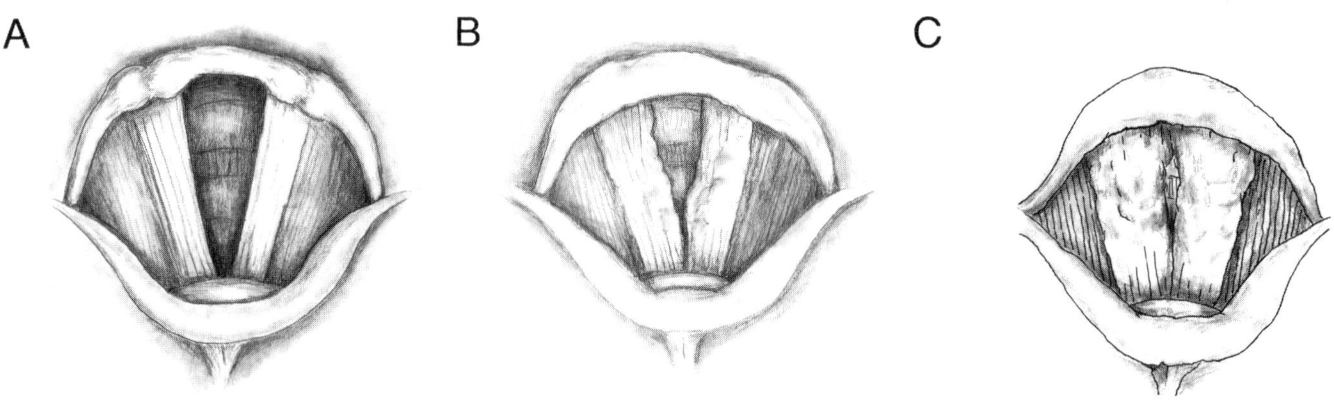

FIG 5–10.
A, normal appearance of vocal cords during laryngoscopy. **B,** appearance of vocal cords during laryngoscopy in a patient with RA who has laryngeal involvement. **C,** appearance of vocal cords during laryngoscopy in a patient with RA who has *severe* laryngeal involvement.

CONCLUSIONS

Patients with RA require a thorough preoperative evaluation of medical problems and physical deformities that may increase the difficulty of regional anesthesia and monitoring techniques, as well as airway abnormalities. Regional anesthesia is usually preferred, but sedation and systemic analgesia is frequently necessary for comfortable positioning. General anesthesia should be undertaken only when necessary, and then with extreme caution. Access to the airway may be severely restricted by cervical spine disease, laryngeal deformation, or arthritis of the TMJ. Finally, the anesthesiologist should show compassion, keeping in mind that patients with RA must undergo many operations and suffer almost continuously from pain and loss of function.

REFERENCES

1. Ansell BM, Simkin PA: The heart and rheumatic disease. *Rheumatology* 1984; 2:292.
2. Bernstein R, Rosenberg A: Anesthesia for orthopedic surgery. *Semin Anesth.* 1987; 6:36–43.
3. Brewer E: Juvenile rheumatoid arthritis—cardiac involvement. *Arthritis Rheum.* 1977; 20(supp2):231–236.
4. Brooker D: Rheumatoid arthritis: Otorhinolaryngological manifestations. *Clin Otolaryngol* 1988; 13:239–246.
5. Cabot A, Becker A: The cervical spine in rheumatoid arthritis. *Clin Orthop* 1978; 131:130–140.
6. Carmel R, Shulman IA: Blood transfusion in medically treatable chronic anemia. Pernicious anemia as a model for transfusion overuse. *Arch Pathol Lab Med* 1989; 113:995–997.
7. Cathcart ES, Spodick DH: Rheumatoid heart disease—a study of the incidence and nature of cardiac lesions in rheumatoid arthritis. *N Engl J Med* 1962; 266:959–964.
8. Creed F, Murphy S, Jayson M: Measurement of psychiatric disorder in rheumatoid arthritis. *J Psychosom Res* 1990; 34:79–87.
9. Edelist G: Principles of anesthetic management in rheumatoid arthritic patients. *Anesth Analg* 1964; 43:227–231.
10. Ekberg O, Redland-Johnell I, Sjoblum KG: Pharyngeal function in patients with rheumatoid arthritis of the cervical spine and temporomandibular joint. *Acta Radiol* 1987; 28:35–39.
11. Funk D, Raymon F: Rheumatoid arthritis of the cricoarytenoid joints: An airway hazard. *Anesth Analg* 1975; 54:742–745.
12. Gorini M, Ginanni R, Spinelli A, et al: Inspiratory muscle strength and respiratory drive in patients with rheumatoid arthritis. *Am Rev Respir Dis* 1990; 142:289–294.
13. Hyland RH, Gordon DA, Broder I, et al: A systematic controlled study of pulmonary abnormalities in rheumatoid arthritis. *J Rheumatol* 1983; 10:395–405.
14. Keenan MA, Stiles CM, Kaufman RL: Acquired laryngeal deviation associated with cervical spine disease in erosive polyarticular arthritis. *Anesthesiology.* 1983; 58:441–449.
15. Krisher JA: The anesthetist surveys the arthritic patient. *Surg Clin North Am* 1969; 49:757–761.
16. Lofgren RH, Montgomery WW: Incidence of laryngeal involvement in rheumatoid arthritis. *N Engl J Med* 1962; 267:193–195.
17. Marin-Garcia J, Sheridan R, Hanissan AS: Echocardiographic detection of early cardiac involvement in juvenile rheumatoid arthritis. *Pediatrics* 1984; 73:394–397.
18. Mody GM, Stevens JE, Meyers OL: The heart in rheumatoid arthritis—a clinical and echocardiographic study. *Q J Med* 1987; 65:921–928.
19. Murphy S, Creed F, Jayson M: Pyschiatric disorder and illness behaviour in rheumatoid arthritis. *Br J Rheumatol* 1988; 27:357–363.
20. Ogus H: Rheumatoid arthritis of the temporomandibular joint. *J Oral Surg* 1975; 12:275–284.
21. Payne CR: Pulmonary manifestations of rheumatoid arthritis. *Br J Hosp Med* 1984; 32:192–197.
22. Pellicci PM, Ranawat CS, Tsaris P, et al: Progression of rheumatoid arthritis of the cervical spine. *J Bone Joint Surg [Am]* 1981; 63:342–350.
23. Pizzarello RA, Goldberg J: The heart in rheumatoid arthritis, in Utsinger PD (ed): *Rheumatoid Arthritis. Etiology, Diagnosis and Management.* Philadelphia, JB Lippincott Co, 1985, pp 431–440.
24. Plumpton FS, Besser GM, Cole PV: Corticosteroid treatment and surgery. *Anaesthesia* 1969; 24:3–17.
25. Puente AE: Personality characteristics of individuals with chronic rheumatoid arthritis. *Percept Mot Skills* 1988; 66:639–642.
26. Redick L: The temporomandibular joint and tracheal intubation. *Anesth Analg* 1987; 66:675–676.
27. Redlund-Johnell I: Upper airway obstruction in patients with rheumatoid arthritis and tempormandibular joint destruction. *Scand J Rheumatol* 1988; 17:273–279.
28. Reginster JY, Damas P, Franchimont P: Specific risks of anesthesia in patients with osteoarticular disease. *Acta Anaesthesiol Belg* 1984; 2:105–121.
29. Rogers MP: Rheumatoid arthritis: Psychiatric aspects and use of psychotropics. *Psychosomatics* 1985; 26:915–925.
30. Roschmann RA, Rothenberg RJ: Pulmonary fibrosis in rheumatoid arthritis: A review of clinical features and therapy. *Semin Arthritis Rheum* 1987; 16:174–185.
31. Salathe M, Johr M: Unsuspected cervical fractures: A common problem in ankylosing spondylitis. *Anesthesiology* 1989; 70:869–870.

32. Sanborn KV, Sharrock NE: Axillary brachial plexus block provides reliable anesthesia for elbow surgery. *Anesthesiology* 1989; 71:A727.
33. Sharrock NE, Savarese JJ: Anesthesia for orthopedic surgery, in Miller RD (ed): *Anesthesia.* New York, Churchill Livingstone Inc, 1990, pp. 1952–1967.
34. Sharrock NE: Perioperative mortality following total knee and hip arthroplasty—The role of anesthesia care? *Anesthesiology*1991; 75:A868.
35. Sukenik S, Pras A, Buskila D, et al: Cardiovascular manifestations of ankylosing spondylitis. *Clin Rheumatol* 1987; 6:588–592.
36. Symreng T, Karlberg BE, Kagedal B, et al: Physiological cortisol substitution of long-term steroid-treated patients undergoing major surgery. *Br J Anaesth* 1981; 53:949–953.
37. Tegelberg A, Kopp S: Clinical findings in the stomatognathic system for individuals with rheumatoid arthritis and osteoarthritis. *Acta Odontol Scand* 1987; 45:65–75.
38. Thompson GE, Miller RD, Stephens WC, et al: Hypotensive anesthesia for total hip arthroplasty. *Anesthesiology* 1978; 48:91.
39. Touger-Decker R: Nutritional considerations in rheumatoid arthritis. *J Am Diet Assoc* 1988; 88:327–331.
40. Turner-Warwick M, Evans RC: Pulmonary manifestations of rheumatoid disease. *Clin Rheum Dis* 1977; 3:549–564.
41. Udelsman R, Ramp J, Gallucci WT, et al: Adaptation during surgical stress. *J Clin Invest* 1986; 77:1377–1381.
42. Vazeery AK, Lunde O: Controlled hypotension in hip surgery. *Acta Orthop Scand* 1979; 50:433.
43. Young ID, Ford SE, Ford PM: The association of pulmonary hypertension with rheumatoid arthritis. *J Rheumatol* 1989; 16:1266–1269.

CHAPTER 6

The Temporomandibular Joint

Barry M. Libin, D.D.S., M.S.D.

David A. Behrman, D.M.D.

INTRODUCTION

Fifty percent to 75% of rheumatoid arthritis (RA) patients have temporomandibular joint (TMJ) involvement.[6, 10, 12, 24, 29] The decision as to which of these patients need treatment, and the method of therapeutic intervention depends to a great extent on the severity of symptoms, degree of functional loss, and the extent to which the symptoms can be controlled. This chapter reviews the anatomy and biomechanics of the TMJ and the specific pathologic features and differential diagnosis of RA in the TMJ. We discuss nonsurgical or presurgical therapy for these patients, and outline a surgical approach to treatment. TMJ dysfunction can be a severely debilitating aspect in the total management of the RA patient. The emphasis must be on the need for both medical and dental coordination of treatment. As imperative as it is for the dental practitioner to refer the patient to a rheumatologist when RA is suspected, so is it necessary for the physician to seek the opinion of the dentist trained in treatment of the TMJ when that diagnosis considered.

ANATOMY

The TMJ is a synovial joint composed of the condylar head of the mandible, the temporal bone, an articular disc interposed between the articulating surfaces of these bones, and a surrounding joint capsule (Fig 6–1). The moving joint is powered by muscles that insert onto the mandible from the cranial and cervical regions (Fig 6–2). The mandible is limited in all ranges of motion by ligaments that join the mandible to the temporal and sphenoid bones (Fig 6–3,A and B).

The articular surface of the TMJ, including the articular disc, is composed of dense fibrous tissue that is neither vascular nor innervated. Thus, with the exception of the clavicles, the TMJ is the only synovial joint that is not composed of hyaline cartilage. This is of prognostic significance as the repair potential of fibrous tissue is much greater than that of hyaline cartilage.

BIOMECHANICS

The TMJ actually functions as two specific joints (Fig 6–4). During the first phase of jaw opening (28–32 mm between the incisor teeth) there is a rotational movement of the mandibular condyle against the articular disc, which remains positioned against the temporal bone. In the second phase of opening, full range of motion (40–50 mm) is achieved by the mandibular condyle and the articular disc acting as a unit and sliding forward against the temporal bone. Mandibular opening and closing is a friction-free and pain-free movement. All articular surfaces are well lubricated with synovial fluid originating in the

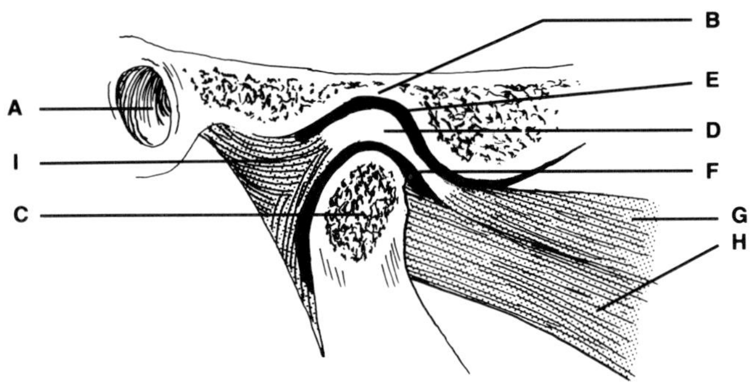

FIG 6–1.
The temporomandibular joint in health. *A* = external auditory meatus; *B* = temporal bone; *C* = head of the mandibular condyle; *D* = articular "disc" of the joint; *E* = superior joint space containing synovial fluid; *F* = inferior joint space containing synovial fluid; *G* = superior head of the external (lateral) pterygoid muscle; *H* = inferior head of the external (lateral) pterygoid muscle; *I* = posterior elastic tissue disc attachment.

synovial tissues lining the peripheral portions of the articular surfaces. The precise coordination of the mandibular condyle moving under its disc, in conjunction with the articular surface of the temporal bone, is essential for normal joint operation. Any dislocation of the disc from its position directly superior to the articular surface of the condyle can result in clicking or locking during jaw opening or closing (Fig 6–5).

RHEUMATOID ARTHRITIS OF THE TEMPOROMANDIBULAR JOINT

Pathology

In the RA patient the TMJ is usually one of the last joints to be affected, although symptoms may originate there. As in other joints, the disease process begins at the periphery with inflammation and hypertrophy of the synovium (Fig 6–6). The synovial tissue of the lower joint compartment is initially affected,[4] resulting in abnormal growth of the one-cell layer of synovial tissue into a 10- or 12-layer thickness that grows onto the articulating surfaces. With even slight function the presence of such highly vascular and innervated synovial tissue on the pressure-bearing joint results in pain. With the growth of villi, the synovial tissue is converted into pannus cells that erode the condyle, temporal bone, articular capsule, and ligaments from the periphery and extend inward toward the middle of the articular surfaces. Following resorption of the condylar head (Fig 6–7) there is a superior movement of the remaining condylar portion into the temporal fossa. This may result in a decreased closing radius causing premature contact of the last molar teeth and an open bite (Figs 6–8 and 6–9). The severe inflammation may also result in fibrous adhesions between the articu-

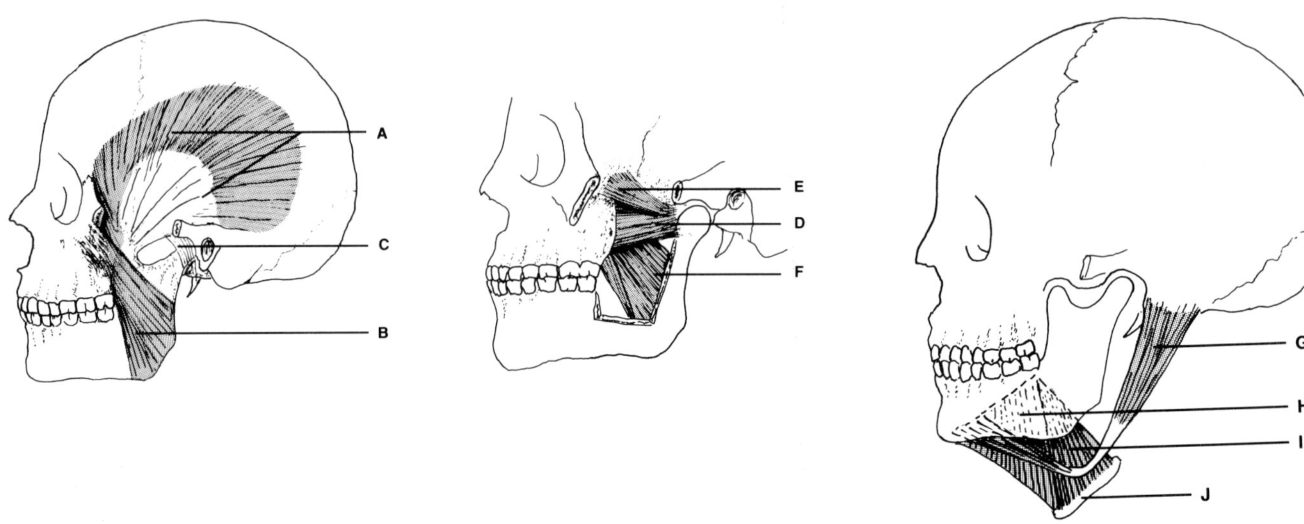

FIG 6–2.
The relationship of the cranial and cervical areas to the jaw is most apparent when observing their muscular attachments. Improper jaw position often results in symptoms of the head and neck. *A* = temporalis muscle; *B* = masseter muscle; *C* = temporomandibular ligament; *D* = inferior belly of the external pterygoid muscle; *E* = superior belly of the external pterygoid muscle; *F* = internal pterygoid muscle; *G* = posterior belly of the digastric, connecting the chin to the hyoid bone; *H* = mylohyoid muscle; *I* = anterior belly of the digastric; *J* = hyoid bone, whose connections to the mandible influence laryngeal position and other infrahyoid structures.

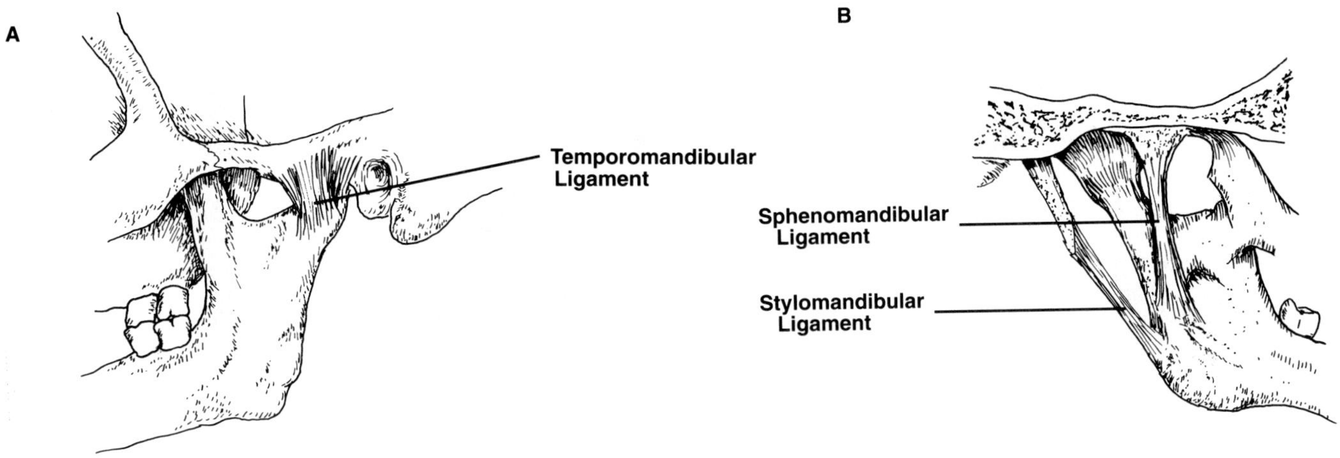

FIG 6–3.
A, temporomandibular ligament limiting medial movement of the mandible. **B,** stylomandibular ligament limiting anterior mandibular movement; sphenomandibular ligament limiting inferior mandibular movement.

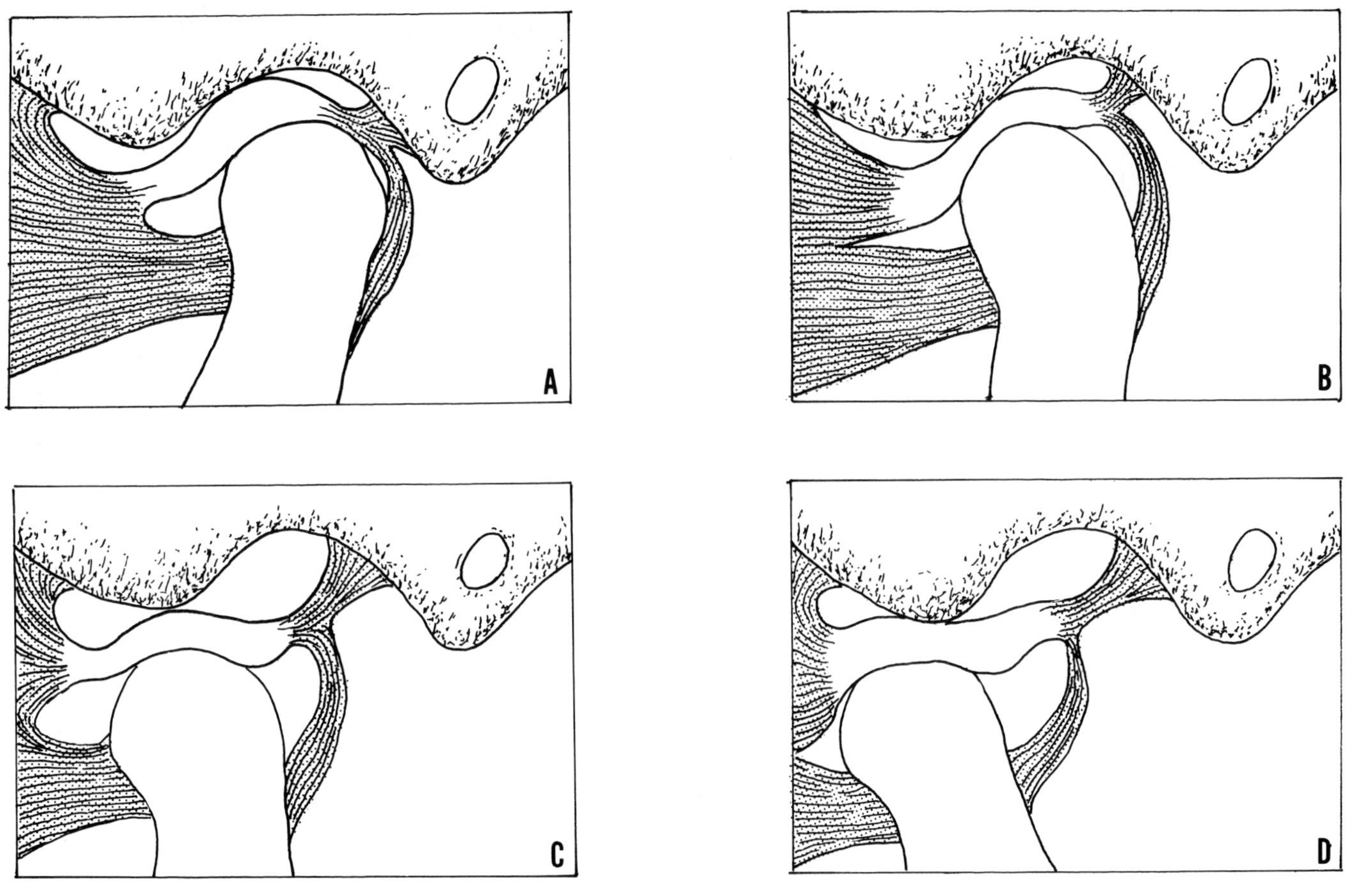

FIG 6–4.
Jaw opening in health. **A,** phase I. Rotation: The head of the mandibular condyle lies beneath the central or thicker portion of the articular disc. Powered mainly by the inferior belly of the external pterygoid muscle, the condylar head rotates in place against the articular disc. This achieves an opening of approximately 28 to 32 mm, or about the distance between the maxillary and mandibular incisor teeth of the patient's middle two fingers. **B–D,** phase II. Translation: The head of the mandibular condyle moves forward and downward along the articular eminence with further contraction of the external pterygoid muscle. This lowers the mandible to achieve full opening of the mouth, about 40 to 50 mm, a minimum distance of the patient's three middle fingers.

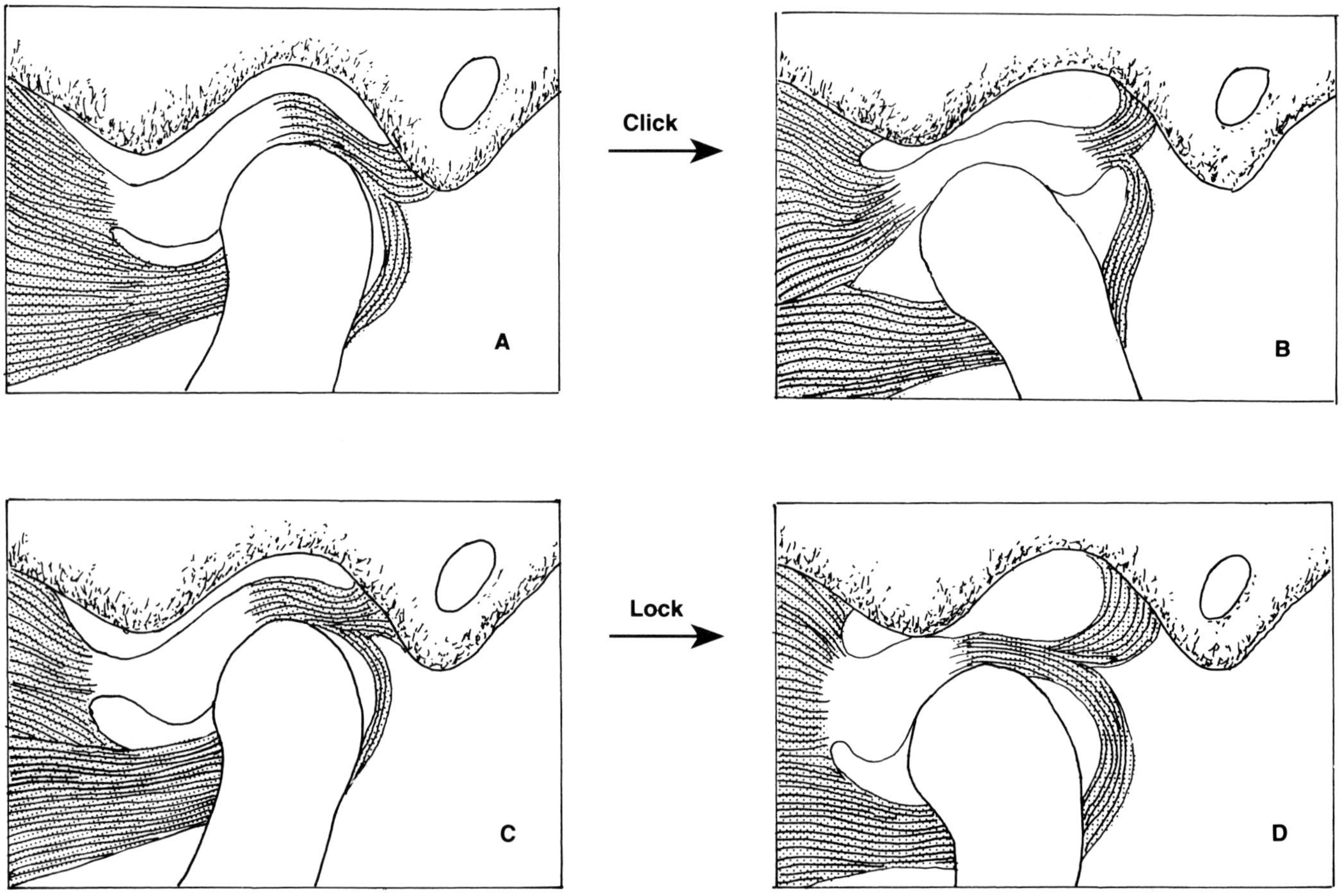

FIG 6–5.
A, B, anteriorly displaced disc with reduction. The disc is located partially in front of the mandibular condyle. This may be due to the condyle being thrust backward from traumatic episodes. As the condyle moves it may engage the disc and jump over it, producing a "click" on its continuous path toward full opening. **C, D,** anteriorly displaced disc without reduction. The disc is so thickened, perhaps due to repeated traumas, that the condyle is unable to negotiate past it during its forward translation. With the mandible unable to open fully, an "open locked" jaw results.

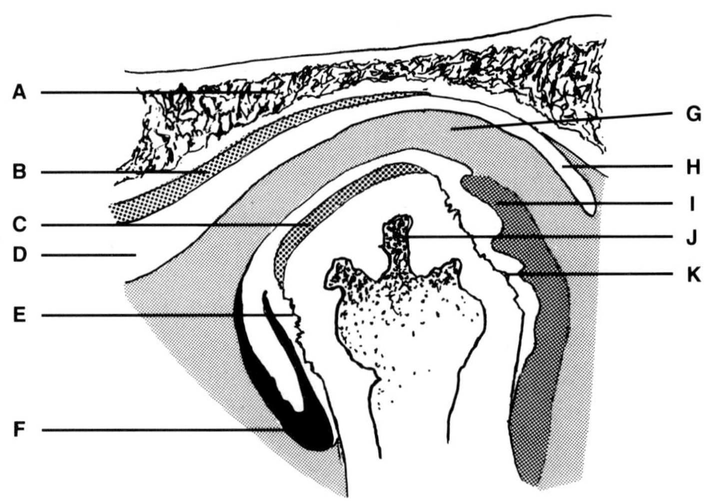

FIG 6–6.
Rheumatoid arthritis of the TMJ. *A* = temporal bone, normal appearance; *B* = articular surface of the articular eminence; *C* = section of mandibular condyle with healthy articular collagen still present; *D* = superior joint space; *E* = erosive head of the mandibular condyle; *F* = pannus cells eroding the condyle; *G* = unaffected collagenous disc; *H* = synovial lining of the superior cavity; *I* = repair collagen; *J* = site of acute inflammation; *K* = posterior condylar resorption.

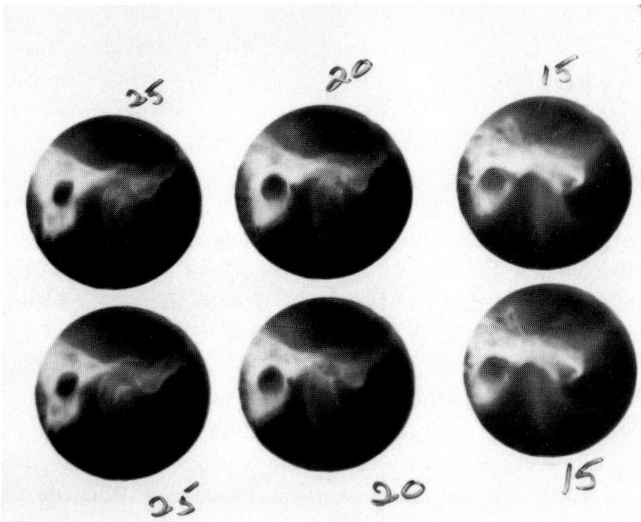

FIG 6–7.
Radiographic changes of the TMJ in the RA patient. Bone resorption of the head of the mandibular condyle. (Courtesy of J. Gibilisco, D.D.S., Mayo Clinic, Rochester, Minn.)

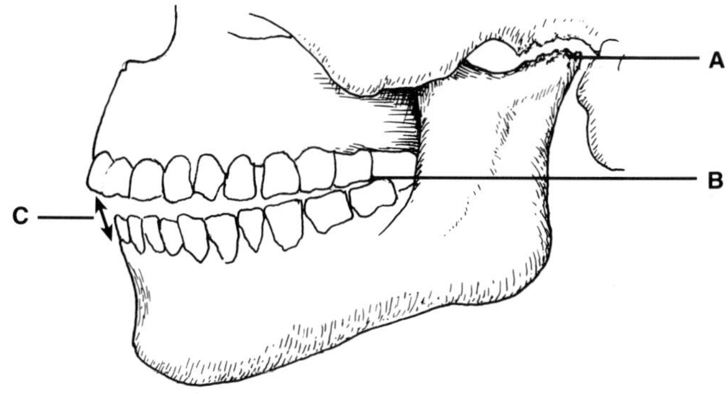

FIG 6–8.
Anterior open bite. With resorption of the mandibular condyle *(A)* the fulcrum for jaw opening moves to the last molar teeth *(B)*, resulting in an anteriorly opened bite *(C)*. Mobility and wear of the molar teeth may also occur as a result of these teeth bearing all of the mandibular forces.

lating parts, producing limited joint movement, and on occasion, complete joint ankylosis. Furthermore, as condylar resorption progresses and the mandible and the attached soft tissues move posteriorly, dysphagia may occur and sleep apnea ensues as the upper airway is infringed upon (see Chapter 5).

Differential Diagnosis

Frequently, patients with RA of the TMJ are not aware that the symptoms are arising from the joints themselves. Rather, as in the case of other patients with TMJ involvement, they will complain of ear, temporal, or facial symptoms. In a radiographic and clinical evaluation of 100 RA patients, 86% had TMJ involvement.[24] In over half the cases symptoms occur bilaterally. Pain and limitation of motion during jaw movement are the two major symptoms. Tenderness upon palpation of the joints posteriorly or laterally is most often present. The most frequent sign of the chronic disorder is crepitus of the TMJ during joint movement. This crepitus is most effectively heard with the use of a stethoscope. Tenderness to palpation of the joints posteriorly and laterally is the most common symptom in the acute phase. Ogus[26] found that 48% of patients with de-

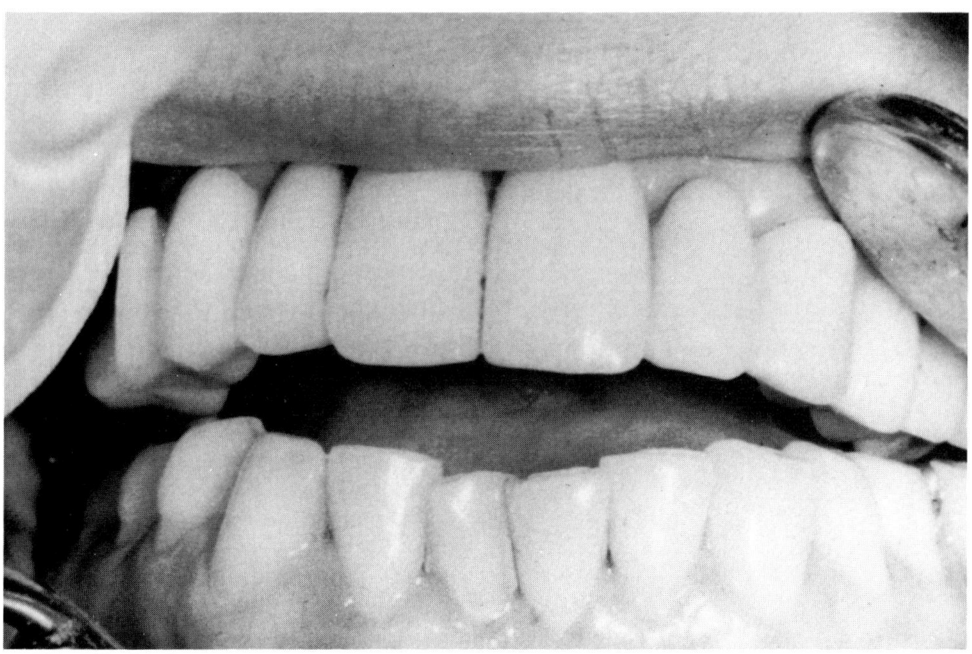

FIG 6–9.
Anterior open bite. Clinical appearance of patient with condylar resorption observed radiographically in Figure 6–7. Only molar teeth are in contact.

generative arthritis of the TMJ had tenderness at one lateral pole of the condyle, with almost all of the RA patients having bilateral condylar pole tenderness. Without the systemic diagnosis it can be difficult at times to make the differential diagnosis of rheumatoid or osteoarthritic changes. Indeed, both types of arthritic degeneration may be present in the TMJ at the same time, as the untoward forces resulting from condylar resorption of RA will often result in osteoarthritic remodeling.

The RA symptoms of the TMJ must also be differentiated from the pain and limitation of mandibular movement that occurs in craniomandibular muscular dysfunction. In these cases myalgia is the cause of pain. This occurs most frequently from muscular fatigue caused by extensive contraction of the masticatory muscles during tooth clenching or other untoward habitual mandibular movements (microtraumas), or overt physical (macro) traumas to the jaw. Craniomandibular myalgia most often occurs unilaterally, and is extremely common in the general population. Headaches; ear, jaw, sinus, and facial pain; tinnitus; and dizziness are the most common symptoms. Tenderness to palpation of the external pterygoid and tendon of the temporalis muscles intraorally give a high degree of accuracy in the differential diagnosis.[20] Placing the ball of the fifth finger behind the maxillary third molar region, curving around the distal portion of the maxilla, and feeling the flat pterygoid plate gives the attachment of the external pterygoid muscle. Rotating the finger pad to face laterally, one will feel the coronoid process of the mandible, the insertion for the temporalis muscle. In the normal person there should be no tenderness to moderate pressure. Often RA-TMJ patients will have a concomitant myalgia of these muscles, and relaxation of them will often reduce pain symptoms significantly.

Radiographic Evaluation

Radiographic erosive changes of the TMJ, most commonly of the mandibular condyles, can be observed in about 65% to 75% of all RA patients (see Fig 6–7), and are most often bilaterally distributed.[1] Marginal proliferation and condylar flattening are often observed. There is good correlation between the grade of RA and the degree of radiographic changes. The degree of pathologic changes observed rediographically is significantly greater in females, as are the clinical incidence and extent of disease.

NONSURGICAL AND PRESURGICAL TREATMENT

Dental treatment objectives in RA patients with TMJ symptoms are to maintain the patient free of pain, minimize further destruction of the joint, and maintain mandibular function. Surgical therapy of the TMJ in RA patients is avoided for as long as possible because of the tendency for recurrence of joint destruction. Only 20% of adult RA patients have complete remission. Although the acute phase of the disease is a medical problem treated with antirheumatoid drug therapy, the dentist's role is to treat it as a unique biomechanical problem. Minimizing mandibular function and avoiding an increased workload is an essential ingredient of treatment in all RA patients. The importance of maintaining a functional occlusion, with forces distributed over as many of the teeth as possible, is extremely important. It has been shown by several authors[1, 19] that the greater the radiologic grade of joint destruction, the poorer the dental health, including a decreased number of occluding teeth, and a greater number of occlusal interferences. As a result of these dental relationships there are several steps that can be taken by the TMJ dentist to maintain the oral health of patients and reduce any possible traumatic stress to the joint region.

DENTAL TREATMENT FOR THE RA-TMJ PATIENT

The patients are instructed to avoid habitual tooth contact, maintaining the jaw in a relaxed posture. The patient repeats "lips together, teeth apart." Most people are not aware that the maxillary and mandibular teeth should only contact during swallowing or mastication. Teeth rarely touch. An increased workload on the joint and musculature can be avoided by a softer diet and limiting eccentric jaw movements.

Physical Therapy

Physical therapy is essential for patients with TMJ disturbances to limit pain and increase joint mobility. This can be accomplished through exercises that help the jaw relax, and manual procedures to maintain capsular extensibility and improve joint mobility. Patients who already experience limitation of movement are instructed to move the jaw into all excursions several times a day for 3 minutes each time. Care is taken to limit the movements to within a pain-free range. Physical therapy is also necessary for treatment of craniomandibular-cervical myalgia that often is associated with the RA patient. In these cases I have used specifically designed nonforce manual techniques to effectively relax the musculature, and aided by physical therapy modalities, to maintain the masticatory and cervical muscles in a relaxed state. Emphasis is placed on posture. The use of a mandibular orthopaedic repositioning appliance (Figs 6–10 and 6–11) can be of great help in achieving and maintaining upper-quarter muscular relaxation by freeing the occlusion and preventing tooth contacts during the active phase of physical therapy. Close coordination between the dentist and physical therapist is essential for optimal results, especially with the need for continual balancing of the intraoral appliance following each physical therapy session, as needed. The mandibular orthopaedic appliance is utilized only during the active phase of physical therapy. Following occlusal force distribution, it is utilized only during acute exacerbations of the disorder.

Occlusal Force Distribution

Once symptoms have diminished and the craniomandibular-cervical musculature has been relaxed, occlusal equilibration is then carried out. The number of occluding teeth must be maximized. In cases with significant condylar loss and open-bite formation, there may be limitations as to the number of teeth that can occlude using occlusal reduction techniques. Because of the possibility of continuous condylar changes, the use of extensive permanent restorative or orthodontic therapy must be carefully evaluated. Use of overlay removable partials, processed temporary restorations, or overlay fixed restorations may be part of treatment planning.

Nightguard Appliance

A nightguard (Fig 6–12) is always considered following the establishment of the occlusion. The TMJ in RA patients appears most susceptible to mechanical forces, and the known preponderance and destructiveness of clenching during sleep must be minimized. I prefer the use of a maxillary soft acrylic appliance that can help absorb muscular forces, and further distribute force vectors from the joint and occluding teeth. It can also help to prevent tooth shifting and overeruption of nonoccluding teeth.

Evaluation of these patients must be made on a periodic basis, usually every 3 months, to check for a balanced occlusion of the natural dentition and of any intraoral appliances used. Imbalances may result in further joint destruction. Furthermore, with destruction of the mandibular condyle occlusal prematurities on one tooth often occur, which can result in mobility and possible loss of that tooth. The use of splinting to maintain tooth stability may be necessary. Reevaluation must include masticatory muscle palpation, and, if necessary, further relaxation techniques to insure a physiologic muscular relationship.

The use of corticosteroid injections into the joint

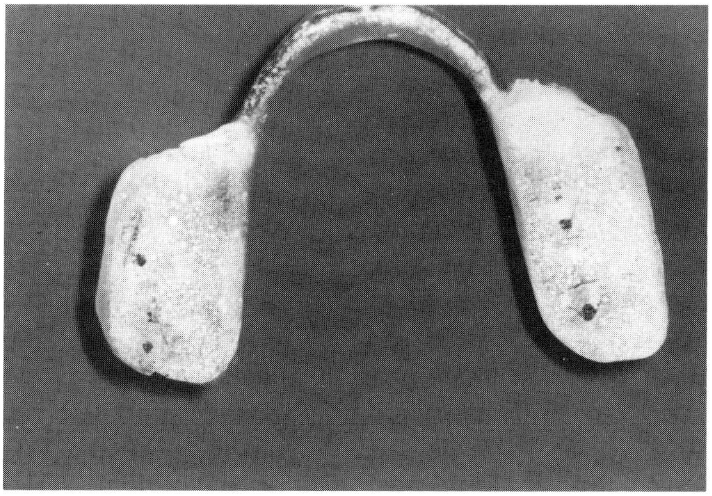

FIG 6–10.
A mandibular orthopaedic appliance, or "splint."

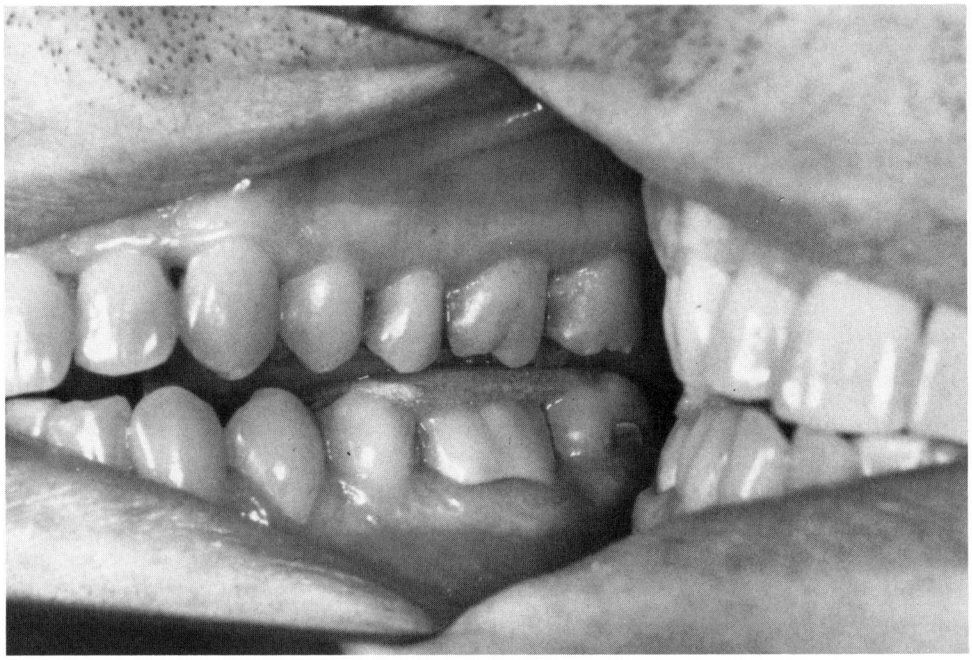

FIG 6–11.
Intraoral view. The splint covers the lower posterior teeth with a flat, smooth plane. With contact only on molar teeth bilaterally, the lower jaw is free to glide to a more relaxed posture without the influence of upper interdigitating teeth. Following complete muscular relaxation the splint is removed and a new muscularly dictated occlusion can be established by the dentist.

space has been found to be rarely necessary, and must be used with great caution owing to the possibility of further osseous degeneration.

JUVENILE RHEUMATOID ARTHRITIS PATIENTS

Juvenile RA (JRA) patients need close evaluation, and extensive physical therapy is often advised to prevent joint contraction and muscular dysfunction during the active phase of the disease process. Eighty percent of JRA patients go into remission as teenagers and very often minimal dysfunction remains. However, orthodontic intervention, or, as discussed in the following section, orthognathic surgery may be necessary to correct the occlusal and skeletal abnormality.

In instances where TMJ destruction limits mandibular mobility or results in facial skeletal deformity so as to interfere with eating, swallowing, breathing,

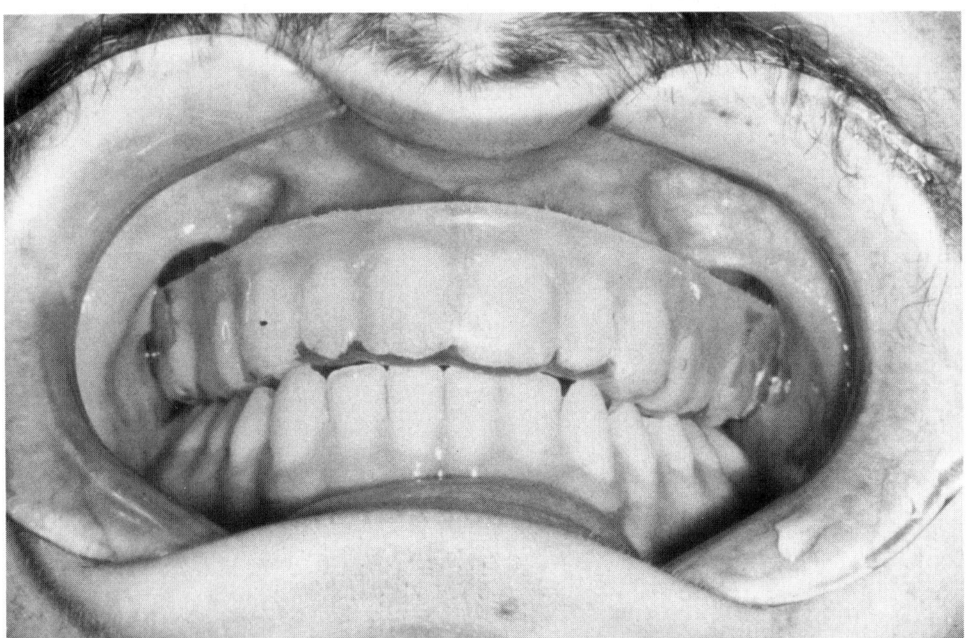

FIG 6–12.
The soft Nightguard appliance. This type of appliance is used to reduce the amount of force applied to the TMJ and teeth by clenching forces. It is used at night or during sports or other exertion activities where jaw forces are initiated. Nightguard flexibility allows for force absorption and distribution.

or speaking, then surgical intervention may be necessary. Once it has been determined by the treating TMJ dentist that nonsurgical therapy will have limited value, consultation with an oral surgeon is essential. The same nonsurgical therapies as outlined above will be needed postsurgically to maintain joint mobility and to prevent destructive forces to the repaired joint in the future.

SURGICAL MANAGEMENT

INDICATIONS FOR SURGERY

The Temporomandibular Joint

Symptoms of internal derangement of the TMJ in the RA patient can include the following:

1. Chronic pain and discomfort in the joint and the associated musculature and soft tissues.
2. Episodes of acute exacerbation of such pain and discomfort.
3. Decreased mandibular range of motion.
4. Crepitus and other joint sounds.

Surgical intervention of the TMJ is appropriate when treatment with other modalities does not provide relief of symptoms. Radiographic and magnetic resonance imaging (MRI) findings such as condylar head degeneration, meniscus degeneration, or meniscus perforation are not in and of themselves specific indications for surgery. Nor does a negative study contraindicate surgery. For example, adhesions within the superior or inferior joint space will not be demonstrable by radiographs or MRI but will require surgical release. However, if surgery is indicated, the presence or absence of radiographic or MRI findings will be a factor in deciding the type of surgical procedure to employ.

The Facial Skeleton

Patients with facial skeletal deformities associated with RA may present with complaints of a poor bite, difficulty in eating and chewing food, pain and discomfort in the TMJs and muscles of mastication, speech impediment, and other functional problems. They certainly may have valid esthetic concerns. Surgical treatment of these deformities is warranted when they adversely affect the quality of life. There are multiple facial skeletal deformities associated with RA. The extent and severity of these deformities will depend upon the age of onset of the disease process.

Juvenile Rheumatoid Arthritis

When the disease process starts early in life, i.e., with JRA, the mandibular condyles will be affected. The end result will be damaged or hypoplastic condylar heads. It is not known whether the disease causes rapid destruction of the developing condyles or induces agenesis or hypoplasia.[2, 9, 16, 17, 21, 27, 30] Damage to this important "growth center" can lead to: (1) poor ramus development with inadequate vertical height; (2) retrognathia with or without an open bite (apertognathia); (3) retrogenia, sometimes with vertical excess; (4) prominent antegonial notching; and (5) multiple impacted posterior mandibular teeth due to inadequate room for eruption (Fig 6–13,A–C).

Adult-Onset Rheumatoid Arthritis

Adult-onset RA can cause slow progressive destruction of the condylar heads in an otherwise normally developed mandible. This may result in some or all of the following[10, 12, 18, 19, 22]: (1) loss of posterior mandibular height; (2) "downward" and "backward" rotation of the mandible; (3) retrognathia; and (4) apertognathia (Fig 6–14,A and B). An appropriate treatment plan can be developed after a complete TMJ and facial skeletal evaluation. This evaluation will determine whether the patient's symptoms and problems stem from (1) pathologic changes intrinsic to the TMJ; (2) the skeletal deformity and consequent malrelationship between the jaws and teeth, or (3) a combination of (1) and (2).

The TMJ can be approached arthroscopically or by open arthroplasty. Skeletal deformities can be treated by orthognathic surgery. A combined or staged orthognathic and TMJ surgical option may be considered as well.

SURGICAL PROCEDURES

The Temporomandibular Joint

Arthroplasty

Surgical findings can include adhesions within the superior and inferior joint spaces; meniscal problems such as displacements, perforations, and morphologic changes; and osseous changes of both the fossa

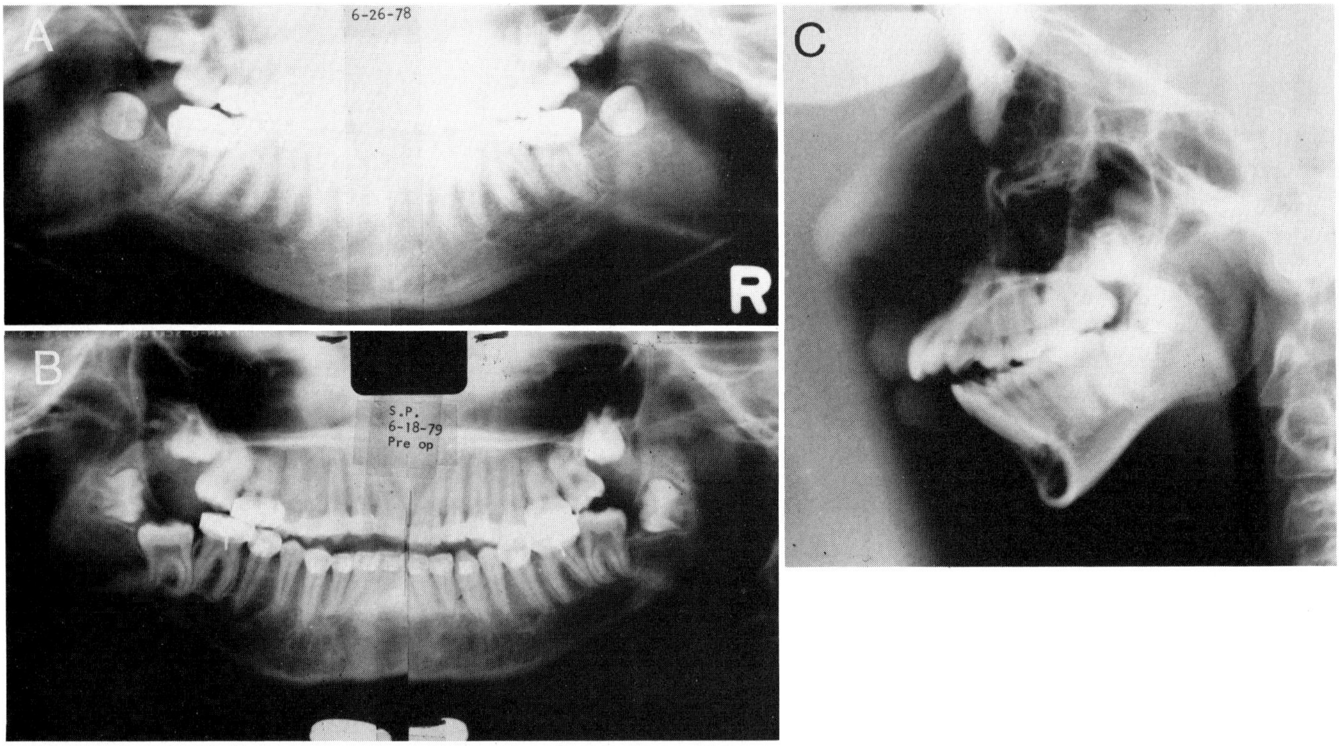

FIG 6–13.
Panoramic radiographs of a 14-year-old girl **(A)** and boy **(B),** both of whom have JRA. Note the absence of mandibular condyles, underdeveloped rami, and the impacted teeth. (Courtesy of Dr. Stanley J. Behrman.) **C,** lateral cephalometric radiograph of the patient in **B** showing the mandibular retrognathia, apertognathia (open bite), and deep antegonial notching.

and condyle. Adhesions can be lysed, allowing for improved meniscal and mandibular range of motion. Plications can be performed along with the excision of redundant tissue or perforations. Osseous changes can be managed by bony contouring. A nonsalvageable meniscus is excised. There are several options available following meniscectomy:

1. Prosthetic replacement with materials such as Teflon-reinforced Silastic:
   a. Permanently secured to the fossa.
   b. Permanently secured to the condylar head.
   c. Placed temporarily to allow capsule formation. The capsule will act as a "pseudomeniscus" after the implant is removed.
2. Allogenic replacement such as freeze-dried dura.
3. Autogenous replacement such as dermis or temporalis fascia.
4. No replacement, employing mandibular myofunctional therapy as necessary to control any deviation secondary to the loss of vertical height.

There are several potential problems with TMJ arthroplasty in the RA patient. The disease process itself and the consequences of long-term steroid therapy place these patients at increased risk for surgical site infection and poor healing. In addition, there is the potential of localized disease exacerbation secondary to surgical manipulation of the synovial and hard tissues. This severely limits the use of standard arthroplasty procedures. Until recently, early surgical intervention was avoided routinely. Treatment was deferred until symptoms and physical findings were of such severity as to justify joint replacement. Today, however, small joint arthroscopy offers a less invasive surgical option from which the RA patient can greatly benefit.

Arthroscopy

Small joint arthroscopic surgery has been adapted to the TMJ by oral and maxillofacial surgeons. Early and frequently less invasive surgical intervention of

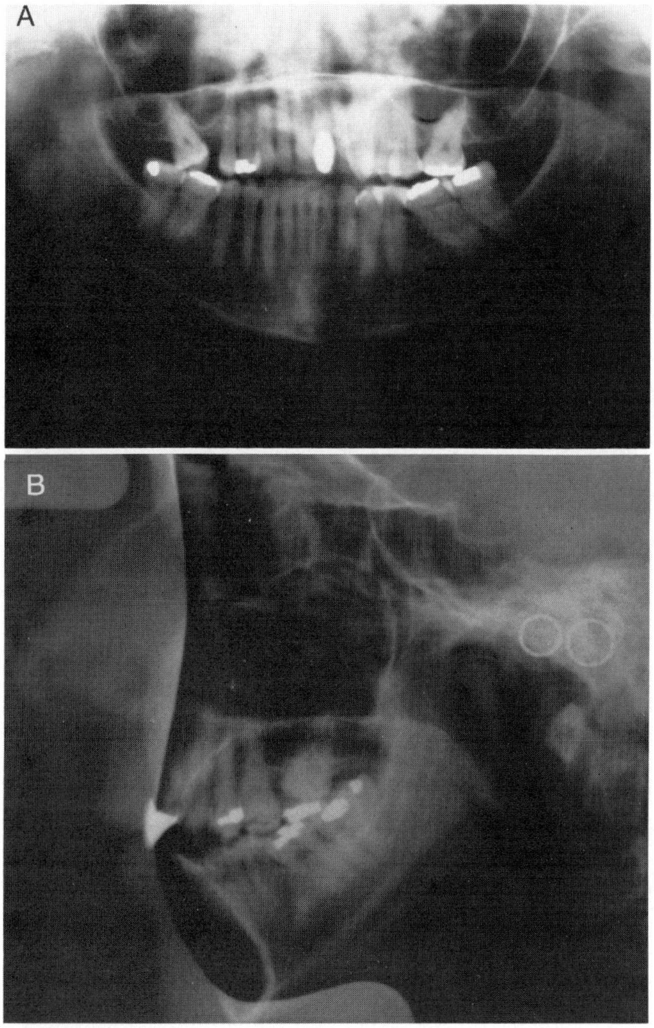

FIG 6–14.
A 36-year-old woman with a 10-year history of RA. **A,** panoramic radiograph showing the resorption of the condyles. **B,** lateral cephalometric radiograph showing the mandibular displacement with retrognathia and apertognathia.

internal derangements is now possible. Koslin has presented well-documented successful arthroscopic management of soft tissue internal derangements in RA.[15] Arthroscopic procedures included:

1. Lysis of adhesions (Fig 6–15).
2. Capsular release.
3. Meniscus release.
4. Synovectomy.
5. Partial meniscectomy.
6. Direct synovial steroid injection under video observation. This is a significant improvement over blind intraarticular steroid "bathing."

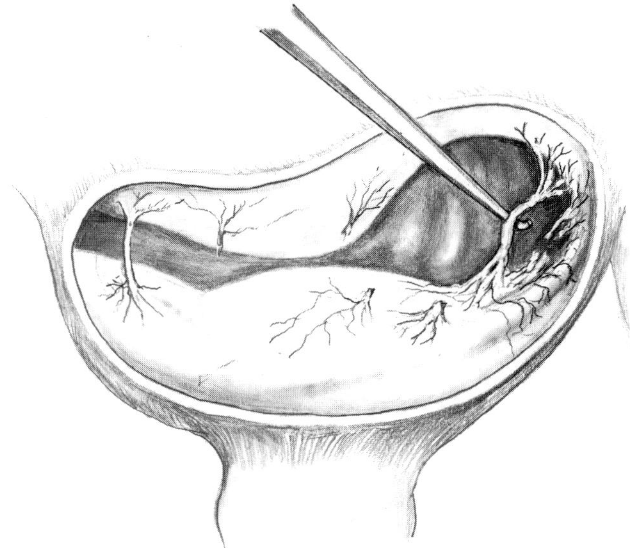

FIG 6–15.
Illustration of lysis of posterior attachment adhesions under direct video observation.

Significant improvement in presenting symptoms was reported. Pain and discomfort were decreased; mandibular range of motion was improved. Immediate postoperative mobilization was facilitated, decreasing the potential for hemarthrosis. Crepitus and other joint sounds were lessened. Most important, there has been no evidence of disease exacerbation or recurrence through 3½ years of follow-up. Koslin's arthroscopic experience with rheumatoid patients compares very favorably with the experience of others, including ours, with patients without RA.

Total Joint Replacement

Numerous materials have been used to replace the TMJ. Autogenous replacements have included sternoclavicular joints, metatarsal joints, and costochondral grafts.[3, 8, 28] Prosthetic joints have been fashioned from Silastic blocks, chrome cobalt, titanium, and Proplast-Teflon laminates. The limiting factor is the ability of the replacement material to withstand the stresses of function. Today, costochondral grafts and total joint prostheses are the two most widely accepted options.

Juvenile Rheumatoid Arthritis

Costochondral grafts are used in managing the mandibular deformities in the young and growing JRA patient.[21–23, 25] Costochondral grafts have the potential for growth and in JRA with loss of condylar height and poor mandibular ramus development, this potential can be quite useful. However, this growth capability is not predictable. Incidences of poor graft growth as well as of exuberant growth are well documented. The need for additional corrective surgery is an accepted possibility which the patient and parents must be informed of preoperatively.

The costochondral graft is secured to the posterior border of the mandible. The cartilagenous cap is positioned so that it can act as a condylar head (Fig 6–16,A–C). Costochondral grafts also have been used with varying success to reposition the mandible. They can increase the ramus height and move the mandible down and forward. Meticulous surgical planning and postoperative management are mandatory. Excessive loading can lead to damage or fracture of the cartilagenous cap. These grafts are also susceptible to ankylosis. The autogenous meniscus or some other interpositional graft is used to minimize this possibility. A balance must be achieved between the necessary immobilization time for graft union and early mobilization to minimize the potential for fibrous ankylosis or hemarthrosis.

Costochondral grafts are susceptible to infection and to destruction by progressing disease or disease exacerbation. Donor site concerns of infection and pulmonary involvement also exist. A recommended

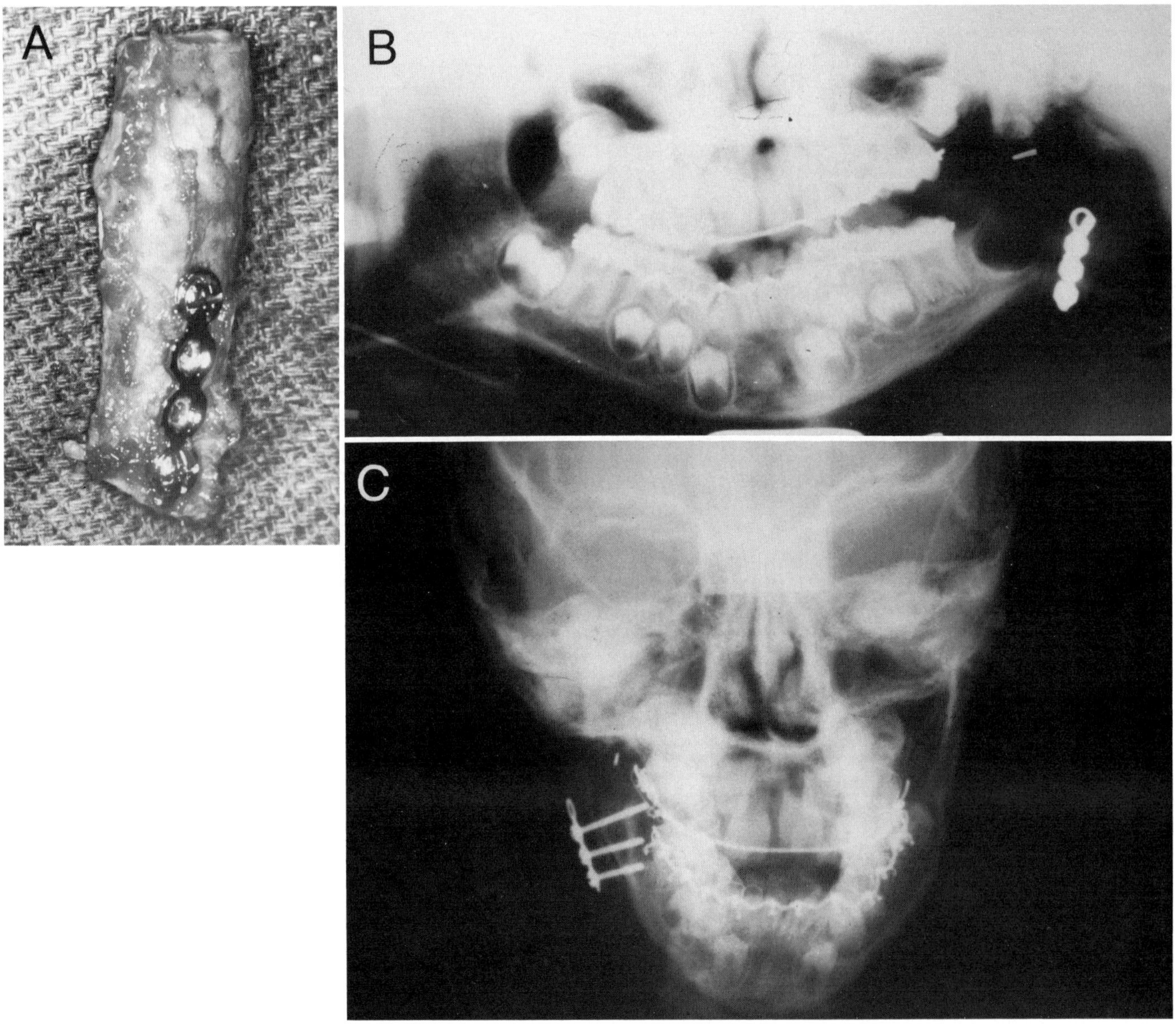

FIG 6–16.
A, a costochondral graft prepared to replace a deformed and ankylosed condyle in an 8-year-old boy. Panoramic **(B)** and anteroposterior skull **(C)** radiographs showing the graft rigidly secured to the posterior mandible allowing early mobilization.

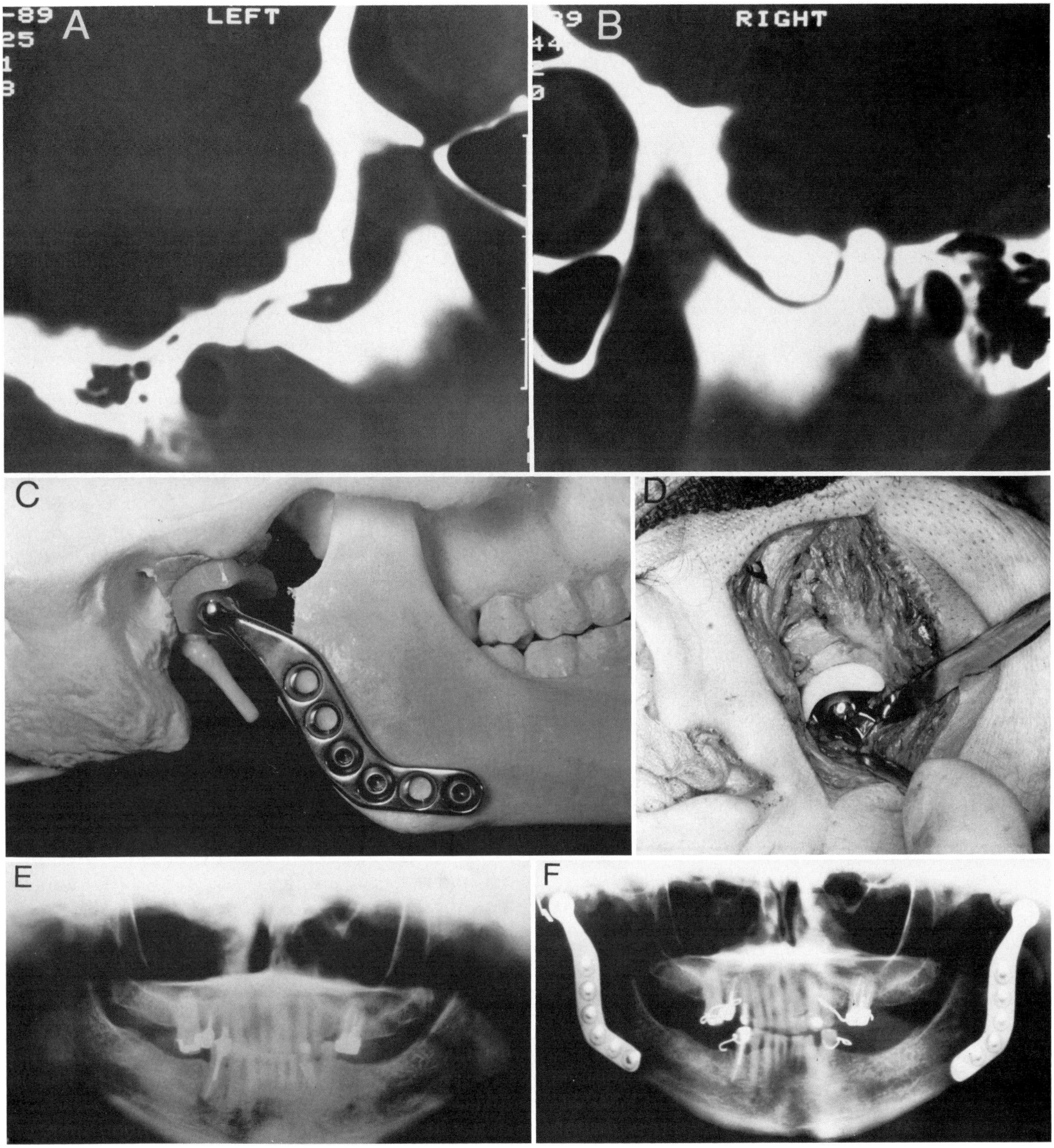

FIG 6–17.
A 59-year-old woman with idiopathic degeneration of the TMJs which led to mandibular displacement with complete ankylosis. CT scans showing the degeneration of the left condylar head **(A)** and right glenoid fossa with perforation and ankylosis of the condyle into the middle cranial fossa **(B)**. **C,** The New York Hospital–The Hospital for Special Surgery TMJ prosthesis. A titanium condyle articulates with an extended-chain ultra-high-molecular-weight polyethylene fossa. **D,** the glenoid fossa insert is cemented in place and is articulating with the condylar process. **E, F,** pre- and postoperative panoramic radiographs.
Continued.

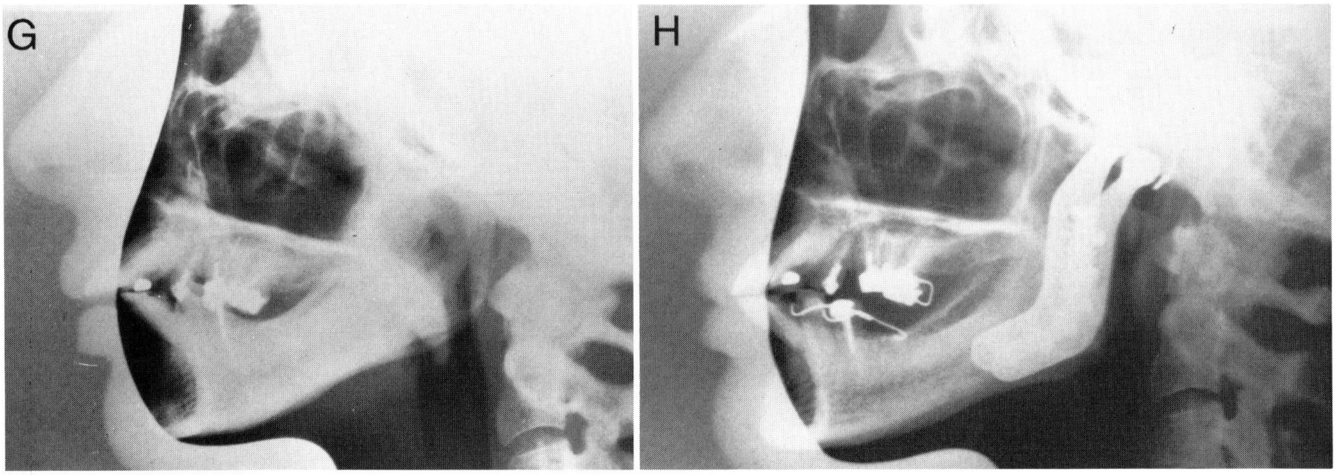

FIG 6-17 cont'd.
G, H, pre- and postoperative lateral cephalometric radiographs. Preoperatively, the mandible was displaced posteriorly with loss of vertical height. The mandible was surgically repositioned down and forward by placement of the TMJ total prostheses. Esthetics were noticeably improved. The patient, 15 months postoperation at the time of writing, has regained excellent function and range of motion; maximal opening without strain is 38 mm, well within accepted normal limits.

protocol has been to defer grafting until the patient has been quiescent for a minimum of 2 years regardless of the existing mandibular position. Nevertheless, disease exacerbation after more than 2 years of quiescence have been reported. If the graft is damaged by such a disease process, or becomes infected or ankylosed, replacement with a prosthetic total joint is indicated.

Adult-Onset Rheumatoid Arthritis

There is no longer any concern for growth or growth potential in the adult with RA. The goals of surgical intervention are now restoration of function and correction of any esthetic deformity. While costochondral grafts are used, use of a prosthetic total joint replacement is a more viable option for several reasons:

1. The mandible can be repositioned with minimal concern over loading damage.
2. There is no concern over graft destruction from exacerbated disease as no autogenous material is used.
3. Patients with active disease can be treated.
4. Immediate mobilization is possible and encouraged, limiting the potential of ankylosis.
5. No donor site surgery is necessary.
6. The prosthesis can be custom-contoured to fit the needs of the individual patient.

As with any prosthetic joint replacement, the primary concerns are infection and prosthesis failure. Meticulous surgical management is mandatory. Prosthetic design has been a problem. A commonly used prosthesis[13, 14] made of a Proplast-lined cobalt chrome condylar process articulating with either a Proplast-Teflon laminate lining the glenoid fossa, or a Proplast–ultra-high-molecular-weight polyethylene laminate replacing the glenoid fossa and secured to the zygomatic arch by screws, failed in the short term because of mechanical failure of the Teflon and Proplast.[5, 11] Implant breakdown with severe foreign body giant cell destructive reaction was occurring within the joint space. Many of these prostheses have had to be removed; many more will likely be removed in the future.

A collaborative effort between The New York Hospital Division of Oral and Maxillofacial Surgery and the Department of Biomechanics of The Hospital for Special Surgery (New York City) has led to the development of a new total joint replacement. This prosthesis utilizes a titanium condylar process which articulates with an ultra-high-molecular-weight or extended-chain ultra-high molecular-weight polyethylene fossa. The condylar process is screwed securely to the posteroinferior border of the mandible. The fossa is cemented to the inferior surface of the glenoid fossa to minimize micromovement. Both components are computer-designed and custom-fabricated from a detailed computed tomography (CT) scan. These materials have been used successfully for many years in total knee and hip joint replacements. This prosthesis has shown promising results in patients with various degenerative processes and is readily applicable to the RA patient (Figs 6–17,A–H and 6–18,A–E). Our follow-

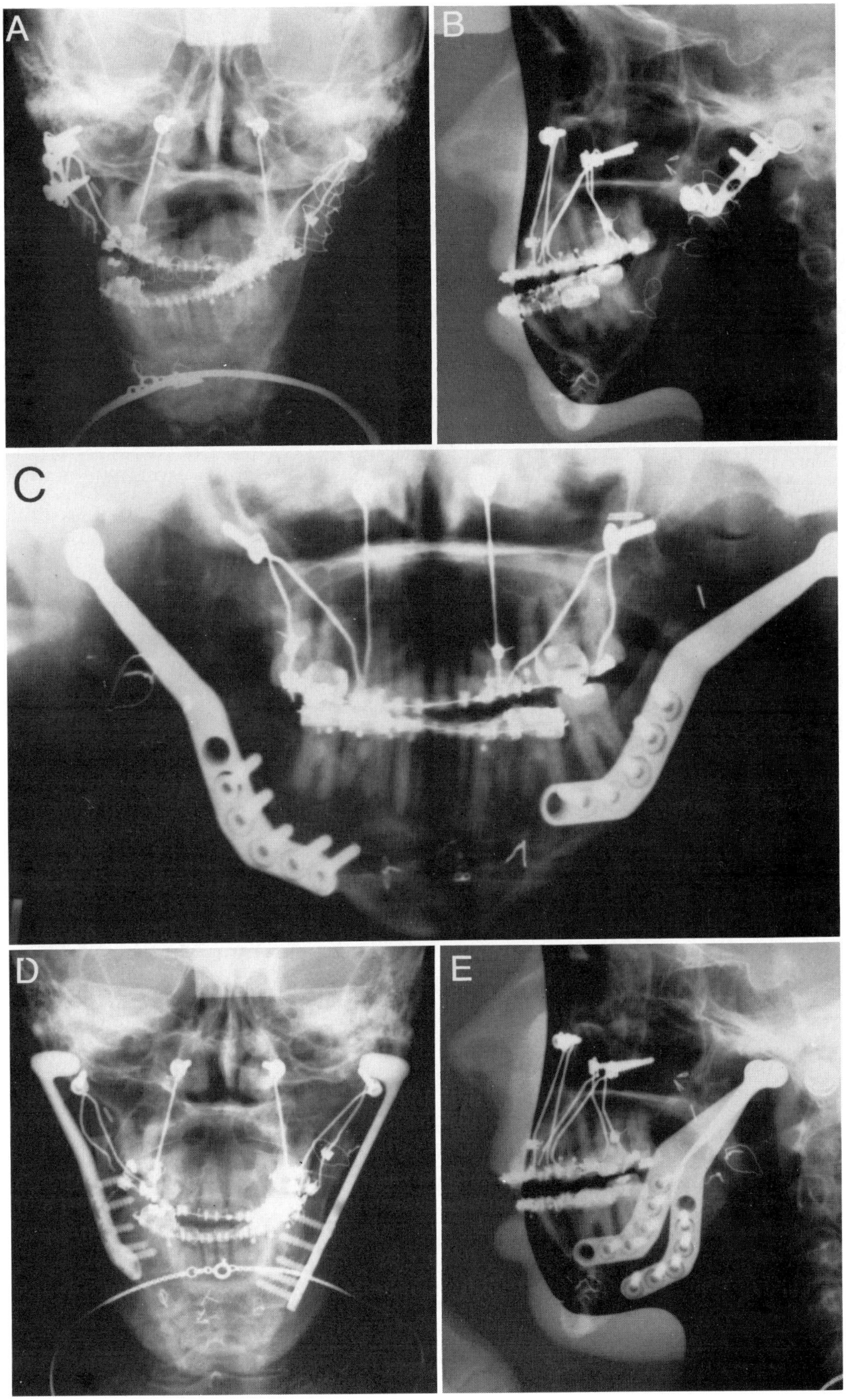

FIG 6–18.
A 41-year-old woman had undergone severe degeneration and loss of the right and left mandibular condyles and rami. Attempts at iliac crest and costochondral reconstruction were unsuccessful. The patient presented with bilateral ankylosis with mandibular laterognathia and an open bite. Preoperative anteroposterior skull **(A)** and lateral cephalometric **(B)** radiographs. Postoperative panoramic **(C),** anteroposterior skull **(D),** and lateral cephalometric **(E)** radiographs. The patient underwent resection of the right and left ankylosed costochondral grafts. The New York Hospital–The Hospital for Special Surgery TMJ prosthesis was placed bilaterally. The mandible was repositioned and immediate mobilization was achieved.

up, however, is short. Prosthetic development continues.

ORTHOGNATHIC SURGERY IN RHEUMATOID ARTHRITIS

For many years facial skeletal deformities have been corrected by orthognathic surgery, usually coupled with orthodontic treatment. It is possible safely and predictably to surgically move the maxilla or mandible, or both, in part or in whole, and in all directions. This surgery can almost always be performed through an intraoral approach.

In the non-RA patient there are few inherent limitations to surgical movements possible and the deformities correctable. The maxilla can be impacted or downgrafted, advanced, set back, rotated, widened, or narrowed. The mandible can also be moved forward or back, rotated, and narrowed or widened within reasonable physiologic limits. Simultaneous maxillary and mandibular surgery is routine at numerous medical centers throughout the United States and Europe. Orthognathic surgery has the potential to provide a patient with a functional occlusion and at the same time improve upon their esthetics as indicated and desired.

The facial skeletal deformities in the RA patient usually can be managed in a similar manner. If the

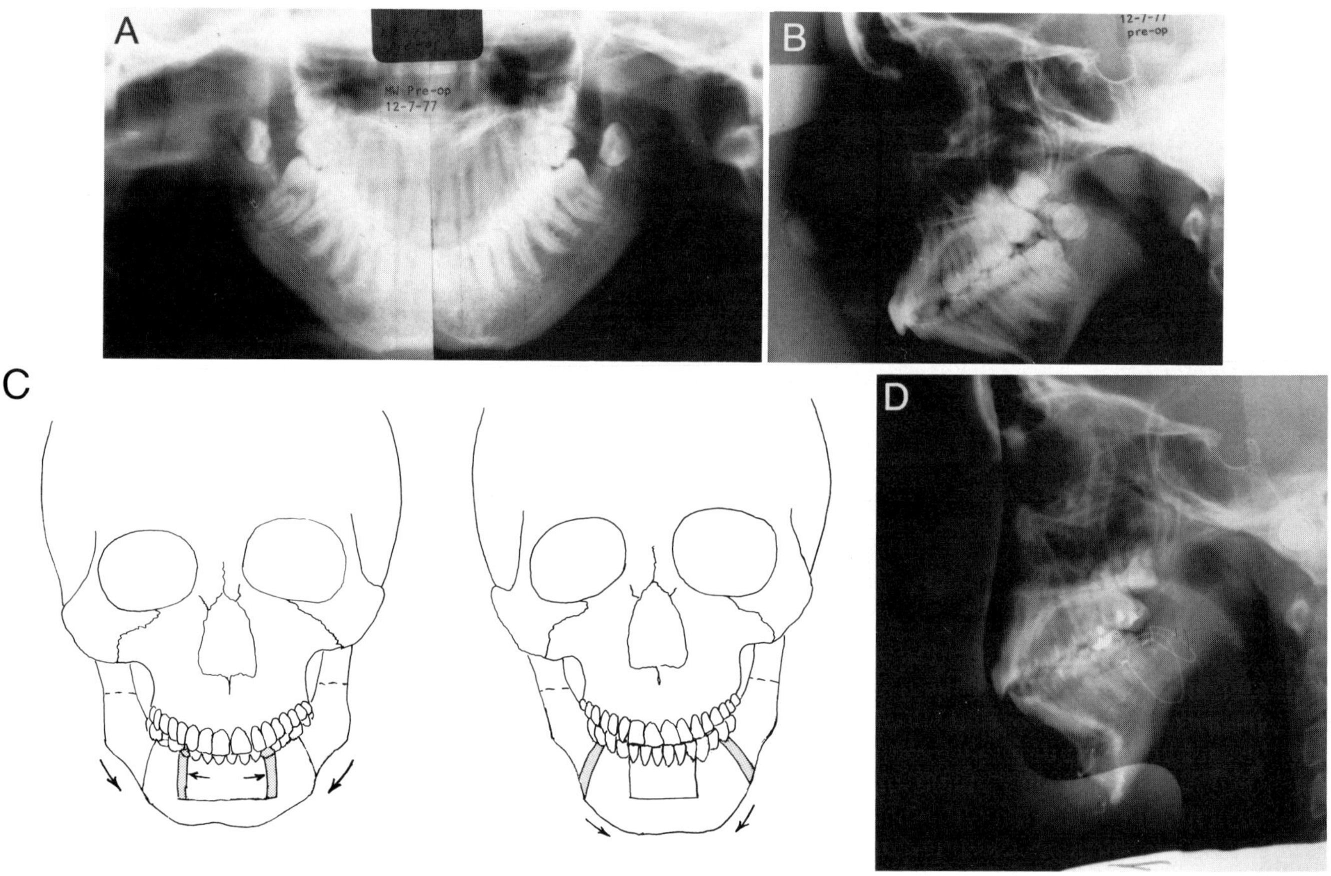

FIG 6–19.
A 14-year-old girl with JRA. (Courtesy of Dr. Stanley J. Behrman.) **A,** preoperative panoramic radiograph showing the absence of condyles and the deep antegonial notching. **B,** preoperative lateral cephalometric radiograph showing the mandibular retrognathia and deep antegonial notching. **C,** surgical plan: (1) Removal of mandibular right and left first premolars and a measured full-thickness segment of bone about the roots of these teeth to below their apices. These vertical ostectomies were connected at their base by a horizontal ostectomy below the apices of the mandibular six anterior teeth. This six-tooth segment is then moved back and secured in this new position. (2) The mandible was advanced by a bilateral sagittal ramusotomy to correct the retrognathia. Additional anterior movement was made possible by first moving the anterior segment back. (3) The anterior mandible was further augmented by placement of a subperiosteal Silastic chin implant. **D,** 4-year postoperative lateral cephalometric radiograph.

RA patient has a functioning, long-term quiescent, albeit damaged or destroyed TMJ, orthognathic surgery can be considered a viable option. Even the JRA patient who has no TMJ but functions on an "articulation" of the mandibular ramus with the temporal bone can be a candidate for orthognathic care. Whether or not a patient will require TMJ reconstruction as well will depend on the degree of TMJ disease and its interference with function.

Maxillary surgery has been shown to be predictable and stable in the RA patient. However, both adult and JRA patients have shown specific limitations with mandibular movements. Mandibular retrognathia without an open bite is surgically correctable in the RA patient by moving the mandible forward (Fig 6–19,A–D). Skeletal open bites require a different approach.

A long-term retrospective review of 77 patients at The New York Hospital who underwent surgical correction of skeletal open bites by mandibular surgery alone was analyzed.[7] The patient population included 55 patients with mandibular setbacks and 22 patients with mandibular advancements. Three of the patients who underwent mandibular advance-

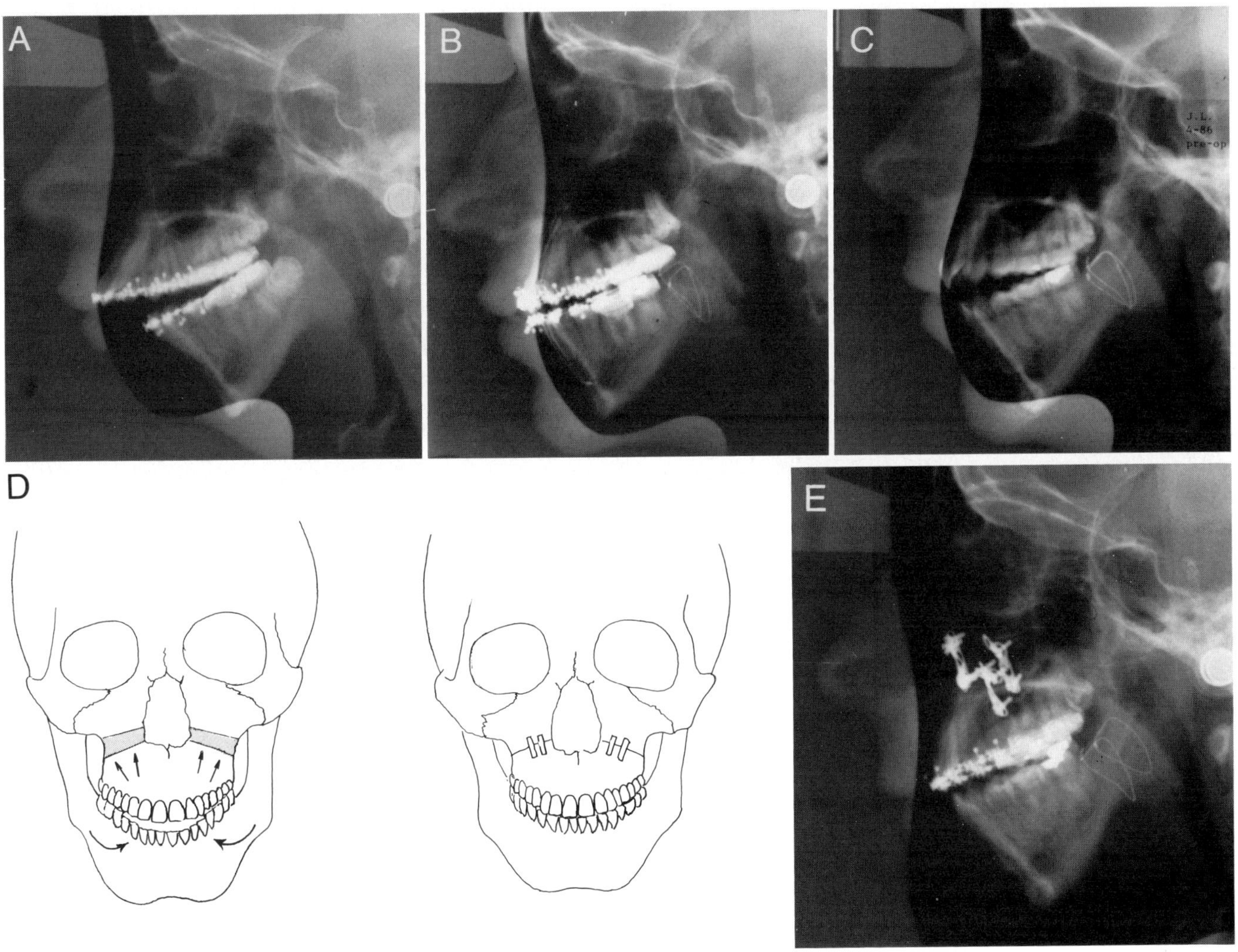

FIG 6–20.
A 15-year-old girl with JRA. (Courtesy of Dr. Stanley J. Behrman.) **A,** preoperative lateral cephalometric radiograph. The patient had undergone preparatory orthodontics. **B,** 1-month postoperative lateral cephalometric radiograph. The patient underwent mandibular advancement and closure of the open bite by a bilateral sagittal ramusotomy. A Silastic chin implant was placed to further augment the anterior mandible. **C,** 3-year postoperative lateral cephalometric radiograph. Significant relapse of the open bite and retrognathia has occurred. **D,** surgical plan: The maxilla was superiorly impacted by a Le Fort I ostectomy. This allowed the mandible to autorotate up anteriorly, closing the open bite and improving the retrognathia. **E,** 2-month postoperative (second surgery) lateral cephalometric radiograph.

ments had JRA. Closure of skeletal open bites through mandibular surgery alone was found to be predictable and stable in all patients except for the three with JRA. A measurable amount of open-bite relapse occurred in these three patients.

The preferred method for managing skeletal open bites in RA involves simultaneous maxillary and mandibular surgery. The maxilla is impacted allowing the mandible to autorotate up anteriorly, closing the open bite. The anteroposterior position of the mandible is then surgically corrected to obtain a stable end result (Figs 6–20,A–E and 6–21,A–D).

Oral and maxillofacial surgeons correct most skeletal chin deformities by an anterior mandibular horizontal osteotomy, also termed a "sliding genioplasty." In this procedure a full-thickness horizontal osteotomy is made through the anterior mandible. The anterior segment, or chin, with its attached soft tissues and musculature, is then moved and rigidly secured in its new position. Rheumatoid arthritis patients will displace the anterior segment inferiorly when it is advanced. This displacement is probably secondary to pull from the suprahyoid musculature and occurs despite suprahyoid myotomies. Placement of a chin implant, either supra- or subperiosteally, is the preferred alternative to managing the retrogenia in these patients after the vertical excess has been corrected through the standard ostectomy.

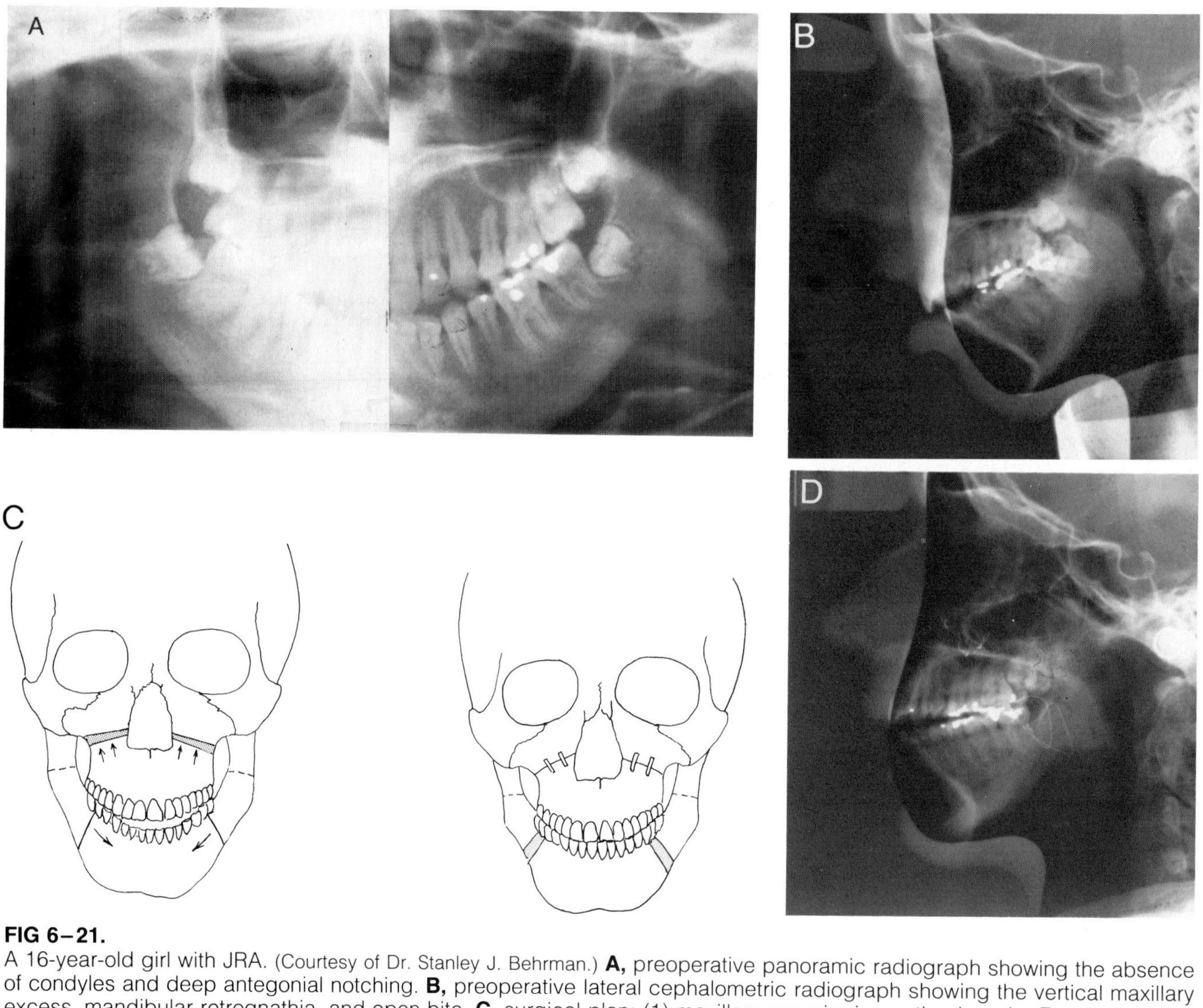

FIG 6–21.
A 16-year-old girl with JRA. (Courtesy of Dr. Stanley J. Behrman.) **A,** preoperative panoramic radiograph showing the absence of condyles and deep antegonial notching. **B,** preoperative lateral cephalometric radiograph showing the vertical maxillary excess, mandibular retrognathia, and open bite. **C,** surgical plan: (1) maxillary superior impaction by a Le Fort I ostectomy to correct the vertical excess and open bite; (2) mandibular advancement by a bilateral sagittal ramusotomy to correct the retrognathia; (3) additional anterior mandibular augmentation by placement of a subperiosteal Silastic chin implant. **D,** 3-year postoperative lateral cephalometric radiograph.

CONCLUSIONS

Advances in TMJ and orthognathic surgery enable the oral and maxillofacial surgeon to offer RA patients several options to ease the effects of their disease and improve the quality of their life.

REFERENCES

1. Akerman S, Nilner S, Petersson A, et al: Relationship between Clinical and Radiologic Findings of TMJ in Rheumatoid Arthritis. *Oral Surg Oral Med Oral Pathol* 1988; 66:639–643.
2. Adair SM, Floyd TP: Temporomandibular joint involvement in juvenile rheumatoid arthritis: Report of two cases. *Pediatr Dent* 1981; 3:271.
3. Barendheuer F, quoted by Lexer E: Joint transplantations and arthroplasty. *Surg Gynecol Obstet* 1925; 40:786.
4. Blackwood H: Pathology of the Temporomandibular Joint. *J Am Dent Assoc* 1969; 79:118.
5. Bronstein SL: Retained alloplastic temporomandibular joint disc implants: A retrospective study. *Oral Surg Oral Med Oral Pathol* 1987; 64:135.
6. Chalmers IM, Blair GS: Rheumatoid arthritis of the temporomandibular joint. *Q J Med* 1973; 42:369–386.
7. Cooney B: *Surgical Correction of Skeletal Anterior Open-Bite by the Bilateral Sagittal Ramusotomy: A Longitudinal Analysis* (thesis). Georgetown University Graduate School, Washington, D.C., 1988.
8. Dingman RO, Grabb WC: Reconstruction of both mandibular condyles with metatarsal bone grafts. *Plast Reconstr Surg* 1964; 34:441.
9. Engel MB, Richmond JB, Brodie A: Mandibular growth disturbance in rheumatoid arthritis in childhood. *Am J Dis Child* 1949; 78:728.
10. Ericsson S, Lundberg M: Alterations in the temporomandibular joint at various stages of rheumatoid arthritis. *Acta Rheumatol Scand* 1967; 13:257.
11. Florini BL, Gatto DJ, Wade ML, et al: Tomographic evaluation of temporomandibular joints following discoplasty or placement of polytetrafluoroethylene implants. *J Oral Maxillofac Surg* 1988; 48:183–188.
12. Franks AST: Temporomandibular joint in adult rheumatoid arthritis: A comparative study of 100 cases. *Ann Rheum Dis* 1969; 28:139.
13. Kent JN, Block MS, Homsy CA, et al: Experience with a polymer glenoid fossa prosthesis for partial or total temporomandibular joint reconstruction. *J Oral Maxillofac Surg* 1986; 44:520.
14. Kent JN, Misiek DJ, Akin RK, et al: Temporomandibular joint condylar prosthesis: A ten year report. *J Oral Maxillofac Surg* 1983; 41:245.
15. Koslin M: Arthroscopic management of soft-tissue internal derangements in rheumatoid arthritics. Presented at the Fifth Annual International Symposium on Arthroscopy of the Human Temporomandibular Joint, New York, Dec 2–4, 1990.
16. Larheim TA, Haanaes HR: Micrognathia, temporomandibular joint changes and dental occlusion in juvenile rheumatoid arthritis of adolescents and adults. *Scand J Dent Res* 1981; 89:329.
17. Larheim TA, Hoyeraal HM, Stabrun AE, et al: The temporomandibular joint in juvenile rheumatoid arthritis. *Scand J Rheumatol* 1982; 11:5.
18. Larheim TA, Johannessen S, Tveito L: Abnormalities of the temporomandibular joint in adults with rheumatic disease: A comparison of panoramic, transcranial and transpharyngeal radiography with tomographraphy. *Dentomaxillofac Radiol* 1988; 17:109.
19. Larheim TA, Storhaug K, Tveito L: Temporomandibular joint involvement and dental occlusion in a group of adults with rheumatoid arthritis. *Acta Odontol Scand* 1983; 41:301.
20. Libin B: Otologic and jaw symptoms of TMJ-MPDS. *Ear Nose Throat J* 1982; 61:49–53.
21. MacIntosh RB: Current spectrum of costochondral grafting, in Bell WH (ed): *Surgical Correction of Dentofacial Deformities*, vol 3; *New Concepts*. Philadelphia, WB Saunders Co, 1985, pp 355–410.
22. MacIntosh RB: Costochondral and dermal grafts in temprormandibular joint reconstruction, in Merrill RG (ed): *Disorders of the TMJ II: Arthrotomy. Oral Maxillofacial Surg Clin North Am.* 1989 (Dec); 363–397.
23. MacIntosh RB, Henny FA: A spectrum of application of autogenous costochondral grafts. *J Maxillofac Surg* 1977; 5:257.
24. Mayne JG, Hatch GS: Arthritis of the temporomandibular joint. *J Am Dent Assoc* 1969; 79:125–130.
25. Obeid G, Guttenberg SA, Connole PW: Costochondral grafting in condylar replacement and mandibular reconstruction. *J Oral Maxillofac Surg* 1988; 48:177.
26. Ogus H: Rheumatoid arthritis of the temporomandibular joint. *J Oral Surg* 1975; 12:275–284.
27. Schaller J: Juvenile rheumatoid arthritis. *Postgrad Med* 1977; 61:177.
28. Snyder CC, Levine GA, Dingman DL: Trial of a sternoclavicular whole joint graft as a substitute for the temporomandibular joint. *Plast Reconstr Surg* 1971; 48:447.
29. Tegelberg A, Kopp S: Clinical findings in the stomatognathic system for individuals with rheumatoid arthritis and osteoarthritis. *Acta Odontol Scand* 1987; 45:65–75.
30. Trenwith A, Beale G: Rheumatoid arthritis in the temporomandibular joint. *N Z Dent J* 1973; 73:195.

SUGGESTED READINGS

Excellent reviews of arthroscopy and arthroplasty are:

Merrill RG (ed): *Disorders of the TMJ I: Diagnosis and Arthroscopy. Oral Maxillofac Surg Clin North Am* 1989 (Sept).

Merrill RG (ed): *Disorders of the TMJ II: Arthrotomy. Oral Maxillofac Surg Clin North Am,* 1989 (Dec).

Selected Readings in Oral and Maxillofacial Surgery. San Francisco, The Guild for Scientific Advancement in Oral and Maxillofacial Surgery.

Braun T (ed): *Temporomandibular Joint Surgery: Part I: Surgical Treatment of Internal Derangement,* vol 1. 1989 (Dec); no. 3.

Braun T, Kent J (eds): *Temporomandibular Joint Surgery: Part II: Partial and Total Joint Reconstruction and Osseous Procedures,* vol 1. 1989; no. 4.

An excellent source on orthognathic surgery is:

Bell WH, Profitt WR, White RP (eds): *Surgical Correction of Dentofacial Deformities, vols 1 and 2.* Philadelphia, WB Saunders Co, 1980.

Bell WH (ed): *Surgical Correction of Dentofacial Deformities: Vol III: New Concepts* Philadelphia, WB Saunders Co, 1985.

CHAPTER 7

The Cervical Spine

Thomas P. Sculco, M.D.

Michael Alexiades, M.D.

INTRODUCTION

The cervical spine is a commonly affected area in rheumatoid arthritis, particularly in patients with moderate to severe polyarticular disease of long duration. The incidence can be as high as 85% in these patients.[13, 49] The disease was first noted in the cervical spine by Garrod in 1890.[24] The inflammatory process affects multiple anatomic structures in the cervical spine and produces a series of diverse clinical and pathologic presentations. Involvement of the diarthrodial joints and supporting ligamentous complexes in the cervical spine can lead to alteration in vertebral alignment both at the occipitocervical junction and in the subaxial area. Inflammatory tissue (pannus) itself can extend from synovial joints to affect the intervertebral disc and produce a spondylodiscitis. This pannus can also compromise the neural canal producing spinal cord compression both at the atlantoaxial articulation and in the subaxial area. Depending upon the specific structures involved, patients may present with occipital and neck pain or frank myelopathy with both upper and lower extremity weakness.

This chapter reviews the pathologic manifestations of the disease as it affects the cervical spine and its clinical presentations. The radiographic criteria for diagnosis are treated at length as are the nonsurgical and surgical treatment.

MANIFESTATIONS OF CERVICAL SPINE INVOLVEMENT

Involvement of the cervical spine in rheumatoid arthritis occurs in three basic patterns: (1) atlantoaxial subluxation, generally with concomitant instability; (2) atlantoaxial impaction or cranial settling; and (3) subaxial subluxation with or without instability. In the most severely affected rheumatoid patients these cervical spine disease patterns may be present singly or in combination.

Atlantoaxial Subluxation

Atlantoaxial subluxation is the most common cervical spine manifestation of rheumatoid disease. There normally exists an interval of 2 to 3 mm between the anterior ring of the atlas and the odontoid. Atlantoaxial distance greater than 3.5 mm is considered abnormal in the adult patient. Displacement beyond this limit is produced by destruction of the supporting ligamentous complex stabilizing the odontoid process to the anterior arch of the atlas. These ligamentous structures are damaged by extension of the synovial disease from the joint between the anterior arch of the atlas and the odontoid and the synovia-lined bursa behind the odontoid which is anterior to the transverse ligament. Additionally, the transverse, apical, and alar ligaments may be damaged by

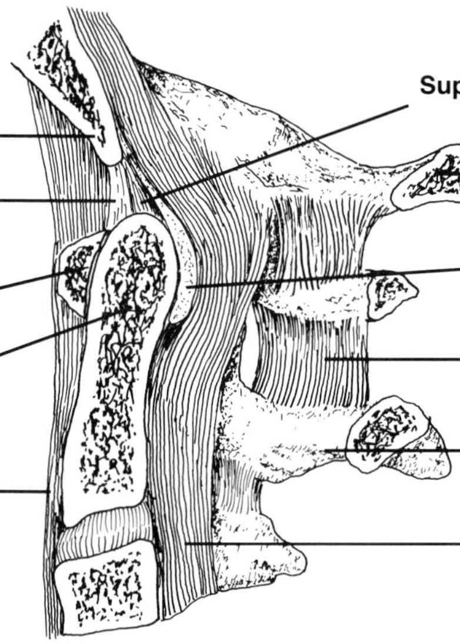

FIG 7–1.
Sagittal section through the cervico-occipital junction.

direct involvement of their collagen matrix by inflammatory mononuclear cells. The transverse ligament is the most important stabilizing structure to the odontoid during flexion-extension of the upper cervical spine. Bland[5] has demonstrated a translation of 5 mm between the odontoid and atlas with transection of this ligament alone. The apical ligament is a minor supporting ligament and the alar ligaments tend to limit rotation of the odontoid. Fielding et al.[21] reported that subluxation beyond 10 mm implies disruption of all ligamentous structures between odontoid and atlas (Figs 7–1 and 7–2). Along with ligamentous damage, synovial disease infiltrates the odontoid, and bony erosion occurs (Fig 7–3,A–D). The odontoid may become quite atrophic and pyramidal in shape. In the most severe cases of odontoid erosion complete absence of the odontoid may occur. Although atlantoaxial and atlanto-odontoid destruction and damage to the odontoid generally occur with ligamentous loss in atlantoaxial subluxation, Kontinnen et al.[30] have reported on 14 patients in whom atlantoaxial subluxation developed without radiographic changes of joint destruction.

As instability and subluxation of the odontoid progresses, the neural canal of the upper cervical spine is compromised and spinal cord compromise may occur. The overall diameter of the neural canal at the atlantoaxial level approximates 30 mm with the spinal cord and the odontoid each occupying about 10 mm. For this reason subluxation beyond 9 to 10 mm produces a potential encroachment of the odontoid on the spinal cord (Fig 7–4). Weissman et al.[55] have demonstrated a correlation between cord compression and degree of subluxation at the atlantoaxial interval with the critical preodontoid space being 9 mm (Fig 7–5,A–C). Atlantoaxial subluxation greater than 9 mm and associated with any degree of atlantoaxial impaction increased the risk of cord compression. Marked degrees of atlantoaxial impac-

FIG 7–2.
Posterior view of the ligamentous complex at the atlantoaxial level.

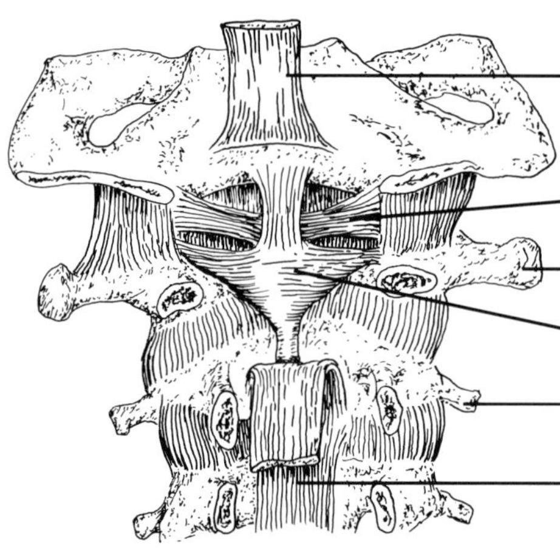

tion (cranial settling) will reduce anteroposterior instability at the atlantoaxial level by locking in the broad base of the odontoid into the ring of the atlas.

The incidence of atlantoaxial subluxation is reported to be as high as 70% in patients with advanced rheumatoid arthritis.[13] Association of atlantoaxial subluxation with male patients, erosive disease, subcutaneous nodules, and seropositivity has been reported by Matthews.[34] Posterior atlantoaxial subluxation may occur but is uncommon. It is seen in patients in whom there has been severe erosion of the odontoid which allows the remaining odontoid to slip anterior to the arch of the atlas. Weissman et al.[55], and more recently Halla, Hardin, and co-workers[25–27] have reported the occurrence of a lateral atlantoaxial subluxation which was noted in 10% of 126 hospitalized patients with rheumatoid arthritis.[25] In these patients the subluxation of the lateral masses at the C1–2 level is greater than 2 mm. Patients may present with nonreducible rotational head tilt and severe pain in the neck–shoulder girdle region.

Atlantoaxial Impaction

Atlantoaxial impaction has been variously termed cranial settling, pseudobasilar invagination, and vertical migration of the odontoid. It occurs as the result of advanced destruction of the atlanto-occipital, atlanto-odontoid, and atlantoaxial joints. Collapse occurs through these bilateral lateral facet joint masses and the resultant progressive vertical translation of the odontoid occurs in combination with settling of the occiput on the upper cervical segments. In severe cases the body of the axis may completely enter the ring of the atlas. As this process unfolds, the odontoid compresses the spinal cord as it enters the foramen magnum. The tip of the odontoid may in fact compress the medulla oblongata as well as the spinal cord and lead to progressive myelopathy. In the most severe cases death may occur due to compression of the medulla oblongata or occlusion of the vertebral arteries[18, 33, 54] (Fig 7–6,A and B). Dysphagia may be noted from pressure on the nucleus of the glossopharyngeal nerve. Cranial sublux-

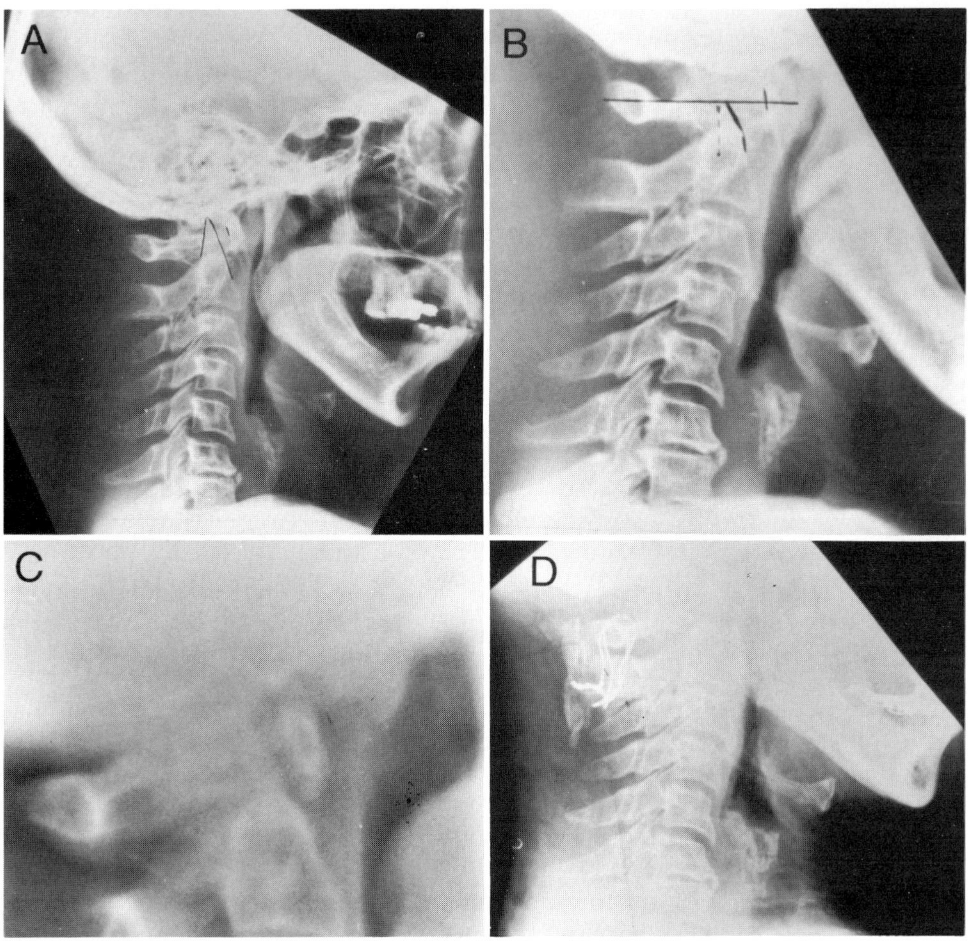

FIG 7–3.
A, lateral radiograph demonstrating C1–2 subluxation at 5 mm. **B,** lateral radiograph 3 years later showing increased subluxation at the atlantoaxial junction to 11 mm. Note odontoid erosion. **C,** lateral tomogram illustrates marked odontoid erosion. **D,** 2 years after C1–2 fusion.

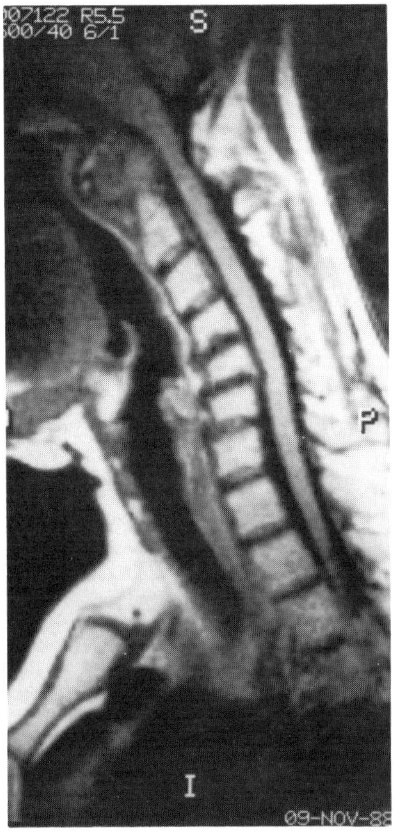

FIG 7–4.
Flexion MRI demonstrates spinal cord compression in a patient with advanced atlantoaxial subluxation.

ation of the odontoid may also occlude flow of cerebrospinal fluid and lead to increased intracranial pressure and hydrocephalus.[53]

Fortunately, erosion of the odontoid is marked in many of these patients and this lessens the spinal cord and brainstem compression and therefore the neurologic deficits. Superior migration of the odontoid will eventually become fixed and further progression will not occur. This is seen when there is bony impingement between the vertebral body of the axis and the ring of the atlas and further cephalad migration is not possible. Attempts to reduce the superior migration of the odontoid with skeletal traction are unsuccessful in these patients as the deformity is rigid and not flexible.

The most severe degree of atlantoaxial impaction, as in atlantoaxial subluxation, is present in the rheumatoid patient with advanced and chronic disease.[32, 41, 49] The overall incidence of atlantoaxial impaction is reported to be as high as 37% of patients undergoing surgical treatment for rheumatoid arthritis affecting the cervical spine.[11] Overlap radiographic patterns may be encountered in which subaxial or atlantoaxial subluxation is seen in combination with atlantoaxial impaction.

Subaxial Subluxation

Subaxial subluxation of the cervical spine in rheumatoid arthritis results from a widespread involvement of supporting vertebral structures. Synovial disease affects both the facet joints and the uncovertebral joints of Luschka. Extension of the synovitis to involve the intervertebral disc leads to a spondylodiscitis which will compromise the stabilizing integrity of the disc and its anterior and posterior longitudinal ligaments. Erosion of the subchondral end plates and osteopenia weaken the bony support to the cervical spine. Thus pathologic involvement encompasses ligamentous support, facet and intervertebral disc stability, and bony integrity, all contributing to ultimate subaxial vertebral subluxation (Fig 7–7). Although the middle segments of the cervical spine are most affected, the entire cervical spine may demonstrate relative levels of anterior subluxation. Instability is usually present and alignment can be improved when the neck is extended. In the most advanced and longstanding cases, however, the subluxation may be fixed and not mobile with either traction or alteration in neck position. Anterior subluxation in these more advanced patients may be accompanied by an element of inferior displacement of the upper subluxing vertebra and severe posterior angulation can result in these patients.

The spinal cord is at great risk in these patients. The neural canal is more narrowed in the subaxial area when compared to the C1–2 level and therefore lesser degrees of subluxation (2–3 mm) may be associated with myelopathic findings. Three possible causes for myelopathy in subaxial disease have been defined: firstly, the spinal cord may be under compression because of the degree of subluxation itself; secondly, there may be anterior pressure on the spinal cord because of discitis; and thirdly, there may be posterior compression of the spinal cord as a result of granulation and pannus extending from rheumatoid involvement of the facet joints.[31]

In degenerative spondylolytic cervical disease, osteophyte formation is common arising from the vertebral end plates and the uncovertebral joints. Compromise of the neural foramina leads to radicular pain. This presentation is uncommon in rheumatoid arthritis in which osteophytes tend to be rare and subchondral erosions are present. Subluxation is the most prevalent manifestation in the rheumatoid patient and this is seen in the osteoarthritic pa-

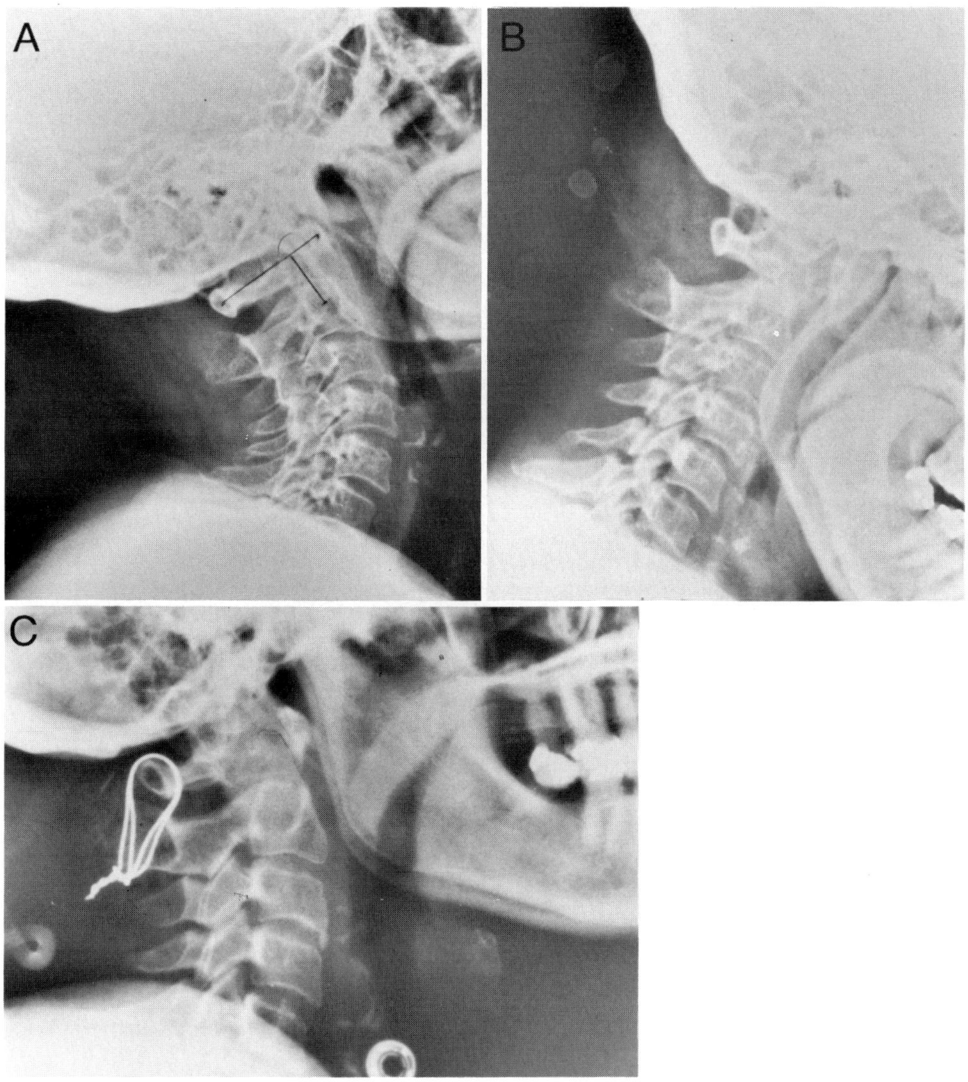

FIG 7–5.
A,B, flexion-extension lateral cervical radiographs in a 42-year-old woman with atlantoaxial subluxation of 11 mm. Patient had myelopathy. **C,** patient treated with reduction of atlantoaxial subluxation and arthrodesis of C1–2. The myelopathy resolved.

tient only if associated with trauma. Subaxial subluxation may also be seen after cervical fusions at levels just below the fusion mass. This entity is discussed in more detail in the surgical treatment section.

CLINICAL CHARACTERISTICS OF THE RHEUMATOID CERVICAL SPINE

Patients with rheumatoid involvement of the cervical spine are the more severely afflicted patients with the disease. Therefore polyarticular involvement is common, and most patients are receiving corticosteroids or immunosuppressive medication. Duration of the disease is usually greater than 5 years although in one series patients who ultimately developed atlantoaxial subluxation demonstrated evidence of the lesion 2 years after the onset of their disease.[58]

Local symptoms are common and include headache, occipital pain, and shoulder and neck pain. In the most severely disabled patients, particularly those with atlantoaxial impaction, sitting in the upright position will bring on severe occipital pain. This is due to the weight of the cranium on the upper cervical spine and compression of the C2 nerve root. Radicular symptoms may be present with paresthesias. In patients with cervical myelopathy the patient may complain of a subtle loss of function of the upper and lower extremities. They may complain of weakness when lifting objects and fine coordination may become impaired. They also may note that their ambulatory status has deteriorated. Wheelchair use becomes necessary in these patients. Lhermitte's sign, electric shock sensations into the

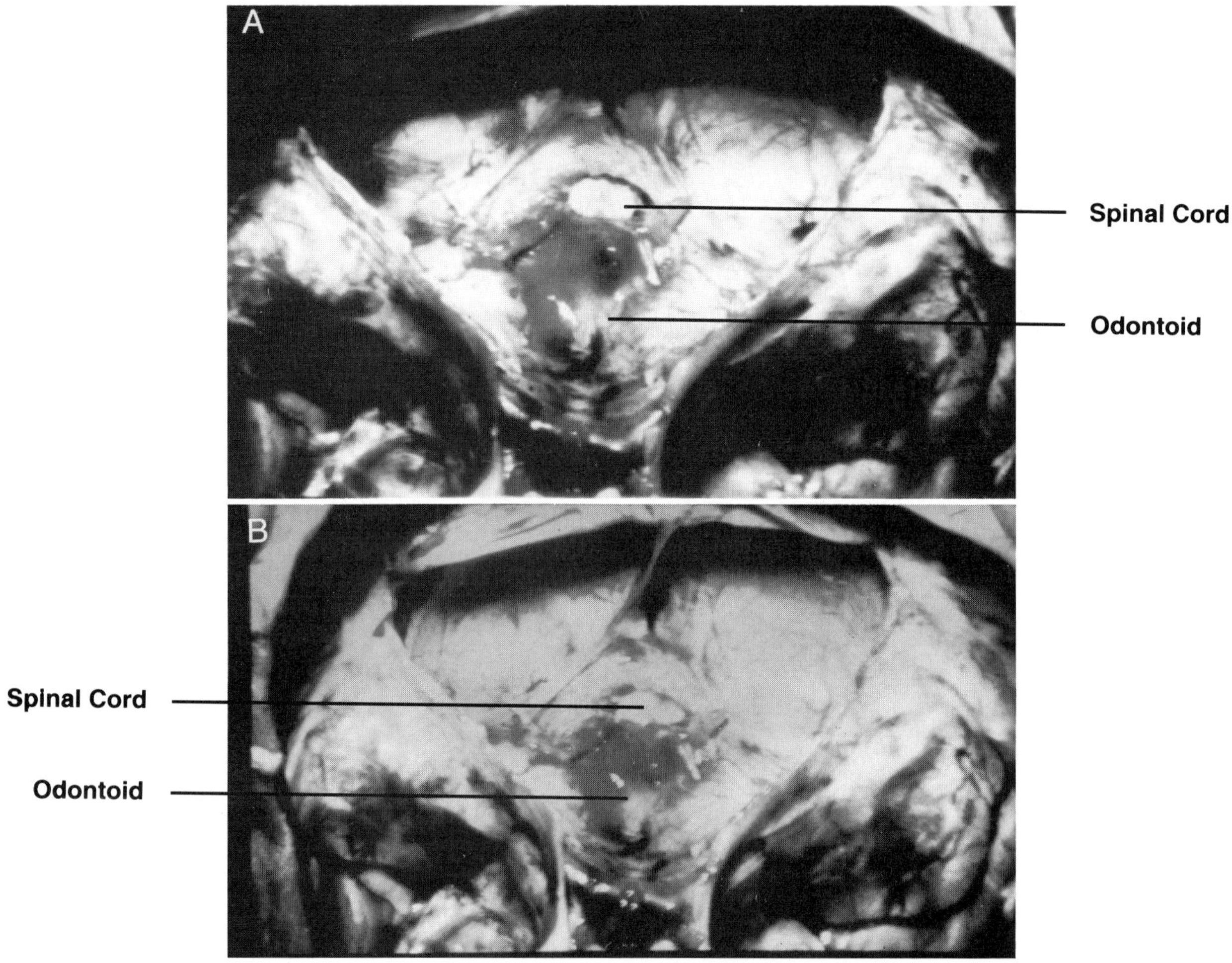

FIG 7–6.
A, autopsy specimen of a rheumatoid patient with atlantoaxial impaction. The spinal cord is not compressed with the neck extended. **B,** spinal cord compression by the odontoid is noted with neck flexion.

FIG 7–7.
Multiple-level subaxial subluxation of C3–4 and C4–5.

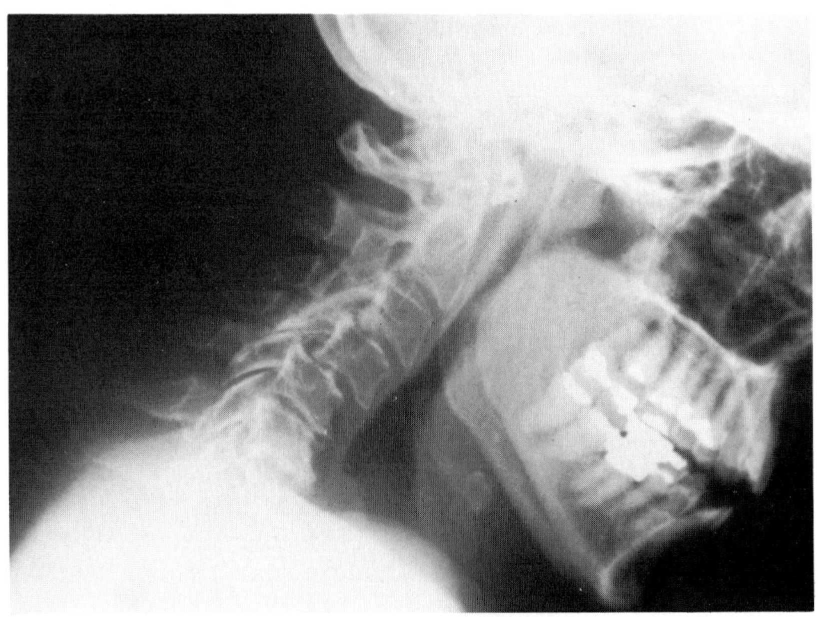

limbs with neck rotation, may be described by these patients. Myelopathic patients can also present with urinary retention and later urinary incontinence.

Physical examination will demonstrate a reduction in cervical spine motion with lateral bending and rotation being lost before flexion and extension. Local muscle tenderness and spasm may be present in the upper cervical spine musculature. Neurologic examination must be carefully performed. Along with a careful motor and sensory examination, findings consistent with upper motor neuron involvement must be evaluated. A positive Babinski's sign or hyperreflexia must alert the surgeon to the presence of possible spinal cord compromise. Some patients with atlantoaxial subluxation have vertebral artery insufficiency resulting in symptoms of equilibrium loss; cranial nerve dysfunction, especially the trigeminal nerve[41]; and visual deficits. Impaired blood flow to the cerebellum, brainstem, and posterior cerebrum will produce these findings. Motor testing to differentiate a peripheral joint severely involved by myelopathy from a weakened limb resulting from joint destruction, tenosynovitis, myopathy, or peripheral neuropathy may be difficult. Floyd et al.[23] have emphasized the problems with neurologic evaluation in the rheumatoid patient with stiff and painful joints. They found no increased incidence of abnormal neurologic findings in comparing two groups of patients, one with abnormal radiographs and the other with normal radiographs. Only in the patients most severely impaired neurologically was there a positive correlation with radiographs. Hyperreflexia was particularly noted to be an unreliable finding.

RADIOGRAPHIC FEATURES OF THE RHEUMATOID CERVICAL SPINE

In following patients who have radiographic evidence of cervical spine involvement in rheumatoid arthritis, progression of subluxation is noted over time. Conlon et al.[13], in a series of 333 patients with rheumatoid arthritis, noted that 50% had radiographic changes and 23% had atlantoaxial subluxation. The authors followed 171 of the original 333 patients greater than 6 years and noted that the number of patients in the atlantoaxial subluxation group had doubled.[29] Smith et al.[50, 51] evaluated 962 patients with rheumatoid arthritis and found that 15% had vertebral subluxations, while 68% were atlantoaxial subluxations. At 5- to 14-year follow-up neurologic deterioration had increased in 130 of their original 150 patients available for follow-up examination. Pellicci et al.[40] demonstrated an 81% progression in radiographic deterioration in patients at long-term follow-up. Thirty-six percent had developed increased neurologic abnormality.

Since the incidence of cervical spine disease is high in the rheumatoid patient, routine cervical radiographs should be obtained, particularly if neck symptoms are present. An anteroposterior radiograph of the cervical spine is recommended with a lateral radiograph taken in neck flexion and extension. An open mouth odontoid view will also provide information concerning the status of the odontoid and the lateral masses (Fig 7–8). Plain radiographs will reveal the site of involvement, the extent and severity of disease, and the degree of instability with neck motion. Serial radiographs may be taken to follow progression of the disease.

Anteroposterior radiographs reveal abnormality in the uncovertebral joints, the width of the spinal canal, and the relative thickness of the intervertebral disc. Lateral radiographs of the atlantoaxial area will demonstrate subluxation or impaction in this area. The relationship of the anterior arch of the atlas to the odontoid should be measured and this will give the preodontoid interval (Fig 7–9). Measurements in flexion and extension of this interval will demonstrate if there is abnormal motion and its extent. An interval greater than 3.5 to 4 mm is considered abnormal. The degree of odontoid erosion may also be

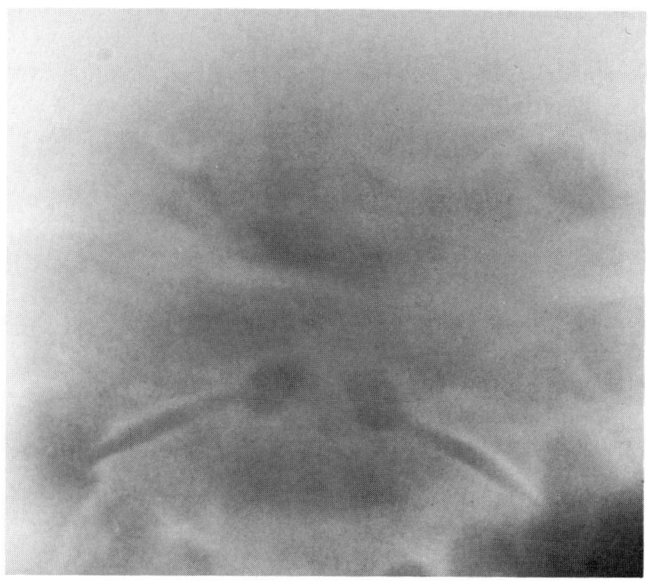

FIG 7–8.
Open mouth radiograph demonstrates severe odontoid erosion and intact lateral facet joints.

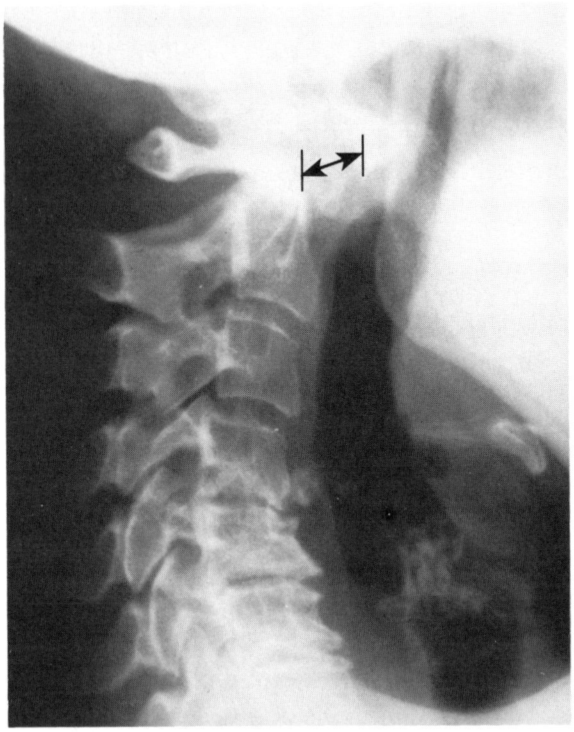

FIG 7–9.
The degree of atlantoaxial subluxation measured from the odontoid to the anterior arch of the atlas.

seen on the lateral radiograph. In the subaxial area, subluxation can be evaluated and the degree of intervertebral disc degeneration and narrowing.

There are a number of radiographic measurements taken on the lateral view of the occipitocervical junction to determine the degree of atlantoaxial impaction. Chamberlain's line projects from the posterior margin of the hard palate to the posterior part of the foramen magnum. The odontoid should not extend cephalad to this line greater than 3 mm. Macgregors's line is drawn from the posterior margin of the hard palate to the base of the occiput on the lateral radiograph. The tip of the odontoid should not project more than 4.5 mm above this line.[55] On the odontoid open mouth radiograph the Fischgold-Metzger measurement can be made. A line is drawn from the base of the mastoid where it joins the skull; the tip of the odontoid should lie 1 cm below this line. These measurements may be difficult and inaccurate because of erosion of the odontoid and destruction of bony anatomy. Often the hard palate is not well visualized and therefore lines are estimations of true relationships. The Ranawat measurement more accurately determines the alteration in relationship between the axis and the atlas and avoids the need for using the hard palate or odontoid as landmarks.[42] In this index a line is drawn from the midpoints of the anterior and posterior arches of the atlas on the lateral radiograph. The midpoint of the pedicles of the axis can be easily determined on the lateral radiograph and a perpendicular line is drawn from this point to the midatlantal line. Normally the distance from the pedicle of the axis to the transaltlantal line is 17 ±2 mm in males and 15 ±2 mm in females (Fig 7–10). The Redlund-Johnell line is similar to the Ranawat index and the relationship of Macgregor's line to C2 is used.[44]

Lateral multiplanar tomograms provide excellent visualization of the bony framework of the spinal canal. Alterations in relationships of odontoid and vertebral bodies are also easily identified. Pathologic features of the facet joints, uncovertebral joints, and the extent of erosion of bone can be well seen on tomographic studies (Fig 7–11). In the same manner

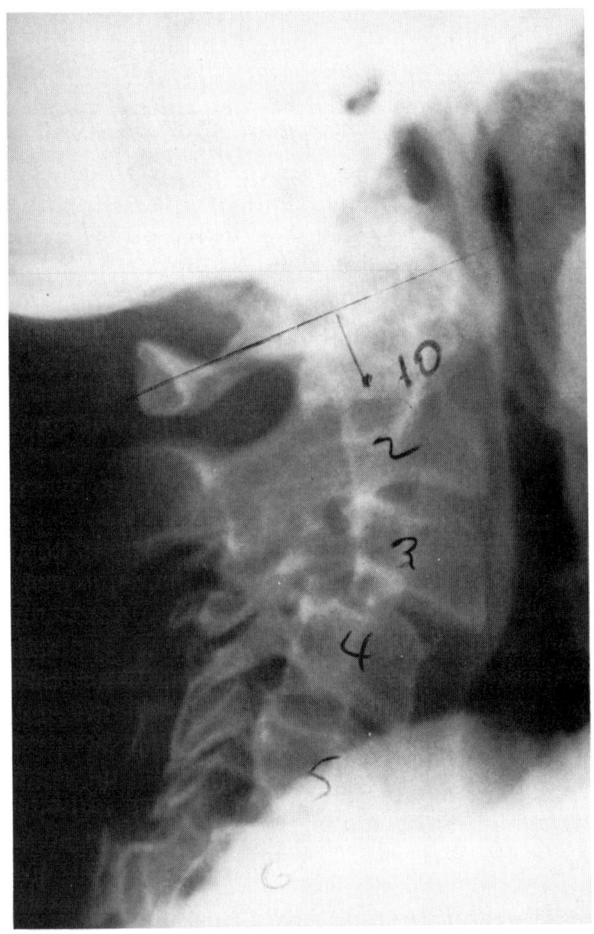

FIG 7–10.
The Ranawat index for atlantoaxial impaction is the distance from the pedicle of C2 to a line traversing the anterior and posterior arch of the atlas. Note subaxial subluxation at C3–4.

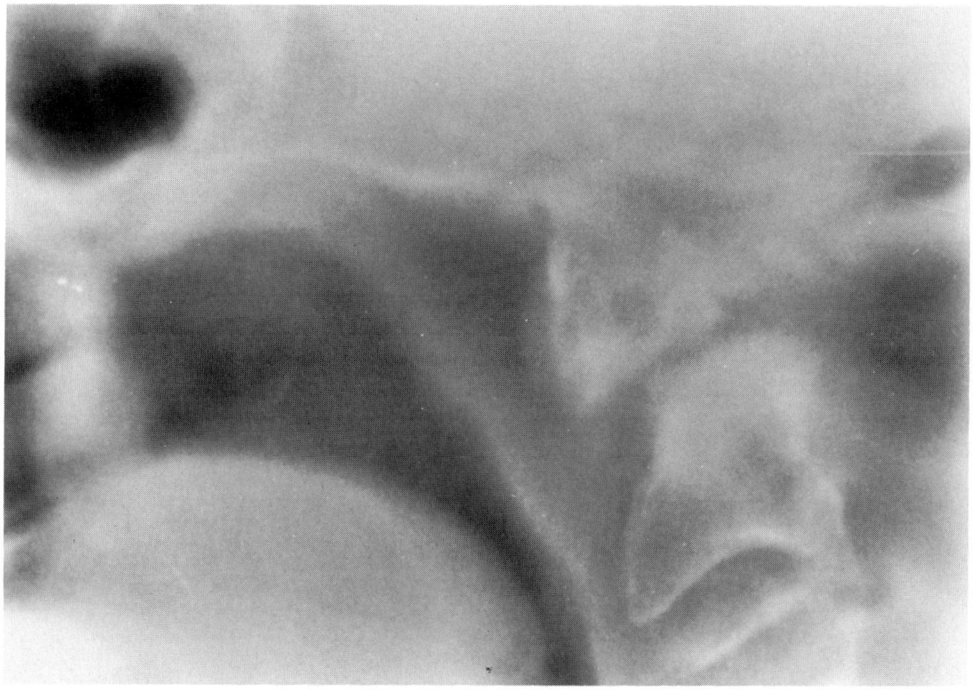

FIG 7–11.
Lateral tomogram demonstrates atlantoaxial subluxation and absence of the tip of the odontoid.

computed tomography (CT) allows for evaluation of not only the bony anatomy but provides some information about the soft tissues. Intrathecal contrast can be used to define the relationship of the spinal cord to the bony neural canal. Compression of the spinal cord or brainstem can be visualized to some extent with this study as well. Spinal cord compression can be appreciated with reformatted studies, but multiplanar tomography is superior for evaluating the atlantoaxial and occipitocervical area.[7] A significant disadvantage to the use of multiplanar tomography and CT is the extent of radiation necessary.

Magnetic resonance imaging (MRI) has been a significant advance in the evaluation of the cervical spine in rheumatoid arthritis. Its major advantages are that it is noninvasive, without ionizing radiation, and provides excellent definition of the soft tissues in the neural canal and cranium. The brainstem, cervical spinal cord, and other neural structures are clearly seen.[37, 38] In addition, axial and sagittal sections can be performed easily and flexion-extension studies can be performed to evaluate bony changes and spinal cord and brainstem compression with alteration in head position. Both T1- and T2-weighted images are utilized. T1-weighted images demonstrate the spinal cord and brainstem. T2-weighted images display a myelogram-type effect which shows encroachment of the dura by pannus, bony malalignment, or facet joint disease. T2-weighted images are also excellent in showing abnormal signal from pannus and erosive tissue around the odontoid.[4, 38] Compression of the spinal cord or brain stem demonstrated on MRI has correlated with myelopathy.[1, 8] Breedveld et al.[8] divided patients into classes depending upon neurologic involvement and noted that atlantoaxial subluxation and impaction could be detected equally by plain radiographs or MRI. However, in all patients with advanced evidence of myelopathy, there was distortion of the spinal cord best seen with the MRI.[8]

At The Hospital for Special Surgery in New York City, 45 consecutive patients with rheumatoid arthritis affecting the cervical spine have undergone evaluation with MRI scanning utilizing T1- and T2-weighted images in both flexion and extension. Most patients with atlantoaxial subluxation and instability do not show spinal cord compression until subluxation of 9 mm or greater has occurred. However, a few patients with as little as 5 to 6 mm of subluxation did show mild cord compression, primarily from soft tissue and pannus in the epidural space. Patients with atlantoaxial impaction showed evidence of brainstem compression in most cases (Fig 7–12,A and B). Combined atlantoaxial subluxation and atlantoaxial impaction almost always demonstrated spinal cord or brainstem compression and were most often myelopathic. Patients with subaxial disease were noted to have cord compression with as little as 3 mm of instability (Fig 7–13). MRI scan-

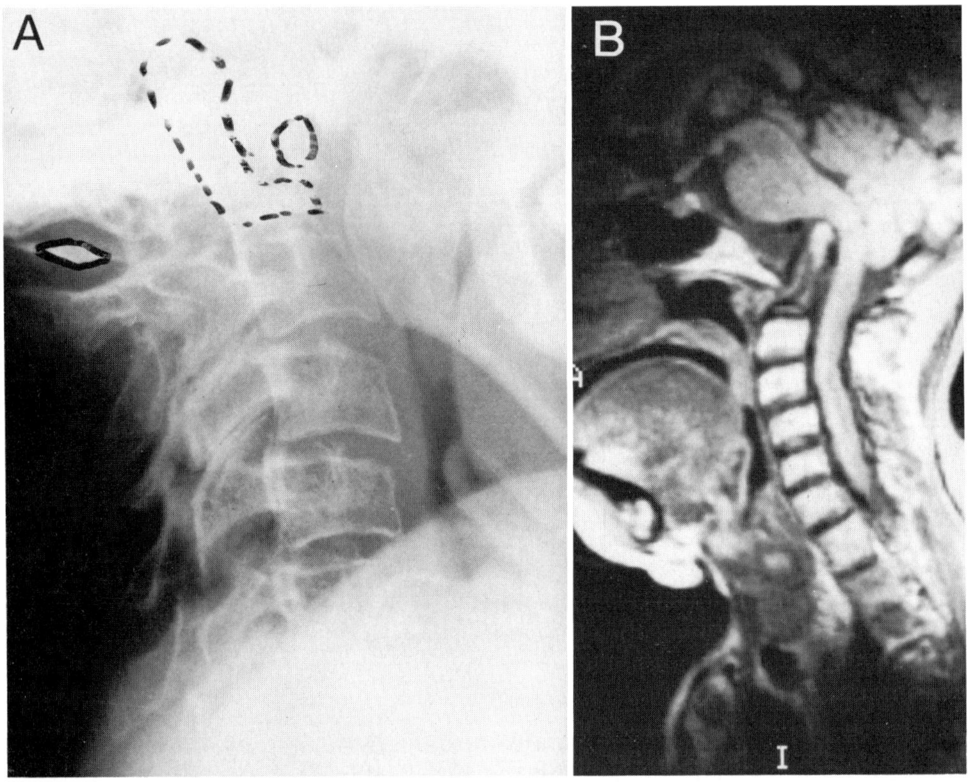

FIG 7–12.
A, severe atlantoaxial impaction with myelopathy. **B,** MRI demonstrates the marked degree of spinal cord and brainstem compression by the odontoid.

ning is routinely performed at this time when there is subluxation greater than 5 mm at the atlantoaxial junction, in all patients with atlantoaxial impaction, and in patients with subaxial subluxation of greater than 2 mm. MRI is also extremely useful in defining the level of spinal cord compression in patients with mixed cervical involvement. In a patient with myelopathy and evidence of both atlantoaxial and subaxial subluxation, MRI can demonstrate if the level of spinal cord compromise is at the upper, lower, or at both levels of cervical spine disease (Fig 7–14). MRI can also document the degree and extent of disease and if followed serially can facilitate the surgical decision based on the progression and severity of the spinal cord compression.

NONSURGICAL MANAGEMENT

There exists significant controversy as to whether surgical treatment with its risk of morbidity and mortality is indicated in the patient with cervical spine disease. Nonsurgical treatment is appropriate in the patient who is symptomatic with local nondisabling pain and who is neurologically intact. These patients must also have radiographic findings which do not demonstrate an advanced degree of atlantoaxial subluxation, atlantoaxial impaction, or subaxial disease. Since it has been shown that cervical spine involvement in rheumatoid arthritis occurs early and correlates with the severity of the disease, it is important that continual monitoring of the cervical spine with radiographic studies and neurologic examination be regularly performed. Nonsurgical treatment is primarily supportive consisting of cervical collars, physical therapy, and medication to relieve pain and relax inflamed and spastic muscle.

Cervical collars are available in a variety of configurations and may provide some relief from local neck discomfort. No collar will prevent progression of subluxation. Althoff and Goldie[3] have confirmed this, showing in fact that more restrictive collars may increase atlantoaxial subluxation. The soft foam collar is the least restrictive but also provides little in the way of support to the neck. A firm plastic collar is probably the most supportive of the simpler collars and is the best tolerated. The Philadelphia-type collar, which provides support to the occiput and supports the chin, will immobilize the neck to a greater extent but is somewhat bulky and cumbersome to put on and remove.

Physical therapy can palliate muscle spasm and thereby relieve pain. Cervical traction is not recom-

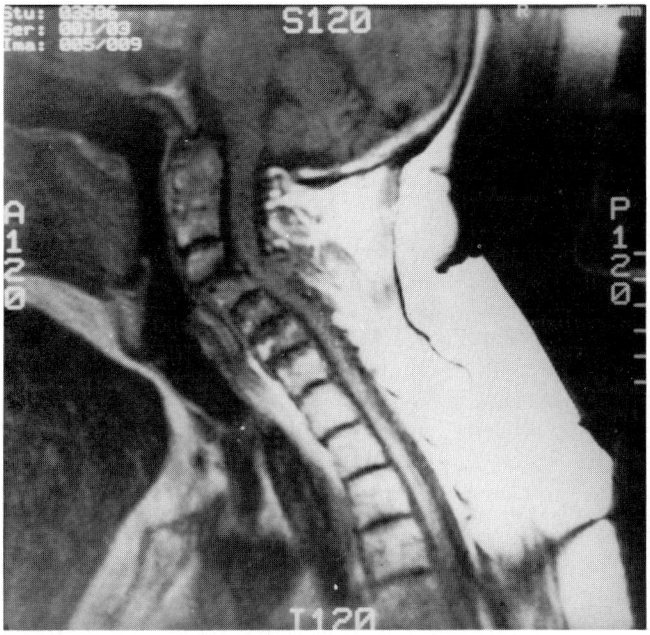

FIG 7–13.
Subaxial subluxation with MRI findings of spinal cord compression.

mended in the rheumatoid patient in that many have an inherently unstable spine which may be decompensated with traction. Local massage, deep heat, transcutaneous electrical nerve stimulation, and gentle range-of-motion and isometric exercises may all provide some relief to the patient. Modifying analgesic and anti-inflammatory medication and adding a muscle relaxant may reduce the acute pain and relieve the muscle irritability.

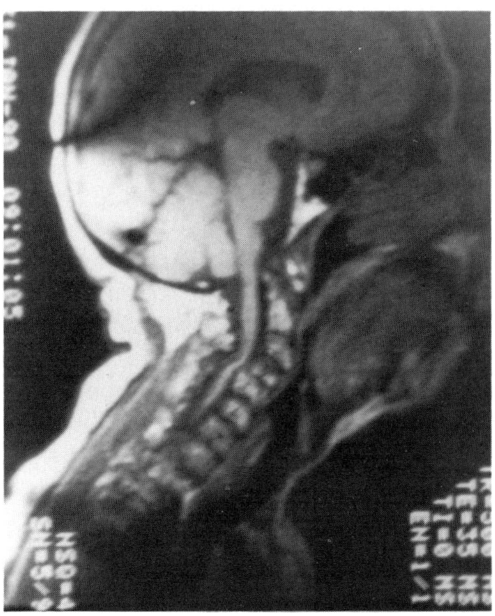

FIG 7–14.
A 35-year-old woman with atlantoaxial and subaxial subluxation. Spinal cord compression is at the subaxial level only.

SURGICAL TREATMENT

EVALUATION OF THE SURGICAL PATIENT

The need for surgical treatment in the rheumatoid cervical spine tends to be uncommon, being indicated in 10% to 15% of patients.[40] This number will be influenced by the criteria used for proceeding with surgical treatment. Many factors in the surgical treatment of the rheumatoid neck can increase the morbidity and mortality associated with the procedures.[14, 15, 42, 46, 52] Since these patients tend to be the most severely affected polyarticular patients, many will have the more serious systemic manifestations of the disease. They are quite debilitated and frail, and many have not been ambulatory either because of the severity of their disease or the myelopathy which accompanies their cervical disease. Anesthetic risks are greater because of airway problems and interstitial pulmonary disease. In the most severe cases elective preoperative tracheostomy may be indicated. Awake nasotracheal intubation using a fiberoptic laryngoscope, positioning the patient while still awake and intubated, has been the method of choice in these patients (Fig 7–15). Neurologic function can then be checked after placing the patient in the prone position and, if unchanged, anesthesia can be administered.

Careful preoperative planning is necessary for these procedures and internal fixation devices must be available prior to surgery. Intraoperative somatosensory monitoring should be used, especially if neurologic status is compromised. Postoperatively, wound healing may be delayed and in our earlier series wound dehiscence was noted because of the excessive use of methylmethacrylate, which increased the bulk within the wound and produced excessive tension on the wound edges.[9]

Attention must be given to the method of rehabilitation to be used postoperatively. This planning must include the type of immobilization and these devices must be available in the operating room. If a

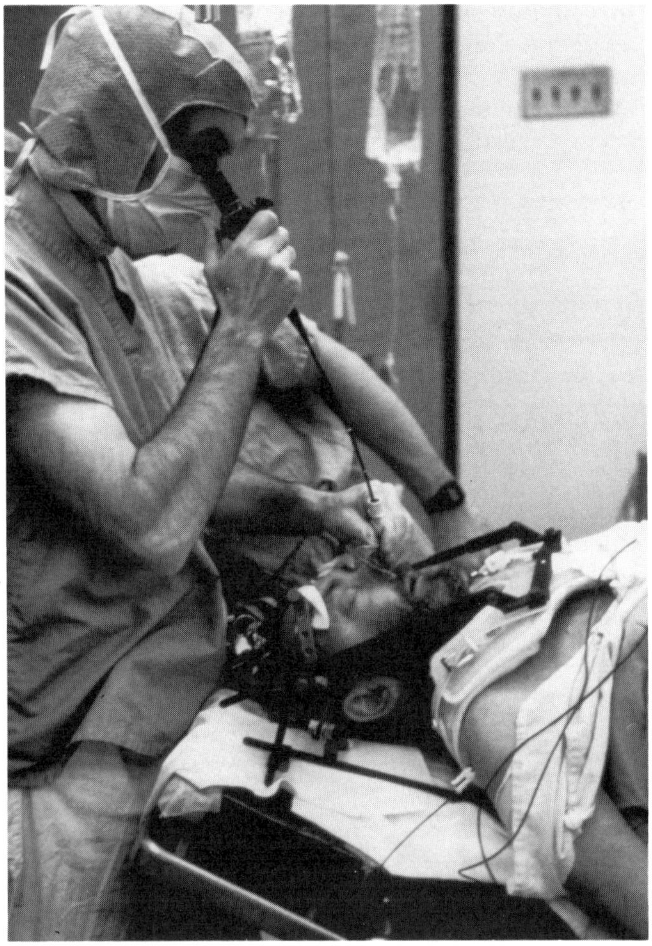

FIG 7–15.
Nasotracheal intubation with mild sedation.

halo is to be used and incorporated into a polyethylene vest postoperatively, this also should be ready in the operating room at the conclusion of the procedure. The rehabilitation of these patients can be quite difficult not only because of their recent neck surgery but because of the severe nature of their underlying disease. Early mobilization from bed is necessary to prevent the pulmonary problems which can prove fatal to these patients in the perioperative period. Skin breakdown, urinary retention and infection, constipation, and impaction aside from pulmonary problems will develop if the patient is kept in bed for more than 48 hours postoperatively. The complex nature of the rheumatoid cervical spine necessitates that the surgeon meet with physical and occupational therapists preoperatively to review the potential and real difficulties anticipated postoperatively and that solutions to these problems be devised.

SURGICAL INDICATIONS

Surgical treatment of the cervical spine in rheumatoid arthritis is indicated when (1) neck and occipital pain is intractable despite all attempts at conservative management, (2) a significant neurologic deficit exists in association with atlantoaxial subluxation, impaction, or subaxial subluxation and (3) there exist symptoms and objective findings indicative of vertebral artery compromise. Although instability by itself does not warrant surgical intervention, the spinal cord is put at risk when advanced degrees of subluxation and instability are present. There is also ample evidence that mortality is greater if cervical myelopathy is allowed to occur.[10, 12, 31, 35, 36, 39, 42, 56, 59] Additionally, once neurologic dysfunction is present, recovery is less predictable. For these reasons surgical treatment is also recommended in cervical spine disease where the spinal cord or brainstem may be at risk. More specifically, atlantoaxial subluxation and instability of greater than 9 mm is considered a surgical indication. Atlantoaxial impaction that demonstrates any compromise of the foramen magnum by the odontoid and spinal cord, or brainstem compression as demonstrated on MRI even in the absence of neurologic symptoms, is an indication for surgical treatment. Subaxial instability of greater than 4 mm with MRI evidence of spinal cord compression also qualifies as a surgical indication in these patients.

SURGICAL TREATMENT OF ATLANTOAXIAL SUBLUXATION

Atlantoaxial subluxation is usually mobile and reduces as the neck is extended. In longstanding cases the subluxation may become fixed but this is uncommon. The surgical treatment is directed toward reducing the unstable segment, stabilizing the atlantoaxial articulation in the reduced position by fusion, and in patients in whom neural compression is demonstrated by MRI, utilizing anterior or posterior decompression depending upon the area of compression.

C1–C2 Arthrodesis

The patient is intubated awake and placed into the prone position. Prior to the induction of anesthesia the patient is asked to move the upper and lower extremities. Skeletal traction is not used routinely intraoperatively if the atlantoaxial subluxation is mobile. A head support is used which allows the neck to be positioned in the neutral position. Positioning of the neck in extension will make exposure difficult, particularly if the patient has a short, heavy neck. Skin folds over the incision area will also interfere with spinal exposure when the neck is extended. Care must be taken not to flex the neck excessively when positioning. A midline incision is used and dissection continued in the midline until the spinous process of C2 is identified. Subperiosteal stripping of muscle from the spinous processes and the laminae of C2 and C3 should be performed to allow adequate exposure. The posterior lamina of the atlas should be exposed next using cautery to remove muscle and fibrous attachments to its bony surface. The arch of the atlas will be anteriorly displaced and depending upon whether there is an element of atlantoaxial impaction it may or may not be difficult to define the superior and inferior margins of the atlas. Using an angled elevator, the ligamentum flavum is dissected from the undersurface of the atlas. This must be done cautiously to prevent anterior slipping into the neural canal. Because of the position of the vertebral arteries, dissection should not extend lateral to the facet joints. It is necessary to clear all ligamentous and fibrous tissue from the undersurface of the posterior arch of the atlas to allow passage of an 18-gauge wire loop from inferior to superior. Two 20-gauge wires may be used if preferred. The passage of the this wire loop is easier if a hook configuration is placed on the wire when passing it from inferior to superior.

Once the loop is visualized superior to the arch it is pulled through and passed around the spinous process of C2. A notch may be made at the base of the spinous process of C2 to fix the wire loop at the base of the process. It is important to have cleared all soft tissues from the base of the spinous process to insure that the wire loop will be at its base. The neck is then extended by the anesthesiologist and the wire ends are tied over the looped wire which is now anterior to the knotted wire. The inferior margin of the atlas should closely approximate the superior margin of the lamina of C2 once the wire has been tied. The anesthesiologist then repositions the head on the frame but in a more extended position.

Decortication of the lamina of the atlas and of C2 is generally performed with a burr prior to the final tying of the wire around the spinous process. The outer cortical surface only should be removed during this procedure. Cancellous iliac crest grafts are used in the lateral gutters and along the decorticated laminae. It is important not to place the grafts under the wire and then tighten the wire over the bone grafts. Graft resorption may occur or the graft may dislodge and fixation by the wire will be lost as it will then be quite lax. A suction drain is used. The wound is closed in layers with interrupted sutures or staples being used for the skin.

If there is evidence of spinal cord compression from the posterior arch of the atlas, laminectomy of this arch should be performed. There is often a constricting fibrous band beneath the lamina which is compressing the dura and an indentation in the dura may be seen. This must be released as part of the decompression procedure. In instances where posterior decompression is necessary, fusion should be extended to the occiput.

If spinal cord compression is anterior by the odontoid, decompression may be performed anteriorly. Crockard et al.[16, 17] have recommended transoral decompression by removal of the anterior arch of the atlas and complete removal of the odontoid and posterior fusion at the same operative setting. Their indications for the procedure are spinal cord or brainstem compression due to: (1) irreducible atlantoaxial subluxation, (2) significant anterior soft tissue (pannus) mass, and (3) vertical migration of the odontoid. The authors reported their results in 68 patients with an early (1 month) operative mortality of 6%. The four deaths were attributed to cord damage at surgery in 1 patient, mesenteric artery thrombosis in 2 patients, and 1 patient died of septicemia. There were cerebrospinal fluid leaks in 6 patients with nonfatal meningitis in 2. Three patients were neurologically worse. Of the remaining 61 patients one third demonstrated a striking improvement and the remainder were improved, although only slightly. The procedure has great merit in that anterior decompression is effected but it should be reserved for those with experience in this approach. Complications are serious and perioperative mortality can occur in this neurologically compromised group of patients.

Nonunion in C1–C2 arthrodesis has been reported in 15% to 33% of patients[10, 20] and has been attributed to the poor-quality bone on the posterior surface of the arch of C1. Clark et al.[10] recommend that halo immobilization be used if bone quality is poor. Methylmethacrylate has been used but improvement in fusion rates is unclear at this time if it is used to augment the fusion site.

A Philadelphia collar worn for 8 to 12 weeks is

used for postoperative immobilization depending upon the progression of the fusion. The patients are mobilized from bed the day after surgery and leave the hospital on the third or fourth postoperative day.

THE SURGICAL TREATMENT OF ATLANTOAXIAL IMPACTION

Surgical stabilization of the occipitocervical junction is necessary in patients with atlantoaxial impaction. Depending upon the degree of superior migration of the odontoid and the degree of spinal cord and brainstem encroachment, decompression may be indicated. Posterior decompression of the foramen magnum and the posterior arch of the atlas is most commonly employed, but transoral anterior decompression by removal of the odontoid may also be considered if compression is primarily anterior. Atlantoaxial impaction is usually fixed and skeletal traction preoperatively is not helpful. The atlas itself may migrate into the foramen magnum making decompression difficult without ample removal of foramen magnum. Many different types of fixation have been employed at this level[8, 22, 28, 43, 45, 56] to augment fixation and facilitate fusion.[47]

Occiput–C2 Arthrodesis

The patient is positioned prone after awake nasotracheal intubation. Neurologic status is checked after final positioning of the neck and then the patient is anesthetized. Positioning of the head on the cervical frame must be in the neutral position to allow ample exposure. A midline incision is used extending from the external occipital protuberance to the spinous process of C3. Dissection is continued in the midline and subperiosteal dissection is performed to remove all soft tissue and muscle from the spinous process of C2 and the posterior arch of the atlas. Dissection is continued onto the occiput and all soft tissue is removed to allow visualization of the foramen magnum and the lower occiput.

If there is posterior compression of the spinal cord or brainstem the foramen magnum is opened using Kerrison rongeurs and a burr. The posterior arch of the atlas also can be removed at this time if it is compressing neural structures anteriorly. Decortication of the occiput, the arch of the atlas if it is not removed, and the lamina of C2 is performed next. Using a heavy titanium fenestrated sheet a dumbbell-shaped plate is fabricated. The broad upper portion of this plate is placed against the occiput and drill holes are made through the outer table of the cranium. Heywood and Learmonth[28] have demonstrated in cadavers that maximum skull thickness is in the region under the external occipital protuberance where it is 11 to 17 mm thick. It remains at least 9 mm thick extending caudad as far as 20 mm from the foramen magnum. The venous sinuses lie under the thick bone caudad to the external occipital protuberance. Drill holes are made using a drill guard to prevent penetration of the cranium of greater than 8 mm. Two 8-mm titanium screws are placed through the fenestrated titanium sheet and this fixes the molded rigid mesh to the occiput. The lower portion of the plate is then molded over the spinous process of C2. A drill hole is placed through the base of the spinous process of C2 and an 18- or 20-gauge wire is placed through the spinous process and the fenestrations on the titanium mesh. By tying this wire over the molded mesh it is fixed to the spinous process (Fig 7–16,A–C).

The construct now supports the occiput and provides a rigid and stable framework incorporating the occiput to the spinous process of C2 (Fig 7–16,D). If decompression has been performed either at the foramen magnum or the posterior lamina of the atlas, the flat portion of the mesh will extend over this area and protect it. Methylmethacrylate is then placed over the construct to improve the rigidity of the titanium and consolidate the screw-mesh-wire complex to the bone. Only a small amount of methylmethacrylate is needed and care should be taken not to make the cement too bulky (Fig 7–16,E). If excess cement is used, wound closure may be under excessive tension and healing may be complicated. An iliac crest graft is used and placed in the lateral gutters along the lamina of C2 extending to the occiput (Fig 7–16,F). A suction drain is usually placed beneath the fascia. The wound is closed in layers and interrupted sutures or staples may be used for the skin (Fig 7–17,A–C).

Postoperatively, a molded Philadelphia collar is used and the patient is quickly mobilized from bed. The collar is used for 8 to 12 weeks depending upon the quality of bone consolidation. In six patients in whom this technique has been used, all have fused. Pain relief has been excellent in all patients. Two patients had neurologic deficits preoperatively, including one with tetraparesis. This last patient improved to become ambulatory and independent of his wheelchair. In this group wound problems did not occur. One patient complained of frontal headaches postoperatively for several months and CT imaging demonstrated that the screws had penetrated the in-

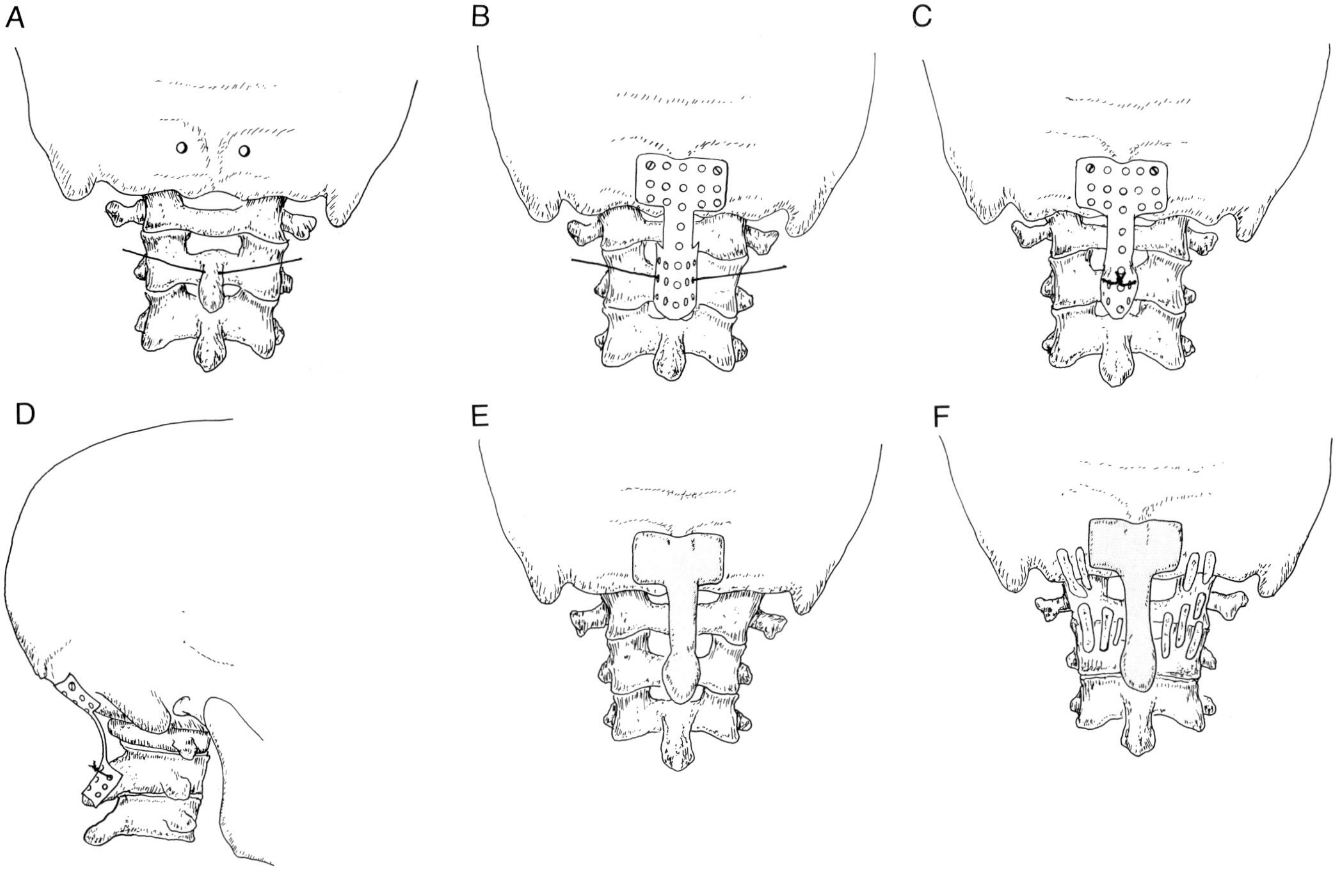

FIG 7–16.
A, the occiput and C2 spinous process exposed. Drill holes are made through the base of the spinous process of C2 and a wire is passed. **B,** titanium mesh plate in place with two screws into the occiput (outer table). The wire through the spinous process of C2 is passed through the mesh. **C,** the wire is tied over the mesh which is molded around the spinous process of C2. **D,** the mesh plate in position supporting the occiput and incorporated into C2. **E,** methylmethacrylate placed around the mesh-wire construct. **F,** an iliac crest bone graft is placed along the lamina and spinous process of C2 and extending to the occiput.

ner table of the cranium. These headaches gradually resolved and were felt to be of frontal sinus origin and no relationship to the screws could be established.

Heywood and Learmonth[28] utilize a similar technique for stabilization of the occipitocervical area. They employ a T-plate which is molded to the occiput and three screws are inserted into the occiput. The plate is screwed and wired to the spinous process of C2. Of 14 patients treated with this technique, 12 fused. One patient died 4 weeks after surgery from sudden respiratory arrest. There was only one pseudarthrosis in this group. Of 8 patients with evidence of cord compression and neurologic deficit, 7 improved. A halo-body orthosis was used in 8 patients. In 1 patient the plate pulled from the occiput after a fall and this was also the patient who went on to pseudarthrosis.

Sakou et al.[45] reported on 16 patients undergoing occipitoatlantoaxial fusion using a rectangular rod for fixation. All patients had atlantoaxial subluxation with 5 of these patients having associated atlantoaxial impaction. Sublaminar wires and wires through the occiput were fixed to the rectangular rod to improve stability. Improvement in pain in the neck and occipital area was noted in all patients. Bone fusion was noted in all patients and there was improvement in those with neurologic symptoms. Paralysis increased in 1 patient which was probably related to use of the sublaminar wire in an already stenotic vertebral canal.

Wertheim and Bohlman[56] described an onlay grafting technique for occipitocervical fusion in which wires are placed through the external occipital protuberance, around the arch of the atlas, and through the spinous process of C2. Two large iliac crest onlay grafts are fashioned and wired from occi-

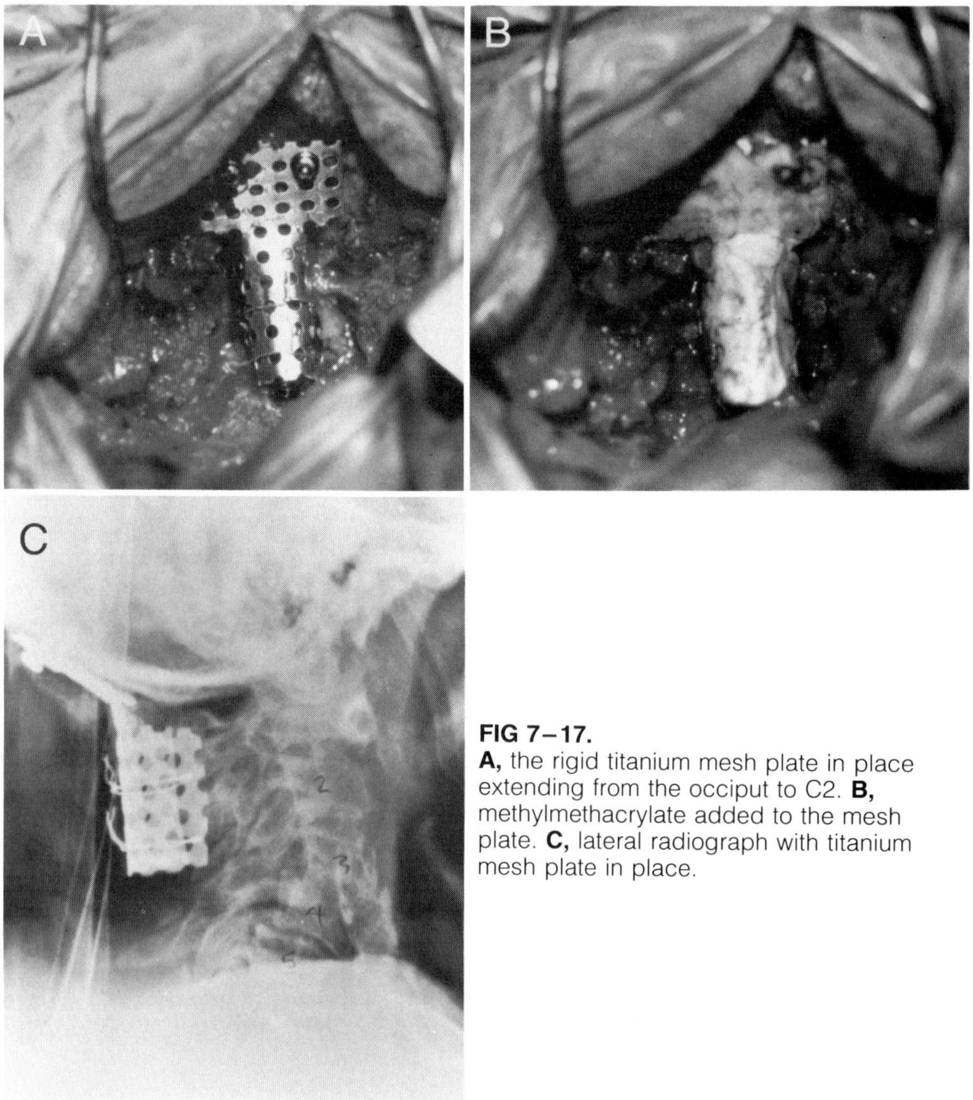

FIG 7–17.
A, the rigid titanium mesh plate in place extending from the occiput to C2. **B,** methylmethacrylate added to the mesh plate. **C,** lateral radiograph with titanium mesh plate in place.

put to C2 on each side of the spinous process. They reported on 13 patients undergoing this technique, 8 with rheumatoid arthritis. All went on to fusion. Ten patients had findings of myelopathy preoperatively, and all improved although 3 with severe motor weakness were only slightly improved and remained nonambulatory. Methylmethacrylate was not used in this series. Patients were immobilized postoperatively in either a rigid two-poster orthosis or a halo cast for 6 to 16 weeks. A soft collar was used for 6 weeks after removal of the orthosis or cast. Ten patients had a satisfactory result, the 3 patients with unsatisfactory results being those with persistent weakness and inability to walk. There were two minor wound complications which resolved on antibiotics and dressing changes.

Slatis et al.[49] reported on 18 patients with atlantoaxial impaction; 6 were treated by fusion and 12 were treated conservatively. Of the 6 fusion patients, 3 required laminectomy of the atlas because of spinal cord compression. The subluxation was arrested with the fusion, but only 4 of the 6 patients had significant functional improvement. The 12 conservatively treated patients demonstrated a progression in their cranial subluxation of the odontoid of 8.6 to 10.5 mm. Two of the conservatively treated patients died during the follow-up period from cardiac causes. In 6 of the remaining 10 patients treated conservatively, their overall condition had deteriorated. Complaints of severe dizziness and chronic occipitocervical pain were common. Four of the 6 patients demonstrated a decreased ability to walk. Neurologic assessment in the nonsurgical group showed a deterioration in class grade in 4 of the 10 patients, with the others remaining unchanged. In the 6 operatively treated patients the neurologic assessment revealed improvement by class grade in 2 patients. Two other patients had improved upper extremity strength and 2 were unchanged.

Surgical treatment is indicated early in patients with atlantoaxial impaction. Vertical migration of the odontoid and progressive destruction of the occipitocervical and atlantoaxial joints and spinal cord and brainstem compromise occur frequently. Mortality and morbidity are significantly reduced if neurologic dysfunction is not severe at the time of surgical intervention. Neurologic recovery is more predictable if irreversible spinal cord and brainstem damage has not occurred. Stabilization procedures have improved significantly to insure high fusion rates with low perioperative morbidity.

THE SURGICAL TREATMENT OF SUBAXIAL SUBLUXATION

Subaxial instability in rheumatoid arthritis occurs in the same population as atlantoaxial subluxation and impaction, namely, those patients most severely affected by the disease. Additionally, subaxial instability is seen in combination with cervical involvement at the occipitocervical and atlantoaxial levels. In a review of 33 patients undergoing surgical stabilization[42] at The Hospital for Special Surgery, 70% had evidence of atlantoaxial subluxation, 60% demonstrated subaxial instability, and 16% had atlantoaxial impaction. The questions that arise in the treatment of subaxial instability are (1) whom to fuse, (2) where to fuse, (3) how to fuse, (4) whether to decompress or not, and (5) what immobilization to use postoperatively.

The indications for surgical stabilization in subaxial subluxation are similar to those for upper cervical subluxation: pain unrelieved by other nonsurgical measures, neurologic deficit, and evidence of significant subluxation (>3–4 mm), with evidence of spinal cord compression on MRI. The difficulty in surgical planning arises when there are multiple levels of subluxation both in the subaxial area and concomitant subluxation or impaction is present at the atlantoaxial level. As a rule, once the decision has been made to progress with surgical stabilization, all levels demonstrating instability should be included in the fusion. The primary reason for this is that if the fusion mass ends at a level above an unstable segment, progression will occur below the fusion mass. If there is disease at the atlantoaxial level that indicates surgical treatment, it should be addressed during the same operative setting as the subaxial fusion. Because of the tendency for subluxation to occur and progress below the level of a fusion, it is recommended that one level should not be left open between two fusion masses, as the interface forces at the open segment will be sufficient to produce major subluxation at the one open segment. At least two open segments should exist between two levels of fusion mass. In the lower cervical spine, if fusion is to be performed to the C6–7 level, it is recommended that the fusion be extended to T1. By fusing to this first rib-bearing vertebra, which has additional stability anteriorly from the rib as an anterior strut, the chance of subluxation may be reduced.

Subaxial Arthrodesis

Once the levels for fusion have been decided on, based on the radiographic and MRI findings, awake nasotracheal intubation is performed and anesthesia administered only after positioning and a neurologic examination. A midline skin incision is made and the fascia overlying the cervical spinous processes incised. Subperiosteal dissection continues along the spinous processes of the cervical vertebra and along the laminae lateral to the level of the facet joints. An intraoperative lateral radiograph is taken to verify the level of dissection. Decortication is performed along the spinous processes and laminae of the affected vertebral levels. Drill holes are made through the bases of the spinous processes to be fused (Fig 7–18,A). Twenty gauge wire is passed through these drill holes with individual wires being placed at each level. A rigid fenestrated titanium mesh rectangular plate is fashioned that is approximately 2 cm wide and the length of the fusion site (Fig 7–18,B). This is molded like a cupola over the spinous processes to the full extent of the area to be fused and the wires are passed through the fenestrations at each level. The wires are then tied over the titanium mesh and the mesh is compressed so that it adheres to the surface of the spinous processes (Fig 7–18,C). Most subaxial subluxations cannot be reduced and are fused in situ. If there is mobility and improvement with neck extension, wires are tightened with the neck extended by the anesthesiologist and the neck is repositioned in its frame in an extended position. Methylmethacrylate is placed into the mesh-wire-spinous process composite and allowed to harden (Fig 7–18,D). This consolidates the fusion segments and provides immediate immobilization. An iliac crest bone graft is used along the lateral gutters of the spinous processes and laminae traversing the levels to be fused (Fig 7–18,E). A suction drain is

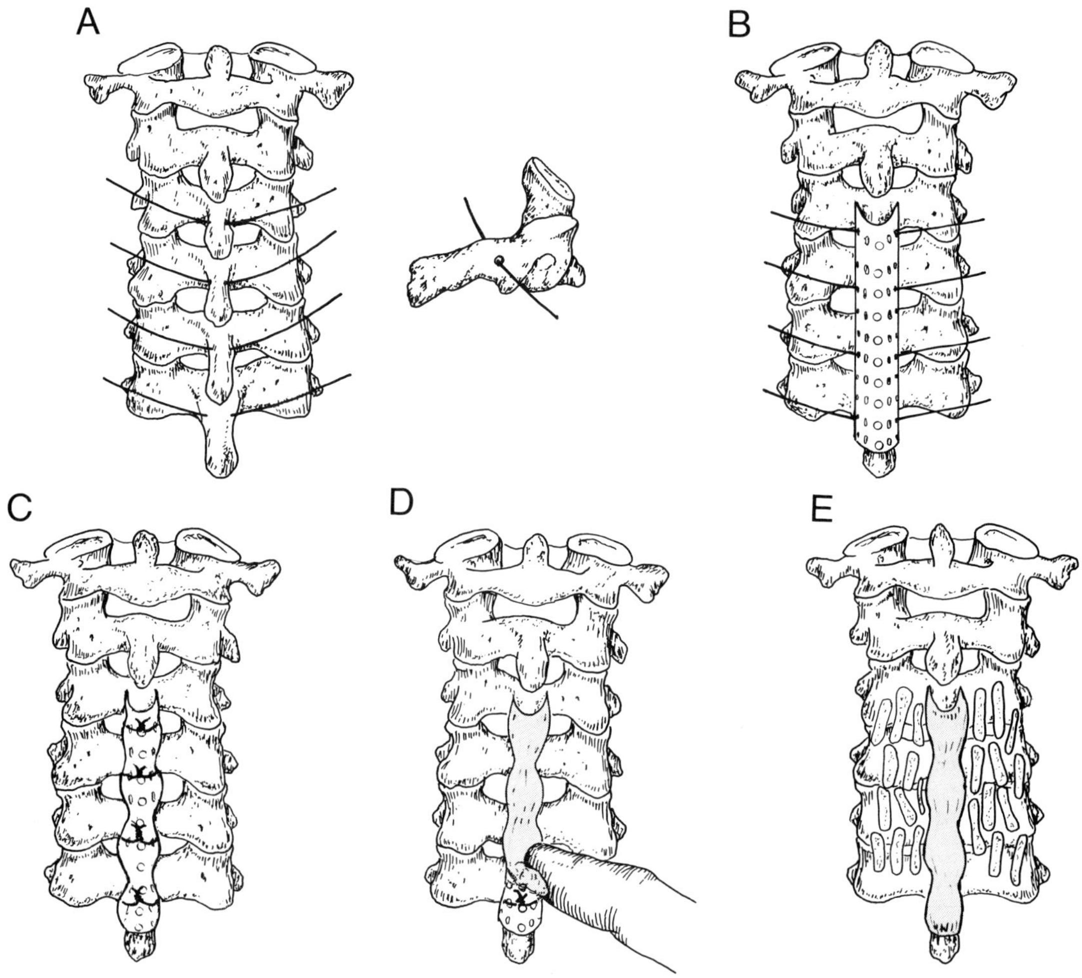

FIG 7–18.
A, wires placed through the base of spinous processes. **B,** wires passed through the fenestration in the titanium mesh. **C,** mesh plate molded to the spinous processes and wire tied over the mesh. **D,** methylmethacrylate added to the mesh-wire composite. **E,** iliac crest bone graft placed along the laminae of the fusion site.

used below the fascia and the wound is closed in layers (Fig 7–19,A–E).

Decompression may be indicated if there is neurologic deficit and evidence of spinal cord compression on MRI. If the area of compression is posterior, then laminectomy should be performed and the fusion should extend one level above and below the area of decompression, particularly if the facet joints are involved in the decompression. Anterior decompression may be performed if spinal cord compromise is anterior. Excision of the vertebral body may be performed with bone grafting, or internal fixation cages may be used to fill the void after decompression. Posterior fusion should always be performed after anterior decompression whether or not there has been anterior fusion or stabilization. Four of five patients treated by anterior fusion went on to poor results in a series of patients from our institution, with collapse and resorption of the graft and pseudarthrosis. Kudo[31] reported recurrent myelopathy in four of six patients treated anteriorly by decompression and anterior fusion alone.

Postoperatively, a molded Philadelphia collar is used for 8 to 12 weeks. Halo orthoses have not been used in these patients. Preoperative skeletal traction has not been helpful in these patients and the prolonged bed rest can result in serious pressure ulcerations or systemic complications.

Santavirta et al.[47] reported on 16 patients with subaxial instability. Three patients had associated atlantoaxial subluxation. Nine of the patients had evidence of neurologic deficit and 5 had severe tetraparesis. All patients with neurologic deficit underwent decompression and posterior fusion. All other

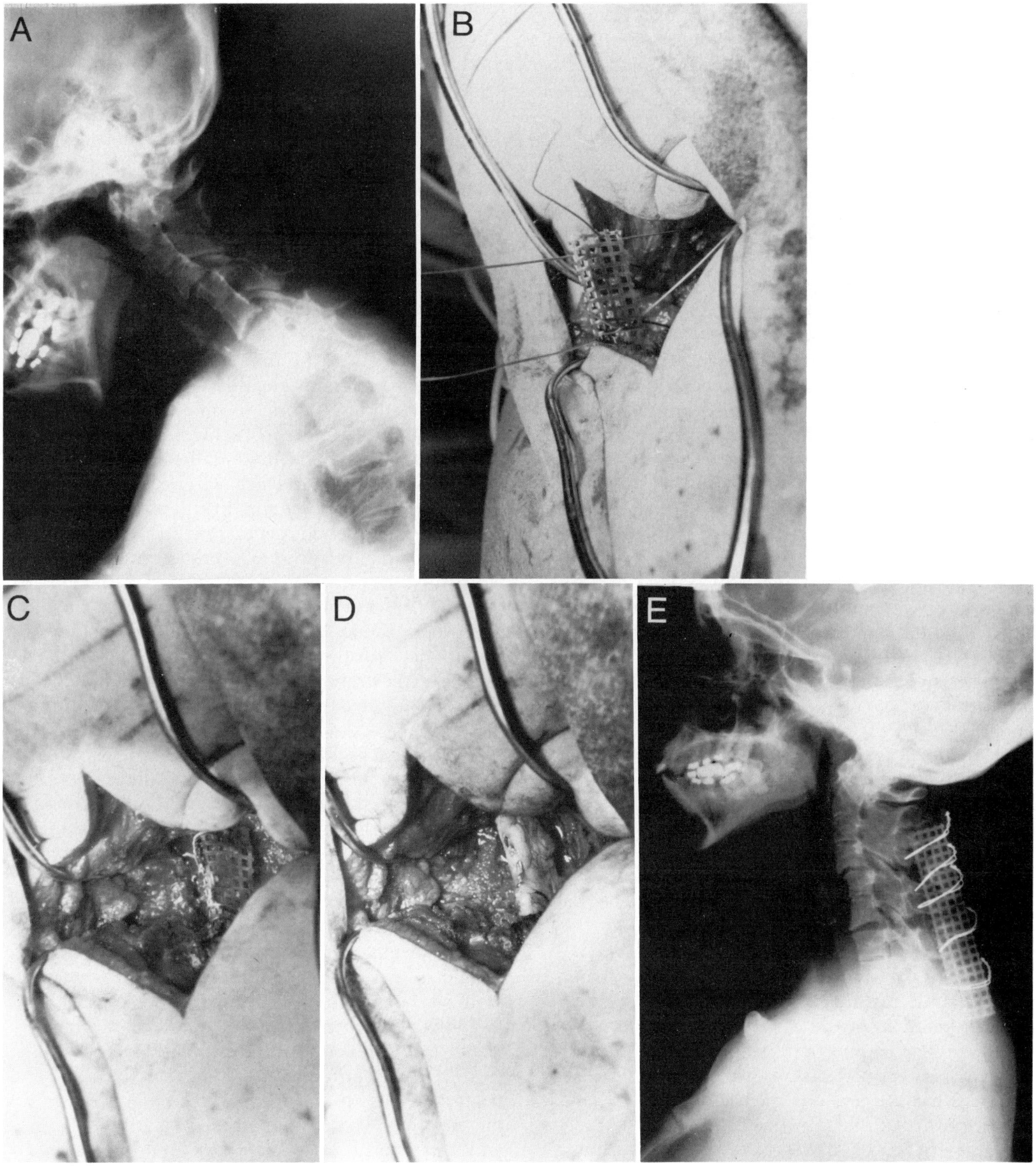

FIG 7–19.
A, a 38-year-old woman with multiple-level subaxial subluxation. **B,** wires being passed through the mesh plate. **C,** mesh "cupola" in place with wires tied over the mesh. **D,** methylmethacrylate incorporating the mesh-wire composite. **E,** postoperative lateral radiograph.

patients underwent posterior fusion alone. Two patients died in the postoperative period, 1 with a myocardial infarction on postoperative day 15 and the other from staphylococcus septicemia and pneumonia. Skeletal traction was used postoperatively in 8 patients for periods ranging from 2 to 8 weeks. Tetraparesis was relieved in 8 of 9 patients with the remaining patient being one of the reported deaths. There were 3 patients who at follow-up evaluation developed new subluxations below the level of fusion, 2 of whom underwent further stabilization.

Kudo[31] reported on 27 procedures for subaxial subluxation, all with evidence of myelopathy. Surgical fusion was performed in all patients. Eighteen patients had good recovery of neurologic function after surgery, five were fair, three poor, and one patient was worse. Two patients died of cause related to their surgery. Treatment was based on localization of disease, and anterior decompression and fusion was performed if compression of the cord was anterior. Anterior interbody fusion was unsuccessful in four patients who had recurrence of their myelopathy.

Bryan, Inglis, Sculco, et al.[9] described the early experience with methylmethacrylate-augmented fusions done primarily for subaxial disease. Eleven patients were treated with wiring or mesh and methylmethacrylate. Bone grafting was performed in all patients. Ten patients demonstrated relief of pain and resolution of neurologic dysfunction. One patient demonstrated subluxation below the fusion mass and died. There were two pseudarthroses and both required further surgery.

METHYLMETHACRYLATE-AUGMENTED CERVICAL FUSIONS

Spinal arthrodesis for subluxation in the rheumatoid cervical spine requires immobilization in the postoperative period to insure a solid fusion. External immobilizing techniques have been employed most frequently after cervical fusion in these patients. These external fixation methods include the use of a halo device with multiple pin fixation into the skull. The halo may be attached with side struts to a thoracic polyethylene jacket or it may be incorporated into a plaster vest. This provides secure immobilization to the cervical spine. The problem with these devices in rheumatoid patients, however, is their inability to tolerate them for extended periods. The outer table of the skull into which these fixation pins are inserted tends to be osteopenic, as is the rest of the rheumatoid skeleton. Migration of these pins can occur as well as disengagement. Pressure areas beneath the immobilizing vest can lead to skin breakdown and ulceration. The constricting nature of these orthoses may limit chest excursion, and pulmonary complications may ensue. The cumbersome nature of these devices and their weight may limit the ability of the rheumatoid patient to ambulate and be mobilized from bed or wheelchair. For all these reasons it is important to attempt improved internal fixation in the rheumatoid patient and reserve use of these external immobilizing orthoses for the most extreme situations.

Bone quality at the time of cervical fusion is frequently poor and may not allow secure stabilization with conventional wiring techniques alone. Therefore, with the success of methylmethacrylate as an adjunct to internal fixation in the management of pathologic fractures, its use was reasonable in the rheumatoid spine. Alsharif[2] first reported its use in children with juvenile rheumatoid arthritis and atlantoaxial subluxation in 1969. Brattstrom and Granholm in 1976 reported the first large series utilizing fixation with wire and methylmethacrylate. Twenty-eight patients underwent occipitocervical fusions using this technique, with all patients but one experiencing improvement in their symptoms. Five patients still had some pain or weakness but described themselves as improved. There were no perioperative deaths. Two patients developed wound infections which were treated with antibiotics and resolved. The spinous process of C2 broke in two patients, and both required reoperation. In two patients there was breakage of the wire and lost of position which required further surgical treatment.

Wound dehiscence and infection occurred in 4 of the 11 patients treated with a wiring and methylmethacrylate technique in our early series.[9] This was related to the excessive bulk and amount of methylmethacrylate used and these wounds all healed with debulking of the bone cement and antibiotics. One of these infections occurred 3 months after surgical treatment and at reexploration of the wound a solid posterior fusion was present. Since this early report this technique has been used 13 additional times with one wound infection. Clark et al.[10] described 1 patient who incurred an occiptal erosion from the methylmethacrylate and three superficial wound infections that responded to local wound care and antibiotics in 41 patients in their study.

Despite the clinical success with methylmethacrylate as an augmentative agent for internal stabilization, Whitehill et al.[57] have raised doubts as to its efficacy. In studies where methylmethacrylate was implanted into the cervical spine of the dog, they noted significant fibrous tissue layering around the bone-cement interface. This was morphologically similar but not identical to the tissue seen at the bone-cement interface in loose mechanically failed joint replacements. Bone graft, however, was not used in this study. Whitehill et al. also question whether the stabilizing effect of the methylmethacrylate is present long enough to allow consolidation of the bone graft, if used. The bone, therefore, is not mature enough to stabilize the spine once the methylmethacrylate has lost its effectiveness. One additional concern is that the cement-bone interface, as loosening occurs, may lead to resorption of bone by activation of collagenases. These are theoretical considerations of concern, but clinical experience has not demonstrated loosening of cement or failure to fuse when methylmethacrylate is employed.[6, 9–11, 19]

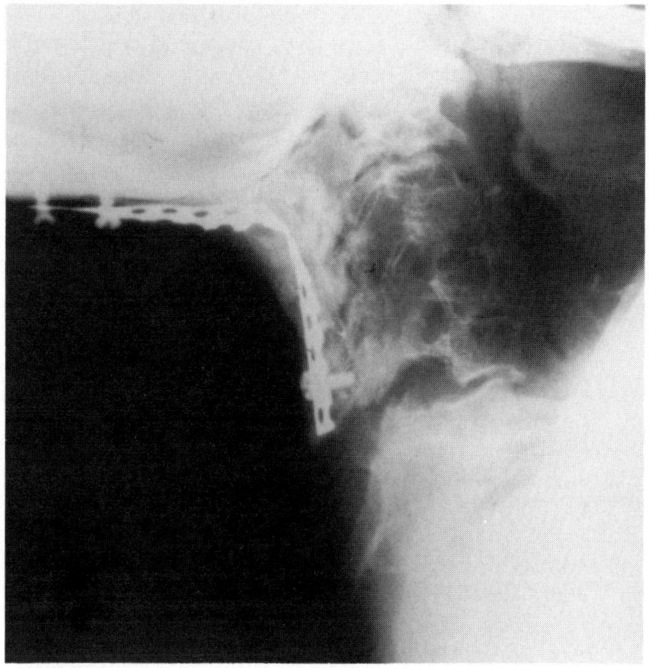

FIG 7–20.
Subaxial subluxation after spinal fusion.

SUBLUXATION BELOW THE CERVICAL ARTHRODESIS SITE

Multiple reports[9, 10, 12, 47] have demonstrated the incidence of subluxation and instability below the fusion mass. This has occurred in the upper cervical spine after atlantoaxial fusion as well as in the subaxial area. Since the disease is diffuse and involves to varying degrees the entire cervical spine, pathologic changes are usually present below the level of cervical fusion. The additional stresses on the interface joints and intervertebral disc below a rigid fusion mass are considerable. This combination of circumstances, the abnormal anatomy and increased stress across this site, provides a setting for subluxation at this interface level. The greater the length of the fusion mass, the greater the rigidity and the more marked the stresses at the interface joint between the fusion and the remaining cervical spine (Fig 7–20). These interface subluxations can be quite marked, produce spinal cord compromise, and require further surgical treatment.

Treatment options to prevent this are limited in that stabilization must resolve the subluxed zone. To lessen the chance of subluxation in the subaxial area, fusion of all abnormal segments is recommended. Avoidance of a single level between two fused areas is also important as the stresses on this open level will certainly lead to subluxation at this level. Careful follow-up examinations with radiographs should be routinely performed in all patients after cervical spine surgery. If evidence of subluxation below a fusion mass is identified, frequent radiographs are necessary and MRI scanning should be performed to define impending or present neural compression. If subluxation is severe and neural compromise occurs, extension of the fusion is necessary.

CONCLUSIONS

Cervical spine involvement in rheumatoid arthritis is the most potentially debilitating and life-threatening of all the skeletal manifestations of the disease. Profound cervical myelopathy superimposed on a debilitated patient with polyarticular rheumatoid disease will produce a catastrophic loss of function and jeopardize life. Too often the subtle alterations in function which herald a myelopathy are missed and only when neurologic function is severely impaired is attention paid to these findings. Surgical treatment at these more advanced stages of myelopathy are less predictable in their ability to reverse neurologic loss. Mortality increases in the perioperative period as neurologic impairment progresses. Early surgical treatment in the rheumatoid patient is recommended when instability is advanced and if there is evidence of spinal cord or brainstem compromise. Procedures performed at this stage will produce a better functional result for the patient and provide excellent relief of pain. Perioperative complications will be less and the risk of surgical mortality will be minimal.

REFERENCES

1. Alexiades MM, Inglis AE: Use of the MRI in evaluation of atlantoaxial subluxation in rheumatoid arthritis. *Orthop Trans* 1990; 14:109–110.
2. Alsharif H: Methylmethacrylate spinal fusion. Its use in spontaneous atlantoaxial subluxation in children. *Egypt Orthop J* 1969; 4:11–16.
3. Althoff B, Goldie E: Cervical collars in rheumatoid atlantoaxial subluxation: A radiographic comparison. *Ann Rheum Dis* 1980; 39:485–489.
4. Anda S, Nilsen G, Roysland P: Periodontoid changes in rheumatoid arthritis, MRI observations . *Scand J Rheumatol* 1988; 17:59–62.
5. Bland JH: Rheumatoid arthritis of the cervical spine. *J Rheumatol* 1974; 1:319–41.
6. Brattstrom H, Granholm L: Atlantoaxial fusion in rheumatoid arthritis: A new method of fixation with wire and bone cement. *Acta Orthop Scand* 1976; 47:619–628.
7. Braunstein EM, Weissman BN, Seltzer SE, et al: Computed tomography and conventional radiographs of the craniocervical region in rheumatoid arthritis. *Arthritis Rheum* 1984; 27:26–31.
8. Breedveld FC, Algra PR, Vielvoye CJ, et al: Magnetic resonance imaging in the evaluation of patients with rheumatoid arthritis and subluxation of the cervical spine. *Arthritis Rheum* 1987; 30:624–629.
9. Bryan WJ, Inglis AE, Sculco TP, et al: Methylmethacrylate stabilization for enhancement of posterior cervical arthrodesis in rheumatoid arthritis. *J Bone Joint Surg [Am]* 1982; 64:1045–1049.
10. Clark CR, Goetz DD, Menezes AH: Arthrodesis of the cervical spine in rheumatoid arthritis. *J Bone Joint Surg [Am]* 1989; 71:381–391.
11. Clark CR, Keggi KJ, Panjabi MM: Methylmethacrylate stabilization of the cervical spine. *J Bone Joint Surg [Am]* 1984; 66A:40–46.
12. Conaty JP, Mongan ES: Cervical fusions in rheumatoid arthritis. *J Bone Joint Surg [Am]* 1981; 63:1218–1227.
13. Conlon PN, Isdale IC, Rose BS: Rheumatoid arthritis of the cervical spine. *Ann Rheum Dis* 1966; 25:120–128.
14. Cregan JCF: Internal fixation of the unstable rheumatoid cervical spine. *Ann Rheum Dis* 1966; 25:242–252.
15. Crellin RQ, Maccabe JJ, Hamilton EB: Severe subluxation of the cervical spine in rheumatoid arthritis. *J Bone Joint Surg [Br]* 1970; 52:244–251.
16. Crockard HA, Calder I, Ransford AO: One stage transoral decompression and posterior fixation in rheumatoid atlantoaxial subluxation. *J Bone Joint Surg [Br]* 1990; 72:682–685.
17. Crockard HA, Essigman WK, Stevens JM, et al: Surgical treatment of cervical cord compression in rheumatoid arthritis. *Ann Rheum Dis* 1985; 44:809–816.
18. Davis FW, Markley HE: Rheumatoid arthritis with death from medullary compression. *Ann Intern Med* 1951; 35:451–455.
19. Dugdale TW, Raycroft JF: The use of cement forms to control methylmethacrylate in immediate posterior stabilization of the cervical spine. *Orthopedics* 1988; 5:707–711.
20. Fehring TK, Brooks AL: Upper cervical instability in rheumatoid arthritis. *Clin Orthop* 1987; 221:137–148.
21. Fielding JW, Cochran GV, Lawsing JF, et al: Tears of the transverse ligament of the atlas. A clinical and biomechanical study. *J Bone Joint Surg [Am]* 1974; 56:1683–1690.
22. Ferlic DS, Clayton ML, Leidholt JD, et al: Surgical treatment of the symptomatic unstable cervical spine in rheumatoid arthritis. *J Bone Joint Surg [Am]* 1975; 57:349–354.
23. Floyd AS, Learmonth ID, Mody G, et al: Atlantoaxial instability and neurologic indicators in rheumatoid arthritis. *Clin Orthop* 1989; 241:177–182.
24. Garrod AE: *A Treatise on Rheumatism and Rheumatoid Arthritis.* London, C Griffin, 1890.
25. Halla JT, Fallahi S, Hardin JG: Nonreducible rotational head tilt and lateral mass collapse: a prospective study of frequency, radiographic findings and clinical features in patients with rheumatoid arthritis. *Arthritis Rheum* 1982; 25:1316–1324.
26. Halla JT, Hardin JG: The spectrum of atlantoaxial facet joint involvement in rheumatoid arthritis. *Arthritis Rheum* 1990; 33:325–329.
27. Halla JT, Hardin JG, Vitek J, et al: Involvement of the cervical spine in rheumatoid arthritis. *Arthritis Rheum* 1989; 32:652–659.
28. Heywood AW, Learmonth MT: Internal fixation for occipitocervical fusion. *J Bone Joint Surg [Br]* 1988; 70:708–711.
29. Isdale IC, Conlon PW: Atlantoaxial subluxation. A six year follow-up report. *Ann Rheum Dis* 1971; 30:387–391.
30. Kontinnen YT, Santavirta S, Kauppi M, et al: Atlantoaxial laxity in rheumatoid arthritis. *Acta Orthop Scand* 1989; 60:379–382.
31. Kudo H: Surgical treatment of subaxial cervical myelopathy in rheumatoid arthritis. *J Bone Joint Surg* 1991; 73:474–480.
32. Lipson S: Rheumatoid arthritis in the cervical spine. *Clin Orthop* 1989; 239:121–127.
33. Martel W, Abell MR: Fatal atlantoaxial subluxation in rheumatoid arthritis. *Arthritis Rheum* 1963; 6:224–231.

34. Matthews J: Atlantoaxial subluxation in rheumatoid arthritis. *Ann Rheum Dis* 1974; 30:526–531.
35. Meijers KAE, Cats A, Kremer HPH, et al: Cervical myelopathy in rheumatoid arthritis. *Clin Exp Rheumatol* 1984; 2:239–245.
36. Meijers KA, Van Beusekom GT, Luyendijk W, et al: Dislocation of the cervical spine with cord compression in rheumatoid arthritis. *J Bone Joint Surg [Br]* 1974; 56:668–675.
37. Modic MT, Weinstein MA, Pavlicek W: Magnetic resonance imaging of the cervical spine: Technical and clinical observation. *AJR* 1983; 141:1129–1136.
38. Modic MT, Rose SS, Masaryk TJ: Imaging of degenerative disease of the cervical spine. *Clin Orthop* 1989; 239:109–110.
39. Morizono Y, Sakou T, Kawaida H: Upper cervical involvement in rheumatoid arthritis. *Spine* 1986; 12:721–725.
40. Pellicci PM, Ranawat CS, Tsairis P, et al: The natural history of rheumatoid arthritis of the cervical spine. *J Bone Joint Surg [Am]* 1981; 63:342–350.
41. Rana NA, Hancock DO, Taylor AR, et al: Upward translocation of the dens in rheumatoid arthritis. *J Bone Joint Surg [Br]* 1973; 55:471–479.
42. Ranawat CS, O'Leary P, Pellicci P, et al: Cervical spine fusion in rheumatoid arthritis. *J Bone Joint Surg [Am]* 1979; 61:1003–1010.
43. Ransford AO, Crockard HA, Pozo JL, et al: Craniocervical instability treated by contoured loop fixation. *J Bone Joint Surg [Br]* 1986; 68:173–177.
44. Redlund-Johnell I, Petterson H: Radiographic measurements of the cranio-vertebral region. *Acta Radiol* 1984; 25:23–29.
45. Sakou T, Kawaida H, Morizono Y, et al: Occiptioatlantoaxial fusion utilizing a rectangular rod. *Clin Orthop* 1989; 239:136–148.
46. Santavirta S, Kontinnen YT, Laasonen E, et al: Ten year results of operations for rheumatoid cervical spine disorders. *J Bone Joint Surg [Br]* 1991; 73:116–120.
47. Santavirta S, Kontinnen YT, Sandelin J, et al: Operations for the unstable cervical spine in rheumatoid arthritis. *Acta Orthop Scand* 1990; 61:106–116.
48. Sharp J, Purser DW, Lausanne JS: Rheumatoid arthritis of the cervical spine in adults. *Ann Rheum Dis* 1958; 17:303–313.
49. Slatis P, Santavirta S, Sandelin J, et al: Cranial subluxation of the odontoid process in rheumatoid arthritis. *J Bone Joint Surg [Am]* 1989; 71:189–195.
50. Smith PA, Benn RT, Sharp J: Natural history of rheumatoid cervical subluxations. *Ann Rheum Dis* 1972; 31:431–438.
51. Smith PA, Sharp J, Kellgren JH: Natural history of rheumatoid arthritis cervical subluxations (abstract). *Ann Rheum Dis* 1972; 31:222.
52. Surnion DR, Hamilton EB, Mathews JA, et al: Vertebral subluxation of the axis in rheumatoid arthritis. *Ann Rheum* 1972; 31:359–363.
53. Toolanen G, Kniebestol M, Larsson SE: Dilatation of cervical ventricles in patients with rheumatoid vertebral atlanto-axial subluxation. *Scand J Rheumatol* 1985; 14:298–302.
54. Webb FW, Hickman JA, Brew D: Death from vertebral artery. *Br Med J* 1968; 2:537–539.
55. Weissman BN, Aliabadi P, Weinfeld MS, et al: Prognostic features of atlantoaxial subluxation in rheumatoid arthritis patients. *Radiology* 1982; 144:745–751.
56. Wertheim SB, Bohlman HH: Occipitocervical fusion. *J Bone Joint Surg [Am]* 1987; 69:833–836.
57. Whitehill R, Drucker S, McCoig JA, et al: Indications and characterization of an interface tissue by implantation of methylmethacrylate cement into the posterior part of the cervical spine of the dog. *J Bone Joint Surg [Am]* 1988; 70:51–59.
58. Winfield J, Cooke D, Brook AS, et al: A prospective study of the radiological changes in the cervical spine in early rheumatoid disease. *Ann Rheum Dis* 1981; 40:109–114.
59. Zoma A, Sturrock RD, Fisher WD, et al: Surgical stabilization of the rheumatoid cervical spine. *J Bone Joint Surg [Br]* 1987; 69:8–12.

CHAPTER 8

The Shoulder

Matthew J. Kraay, M.D.

Mark P. Figgie, M.D.

INTRODUCTION

Rheumatoid arthritis and other inflammatory arthropathies frequently involve the shoulder joint, resulting in pain and contributing to the overall disability of affected patients. Although shoulder involvement rarely occurs during the initial or early presentation of rheumatoid arthritis, the majority of patients will develop some manifestation of rheumatoid arthritis in the shoulder during the later course of their disease.[4, 33] The broad spectrum of potential rheumatoid involvement about the shoulder and the diffuse, systemic nature of the disease often make precise anatomic localization of these problems difficult. This difficulty is further compounded by the typically observed variations in the activity of the underlying inflammatory disease and the frequent simultaneous involvement of several discrete anatomic locations about the shoulder. These factors make both the diagnosis and the treatment of shoulder problems in the patient with rheumatoid arthritis a challenge to the orthopaedic surgeon and rheumatologist. Nevertheless, a relatively pain-free, mobile shoulder in the rheumatoid patient with upper or lower extremity involvement is critical to maintenance of the most basic activities of daily living. Frequently, this goal can only be achieved with appropriate surgical treatment, after an adequate trial of conservative management has failed.

BIOMECHANICAL AND FUNCTIONAL CONSIDERATIONS

A painless, stable, and satisfactorily mobile shoulder is a critical determinant of the overall function of the upper extremity. In the rheumatoid patient with functional limitations of other joints in the upper extremity, maintenance of adequate shoulder function can be essential for the independence of the patient. Significant functional limitation of the shoulder and the ipsilateral elbow occurs frequently, and can be most disabling. Although the range-of-motion requirements for most activities of daily living have been established for the elbow,[23] similar requirements for the shoulder are more difficult to determine. Fortunately, the shoulder has a generous reserve of possible motion, as a result of its relatively unconstrained glenohumeral joint, and contributions from the scapulothoracic, acromioclavicular, and sternoclavicular articulations.

In general, motion at the glenohumeral joint appears to predominate during the first 30 degrees of elevation, while both glenohumeral and scapulothoracic motion appear to contribute equally to the last 60 degrees of elevation.[5] Throughout the entire arc of shoulder movement, the overall ratio of glenohumeral to scapulothoracic motion is approximately 2 to 1. Frequently, range of motion of the shoulder is severely limited in the patient with rheumatoid arthritis. Despite this, satisfactory function of the extremity may be maintained, provided the shoulder is relatively painless and the limited arc of shoulder motion occurs in a functional range.

In the normal shoulder, glenohumeral motion approximates the situation of pure rotation around a relatively fixed center of rotation. In actuality, some limited gliding and rolling motion does occur in the glenohumeral joint under normal circumstances. The instant center of rotation of the normal shoulder has been estimated to be contained within a locus of points 6 ± 2 mm from the geometric center of the humeral head, which supports this approximation.[27, 28] For this relatively pure rotation to occur, translation of the humeral head on the glenoid must be restrained.

In many joints, such as the hip, the conformity of the articular surface limits translation that may occur from rolling or gliding. Since the glenohumeral articular surface lacks the inherent constraint for restriction of this translation, it is provided instead by the dynamic stabilizing effect of the rotator cuff muscles. With active movement of the shoulder, the rotator cuff muscles act in concert to stabilize the humeral head against the glenoid, and provide a fulcrum for rotation to occur. Normally, during the first 30 degrees of elevation of the arm, an associated superior translation of the humeral head of 3 mm occurs. It is theorized that this superior translation of the humeral head in the glenoid occurs as a result of the upwardly directed pull of the deltoid during initiation of abduction. During the remainder of arm elevation, additional translation is limited to only 1 mm in the superior or inferior direction.[27, 28] Patients with rotator cuff deficiencies, which occur frequently in the rheumatoid patient, or with altered shoulder mechanics for other reasons, can have abnormal superior translation of up to 1 cm. Instant center analysis has demonstrated considerable variation of the center of rotation in these patients, indicating that a greater degree of gliding and rolling motion is occurring at the joint surface. Loss of the soft tissue interposition of the rotator cuff and unbalanced pull of the deltoid during initiation of arm elevation are possible explanations for this excessive superior translation.

Because its line of action is orientated parallel to the glenoid at low angles of elevation, deltoid activation tends to cause peripheral loading of the glenoid. This results in a joint reaction force which is directed superiorly. The line of action of the other principal elevator of the shoulder, the supraspinatus, is orientated approximately perpendicular to the glenoid surface at low angles of elevation. This results in a more centrally directed joint reaction force. The magnitude of forces across the shoulder joint with simple arm elevation has been estimated to approach one half to one times body weight.[20, 28] These factors have important implications for the design, fixation, stability, and loading of the glenoid component of a total shoulder arthroplasty. The patient with rotator cuff deficiency typically not only loses the balancing force of the supraspinatus, resulting in an upwardly directed joint reaction force, but also experiences superior translation of the point of application of this force. The result of these alterations in normal mechanics is eccentric loading of the glenoid which can, post arthroplasty, lead to instability, component loosening, and accelerated polyethylene wear. Frequently, when ambulation requires the use of assistive devices, weightbearing through the shoulder is required in the rheumatoid patient. The magnitudes and directions of these externally applied forces can have a further adverse effect on shoulder implant function and longevity.

ROTATOR CUFF DISEASE AND IMPINGEMENT SYNDROME

The continuum of subacromial impingement and rotator cuff disease in the rheumatoid patient can present in much the same way as it does in the patient with degenerative joint disease. In the rheumatoid patient, however, inflammatory synovitis of the glenohumeral joint and periarticular bursae play the primary role in the initiation of these syndromes. This differs from the typical etiology of degenerative rotator cuff disease, in which inflammation occurs secondarily from impingement underneath the subacromial arch. The consequences of these different mechanisms have implications regarding both the presentation and treatment of rotator cuff disease in the rheumatoid patient.

Rheumatoid synovitis involving the glenohumeral joint results not only in the typical loss of articular cartilage from the joint but also compromises the integrity and function of the surrounding soft tissues. Attenuation of the joint capsule and tendons of the rotator cuff, caused by chronic intraarticular synovial proliferation, results in relative instability and weakness about the shoulder. This rotator cuff deficiency may lead to superior migration of the humeral head against the undersurface of the acromion. Frequently, this resulting impingement is located laterally, rather than anterolaterally, as is typically seen with subacromial arch impingement. The classically described "impingement sign" seen in degenerative rotator cuff disease may be absent in these situations.

Chronic attenuation of all of the rotator cuff tendons also typically occurs in the setting of rheumatoid arthritis (Fig 8–1). This differs from the usual isolated attrition, and possible tearing of only one or two tendons that occurs with rotator cuff disease in the nonrheumatoid patient. Often, despite significant attenuation or thinning of the rotator cuff tendons, discontinuity or frank tearing of the rotator cuff is absent in the rheumatoid patient. The reported incidence of full-thickness rotator cuff tears in rheumatoid patients with shoulder pain has been estimated to be 26.5%.[14] Functional insufficiency of the rotator cuff in these patients is nevertheless present, and is the source of considerable disability for the patient. Clinical tests considered to be diagnostic for rotator cuff tearing ("drop arm test") are difficult to interpret in the rheumatoid patient with intraarticular disease and secondary rotator cuff thinning. Similarly, inference regarding possible tearing of the rotator cuff using plain radiography (decreased acromiohumeral interval) can be difficult to interpret in the patient with diffuse thinning of the rotator cuff tendons.

Obviously, surgical treatment of a diffusely thinned, deficient rotator cuff, whether discontinuous or even when still in continuity, has its limitations. The prognosis for successful healing of a full-thickness rotator cuff tear that has been attenuated by chronic synovitis is guarded. Since the underlying mechanism responsible for the development of rotator cuff disease in rheumatoid arthritis differs from that in the nonrheumatoid patient, procedures directed at decompression of the subacromial arch (acromioplasty, coracoacromial ligament and acromioclavicular joint resection) are of limited value. Early glenohumeral synovectomy or subacromial-subdeltoid bursectomy may slow the development of rotator cuff deficiency in the occasional patient in whom these procedures are indicated. In general, however, conservative treatment with medical management, physical therapy, and corticosteroid injections form the mainstay of treatment for disorders of the rotator cuff in rheumatoid arthritis.

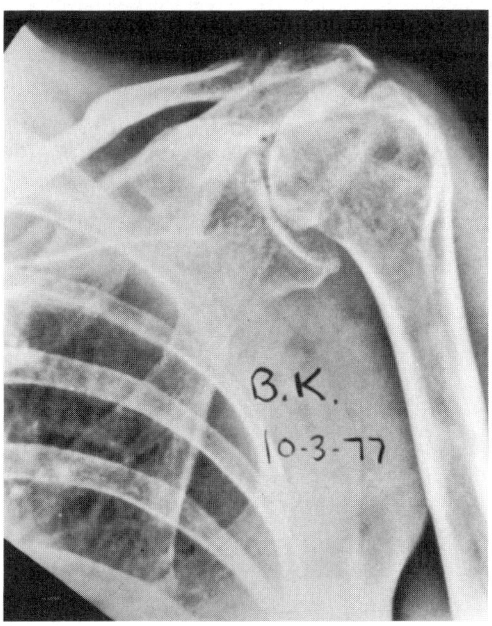

FIG 8–1.
Chronic rotator cuff tears may result in superior subluxation of the shoulder.

OTHER BURSITIS AND TENDONITIS SYNDROMES

Subdeltoid Bursitis

Chronic inflammation and proliferation of synovitis often occurs in the subdeltoid bursa in patients with rheumatoid arthritis (Fig 8–2). Because of its anatomic connection with the subacromial bursa, the integrity of the rotator cuff can be further compromised by inflammation in this area.

Clinically, the patient with subdeltoid bursitis typically presents with chronic shoulder pain which is often constant in duration and frequently referred to the deltoid tuberosity. In some, the pain may be worse at night and exacerbated with abduction or internal rotation of the shoulder. Physical findings consist of localized swelling, tenderness, and crepitations in the subdeltoid area with range of motion of the shoulder.

Fortunately, the course of this inflammatory manifestation of rheumatoid arthritis is generally limited and responsive to conservative management. Brief periods of immobilization with a sling, nonsteroidal anti-inflammatory medications, and cold packs during episodes of acute inflammation provide symptomatic relief for many patients. Injection of local anesthetic and corticosteroids into the inflamed bursa can also provide relief in many patients.

Surgical subdeltoid bursectomy is rarely necessary, and is indicated only for patients with persistent bursitis lasting greater than 6 months that are

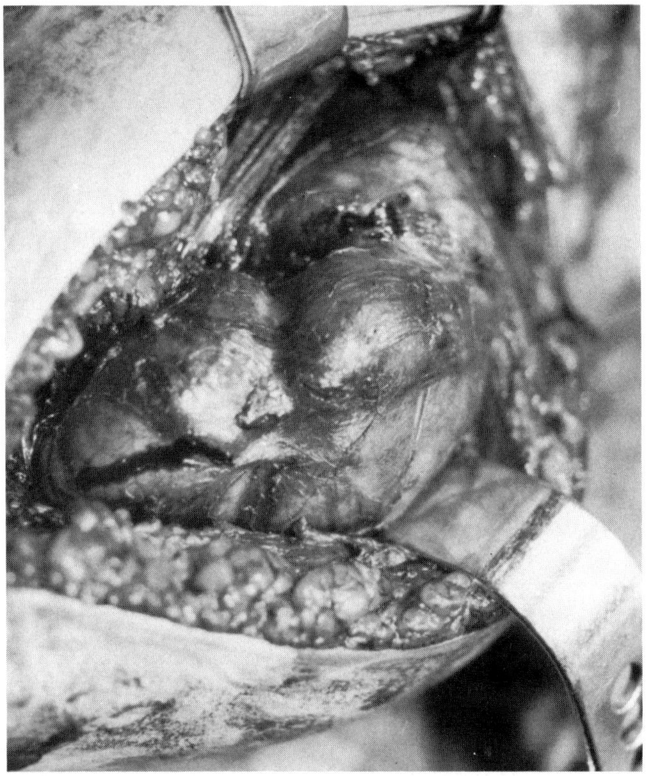

FIG 8–2.
Frank subdeltoid bursitis with chronic inflammation and rice bodies.

refractory to conservative management. Usually, a deltopectoral approach, allowing for debridement of the subacromial and subdeltoid spaces, is used. Care must be exercised during subdeltoid bursectomy to avoid injury to the axillary nerve in its vulnerable location on the undersurface of the deltoid muscle.

Bicipital Tenosynovitis

Bicipital tenosynovitis occurs frequently in the rheumatoid patient. Although this condition in the nonrheumatoid patient typically develops in association with rotator cuff or other degenerative shoulder lesions, direct involvement of the tendon sheath with synovitis occurs in the patient with rheumatoid arthritis. The anatomic continuity of the tendon sheath with the glenohumeral joint and the intraarticular course of the tendon of the long head of the biceps contributes to the frequent occurrence of bicipital tenosynovitis in these patients.

The patient with bicipital tenosynovitis usually presents with chronic dull, aching pain about the shoulder which is often aggravated by movement of the arm. Generally, tenderness, and occasionally swelling, can be localized over the bicipital groove, which is directly anterior and distal to the acromion with the shoulder in 10 degrees of internal rotation. Movement of this point of tenderness with rotation of the arm is a useful finding which differentiates bicipital tendonitis from subdeltoid bursitis and impingement syndrome. In these latter two conditions, tenderness is more diffuse and does not move with rotation of the arm. Several other diagnostic maneuvers, such as Speed's test and Yergason's sign, can be helpful in establishing the diagnosis of bicipital tenosynovitis. Injection of the tendon sheath with local anesthetic and corticosteroids is helpful in confirming the diagnosis and providing long-lasting relief of symptoms. Direct intratendinous steroid injection is to be avoided since it further predisposes the inflamed tendon to rupture. Rarely, conservative measures such as local heat, anti-inflammatory medications, and local injections fail to satisfactorily control the tenosynovitis surrounding the biceps tendon. In these patients, synovectomy of the biceps tendon sheath, often in conjunction with glenohumeral synovectomy, can be considered. Guidelines for treatment of ruptures of the long head of the biceps tendon are similar to the recommendations for tendon rupture in nonrheumatoid patients.

Other bursitis and tendonitis syndromes can affect the shoulder in the rheumatoid patient, as they commonly occur in the nonrheumatoid patient. In general, the diagnosis and principles of treatment are similar in both groups. Again, conservative modalities remain the mainstay of treatment in these situations. Certainly, the painful rheumatoid shoulder with deficiency of the rotator cuff, glenohumeral arthritis, or subdeltoid bursitis is susceptible to development of a secondary frozen shoulder syndrome. A routine program of active and passive range-of-motion exercises and gentle stretching can minimize occurrence of this complication.

RHEUMATOID ARTHROPATHY

Pathophysiology

As in other joints affected with rheumatoid arthritis, the immunologically mediated mechanisms resulting in chronic synovial inflammation and pannus formation are responsible for the articular damage seen in the rheumatoid shoulder. As mentioned previously, the effects of this process on the periarticular soft tissues, which provide the static and dynamic stability of this relatively unconstrained articulation, are also significant. Progression of rheumatoid synovitis involving the glenohumeral joint can thus result in a broad spectrum of clinical manifestations including arthritis due to loss of articular cartilage, rotator cuff deficiency, and subacromial impingement. Avascular necrosis of the humeral head, while frequently seen in systemic lupus erythematosus, can also occur secondary to chronic steroid therapy in the patient with rheumatoid arthritis (Fig 8–3). Not surprisingly, the clinical presentations of these related conditions frequently overlap and are often indistinguishable.

Since glenohumeral joint synovitis is the primary event responsible for the development of these related conditions, treatment directed toward controlling or eradicating any active synovitis within this joint is warranted. Usually, this consists of appropriate rheumatologic management, including the judicious use of intraarticular steroid injections. Fortunately, conservative modalities are effective in controlling active synovitis in the majority of patients. Slow progression of articular cartilage loss occurs in many patients, with resultant development of glenohumeral arthritis (Fig 8–4).

Occasionally, significant synovitis will persist despite adequate medical management. In these patients, pain, boggy swelling about the shoulder, and soft crepitations with range of motion are frequently present. Similar findings can occur from synovial hypertrophy within the subdeltoid bursa, or from synovial fluid extravasation and synovial tissue extension through a torn rotator cuff. Double contrast shoulder arthrography has been useful in providing information regarding the extent and severity of synovitis, and in demonstrating tears of the rotator cuff.

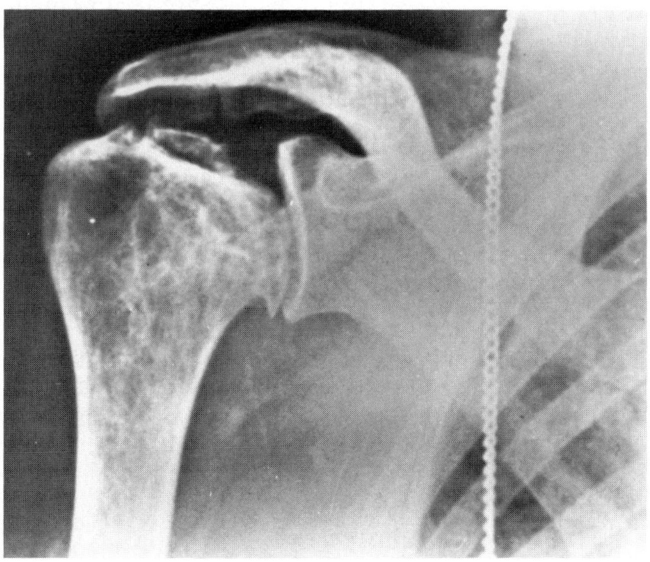

FIG 8–3.
Avascular necrosis secondary to prednisone therapy in a patient with rheumatoid arthritis and systemic lupus erythematosus.

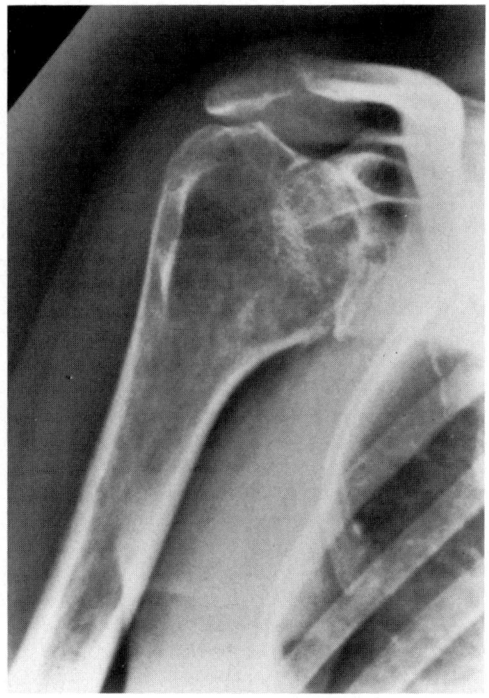

FIG 8–4.
Symmetric joint space loss and periarticular osteopenia are typical in rheumatoid arthritis.

SURGICAL TREATMENT OF THE SHOULDER

GLENOHUMERAL SYNOVECTOMY

In the patient with refractory glenohumeral synovitis of greater than 6 months' duration, synovectomy should be considered. Presence of synovial hypertrophy, as demonstrated by arthrogram, and maintenance of at least one half of the normal articular cartilage thickness are a prerequisite for consideration of this procedure. In patients with an intact rotator cuff and without subdeltoid bursitis, we prefer arthroscopic shoulder synovectomy over the traditional open procedure. Patients with rotator cuff tears and those who require subdeltoid bursectomy are not candidates for the arthroscopic procedure. Open synovectomy utilizing a deltopectoral approach is preferred in these patients. This technique facilitates adequate glenohumeral synovectomy, subdeltoid and subacromial bursectomy, rotator cuff repair, and acromioplasty if necessary. Postoperative management consists of early passive range-of-motion exercises, with later institution of active assisted and active range-of-motion exercises, dependent on the status of the rotator cuff. Clinical reports documenting the effectiveness of these procedures are limited, but, good results apparently occur in the majority of patients.[26, 29]

SHOULDER ARTHROPLASTY

Frequently, as a result of chronic rheumatoid synovitis involving the shoulder, there is progressive loss of articular cartilage and significant glenohumeral arthritis develops. As the severity of these arthritic changes increases, the effectiveness of conservative management in providing even temporary symptomatic relief typically diminishes. Treatment options then become more limited, and these tend to be generally more complex in nature.

Arthrodesis and Resection Arthroplasty

With the development of hemiarthroplasty and total resurfacing arthroplasty of the shoulder, arthrodesis and resection arthroplasty should have a limited role in the treatment of rheumatoid arthritis. In general, the indications for these procedures are similar to those for other joints affected in rheumatoid arthritis. The rheumatoid patient who has, or who may develop, multiple joint arthritis and functional limitation in the future will assuredly have additional disability as a result of loss of shoulder motion following an arthrodesis. An arthrodesis is often difficult to achieve and will result in increased stress on the ipsilateral elbow. This option is mentioned only to be condemned as a treatment for uncomplicated rheumatoid arthritis involving the shoulder. Use of this procedure should be strictly limited to salvage situations in which arthroplasty has either failed because of mechanical reasons or infection, or is technically impossible. Resection arthroplasty of the shoulder, in general, provides less reliable pain relief and function than shoulder arthroplasty. Early instability, late stiffness, and persistent shoulder weakness following resection arthroplasty often render the upper extremity relatively useless in the patient with arthritis affecting other joints. Similar to shoulder arthrodesis, the use of this technique should be limited to salvage situations such as failed total shoulder arthroplasty, deep infection, or unreconstructable bone deficits.

Shoulder Hemiarthroplasty

Hemiarthroplasty of the shoulder has few indications in most patients with rheumatoid arthritis. Total joint resurfacing of the shoulder is preferred in nearly all cases. Pain relief is generally more predictable when both articular surfaces are resurfaced by the procedure. Removal of all articular cartilage at the time of resurfacing arthroplasty has long been considered to be important in eliminating the source of continued inflammatory synovitis in the rheumatoid patient.[29] Occasionally, however, hemiarthroplasty may be indicated. The presence of significant glenoid bone deficiencies, which cannot be reconstructed with bone grafting or custom implants, is the most common indication for hemiarthroplasty (see Fig 8–8,G). These defects can occur as a result of bone erosion by the inflammatory process, or secondarily from glenoid component loosening and associated osteolysis in a revision situation. Rarely, an anatomically small glenoid, in association with a patient of small physical stature, may prohibit glenoid resurfacing. These anatomically deficient glenoids typically occur in the patient with juvenile rheumatoid arthritis and often require use of a custom prosthesis.

The concept of a bipolar shoulder hemiarthroplasty is an attractive alternative to standard hemiarthroplasty, especially in the rheumatoid patient with rotator cuff and glenoid deficiencies. An appropriate biarticular design may allow for optimization of motion, stability, and pain relief in these adverse circumstances. Clinical experience with implants of this type is limited, however.[31] Several previous designs, modeled after bipolar hip prostheses, require significant humeral bone resection for implantation and fail to reestablish the anatomic center of rotation of the glenohumeral joint, resulting in abnormal shoulder mechanics. We are currently investigating alternatives to previous bipolar shoulder implant designs. Fortunately, these difficult reconstructive problems occur infrequently.

Total Shoulder Arthroplasty

The most reliable technique for resurfacing of the arthritic glenohumeral joint is a total shoulder arthroplasty. Both pain relief and functional outcome have been shown to be superior to the results obtainable with arthrodesis, resection arthroplasty, and hemiarthroplasty of the shoulder.[9, 10, 12] Indications for total shoulder arthroplasty include disabling pain associated with significant loss of articular cartilage that persists despite a thorough trial of conservative treatment. Functional limitation and restriction of range of motion of the shoulder, especially rotation, may be secondary indications. Careful clinical evaluation is important to identify those causes of pain and dysfunction about the shoulder which may be amenable to more conservative procedures such as synovectomy or bursectomy. Contraindications to total shoulder arthroplasty include a history of recent sepsis of the shoulder, paralysis of the joint with loss of both deltoid and rotator cuff function, and a painless arthrodesis or resection arthroplasty. Remote joint sepsis is a relative contraindication which mandates a thorough preoperative evaluation for quiescent infection, and careful consideration of the risks by the surgeon and patient.

Preoperative Considerations

Total shoulder arthroplasty warrants careful preoperative consideration of unique problems which can complicate surgery in the rheumatoid patient. Plain radiographs should be carefully studied and templated to insure that appropriately sized implants are available for surgery. The generally small body habitus of the rheumatoid patient, and related small size of the humeral head and glenoid, often requires design and manufacture of custom implants. The axillary view can be helpful in identifying bone deficits in the glenoid which may require either bone grafting or a custom glenoid component, or which may be unreconstructable. Computed tomography is useful to more accurately assess these bone deficiencies, to provide a template for selection of components, and to design a custom implant should this be necessary. Use of a short-stemmed humeral component may be necessary in the patient with an ipsilateral total elbow arthroplasty. This should also be considered in the patient with ipsilateral elbow arthritis who may require total elbow arthroplasty in the future (see Fig 8–9).

Other design considerations which need to be addressed preoperatively relate to the planned method of implant fixation. In general, most rheumatoid patients requiring total shoulder arthroplasty will have at least a moderate amount of osteopenia, because of the typical later onset and slow progression of rheumatoid arthritis involving the glenohumeral joint. In these patients, cemented fixation with polymethyl methacrylate is probably the most appropriate technique. In younger patients and in patients without significant osteopenia, however, we have achieved satisfactory early results with the use of porous-coated,[15, 22] uncemented glenoid and humeral components. Further follow-up is necessary to determine the durability of this biologic fixation in these patients with inflammatory arthritis.

Knowledge regarding the status of the rotator cuff can be important in surgical planning, and useful in advising the patient about the expected outcome and limitations of surgery. The presence of a rotator cuff tear that requires repair increases the complexity of the procedure and modifies the postoperative rehabilitation. The prognosis regarding recovery of function in the patient with a massive rotator cuff deficiency is less favorable. In these patients, specific attention to protect the integrity of the deltoid and restore the anatomy and optimize the mechanics of the glenohumeral joint will improve the results of surgery. The prevalence of full-thickness rotator cuff tears in rheumatoid patients undergoing total shoulder arthroplasty has been reported to be 27% by Cofield[8] and 42% by Neer et al.[25]

Prior to surgery, clinical and radiographic evaluation of the cervical spine should be performed. A careful neurologic and cervical spine examination may, on occasion, identify a problem of a more serious nature, resulting from rheumatoid involvement of the cervical spine. The presence of asymptomatic cervical instability at the basilar, atlantoaxial, or subaxial level can be an important consideration in planning the patient's anesthesia. Use of regional anesthetic techniques, though demanding, can obviate some of the increased risks of anesthesia.

Frequently, there will be significant involvement of both the shoulder and the ipsilateral elbow. In general, the most painful of these should be replaced first. Should involvement of both joints be equally severe, we prefer to replace the elbow first, as this may provide the patient with considerable functional improvement.[18] If the rehabilitation following total elbow arthroplasty would be seriously compromised by a stiff and painful ipsilateral shoulder, however, then shoulder arthroplasty should be performed first. Restoration of shoulder rotation provides protection from rotatory stresses, which may otherwise be transmitted to the elbow arthroplasty and contribute to loosening. In the patient who is to undergo lower extremity total joint arthroplasty, rehabilitation requiring upper extremity weightbearing with assistive devices may be impossible if significant shoulder arthritis is present. Rarely, a patient may require total shoulder arthro-

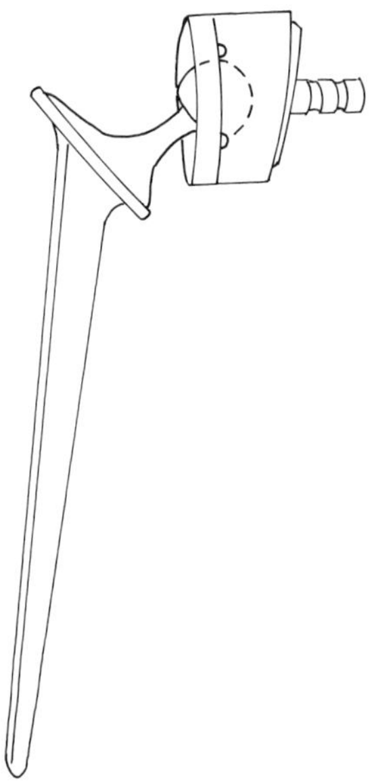

FIG 8–5.
Constrained total shoulder replacements may give early satisfactory results in patients with rotator cuff deficiency, but have high loosening rates.

plasty prior to lower extremity joint replacement to allow the necessary postoperative rehabilitation. Similarly, lower extremity total joint arthroplasty may be beneficial in the patient with a total shoulder arthroplasty who requires assistive devices for ambulation, as this may ultimately eliminate the need for weightbearing at the shoulder.

Surgical Technique

Total shoulder arthroplasty is perhaps the most demanding of all joint arthroplasties that the orthopaedic surgeon performs. Adequate surgical exposure of the glenohumeral joint is critical for success. Based on preoperative planning, the surgeon considering total shoulder arthroplasty should have available the necessary implants that may be required for resurfacing of the glenohumeral joint. Because of the frequent problems with loosening of constrained total shoulder prostheses, we have found few indications for use of these implants in the rheumatoid patient (Fig 8–5). The use of semiconstrained implants with hooded glenoid components, while theoretically attractive in the patient with rotator cuff deficiency, has also been associated with frequent glenoid loosening[13] (Fig 8–6). Both constrained and semiconstrained implant designs have a higher incidence of instability and dislocation than do nonconstrained prostheses.[11] In nearly all patients, we prefer nonconstrained implants (Fig 8–7). Anatomically shaped glenoid components fulfilling these criteria are available in either all-polyethylene or metal-backed polyethylene designs. The addition of metal backing may result in thickening of the glenoid component, and slight lateral displacement of the center of rotation of the shoulder. This disadvantage is probably offset by the enhanced component stability provided by metal keels and base plates, and the provision for supplementary screw fixation.

The technique of total shoulder arthroplasty begins with regional or general anesthesia and proper positioning of the patient. The patient is positioned in the semisitting (modified Fowler's) position, with hips and knees flexed approximately 30 degrees, and as far toward the edge of the operating table as possible to provide for free access to and draping of the area. A well-padded sandbag or blanket roll can be placed behind the scapula, allowing for further free exposure of the extremity. Safety straps are used to secure the patient, as manipulation of the operative extremity tends to pull the patient off the table during the procedure. A kidney rest or other support positioned at the level of the lower rib cage can help in this regard. The head and neck should be gently rotated away from the operative field, with care taken to prevent traction on the brachial plexus or injury to the cervical spine, as these patients frequently have cervical spine instability. The extremity should be prepared and draped in a free fashion, with the hand and forearm excluded from the operative field with a stockinette. An adjustable, sterile-draped, padded Mayo stand can be used to support the arm in the abducted position when necessary.

A gently curving anterior skin incision overlying

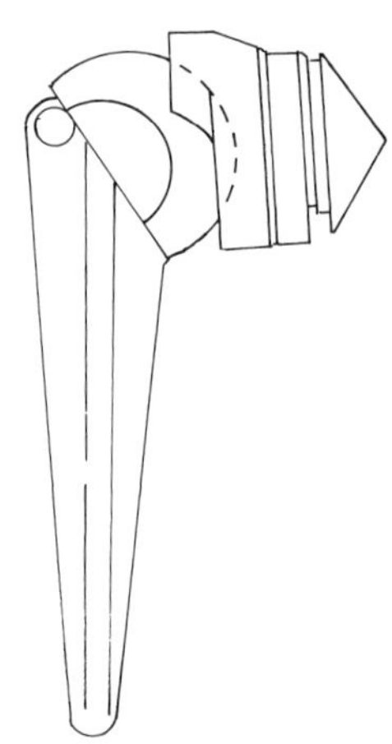

FIG 8–6.
Semiconstrained components with hooded glenoid components have not attained adequate results in the rotator cuff–deficient shoulder.

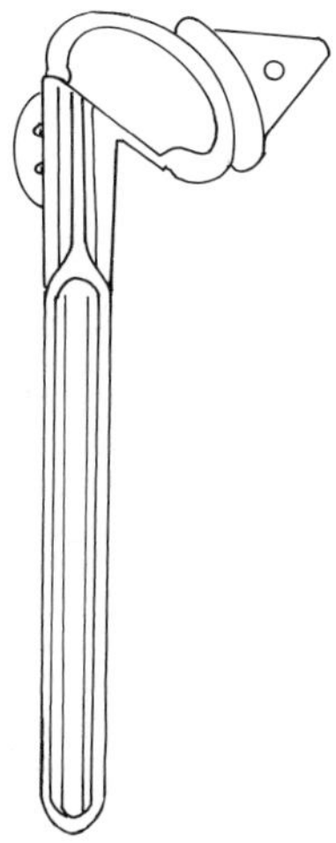

FIG 8–7.
The Neer prosthesis has been widely used but has a fixed offset. The long stem is often a disadvantage in patients with an ipsilateral total elbow replacement.

the deltopectoral interval, extending from the area of the distal clavicle to the anterior aspect of the deltoid tuberosity is made (Fig 8–8,A). Dissection through the subcutaneous layer and superficial fascia is then performed to expose the cephalic vein in the deltopectoral interval. This extends proximally to expose the infraclavicular triangle. Careful hemostasis is maintained throughout. The cephalic vein is then retracted medially and the interval between the deltoid and pectoralis major is developed (Fig 8–8,B). With the deltoid retracted laterally, the proximal 1.0 to 1.5 cm of the pectoralis major insertion is released just medial to the tendon of the long head of the biceps, using electrocautery. The small cuff of tendon insertion on the humerus facilitates later repair of the tendon at the time of wound closure.

The fascia between the underlying subscapularis and the conjoined tendons of the coracobrachialis and the short head of the biceps is then incised, just lateral to the conjoined tendon. If the coracoid process is small, the lateral two thirds of the conjoined tendon can be divided transversely, just distal to the coracoid. In patients with a prominent or overhanging coracoid process, better exposure will be obtained with osteotomy of the tip of the coracoid. Both of these techniques will allow the conjoined tendons to be retracted medially, facilitating exposure of the glenohumeral joint. Abduction of the arm should be avoided during this stage of the surgical exposure, as this positioning brings the underlying musculocutaneous nerve beneath the tip of the coracoid process and into the operative field.

At this point, the subscapularis insertion on the lesser tuberosity should be well exposed. The axillary nerve may be seen entering the quadrangular space anteriorly, just below the subscapularis tendon (Fig 8–8,C). The subscapularis tendon and underlying glenohumeral joint capsule are then incised as a single flap approximately 1 cm medial to the lesser tuberosity. The substantial nature of this strong capsular and tendinous flap allows for secure repair at the time of wound closure, permitting early mobilization. During this stage of the exposure, external rotation of the arm will increase the distance between the incision and the axillary nerve, which must be protected (Fig 8–8,D). The leash of vessels just caudal to the subscapularis tendon defines the inferior limits of the incision through the subscapularis. These vessels are then ligated and the incision is continued superiorly toward the top of the lesser tuberosity, avoiding the tendons of the supraspinatus and the long head of the biceps. As this incision is extended, the arm is able to be externally rotated further (Fig 8–8,E). Additional release of the inferior glenohumeral capsule is usually required for adequate exposure and dislocation of the humeral head. This release should be performed directly on the humeral neck, at the level of the capsular attachment, owing to the close proximity of the axillary nerve. The coracoacromial ligament is generally not incised, as this structure may prevent superior subluxation of the humeral head and is not responsible for rotator cuff deterioration in the rheumatoid patient.

The humeral head is then dislocated by external rotation and extension of the arm, while lifting the proximal humerus anteriorly. Osteophytes are removed with a rongeur, and additional capsular release from the humeral neck can be carefully performed to gain additional exposure of the humeral head. Orientation of the proximal humeral osteotomy is then carefully planned. Depending on the prosthesis and instrumentation used, either a trial prosthesis or a humeral head cutting guide is used to determine the proper resection of the proximal humerus. A humeral head implant which best approximates the size and radius of curvature of the patient's humeral head should usually be selected for implantation. If the humeral head is grossly deformed, it may be difficult to determine the appropriate implant size. The angle of the osteotomy relative to the longitudinal axis of the humerus is determined by the relationship between the stem and the undersurface of the articular portion of the component. This angle is approximately 45 degrees with most implants. The level of the osteotomy, in general, should remove an amount from the proxi-

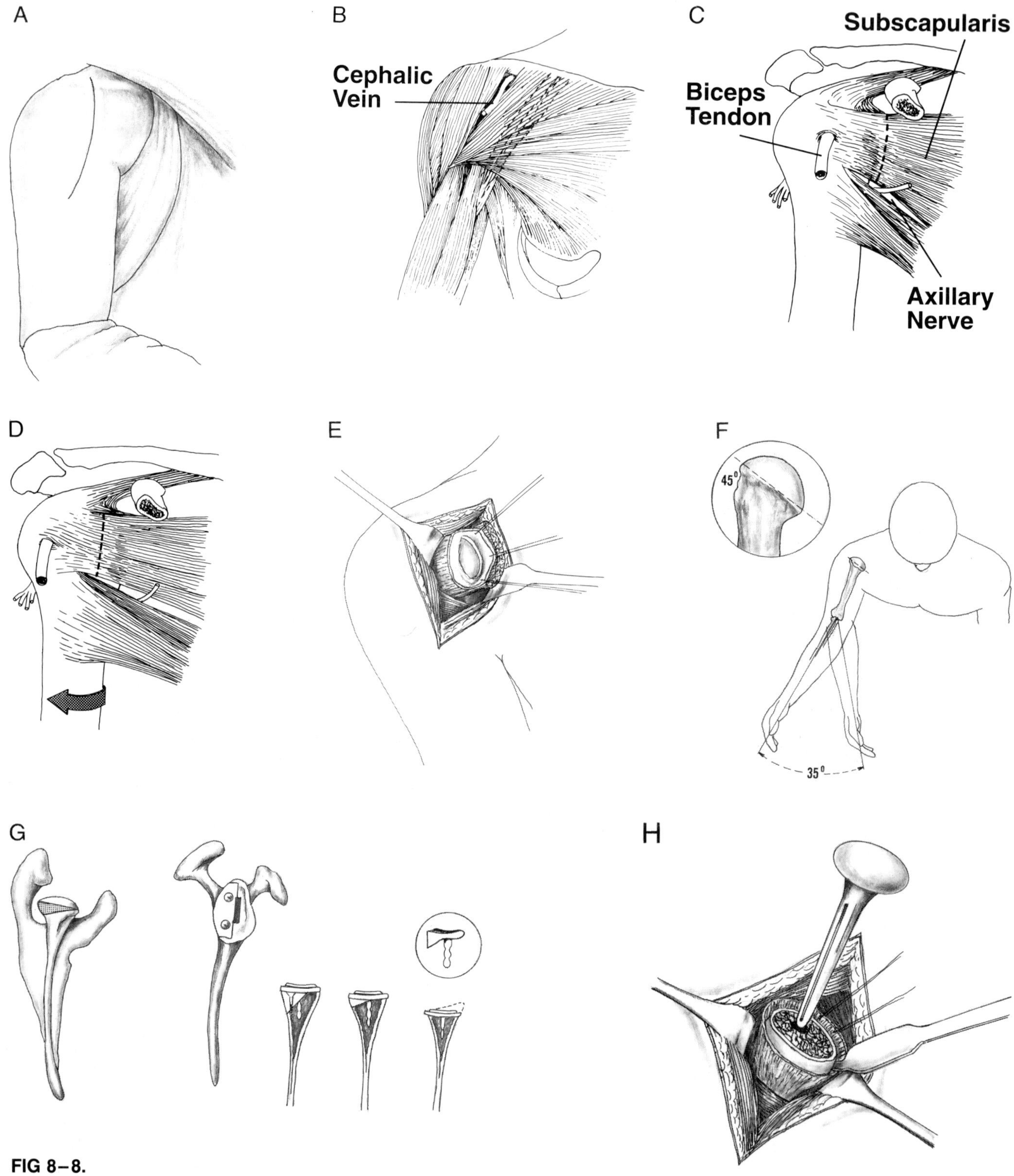

FIG 8–8.
A, a deltopectoral approach is used. **B,** the deltopectoral groove is marked by the cephalic vein. **C,** the axillary nerve enters the quadrangular space. **D,** the axillary nerve can be protected by external rotation of the arm. **E,** the subscapularis and capsule are raised as a single flap. **F,** the humeral osteotomy is usually a 45-degree angle with 35 degrees of retroversion. **G,** bone deficits may be repaired using bone grafts or custom glenoid components. **H,** the humeral component should be positioned such that impingement of the greater tuberosity does not occur.

mal humerus equal to that which will be replaced by the articular surface of the humeral component (Fig 8–8,F).

Usually, an appropriate osteotomy will begin at the superolateral aspect of the articular surface, just above and medial to the rotator cuff insertion on the greater tuberosity. This should allow the articular surface to be slightly above the level of the greater tuberosity, providing clearance between the rotator cuff and the acromion during initiation of abduction. This will prevent impingement of the greater tuberosity on the undersurface of the acromion. Provision for the normal humeral head retroversion of 30 to 45 degrees is determined by first flexing the elbow to 90 degrees. When the arm is then externally rotated 30 to 45 degrees, an osteotomy directed from anterior to posterior should provide the desired amount of humeral head retroversion. After proper orientation is determined, the humeral head is carefully osteotomized with an oscillating saw. Injury to the rotator cuff must be avoided, and this may warrant completion of the osteotomy with small osteotomes. With the arm returned to neutral rotation, the osteotomized surface of the humerus should face directly toward the glenoid.

The status of the rotator cuff is evaluated, and plans for reconstruction of a deficient rotator cuff are formulated. Attention is then directed to preparation of the glenoid. The proximal humerus is retracted posteriorly and laterally with a humeral head retractor. The glenoid is assessed for bone quality and the presence of any deficiency which may need to be reconstructed with bone grafting or prosthetic augmentation.[24] If the glenoid is determined to be amenable to resurfacing, the labrum, if present, is then trimmed to provide exposure of the entire surface of the glenoid. The anterior capsule can be elevated for a short distance toward the glenoid neck, using subperiosteal sharp dissection, to allow secure positioning of a glenoid capsule retractor. The inferior glenohumeral ligament should not be released, however, as this structure provides considerable stability to the shoulder following capsular repair.

The surface of the glenoid is then carefully planed, using high-speed burrs, to provide for intimate apposition of the implant to the bony surface. Bone removal should be minimal, as the subchondral plate, which is already frequently thinned, provides the best support for the glenoid component. Depending on the type of implant used, the subchondral surface will then need to be prepared further to accommodate the keel, stem, or fixation screws incorporated in the implant design. Use of drill guides and templates provided with the implant instrumentation facilitates accurate preparation of these. Significant bone deficiencies which require grafting can be addressed at this time. Structural bone grafts, obtained from the osteotomized humeral head, are shaped to fit in the defects and secured in place with small AO or ASIF screws[24] (Fig 8–8,G).

If cement fixation of the component is planned, the soft cancellous bone within the glenoid should be removed sparingly with a curette to allow for seating of the stem or keel. An angled curette can be used to create a cement recess along the axillary border of the scapula and anteriorly toward the coracoid process. Similarly, the subchondral plate can be undermined to enhance mechanical cement interlock. After adequate preparation of the glenoid, irrigation of the surfaces with pulsatile lavage is performed. The area is then thoroughly packed and dried prior to cementing. Polymethylmethacrylate, in a doughy state, is then forcibly packed into the slot and around the keel and back of the component. The implant is placed and held securely in position, and excess cement is carefully removed. When an uncemented component is used, the component is impacted into position, and secured with screws.

Attention is then redirected to further preparation of the proximal humerus. The medullary canal of the proximal humerus is located by passing a narrow axial reamer distally, in line with the longitudinal axis of the humerus. The starting point for insertion of this reamer is somewhat lateral to the center of the cut surface of the humeral head. Failure to recognize this may result in a varus position of the humeral component. Since the humeral osteotomy is obliquely orientated, this can also result in positioning of the component inferior to its intended location (Fig 8–8,H). In this situation, the greater tuberosity may extend above the articular surface of the component, resulting in impingement during abduction.

For reasons mentioned previously, we generally prefer to use shorter-stemmed humeral implants which require little reaming into the diaphysis (Fig 8–9,A and B). Fixation with polymethyl methacrylate limited to the undersurface of the prosthesis and proximal portion of the stem is generally satisfactory in the patient with good cancellous bone in the proximal humerus. When bone stock is poor, implant fixation requires longer-stemmed components. Depending on the length of the stem, further axial reaming may be necessary to allow passage of the implant into the diaphysis of the proximal humerus.

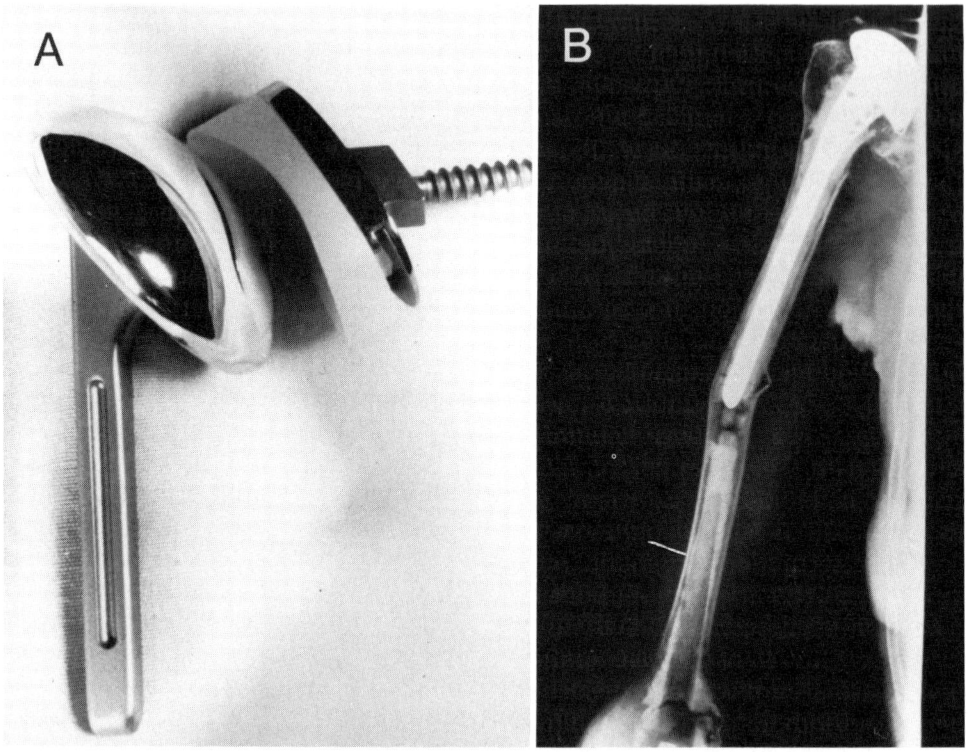

FIG 8–9.
A, a short-stemmed humeral component may be more appropriate in patients with rheumatoid arthritis. **B,** a long-stemmed humeral component combined with an elbow replacement creates a significant stress riser and a fracture may result.

Care should be taken not to ream the diaphyseal cortex excessively. Following reaming of the canal, a trial component is inserted and the shoulder reduced. Soft tissue tension, stability, range of motion, retroversion of the humeral head, and restoration of prosthetic height and offset is then evaluated. The osteotomized surface of the humeral head may need to be further shaped to provide optimal fit and positioning of the prosthesis. Use of a thick glenoid or oversized humeral head component may result in excessive lateral displacement of the humerus and increased tension on the subscapularis tendon. This may contribute to failure of the anterior capsular repair and anterior dislocation of the shoulder.

Following this, the trial implant is removed and rotator cuff repair performed if needed. After reconstruction of a rotator cuff tear, a repeat trial reduction is warranted to insure that the previously selected implant does not place excessive tension on the repair. If an uncemented arthroplasty is to be performed, this implant is inserted at this time and the stability of the component evaluated. Otherwise, the proximal humerus is irrigated with pulsatile lavage and the bone surfaces are thoroughly dried, in preparation for fixation with polymethylmethacrylate. When a tight press fit of the stem is obtained, good fixation can be achieved with restriction of cement to the metaphyseal portion of the implant. Failure to obtain a press fit of the component in the diaphysis necessitates plugging of the medullary canal and cement fixation of the entire component. Cement is injected into the canal with a syringe and manually compressed into the osteotomized metaphyseal surface. The prosthesis is then inserted into the proximal humerus, in the proper orientation, and held securely in place until the cement polymerizes. Excess cement is carefully trimmed from the periphery of the implant. The shoulder is again reduced and the adequacy of the reconstruction evaluated.

Following thorough irrigation, attention is then directed to wound closure. The capsular and subscapularis flap is repaired to the remaining cuff of subscapularis tendon on the lesser tuberosity with no. 0 nonabsorbable sutures. Proximally, the interval between the subscapularis and supraspinatus is reapproximated with no. 0 absorbable and nonabsorbable sutures. The transverse tenotomy of the conjoined tendon is repaired with no. 0 absorbable suture. If the coracoid was osteotomized, the tip is then reapproximated to the remaining process of the coracoid with no. 0 nonabsorbable suture. Predrilling the tip of the coracoid prior to osteotomy facilitates its repair at the time of wound closure. The pectoralis major tendon, which was previously incompletely released, is then reapproximated with no. 0 absorbable sutures. A small suction drain is left in the subcutaneous layer and brought out through a separate stab wound. The skin is closed in routine fashion and a dry sterile dressing applied over the wound. The patient is then placed into a sling and swathe-type shoulder immobilizer.

POSTOPERATIVE REHABILITATION

A carefully formulated and coordinated postoperative rehabilitation program is essential for successful total shoulder arthroplasty. This involves the continued efforts and cooperation of the patient, surgeon, and therapist who is familiar with the principles of upper extremity rehabilitation. Preoperative evaluation and education by the therapist regarding the planned postoperative treatment can facilitate the patient's understanding and cooperation necessary for compliance with an often arduous regimen. Frequently, this therapeutic program will need to be modified according to the intraoperative condition of the surrounding soft tissues and the adequacy of their repair, the stability of the arthroplasty, and the progress of the patient postoperatively.

Initial postoperative therapy for the patient with an intact rotator cuff and without instability is similar to the recommendations of Neer et al.[25] The patient is seen twice daily by the therapist and instructed in pendulum exercises, with the arm in a sling or with the elbow flexed, starting on postoperative day 2 or 3. On postoperative days 3 to 5, passive and active assisted forward flexion in the supine position, and active assisted external rotation to neutral is initiated under the close supervision of the therapist. In addition to these sessions, which normally last 5 to 10 minutes, the patient performs three daily sessions independently. Active assisted extension is begun on postoperative day 5 to 8. Phase 1 continues with initiation of active assisted abduction and adduction in the supine position on day 9 to 11. Active assisted internal rotation with the arm behind the back and isometric exercises for the internal and external rotators and posterior and middle deltoid muscles are also initiated at this time. Overhead pulleys are provided to assist with these exercises. Sling immobilization is continued for 2 to 3 weeks, with gradual discontinuation beginning 10 days postoperatively. This intensive rehabilitation program generally requires continued hospitalization for inpatient therapy for at least 10 to 14 days postoperatively.

Phase 2 of the rehabilitation generally begins between postoperative day 11 and 21, just prior to or immediately following discharge from the hospital. Previously prescribed exercises are continued at home by the patient three or four times daily during this time. Active forward flexion exercises in the supine position, with the elbow flexed, are instituted during twice-weekly outpatient therapy sessions. Active assisted exercises previously performed in the supine position are gradually begun in the vertical position. These activities progress to active flexion, extension, abduction, adduction, and internal and external rotation range-of-motion exercises. During postoperative weeks 3 to 6, active range-of-motion exercises are gradually increased, and light resistive exercises are initiated. A progressive program of daily strengthening exercises is recommended for 6 months after the patient completes the above program.

In patients with significant rotator cuff deficiency or shoulder instability following total shoulder arthroplasty, a "limited goals" rehabilitation program[25] is generally warranted. In these patients, postoperative rehabilitation is directed toward obtaining satisfactory soft tissue healing and stability. Initiation and progression of passive and active range-of-motion exercises are necessarily delayed. External immobilization in a sling and swathe, or occasionally in an abduction orthosis, is generally recommended for 6 weeks in these patients. Appropriate modification of the previously described rehabilitation protocol therefore generally results in a more limited range of motion. Fortunately, satisfactory pain relief and a functional, stable range of motion is still obtained in most patients. In situations of glenohumeral instability, the rehabilitation program can be modified to restrict certain motions in accordance with the "safe zone" of stability determined intraoperatively. Rehabilitation in patients with rotator cuff deficiency should be dictated by the size of the defect, quality of the tissues, and adequacy of the repair. Although pendulum exercises may be started as early as 3 to 5 days postoperatively, activities may be otherwise restricted to passive and gentle active assisted range-of-motion exercises until 4 to 6 weeks postoperatively. Active range-of-motion and strengthening exercises are frequently delayed until 6 weeks postoperatively. Individualized postoperative rehabilitation can optimize the results obtained in the patient with instability or rotator cuff deficiency complicating total shoulder arthroplasty.

RESULTS

Several recent studies have documented good to excellent results in the majority of patients following unconstrained total shoulder arthroplasty. Neer et al.[25] reviewed the results of 194 total shoulder arthroplasties using the Neer prosthesis in patients with a variety of diagnoses. In the 43 patients in this series with rheumatoid arthritis and a minimum 2-year follow-up, excellent results were obtained in 28, and satisfactory results were obtained in 12 patients. Fourteen of these patients had complete rotator cuff tears that were repairable at the time of surgery. Postoperative improvement in forward flexion averaged 57 degrees and external rotation averaged 60 degrees. An additional 7 patients with rheumatoid arthritis and massive rotator cuff deficiencies, who were treated with a limited goals rehabilitation program, all had a successful result. All 50 patients had satisfactory pain relief. The 3 patients with unsatisfactory results failed to obtain 90 degrees of elevation because of muscle weakness.

Cofield[9] reviewed the results of 77 total shoulder arthroplasties using the Neer prosthesis. Pain relief was generally good with only 6 patients having moderate or severe pain postoperatively. Only 6 patients thought that the shoulder was unchanged or worse postoperatively. Rheumatoid arthritis was the primary diagnosis in 29 shoulders. The rotator cuff was normal in 5 and thinned in 17 shoulders. One patient had a minor rotator cuff tear and 6 had a major tear. Postoperative abduction averaged 103 degrees and external rotation averaged 35 degrees in the patients with rheumatoid arthritis.

Barrett et al.[2] reported the results of 50 Neer II total shoulder arthroplasties followed prospectively. Of the 11 patients in their series with rheumatoid arthritis, all obtained satisfactory pain relief. Rotator cuff tears were noted in 3 patients. Active forward elevation of the arm improved an average of 34 degrees postoperatively to 100 degrees. External rotation improved an average of 16 degrees postoperatively. Improvements in internal rotation and overall function were also noted.

Using survivorship analysis, Brenner et al.[7] reviewed their results with the Neer and unconstrained Gristina total shoulder prostheses. Using implant revision or patient dissatisfaction with the procedure as the failure criteria, survivorship was estimated at 92% at 11 years for their 25 patients with rheumatoid arthritis. Postoperative forward flexion averaged 93 degrees, representing an improvement of 28 degrees. Improvement in external rotation averaged 24 degrees. Pain relief, internal rotation, and function were also improved postoperatively.

Reports of the results of total shoulder arthroplasty in patients with inflammatory arthritis exclusively are limited. Friedman et al.[19] recently reviewed the results of unconstrained total shoulder arthroplasty in 20 American Rheumatism Association (ARA) functional class IV patients with rheumatoid arthritis. The rotator cuff was intact in six, and attenuated in nine shoulders. Six patients had minor rotator cuff tears and 3 had major tears. Pain relief was consistently obtained with 18 (92%) patients having absent or only mild pain at a mean follow-up of 4.5 years. Postoperative arm elevation averaged 81 degrees, representing an improvement of 38 degrees. Significant improvements in postoperative internal and external rotation of 22 and 11 degrees, respectively, was noted. Functional outcome also improved significantly, with 15 (75%) patients being able to attend to all activities of daily living involving the shoulder. There was no significant difference in pain relief, range of motion, or functional result between those patients who had a rotator cuff tear and those without a rotator cuff tear.

Barrett et al. retrospectively reviewed the results of 140 total shoulder arthroplasties in 114 patients with polyarticular rheumatoid arthritis.[3] Rotator cuff attenuation was present in 35% of the patients and moderate or massive rotator cuff tears were noted in 45% of the patients. Excellent pain relief was obtained in 93% of the patients. Although postoperative range of motion in these patients was less than reported in other series involving patients with osteoarthritis, significant improvements in range of motion were still obtained. Despite the limitations imposed by arthritic involvement of other multiple joints, significant functional improvement was noted in many patients. Humeral component loosening was not a significant problem with either cemented or press-fit, uncemented fixation. Although no components were revised for loosening, the authors were concerned about the 8% incidence of radiographic glenoid loosening.

Figgie et al.[16] analyzed the results of 50 unconstrained total shoulder arthroplasties in patients with inflammatory arthritis. Pain relief was consis-

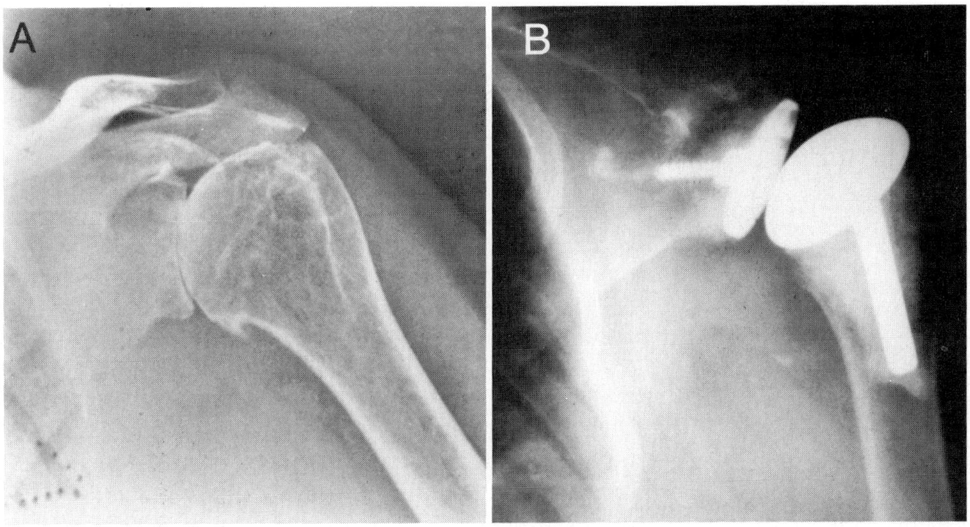

FIG 8–10.
A, preoperative radiograph of a patient with rheumatoid arthritis and secondary degenerative changes. **B,** a total shoulder replacement was performed utilizing a short-stemmed humeral component and a custom-fitted glenoid component.

tently obtained with 48 patients having complete relief or only occasional mild pain postoperatively. Substantial functional improvement with complete independence in activities of daily living was noted in 40 of 50 (80%) patients. Postoperative functional score and range of motion exhibited statistically significant correlations with the status of the rotator cuff. Restoration of the humeral and glenoid alignment and positioning also correlated with functional score, glenoid component migration or loosening, and the need for revision.

Thomas et al.[1, 32] reported their results of 30 DANA total shoulder arthroplasties in patients with rheumatoid arthritis. In 26 shoulders in which unconstrained glenoid components were used, considerable improvement in pain relief, function, flexion, and internal and external rotation were noted. Rotator cuff repairs were performed in 7 of these patients. Four additional patients with massive unrepairable rotator cuff defects had reconstruction with a hooded glenoid component. Although pain relief, function, flexion, and abduction improved in these patients, internal and external rotation decreased postoperatively.

Figgie et al.[15] reviewed the results of 29 custom-fitted unconstrained total shoulder arthroplasties in patients with inflammatory arthritis (Fig 8–10,A and B). These custom implant designs attempted to provide for restoration of anatomic alignment and offset and to optimize glenoid surface coverage. Thirteen patients had major rotator cuff tears with preoperative proximal migration of the humeral head. All patients had improvement in pain scores and external rotation postoperatively. Average flexion improved from 60 to 100 degrees, and average abduction improved from 55 to 100 degrees postoperatively. Radiographic evaluation at an average follow-up of 4 years revealed incomplete glenoid radiolucencies in 6 of 29 (23%) of the custom-fitted metal-backed glenoid components.

COMPLICATIONS

The complications following total shoulder arthroplasty in the rheumatoid patient are similar to those experienced in patients with other diagnoses. The nature and treatment of the chronic inflammatory disease may increase the incidence of certain of these complications.

Neurologic injury is rare following total shoulder arthroplasty. Cofield[11] tabulated the complications occurring in 586 Neer total shoulder arthroplasties, from nine separate clinical series, and estimated the prevalence of neurologic injury to be 0.68%. Most of these have been transient and involve the axillary nerve; however, transient ulnar nerve[21] and musculocutaneous nerve palsy[15] and intraoperative axillary nerve laceration[9] have been reported. Unless intraoperative transection is suspected, treatment should be expectant with recovery of nerve function anticipated. The axillary nerve is most vulnerable to injury as it courses inferior to the glenohumeral joint capsule. Subperiosteal release of the inferior capsule from the proximal humerus may minimize the risk of injury to the axillary nerve, especially when significant capsular contracture is present. The musculocutaneous nerve may be injured by excessive trac-

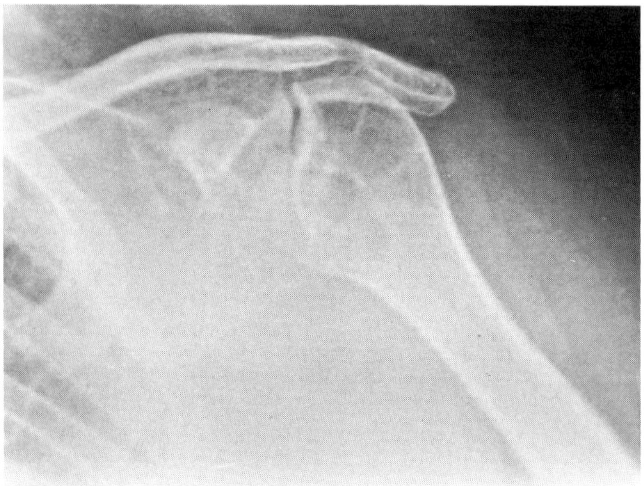

FIG 8–11.
A patient with marked bone loss will have significant capsular contracture requiring anterior and posterior release.

tion along the conjoined tendon and thus careful retraction in this area is warranted.

The overall incidence of deep infection following total shoulder arthroplasty has been estimated to be less than 1%.[11] Infection is an important concern, especially in the rheumatoid patient receiving corticosteroid and immunosuppressive medications. Many of these have been late infections, presumably occurring by hematogenous spread, with *Staphylococcus aureus* as a frequent pathogen. Component removal, debridement, and resection arthroplasty in conjunction with antibiotic therapy is the most appropriate treatment in nearly all cases.

Intraoperative fracture of the humerus was noted by Cofield[11] to occur in 1.4% of 586 Neer total shoulder arthroplasties. The prevalence of this complication may be higher in the rheumatoid patient with osteopenia.[2] Cautious manipulation and retraction of the humerus and adequate surgical exposure may prevent this complication. Fortunately, these fractures are usually minimally displaced and treatment with cerclage wiring and cement fixation of the humeral component is generally sufficient.

Subacromial impingement may develop postop-

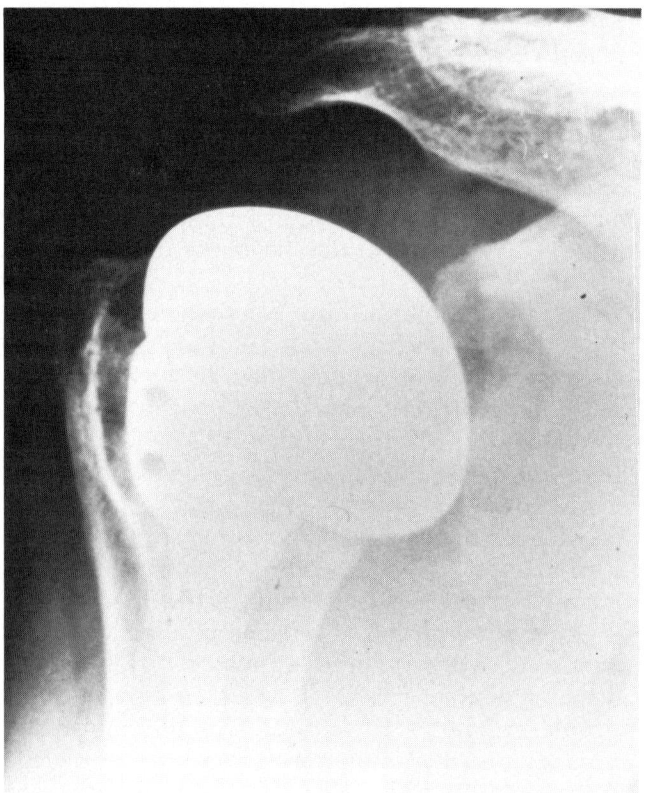

FIG 8–12.
A press-fit humeral component may be prone to rotational instability in patients with marked osteopenia.

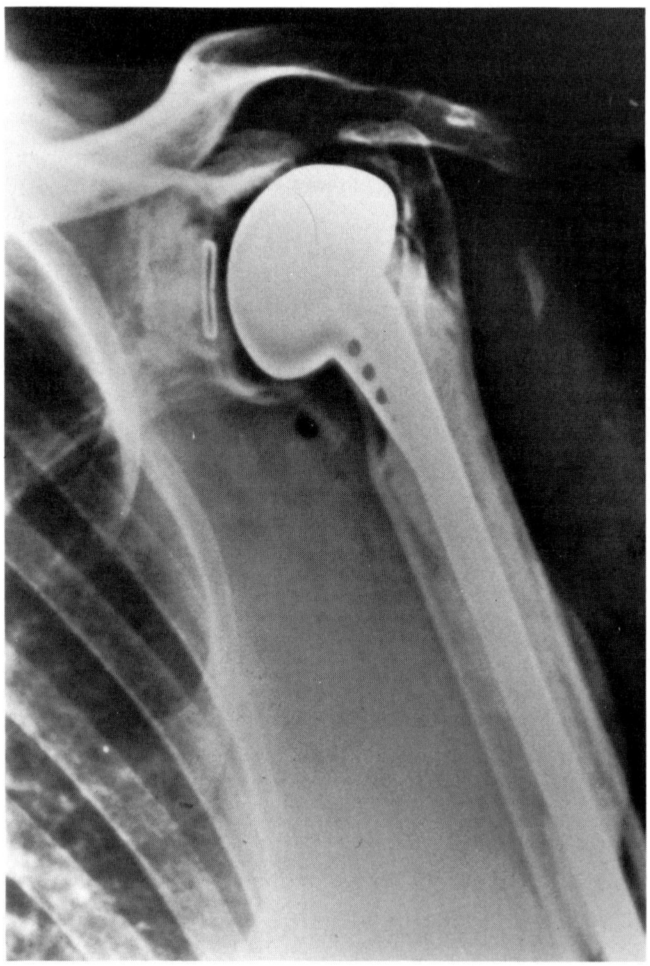

FIG 8–13.
Long-stemmed cemented humeral components may develop proximal bone resorption due to stress shielding.

eratively in approximately 1% of patients.[11] This complication is frequently associated with improper positioning of the humeral component below the level of the greater tuberosity.[16, 25] Osteophytes on the undersurface of the acromion or acromioclavicular joint may also be responsible for rotator cuff impingement. Painful acromioclavicular joint arthritis may exist concurrently and be difficult to distinguish from subacromial impingement. Acromioplasty and acromioclavicular joint resection may be beneficial in these patients.

Instability has been reported in 1% to 2% of patients.[11] This complication is best prevented by careful restoration of humeral and glenoid component version and assessment of implant stability intraoperatively. Failure to reconstruct bone deficits of the anterior or posterior glenoid may result in anterior or posterior instability, respectively. Unless significant component malposition is present, perioperative dislocations can generally be satisfactorily treated with closed reduction and immobilization for 3 to 6 weeks. Following this, rehabilitation can be resumed with satisfactory stability anticipated. If significant component malposition is present, recurrent dislocation frequently occurs, and revision of the malpositioned component is usually necessary.

Instability may also result from soft tissue imbalance or rupture of the repaired soft tissues. This may occur secondary to disruption of the repaired anterior capsule or rotator cuff, or iatrogenic incision of the posterior capsule at the time of proximal humeral osteotomy. Treatment of these specific causes should be directed toward reconstruction of the underlying soft tissue deficiency. Frequently, the patient with significant glenoid or humeral head bone loss will develop a significant capsular contracture due to relative medialization of the humeral head (Fig 8–11). Although lengthening of the subscapularis tendon can allow for anterior capsular and tendinous closure, residual posterior capsular contracture may predispose to failure of this repair and anterior instability. Limited posterior capsular release may be necessary to provide appropriate soft tissue balance and stability.

Recurrent rotator cuff tearing occurs infrequently.[11] Fortunately, most of these tears are asymptomatic and not associated with pain or marked functional limitation. Treatment is nonoperative, with good results.[2, 9] Symptomatic postoperative rotator cuff tears are often traumatic[25] and associated with pain and disability. Rotator cuff repair is indicated in the symptomatic patient, provided the tendons are not attenuated beyond the point that secure repair is still feasible.

Humeral component loosening rarely occurs following total shoulder arthroplasty (Figs 8–12 and 8–13). Cofield[11] estimated the incidence of this complication to be 0.34% in 586 total shoulder arthro-

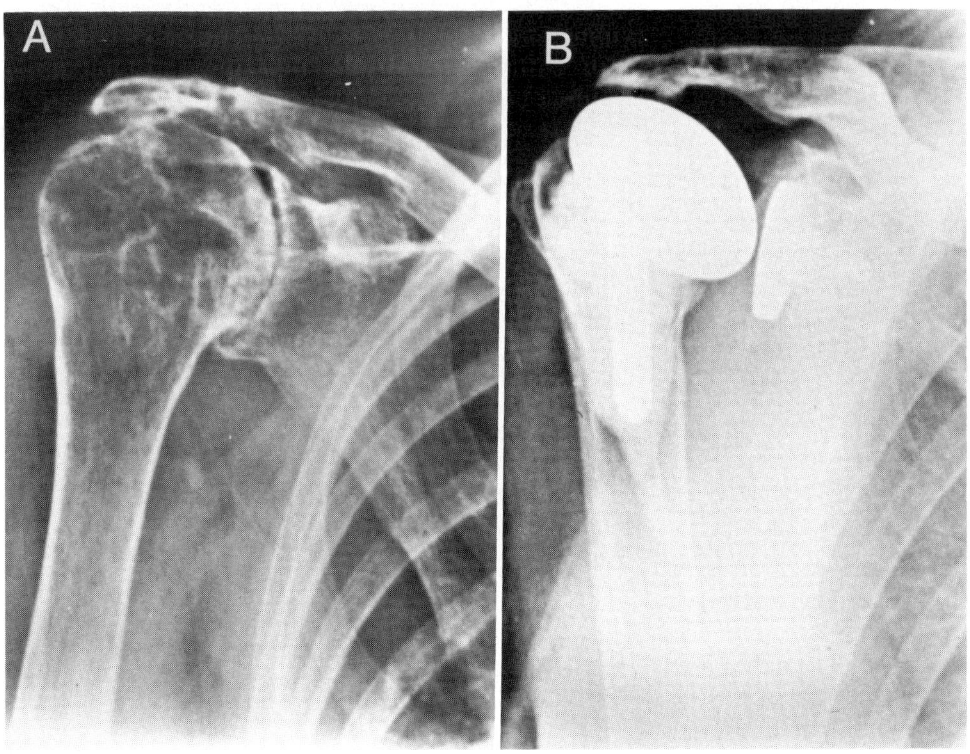

FIG 8–14.
A, a patient with massive rotator cuff deficiency demonstrates superior subluxation of the humerus, and acromial erosion. **B,** postoperatively, the humeral head still demonstrates superior subluxation leading to superior edge loading and an inferior tensile stress on the glenoid. This may result in glenoid loosening due to the "rocking horse" motion.

plasties with the Neer prosthesis. The adequacy and durability of fixation of the glenoid component appears more uncertain, however. Franklin et al.[17] compiled the results of radiographic glenoid loosening and revision for glenoid loosening in 766 unconstrained total shoulder arthroplasties from 12 reported clinical series. Although the radiographic evaluation was not standardized in these studies, partial or complete lucencies around the glenoid components were noted ranging from 30% to 93% of these cases. Radiographic loosening, defined as migration of the glenoid component, occurred in only 25 cases (3.6%) and revision for symptomatic loosening was necessary in only 14 cases (1.8%). Franklin et al. evaluated their 7 cases of glenoid component loosening and noted a statistically significant correlation between upward migration of the humeral component that occurs with rotator cuff deficiency and glenoid component loosening (Fig 8–14,A and B). The authors suggested that the upward migration of the humeral head and muscle imbalance between the rotator cuff and the deltoid results in eccentric loading of the glenoid with resultant glenoid loosening.[17] Brems et al.[6] and Neer et al.[25] have noted that glenoid radiolucencies, if present, are usually detectable perioperatively and have postulated that these are dependent on cement technique. Progression of the lucencies was infrequent and symptomatic component loosening was absent in both these studies. Considering the frequent occurrence of glenoid component interface lucencies, however, further evaluation is necessary to insure that progressive loss of glenoid component fixation does not develop with longer follow-up.

Reflex sympathetic dystrophy occurs rarely following total shoulder arthroplasty and can be a cause of persistent postoperative pain.[25] The classic signs of disproportionate pain, swelling and stiffness of the hands and fingers, and vasomotor instability are typically present. Treatment consists of early recognition of this disorder and intensive physiotherapy.

CONCLUSION

Unconstrained total shoulder arthroplasty is an effective treatment for severe inflammatory arthritis involving the shoulder. The primary objective of pain relief due to glenohumeral arthritis is achieved in nearly all patients. Although the presence of associated soft tissue and bone deficiencies and polyarticular involvement may compromise the results of the procedure, significant functional improvement is obtained in most patients. Carefully planned and executed surgery and postoperative rehabilitation can minimize the complications and maximize the benefits of the procedure in the patient with inflammatory arthritis of the shoulder.

REFERENCES

1. Amstutz HC, Thomas BJ, Kabo JM, et al: The DANA total shoulder arthroplasty. *J Bone Joint Surg [Am]* 1988; 70a:1174–1182.
2. Barrett WP, Franklin JL, Jackins SE, et al: Total shoulder arthroplasty. *J Bone Joint Surg [Am]* 1987; 69a:865–872.
3. Barrett WP, Thornhill TS, Thomas WH, et al: Nonconstrained total shoulder arthroplasty in patients with polyarticular rheumatoid arthritis. *J Arthroplasty* 1989; 4:91–96.
4. Bennett JC: Rheumatoid arthritis: Clinical features, in Schumacher HR (ed): *Primer on the Rheumatic Diseases.* Atlanta, Arthritis Foundation, 1988, p 89.
5. Bergmann G: Biomechanics and pathomechanics of the shoulder joint with reference to prosthetic joint replacement, in Kolbel R, Helbig B, Blauth W (eds): *Shoulder Replacement.* Berlin, Springer-Verlag, 1987.
6. Brems JJ, Wilde AH, Borden LS, et al: Glenoid lucent lines. *Orthop Trans* 1986; 10:231.
7. Brenner BC, Ferlic DC, Clayton ML, et al: Survivorship of unconstrained total shoulder arthroplasty. *J Bone Joint Surg [Am]* 1989; 71a:1289–1296.
8. Cofield RH: Unconstrained total shoulder prostheses. *Clin Orthop* 1983; 173:97–108.
9. Cofield RH: Total shoulder arthroplasty with the Neer prosthesis. *J Bone Joint Surg [Am]* 1984; 66a:899–906.
10. Cofield RH: Shoulder arthrodesis and resection arthroplasty. *Instr Course Lect* 1985; 34:268–277.
11. Cofield RH: Degenerative and arthritic problems of the glenohumeral joint, in Rockwood, CA, Matsen FA III (eds): *The Shoulder.* Philadelphia, WB Saunders Co, 1990, pp 740–745.
12. Cofield RH, Briggs BT: Glenohumeral arthritis. *J Bone Joint Surg [Am]* 1979; 61a:668–677.
13. Engelbrecht E, Heinert K: More than ten years experience with unconstrained shoulder replacement, in Kolbel R, Helbig B, Blauth W (eds): *Shoulder Replacement.* Berlin, Springer-Verlag, 1987, pp 85–91.
14. Ennevaara K: Painful shoulder joint in rheumatoid arthritis: A clinical and radiological study of 200 cases with special reference to arthrography of the glenohumeral joint. *Acta Rheum Scand* 1967; (suppl 11); 1–108.
15. Figgie MP, Inglis AE, Figgie HE III, et al: Custom total shoulder arthroplasty for inflammatory arthritis, in

Post M (ed): *Surgery of the Shoulder*. St Louis, Mosby–Year Book, Inc, 1990, pp 285–288.
16. Figgie HE III, Inglis AE, Goldberg VM, et al: An analysis of factors affecting the long-term results of total shoulder arthroplasty in inflammatory arthritis. *J Arthroplasty* 1988; 3:123–130.
17. Franklin JL, Barrett WP, Jackins SE, et al: Glenoid loosening in total shoulder arthroplasty. *J Arthroplasty* 1988; 3:39–46.
18. Friedman RJ, Ewald FC: Arthroplasty of the ipsilateral shoulder and elbow in patients who have rheumatoid arthritis. *J Bone Joint Surg [Am]* 1987; 69a:661–666.
19. Friedman RJ, Thornhill TS, Thomas WH, et al: Nonconstrained total shoulder replacement in patients who have rheumatoid arthritis and class-IV function. *J Bone Joint Surg [Am]* 1989; 71a:494–498.
20. Inman VT, Saunders JR, Abbott LC: Observations on the function of the shoulder joint. *J Bone Joint Surg [Am]* 1944; 26:1–30.
21. McCoy SR, Warren RF, Bade HA, et al: Total shoulder arthroplasty in rheumatoid arthritis. *J Arthroplasty* 1989; 4:105–113.
22. McElwain JP, English E.: The early results of porous-coated total shoulder arthroplasty. *Clin Orthop* 1987; 218:217–224.
23. Morrey BF, Askew LJ, An KN, et al: A biomechanical study of normal functional elbow motion. *J Bone Joint Surg [Am]* 1981; 63a:872.
24. Neer CS, Morrison DS: Glenoid bone-grafting in total shoulder arthroplasty. *J Bone Joint Surg [Am]* 1988; 70a:1154–1162.
25. Neer CS, Watson KC, Stanton FJ.: Recent experience in total shoulder arthroplasty. *J Bone Joint Surg [Am]* 1982; 64a:319–346.
26. Pahle JA, Kvarnes L: Shoulder synovectomy. *Ann Chir Gynaecol Suppl* 1985; 198:37–39.
27. Poppen NK, Walker PS: Normal and abnormal motion of the shoulder. *J Bone Joint Surg [Am]* 1976; 58a:195–201.
28. Poppen NK, Walker PS: Forces at the glenohumeral joint in abduction. *Clin Orthop* 1978; 135:165–170.
29. Sledge CB, Ewald FC: Total shoulder arthroplasty. Experience at the Robert Breck Brigham Hospital. *Clin Orthop* 1979; 145:78.
30. Smith-Peterson MN, Aufranc OE, Larson CB: Useful surgical procedures for rheumatoid arthritis involving joints of the upper extremity. *Arch Surg* 1943; 46:764–770.
31. Swanson AB, deGroot Swanson G, Maupin BK, et al: Bipolar implant shoulder arthroplasty. *Orthopedics* 1986; 9:343–351.
32. Thomas BJ, Amstutz HC, Cracchiolo A.: Shoulder arthroplasty for rheumatoid arthritis. *Clin Orthop* 1991; 265:125–128.
33. Walch G, Noel E, Guier C, et al: Rheumatoid arthritis of the shoulder: A review of 250 patients, in Post M, Morrey BF, Hawkins RJ (eds): *Surgery of the Shoulder*. St Louis, Mosby–Year Book, Inc, 1990, pp 267–269.

CHAPTER 9

The Elbow

Allan E. Inglis, M.D.

INTRODUCTION

The elbow joint is critical to the function of the upper extremity. The hand must be considered the essential tool of prehension with which we tactually manage and manipulate our environment. The elbow permits the extensile positioning of the hand in space.[1] Even in the presence of a stiffened shoulder the elbow can still position the hand away from the body in an extremely precise manner and at a variety of velocities. It must be recalled that not only does the elbow bring the hand toward and away from the body but it enables the hand to rotate through a 180-degree arc in any position of flexion or extension. As R. J. Last writes in his anatomy text, the biceps brachii "not only inserts the corkscrew, but pulls out the cork as well."[16] And, I might add, pours at any position of flexion or extension as well.

The movements of the normal elbow are of five types: first, there is flexion of approximately 135 degrees; second, there is extension to 0 degrees, i.e., when the elbow is completely straight; third, there is pronation of approximately 80 degrees; fourth, there is supination of approximately 80 degrees; fifth, there is an eccentric or camlike movement of the elbow joint through the flexion-extension arc.[21] In extension, the elbow is in 15 degrees valgus relative to the upper arm, and in full flexion it moves into neutral or 0-degree alignment through the camlike effect produced by the surfaces of the trochlea of the humerus and the semilunar notch of the ulna (Fig 9–1). These surfaces guide the joint through an arc of motion with a high level of precision.

The stability of the elbow joint is achieved through four ligaments. The most essential stabilizing ligament is the anterior medial ligament[16] on the inner aspect of the elbow joint (Fig 9–2). This ligament passes from the medial epicondyle of the humerus to the sublime tubercle of the ulna. The next essential ligament for elbow function is the annular ligament. This ligament stabilizes the radius against the proximal radioulnar joint during rotation. It also stabilizes the radioulnar joint during contraction of the biceps brachii, both in flexion and in supination. The third ligamentous structure is the lateral collateral ligament extending from the orbicular ligament to the lateral epicondyle and to the ulna. The ulnar portion of this ligament is within the anconeus muscle and has only recently been described by Morrey[19, 20] as the major stabilizing ligament on the lateral aspect of the elbow joint.

Additional stability to the elbow articulation is achieved through the muscular origins on the medial and lateral epicondyles. These muscles are sufficiently far from the articular surfaces of the elbow joint to exert a considerable stabilizing effect on the joint.[19] Their protective stabilization during varus and valgus stress forces is not force times distance but force times distance *squared*.[12] Therefore, sudden applied forces to the elbow joint will initiate a stretch reflex in the forearm flexors and extensors, thereby reducing the force applied directly to the joint surfaces. The capsule, fascia, and the epimysium surrounding the muscles also assist in stabilizing the elbow by providing a passive viscoelastic support to the joint. The soft tissue envelope, the stretch reflexes of the flexor and extensor muscles, and the precise geometric design of the joint surfaces provide for a durable, stable articulation. These forces work not only during flexion and extension but in pronation and supination as well.

In the normal activities of daily living, the forces

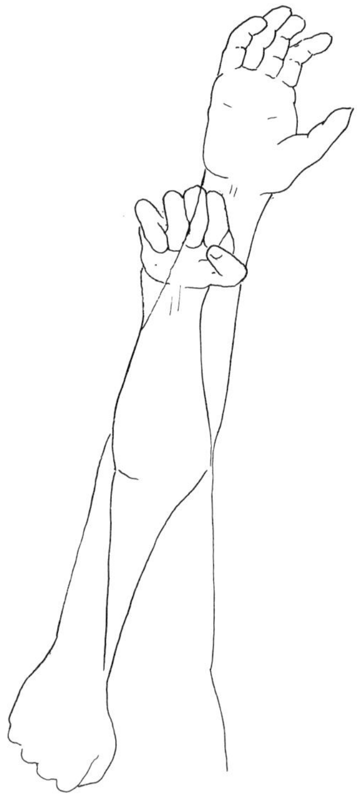

FIG 9–1.
In extension, the elbow is in 15 degrees valgus with respect to the arm. In flexion, the elbow moves into neutral alignment due to the cam effect produced by the shape of the trochlea of the humerus.

across the elbow joint are almost entirely compressional, i.e., say if a person lifts a 40-lb suitcase, the loading across the elbow joint is 40 lb of compression, not 40 lb of tension. Therefore, simple contraction of the muscles about the elbow joints when stabilized by the joint surfaces and the collateral ligaments provides a stable smooth movement during a variety of loading situations. There are a few tensile loads that may be applied across the elbow joint, one of which is rapid unopposed extension of the elbow joint by the triceps muscle. As the elbow joint reaches full extension, the elbow flexors, i.e., the brachioradialis, the brachialis, and the biceps, must contract in sufficient time or a tensile load will be applied across the elbow joint. This unusual tensile loading is important if the ligaments are compromised or the patient has a total elbow replacement.

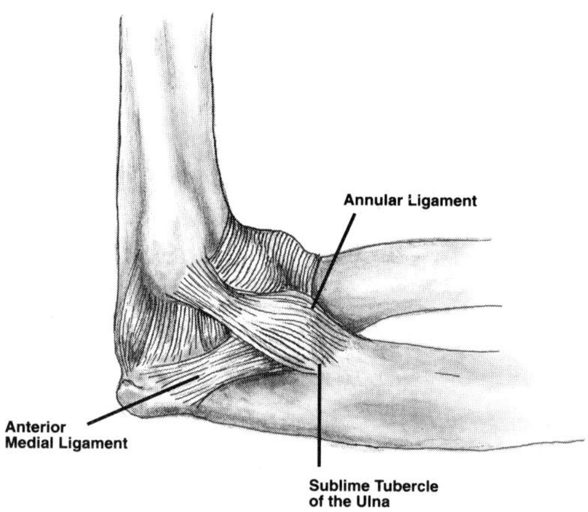

FIG 9–2.
The medial side of the elbow. The anterior medial ligament passes from the medial epicondyle to the sublime tubercle of the ulna.

Rheumatoid or inflammatory arthritis may adversely affect the elbow in a number of ways. It may merely produce a synovitis with accompanying pain and restriction of motion.[18] In this situation, there is mainly a loss of extension and some loss of flexion. As the synovitis progresses there may be joint effusion with swelling, joint destruction, and further pain and limitation of motion. As the synovitis progresses further, there will be proliferation of the synoviocytes with gradual distention of the joint with bulky synovial tissue. A pannus will form at the edges of the articular surfaces, eroding and destroying the hyaline cartilage and bone. Some of the synovial tissue may penetrate the ulna and trochlea, forming cysts. These cysts may become sufficiently large that the overlying articular surfaces become weakened, allowing the joint to collapse. The combination of thinned joint surfaces caused by synovial erosion and the collapsing of the small cysts leads to joint instability. Because of joint foreshortening, the ligaments become relatively lax, permitting abnormal motion with further joint damage. The combination of continuing synovitis and inflammation along with instability frequently results in pain and ultimately poor elbow function.

Normally, the transmission of compression forces across the radiocapitellar joint is modest until significant loads are applied across the radiohumeral joint.[19, 21] These significant loads begin when 50% of the maximum loading occurs across the ulnohumeral joint.[5] These relatively low loads across the radiocapitellar joint in the normal elbow can be radically altered in rheumatoid arthritis. As the joint surfaces of the trochlea and the semilunar notch and the radius and capitellum erode, the loading across the radiocapitellar joint may increase dramatically. The barren radial head will then articulate directly and continuously with the capitellum (Fig 9–3). As the superior radioulnar joint becomes eroded and irregular, pain on pronation and supination may develop. Joint incongruities at the superior radioulnar joint may result in locking during pronation and su-

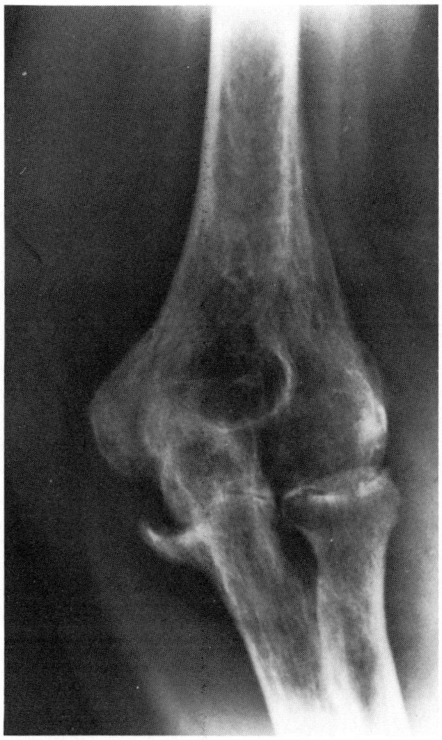

FIG 9–3.
The radiocapitellar joint is narrowed sufficiently so that it is now loading during the entire arc of motion. Note the distribution of the trochlea.

pination as well as in flexion and extension. Therefore joint surface damage with resultant instability and joint incongruities frequently leads to pain and loss of elbow function.[12]

In the treatment of patients with rheumatoid arthritis it is important to determine the priorities of the patient's disease and disabilities.[6, 12] Certainly, painful and disabling articulations take precedence over deformities. The capacity to walk or, in the case of patients with rheumatoid arthritis, perform activities of daily living (ADLs), is essential. Elbow flexion and extension are important to hygiene, the ability to feed oneself, grooming, and the ability to perform useful work. An elbow immobilized by pain or ankylosis at 90 degrees imposes enormous restrictions on these activities.

CONSERVATIVE TREATMENT

Therapeutic measures should be instituted when elbow function becomes sufficiently reduced either by pain or by lack of motion. These patients should be cared for by an orthopaedic surgeon in concert with a rheumatologist.[18] All patients should be followed directly by a rheumatologist so that the other organ systems involved in inflammatory or rheumatoid arthritis can be assessed. Frequently patients will have rheumatoid pulmonary disease, carditis, anemia, renal involvement, and other problems. In addition to supporting the rheumatologist's programs, the orthopaedic surgeon will contribute to the care of the patient with appropriate arthrocenteses, steroid instillations, splint requisitions, exercise programs, and finally, surgical therapy. The management of a painful, disabled elbow should include a complete orthopaedic examination to provide a baseline for treatment of the current problem as well as those problems which may develop in other articulations in the future.[19] The evaluation should include radiographs of the cervical spine in flexion and extension, and of the shoulder, elbow, hand, and wrist, bilaterally. If large cysts are seen on the plain film, a computed tomography (CT) scan is useful in planning therapeutic measures. If the patient has neurologic symptoms such as neck pain, ulnar neuritis, or if brachial plexus involvement is suspected, nerve conduction velocities and electromyelogram (EMG) studies should be obtained. Range of motion, both active and passive, should be measured during each evaluation of the patient. An ADL evaluation by an occupational therapist is useful.

The single most important therapeutic measure that can be brought to bear on the painful rheumatoid elbow is an intraarticular injection of a long-acting corticosteroid.[18] One must be certain that the injection is within the elbow joint and not in the anterior fat pad above the capsule. The injection should be carefully planned and accomplished with a small-bore needle on the lateral aspect of the elbow. The precise joint line is easily identified and marked on the elbow in full extension or in a few degrees of flexion. It is difficult to palpate the radiocapitellar articulation with the elbow at 90 degrees of flexion owing to the overlying extensor muscle origins. Forty milligrams of delayed-action steroid is sufficient. The steroid should be mixed with a small amount of local anesthetic to provide immediate pain relief.

An occasional patient may benefit from a night splint fabricated so that it is in approximately 90 degrees of flexion. Some patients will achieve relief by placing their elbow on a pillow at night. An occasional patient will benefit from a flexible flexion-extension splint adjusted to provide the tension needed for function. Dynamic splints or rubber straps with springs are contraindicated. These splints tend to aggravate the elbow by initiating stretch reflexes both in flexion and in extension so that the elbows actually lose rather than gain motion. Exercises are also contraindicated. If the surgeon is considering synovectomy and debridement or other surgical procedure, it is essential that the rheumatologist be advised so that he or she can be supportive of the need for surgical therapy.

Surgical therapy should be considered only after the patient has been carefully assessed to be certain that there are no other surgical priorities that might take precedence over the elbow problem. The surgeon may consider a concomitant procedure,[18] but it is important that the number of surgical procedures be held to a minimum in these patients. These patients may simply run out of ego reserves to sustain them over the course of many surgical procedures. I prefer to perform two operations during the same anesthesia, when possible, to minimize the psychological and physical trauma of surgery.

SURGICAL CONSIDERATIONS

Large rheumatoid nodules over the olecranon process may become disabling and painful and subject to repeated infections. If there are multiple nodules from the olecranon process distally along the ulna, these should be removed with separate, relatively small incisions. The incisions should be transverse. If there is a single, large nodule over the olecranon process, it should be removed through a transverse incision, which *should not extend beyond the medial border of the olecranon process.* If the incision extends beyond the medial border of the triceps, it may compromise a future incision needed for synovectomy or replacement arthroplasty. Following surgery, the elbow should be placed in a well-padded dressing with an anterior splint. The splint should *not* be placed posteriorly, as this produces pressure on the incisions. Alternatively, the elbow may be placed in a cylinder cast split along both sides or in a bulky compression dressing with an anterior splint split along both sides. The splint is kept in place for 4 to 7 days to be certain that primary wound healing is achieved. Prophylactic antibiotics are not used as this is a soft tissue surgical procedure. Parenteral steroids may be required if the patient is on maintenance corticosteroid therapy. The use of additional corticosteroids should be not more than three times the daily maintenance dose. The dosage can be coordinated with the rheumatologist. The patient should be advised that these nodules may recur, although in my experience the recurrence level is very low.

A synovial mass may arise on the posterior medial aspect of the elbow (Fig 9–4). These masses arise from within the ulnohumeral joint and break through the capsule into the cubital tunnel. Local excision is ineffective. The masses will recur due to underlying elbow synovitis. The treatment for ulnar neuropathy and synovial masses is synovectomy and removal of the mass through the same incision. At times, a median neuropathy may develop with a

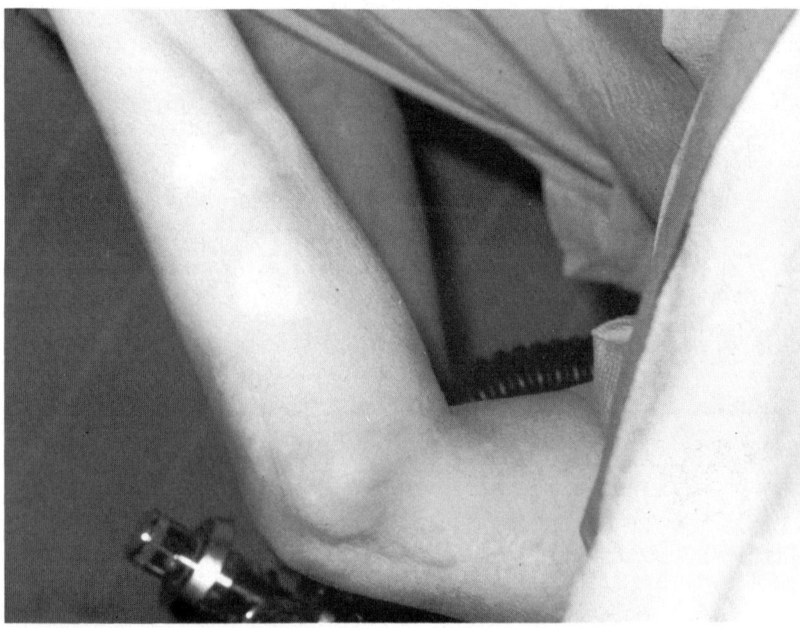

FIG 9–4.
A synovial mass on the medial side of the elbow. The patient had two prior operations (note healing incisions) to release the ulnar neuropathy due to synovial masses. The patient underwent a synovectomy of the elbow and excision of the mass emanating from the elbow joint.

large evagination of synovium from the anterior area of the elbow joint. These are easily palpable in the antecubital fossa just distal to the lacertus fibrosus. Again, removal of just these synovial masses will lead to recurrence because the underlying problem is intraarticular synovitis. *Synovectomy* of the elbow joint is a useful, predictable procedure for uncontrolled synovitis of the elbow joint when the articular surfaces are preserved.[3, 7, 9, 14, 24] However, it will lead to the need for additional surgical procedures if the articular surfaces are severely damaged with resultant joint incongruities and instability (Fig 9–5). The patients should be advised that even with a relatively intact joint, they may still require synovectomy at some time in the future. It has been our experience that the need for implant arthroplasty following synovectomy, although relatively uncommon, will be apparent within 2 years following the initial procedure.

There are four surgical approaches to elbow synovectomy: (1), a lateral incision with removal of the radial head and removal of as much synovium as can be visualized through a lateral approach[17]; (2), olecranon osteotomy with removal of the radial head and debridement of the irregular joint margins and a total synovectomy[15]; (3), an incision along the posterior medial aspect of the elbow with removal of the radial head and a total synovectomy[4, 12]; (4), arthroscopic synovectomy.

Synovectomy through the lateral approach has certain advantages. First, it allows for removal of the radial head and it can be performed relatively quickly.[7] This procedure has been utilized by Nalebuff and others who advocate this type of synovectomy along with reconstructive hand surgery as a single surgical procedure. This has obvious advantages, but allows for only a subtotal synovectomy because of the limited exposure. Nevertheless, good long-term functional results have been reported. It also has a low complication record.

Synovectomy through a posterior approach and osteotomy of the olecranon process has many advantages.[15] It allows for a complete exposure of the posterior aspect of the elbow joint, removal of the radial head, removal of all of the synovium in the anterior and posterior portions of the joint, and removal of all of the synovium beneath the medial and lateral collateral ligaments.

Synovectomy and debridement utilizing the transolecranon approach is relatively uncomplicated. The incision is made in the midline just over the radial aspect of the ulna and extends another 10 cm along the posterior aspect of the humerus (Fig 9–6,A).[15] The dissection is carried down to the periosteum of the ulna and to the epimysium of the triceps. A narrow flap is developed medially and laterally, exposing the entire olecranon process and the superficial surface of the triceps. The ulnar nerve is

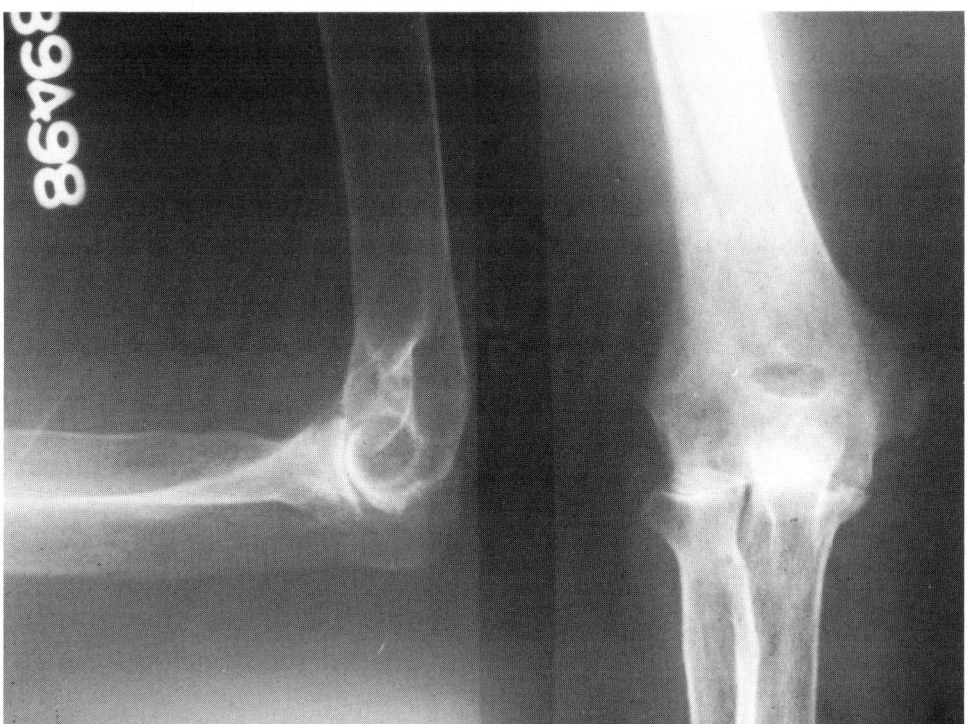

FIG 9–5.
Postoperative radiograph of a patient who underwent a synovectomy. Six months later, a replacement arthroplasty was required due to persistence of pain and irritability.

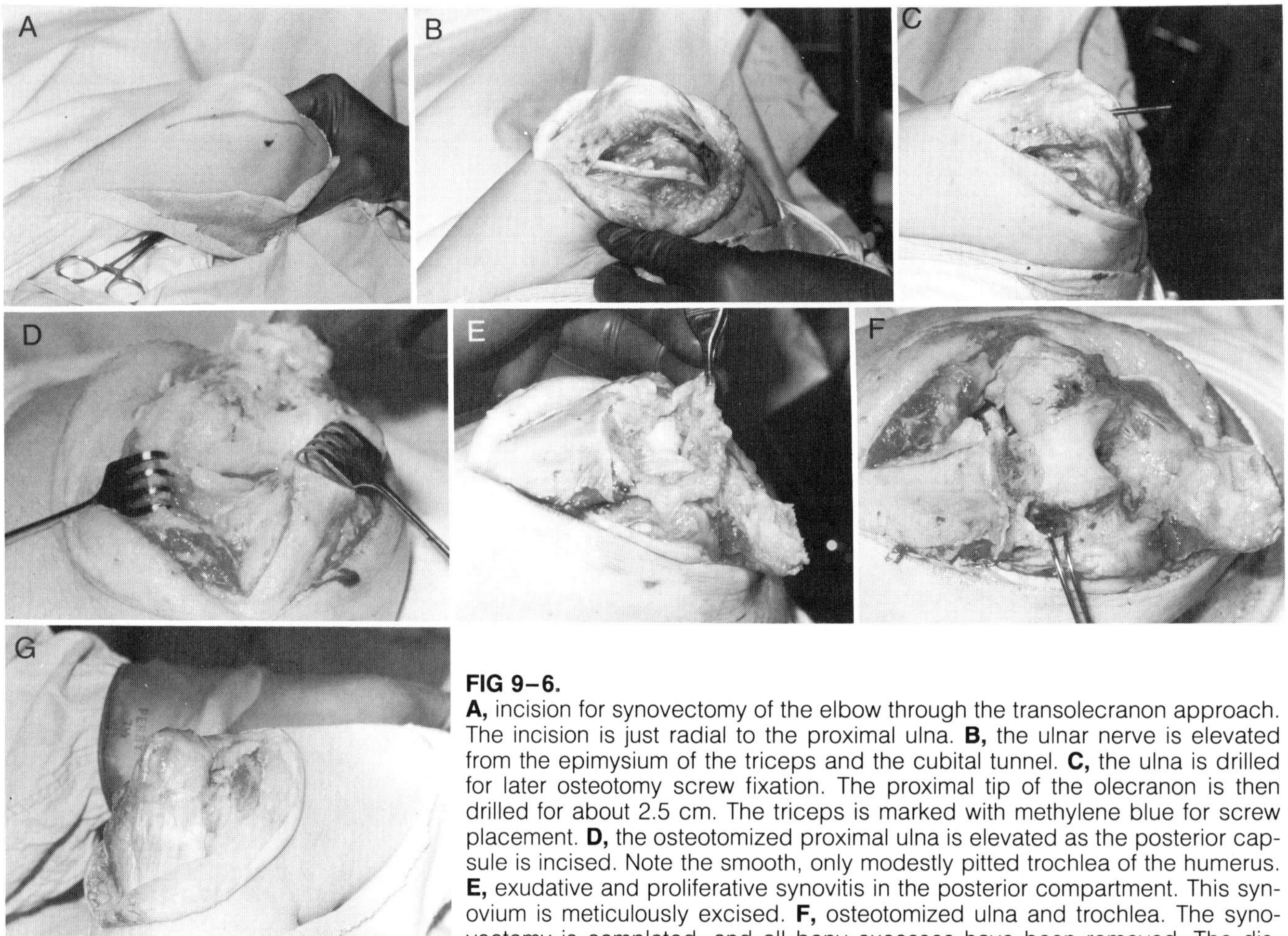

FIG 9–6.
A, incision for synovectomy of the elbow through the transolecranon approach. The incision is just radial to the proximal ulna. **B,** the ulnar nerve is elevated from the epimysium of the triceps and the cubital tunnel. **C,** the ulna is drilled for later osteotomy screw fixation. The proximal tip of the olecranon is then drilled for about 2.5 cm. The triceps is marked with methylene blue for screw placement. **D,** the osteotomized proximal ulna is elevated as the posterior capsule is incised. Note the smooth, only modestly pitted trochlea of the humerus. **E,** exudative and proliferative synovitis in the posterior compartment. This synovium is meticulously excised. **F,** osteotomized ulna and trochlea. The synovectomy is completed, and all bony excesses have been removed. The displaced ulnar nerve is in the foreground beneath the retractor. **G,** the olecranon has been anatomically replaced and secured with a screw. An additional figure-of-eight wire will provide extra support for early mobilization.

identified and elevated from the cubital tunnel (Fig 9–6,B). A small Penrose drain is placed around the nerve and secured with a suture (not a clamp). The nerve is then gently retracted medially. A 1-cm longitudinal incision is made in the insertion of the triceps muscle into the olecranon process. The olecranon process is then drilled for placement of an olecranon screw (Fig 9–6,C). Another larger drilling is then made over the previous hole for approximately 2.5 cm. This allows for subsequent compression of the olecranon osteotomy by the fixation screw. The olecranon osteotomy is carried out with a thin-bladed microsaw in the midportion of the semilunar notch. The tip of the olecranon process can then be elevated and retracted with the entire triceps up and away from the bulging posterior capsule (Fig 9–6,D and E). The radiocapitellar joint is exposed by elevating the anconeus muscle and the origins of the adjacent wrist extensor muscle. The capsule and the bulging synovium from the radiocapitellar joint are then excised. The radial head is exposed and excised. The remaining osteotomized radius should be inspected to be certain that there are no sharp edges remaining after the osteotomy. Through this exposure, the entire anterior capsule can be visualized, and the synovium is removed with rongeurs or sharply excised. All of the synovium must be removed.

The posterior capsule is completely excised along with the synovium. As this posterior capsulectomy and synovectomy is completed, attention is directed to the area along the medial aspect of the elbow joint, i.e., the area beneath the medial collateral ligament and the ulnar nerve (Fig 9–6,F). At times, the synovium from the medial side of the ulnohumeral joint will extrude through the capsule and exert pressure on the ulnar nerve. The area lateral to the trochlea should be explored for hyperplastic synovium beneath the collateral ligament. The margins of the joint should be carefully inspected for small pockets of residual synovium. Following a complete synovectomy, the joint should be inspected and divided for any bony excrescences or ridges that would retard the patient's rehabilitation and convalescence. Following synovectomy and debridement, the tourniquet is deflated and hemostasis secured. An Esmarch's bandage is reapplied and the tourniquet is reinflated. The olecranon screw is passed through the olecranon fragment and the fragment replaced to the remaining ulnar bone (Fig 9–6,G). A small transverse drill hole is then made in the distal ulna approximately 2.5 cm from the osteotomy site. A 20-gauge wire is passed through this drill hole. The wire is then laid in a figure-of-eight fashion across the osteotomy site and around the fixation screw. The wire is then tightened. This provides additional fixation for the olecranon osteotomy. The subcutaneous tissues are closed and the skin approximated with clips or fine sutures. The arm is placed in a large bulk dressing with an anterior splint at 45 degrees of extension. A negative pressure drain is passed out through the skin in the mid–upper arm. Active exercises are begun on the fourth postoperative day.

The lateral subtotal synovectomy is also useful. A lateral incision over and just below the lateral epicondyle is used. The extensor carpi radialis brevis and longus are incised transversely approximately 0.5 cm from their epicondylar origin. These muscles and the lateral collateral ligament are elevated to expose the lateral aspect of the radiocapitellar joint. The radial head is excised and synovectomy is performed. Through the same incision the triceps is elevated from the posterior aspect of the capitellum, exposing the posterior capsule of the elbow joint. The synovectomy is then carried out.

A third method for synovectomy and debridement is the medial approach of Bryan and Morrey.[4, 6] The incision begins 10 cm from the olecranon process over the ulna and continues proximally midway between the olecranon process and the medial epicondyle. It continues another 10 cm medially up the arm along the medial border of the triceps. Flaps are avoided. Here the epimysium of the flexor carpi ulnaris and the periosteum of the ulna as well as the entire triceps, including the insertion to the olecranon process, are reflected as a single flap toward the lateral aspect of the elbow joint. Again, the radial head is excised and a complete anterior and posterior synovectomy is carried out. A debridement should also be performed of any bony ridges or excrescences. At the completion of the procedure, the central tendon of the triceps is sutured to the tip of the olecranon process through two drill holes. This exposure has the advantage of early immobilization without fear of displacement of the osteotomy, as in the transolecranon approach.

The results of synovectomy and debridement have been salutary.[7, 22] Eighty-five percent to 90% of patients undergoing synovectomy and debridement will achieve good to excellent results.[2] Complications and failures have occurred in those patients in whom the arthritis and joint destruction was advanced or in patients who were unable to cooperate in the rehabilitation program. When indicated, this latter group of patients can always be relieved of symptoms with an elbow replacement arthroplasty.

Arthroscopic synovectomy in inflammatory arthritis may have some advantage with small incisions. Difficulty in removing the radial head with complete removal of the synovial pockets beneath the collateral ligaments and cubital tunnel, and of accurately debriding the joint margins, makes this approach less attractive than the conventional technique. Additionally, the remaining radial head may cause problems in the future.

TOTAL ELBOW ARTHROPLASTY

The indications for total elbow replacement in rheumatoid arthritis are similar to those for synovectomy of the elbow: disabling pain, instability, and reduced motion. When the joint is narrowed and the articular surfaces are deficient, or there is bone loss and cyst formation, replacement arthroplasty rather than synovectomy and debridement becomes the procedure of choice.[5, 12] The other indication for replacement is a failed elbow synovectomy or a painless ankylosis in poor position for ADLs.

The modern experience with elbow replacement arthroplasty dates back to 1974 when Ewald and Inglis began their series of patients with Capitellar-condylar and Triaxial total elbow replacements. In 1973 Souter[23] and Dee[8] reported their experience with a constrained elbow implant. Although their results initially appeared encouraging, ultimately the constrained implant used was unsatisfactory. During this same period Coonrad[6] was developing his constrained elbow implant. This implant initially had problems owing to its fully constrained nature. However, it was subsequently redesigned and has since been successfully employed.[6] The Capitellar-condylar implant is a nonconstrained device that utilizes its own joint surface congruity and a retained anterior (medial collateral) ligament for stability. The only problem with the implant has been its tendency for dislocation, the management of which is highly dependent upon exacting surgical technique and patient compliance. It has achieved excellent results in patients with lesser joint damage and initial good joint stability. The Hospital for Special Surgery Triaxial implant initially was designed with a high-density, molecular polyethylene humeral component[14] (Fig 9–7). It provided a 30-degree anterior tilt of the humeral component and a 15-degree valgus alignment of the ulna with 7 degrees of laxity in all planes. One of the high-molecular-weight humeral components broke, so the polyethylene was replaced with stainless steel (Fig 9–8). The two components were corrected with a "snap-fit" articulation. This implant achieved early success, but approximately 5% of patients developed a dislocation due to the "snap-fit" articulation. This was subsequently modified with a nonloaded axle. The long-term results with these implants has been satisfactory.[12]

The Capitellar-condylar total elbow replacement is accomplished through the Kocher incision in which the medial collateral ligament is preserved and retained throughout the procedure. The radial head is excised. The basic articulation is therefore between the ulnar and humeral components. These components are available in various sizes so that the ligaments and soft tissues can be perfectly balanced, thereby avoiding postoperative instability and dislocations.

The Hospital for Special Surgery custom implant has the same geometry and ligament and loading characteristics as the original triaxial implant (Fig 9–9,A), the only notable exception being a variation in the loading mechanism in which the load is transmitted centrally during normal movements and along the two condyles with varus and valgus stresses. The Hospital for Special Surgery custom implant and the Coonrad implant, or the Mayo modification of the Coonrad implant, have the added capacity for a bone ingrowth when this need arises. For general use The Hospital for Special Surgery custom implant is used with cement as loosening has not been a significant problem at long-term follow-up.[19]

Preoperative planning should include templating the patient's radiographs. The presurgical inventory should include both the large and small components and at least one additional high-molecular-weight polyethylene bushing (in case one falls to the

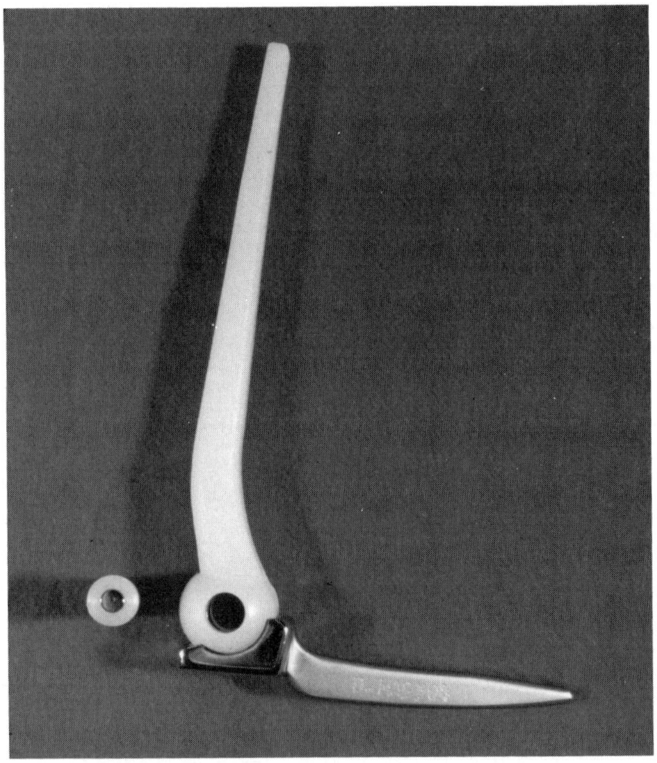

FIG 9–7.
Original Triaxial total elbow replacement. Note the anterior angulation of the distal portion of the humerus.

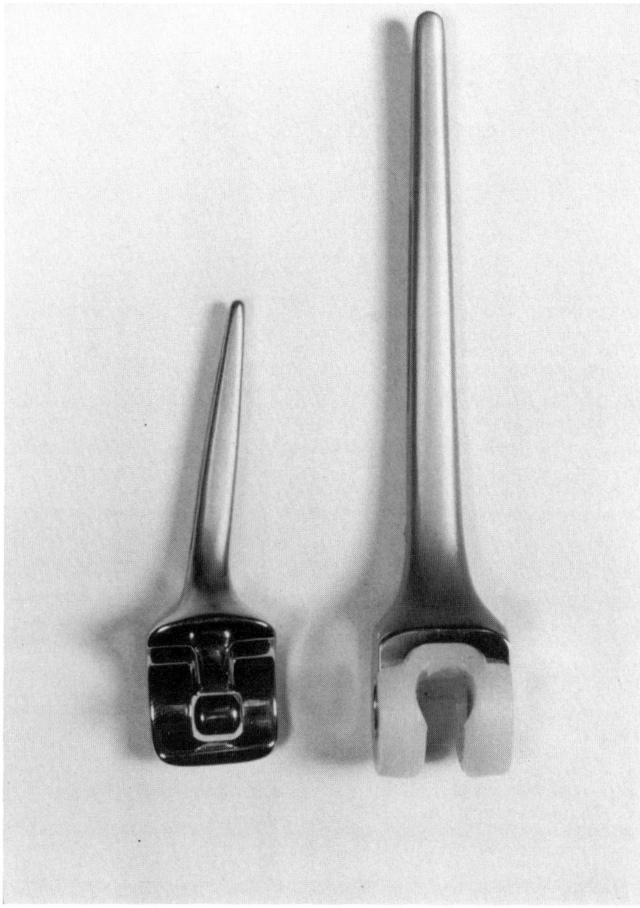

FIG 9–8.
Modified Triaxial implant. Note the valgus alignment of this right-sided total elbow replacement.

floor during surgery). The templating should be for the largest implant that will fit into the humerus and ulna. The surgical technique for implant insertion generally follows the Bryan-Morrey approach.[4, 12] Instruments for making the various bone cuts, reaming, broaching, and testing are available. These alignment jigs correspond precisely to the implants required for the arthroplasty.

The surgical approach is along the posterior aspect of the elbow beginning 10 cm from the tip of olecranon process over the ulna. It is continued to a point equidistant from the medial border of the olecranon process and the medial epicondyle directly over the ulnar nerve and the cubital tunnel. The incision is continued 10 cm further along the medial border of the triceps and carried down to the epimysium of the flexor carpi ulnaris and the epimysium of the triceps (Fig 9–9,B). The ulnar nerve is identified within the cubital tunnel where it passes between the medial epicondyle and the ulna. A nerve muscle hook is passed beneath the medial epicondylar retinaculum and is opened to expose the ulnar nerve. The epimysium is then opened from this point distal to the ulna. The epimysium is lifted as a single layer along with the periosteum of the ulna and the insertion of the central portion of the triceps tendon into the olecranon process. The ulnar nerve is separated from within the triceps and a small Penrose drain is wrapped around the ulnar nerve. A suture is placed in the Penrose drain so that careful retraction of the ulnar nerve may be carried out throughout the procedure. The triceps muscle is elevated away from the posterior aspect of the humerus and separated from the posterior capsule of the elbow joint. The posterior capsule of the elbow joint is not opened until the entire triceps flap is elevated toward the lateral aspect of the elbow. The triceps flap will include most of the substance of the anconeus muscle and the capsule of the radiocapitellar joint. The entire triceps flap is then retracted away from the posterior aspect of the elbow joint, providing excellent exposure of the joint (Fig 9–9,C). The capsule and synovium of the radiocapitellar joint is excised to expose the radial head. The radial head is osteotomized and removed just proximal to the annular ligament. The radius is inspected

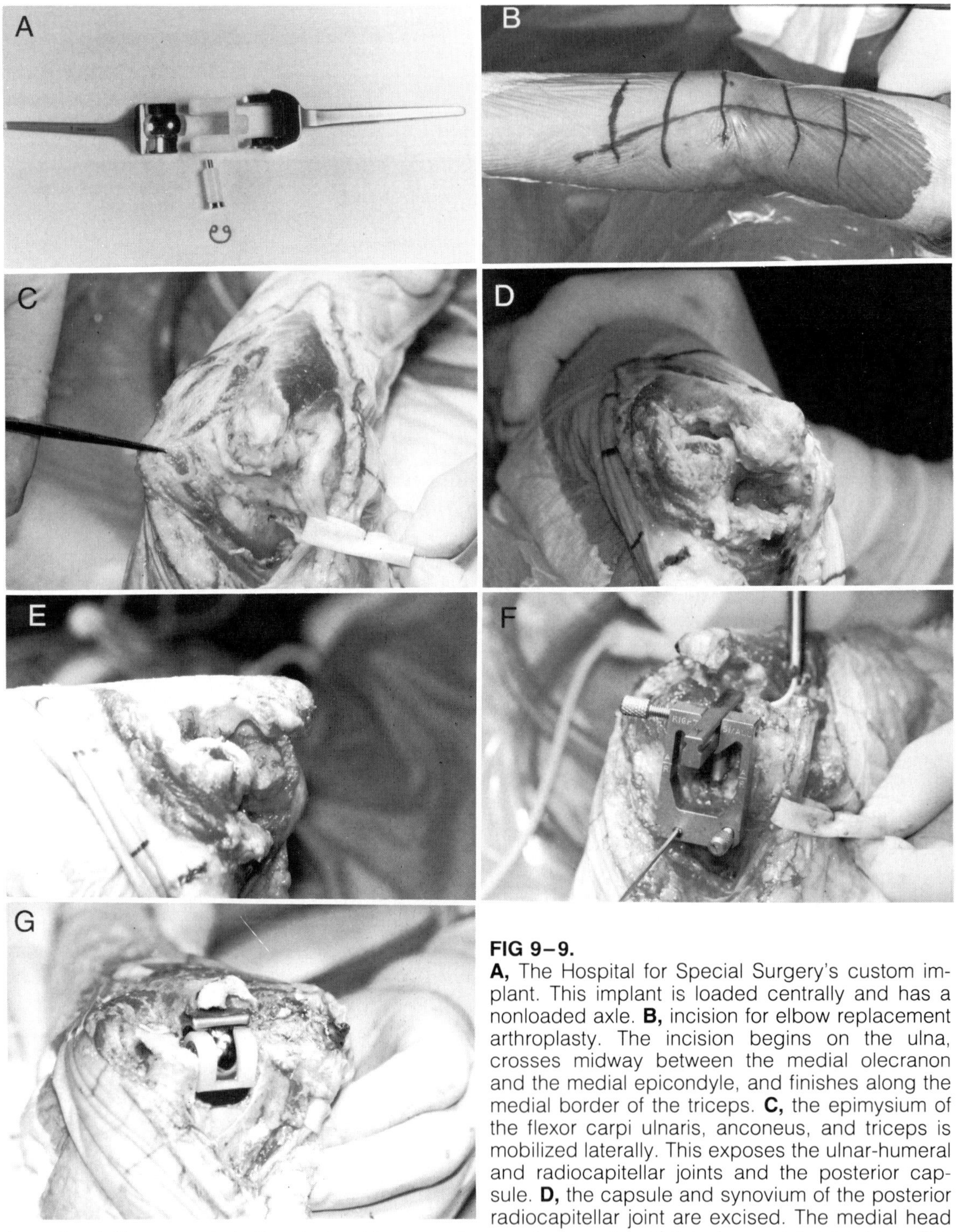

FIG 9–9.
A, The Hospital for Special Surgery's custom implant. This implant is loaded centrally and has a nonloaded axle. **B,** incision for elbow replacement arthroplasty. The incision begins on the ulna, crosses midway between the medial olecranon and the medial epicondyle, and finishes along the medial border of the triceps. **C,** the epimysium of the flexor carpi ulnaris, anconeus, and triceps is mobilized laterally. This exposes the ulnar-humeral and radiocapitellar joints and the posterior capsule. **D,** the capsule and synovium of the posterior radiocapitellar joint are excised. The medial head is excised. The capsule is then incised between the semilunar notch of the ulna and the trochlea. The anterior medial ligament is released. **E,** excellent exposure of the proximal ulna is achieved following release of the capsule and anterior medial ligament. **F,** the humeral cutting jig is inserted to the center of rotation. Note the protected ulnar nerve. The saw is used to cut inside the cutting jig. **G,** the final cemented implant. Remaining bone is excised from the tip of the ulnar component.

to be certain that there are no remaining sharp edges or excrescences to interfere with the ulna during pronation and supination.

The ulnohumeral joint is exposed by incising the capsule between the edges of the trochlea and the ulna. As this dissection proceeds medially it will be necessary to elevate portions of the insertion of the flexor carpi ulnaris away from the ulna to expose the sublime tubercle of the ulna. As the sublime tubercle is exposed,[16] the ulnar origin of the flexor digitorum superficialis will be released along with the anteromedial ligament of the elbow (Fig 9–9,D). At this point the ulna can be lifted up and away from the trochlea to provide a broad exposure of the humerus and the semilunar notch and the coronoid process of the ulna (Fig 9–9,E). The anterior capsule of the elbow joint is incised over a small clamp. If there has been a preoperative elbow flexion contracture, a small portion of the brachialis muscle can be released from the proximal ulna. The center of rotation of the ulna is then noted and marked. A small cutting guide or jig is placed over the ulna and the amount of bone to be resected is marked with methylene blue or another appropriate marker. A fine oscillating saw is used to remove the marked portion of the ulna. Following removal of the semilunar notch, a medium-sized burr is used to identify the intermedullary space of the ulna. The rasp and broach are then used to open up the intermedullary portion of the ulna. There are prescribed broaches for bone preparation. At times a burr will be necessary to remove small corners of the proximal ulna for an optimal fit of the ulnar component. The implant should be able to be inserted such that the center of rotation of the implant matches the marked center of rotation on the olecranon process.

The humeral implant preparation begins by removing the remaining capsule and synovium from the posterior aspect of the elbow joint. These tissues are excised from the olecranon fossa. A sufficient amount of capsule will need to be removed so that the two margins of the humerus are clearly exposed, thereby protecting the two epicondyles during preparation of the humerus. The center of rotation of the humeral articulation is determined and marked. A small alignment guide is inserted and the center of the trochlea of the humerus is marked. This portion of the humerus is removed with the oscillating saw. The proximal portion of this cut may need to be trimmed with rongeurs to provide an entrance to the intermedullary area of the humerus. When this has been completed, a centralizing guide can be inserted into the humerus and adjusted for the marked center of rotation of the humeral component. The guide or jig is then slid over this guide post and stabilized with a 0.62 guage pin. The oscillating saw is used to cut out the proper portion of the humerus for the ulna implant (Fig 9–9,F). Care must be taken not to violate the lateral portions of the epicondyles which may lead to a stress fracture. This device is then removed and the medullary canal is opened so that the component can be inserted easily into the humerus with the two axial holes of the component matching the centers of rotation as previously marked. When this has been completed, the trial humeral and ulnar components are inserted along the bushing and the joint is brought through a range of motion. The surgeon must be assured that there are no bony edges that will interfere with movement of the elbow and that full extension has been achieved.

The elbow is carefully irrigated and the methylmethacrylate cement is prepared in a somewhat liquid form. The cement is packed simultaneously into both the ulna and the humerus. Firm packing is required to be certain that the cement is sufficiently distal and proximal in the humerus and ulna for good fixation. Tobramycin and a small amount of methylene blue may be added to the cement. After the cement has been packed tightly, both implants are inserted and held firmly in place. The cement must be removed meticulously about the *anterior* aspect of the humerus and humeral component to be certain that the ultra high molecular weight bearing will fit tightly. A hole is made in the lateral epicondyle for axle insertion. After the cement has hardened, the drill guide is seated over the humeral component. A small burr is then inserted through the guide window and the cortex of the humerus is opened. A special drill can be inserted through an opening in the guide and the hole in the lateral epicondyle completed. The high-density polyethylene humeral bearing is inserted over the humeral component. One must be certain that the bearing fits tightly onto the humeral component. The ulnar component is brought into position and the components are reduced. The small plastic bearing and pin are then inserted through the hole in the lateral epicondyle and into the humeral component. A small quasi-screwdriver is used to push the small pin into place. The pin is rotated and a definite click is audible as the pin is seated. The pin will back out postoperatively if it is not fully seated (Fig 9–9,G).

The elbow is brought to a full range of motion and the edges are evaluated to be sure that there is no impingement between the ulna and the humerus or between the radius and the capitellum. The tourniquet is then deflated and additional hemostasis secured. The tourniquet is reinflated to aid in closure. Any ulnar bone that extends beyond the tip of the ulnar component is removed by saw. Two holes are then placed in the ulna and two large absorbable sutures are passed with a Keith needle through these holes for attachment of the central tendon of the triceps muscle. The arm is then brought into approximately 45 degrees of extension and the two sutures are brought through the central tendon of the triceps while adjusting the tension. The triceps is *not* tied down at this point. The epimysium of the flexor carpi ulnaris muscle is then carefully sutured with an absorbable suture from distal to proximal. These sutures will continue until the ulnar nerve is in position. Care should be taken not to close the flexor carpi ulnaris too tightly over the ulnar nerve. The nerve is not transposed. The triceps can be pulled into position on the olecranon process and the sutures tied. A negative pressure drain is then inserted into the articulation and brought out through the skin of the upper arm. The subcutaneous margins are closed with fine absorbable sutures and the skin margins are closed with staples or fine nylon sutures. The arm is placed in 45 degrees of extension and a large bulky dressing is applied. The dressing is stabilized with an anterior splint.

The dressings are left in place for 4 days. If the condition of the wound permits, exercises are started on the fourth day postoperatively. The exercises are continued until the patient is able to flex the elbow sufficiently to reach the back of the head. A dynamic flexion-extension splint is worn when the patient is not exercising. The splint is worn for approximately 1 month. It is particularly important that the elbow be splinted in 45 degrees of extension at night to protect the triceps repair.

REHABILITATION

Elbow rehabilitation is a trio performed by the patient, the therapist, and the treating physician. It is essential that the physician be actively involved in the rehabilitation program.[19] It is the physician that knows the quality of the soft tissues, the security of the surgical repair, and the overall condition of the bony tissues. High levels of patient cooperation can be achieved if the physician is supportive of the therapist's efforts and of the progress achieved. With both elbow synovectomy and implant arthroplasty a certain degree of gentle *assisted* exercises will be required. At times these exercises can best be accomplished with the patient in the supine position and the arm directly over the patient's face so that the patient can see the progress of gentle flexion exercises. Passively, elbow extension can be achieved with the elbow placed on a padded surface and a gentle intermittent pressure applied. It is important that no spring-loaded flexion or extension splints be used. These tend to activate flexor or extensor stretch reflexes that pull the arm in the opposite direction intended by the splint. Similarly, walking about with heavy weights activates stretch reflexes and is contraindicated. Gentle exercises with a careful warm-up and ice applications at the end are helpful. Splints that are fixed in extension or flexion do not initiate stretch reflexes and apply gentle pressure to the resistant soft tissues. Appropriate and liberal use of analgesics also will facilitate patient cooperation and compliance. Realistic goals should be established. These goals should be modest. Overoptimistic goals lead to frustration and disappointment and reduced patient compliance with the rehabilitation program. The surgeon should not expect the therapist to achieve more motion and stability than that accomplished in the operating room.

COMPLICATIONS

The most serious complication following elbow replacement arthroplasty is infection[11–13] (Fig 9–10,A and B). Patients with inflammatory or rheumatoid arthritis are particularly at risk because many patients are immunologically compromised or physiologically depressed. Anemia, low total protein, and collagen deficiencies all contribute to alterations in wound healing. It must also be recalled that the elbow joint is in close proximity to the skin surface; hence there is little soft tissue protection between the skin and underlying bony structures.

Two percent of patients will have ulnar neuropathy following replacement arthroplasty.[12] One percent of patients will sustain an epicondylar fracture in the immediate postoperative rehabilitation period or within the first month of surgery. This occurs due to the strong muscular pull of the wrist and hand flexor or extensor muscles. This complication does not affect the overall result but because of pain the rehabilitation is delayed. Less than 1% of patients

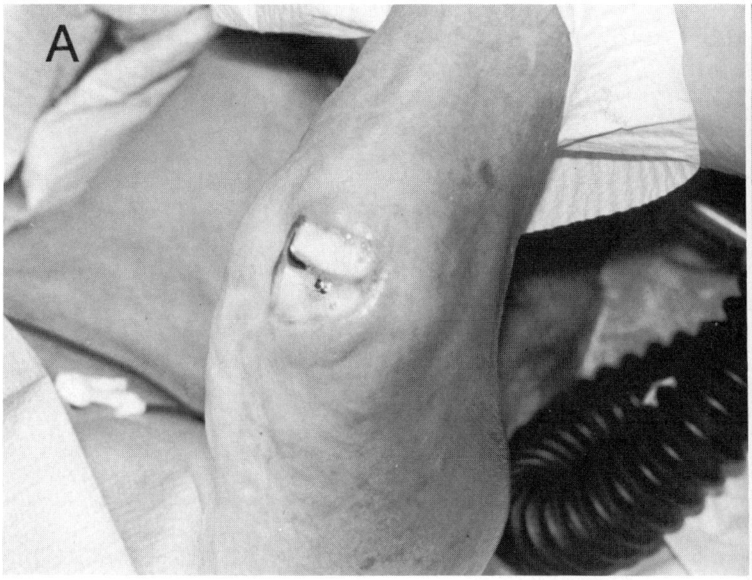

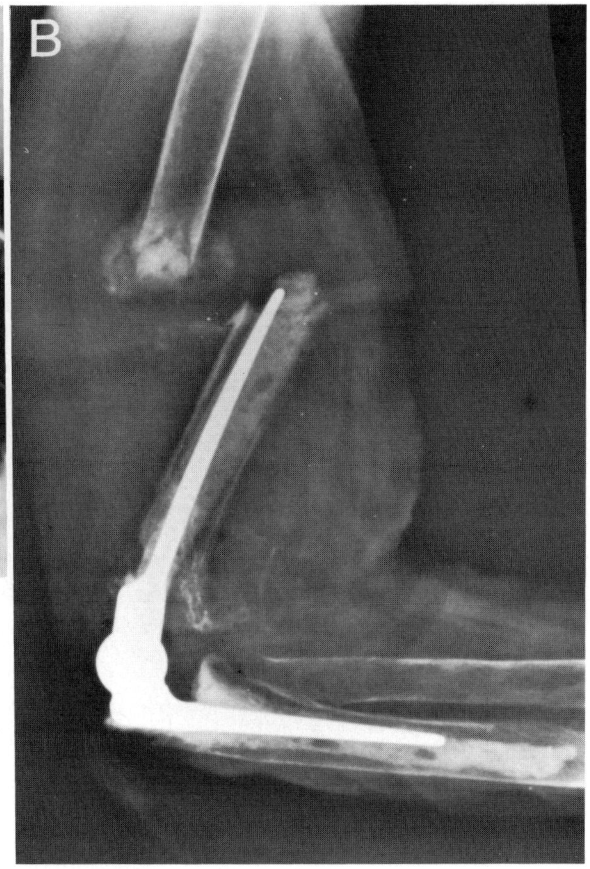

FIG 9–10.
A, a late infection due to a fall and an untended laceration with full bone thickness and soft tissue loss. **B,** radiograph of the humeral fracture caused by a fall.

will have loosening of either the ulnar or humeral component at the cement-bone bond. This loosening becomes apparent within the first 2 years following surgery. These patients have been successfully reimplanted with porous-coated implants.

It is apparent that from this initial 17-year postoperative interval that elbow replacement arthroplasty has achieved an important place in the treatment of severe rheumatoid arthritis of the elbow.

CONCLUSIONS

Patients with rheumatoid arthritis should achieve a good to excellent result in over 90% of cases when the appropriate procedure is selected.[6, 12] Flexion and extension may be only minimally improved. It must be recalled that many of these patients have good flexion and extension preoperatively and that their major disability is pain and instability. The major improvement is in improved stability and relief of pain and therefore an overall improvement in upper extremity function.

REFERENCES

1. Amis AA, Hughes SJ, Miller JH, et al: A functional study of the rheumatoid elbow. *Rheum Rehabil* 1982; 21:151.
2. Anderson LD, Heppenstall M: Synovectomy of the elbow and excision of the radial head in rheumatoid arthritis, in Cruess RL, Mitchell NS (eds): *Surgery of Rheumatoid Arthritis.* Philadelphia, JB Lippincott Co, 1971, pp 127–134.
3. Brattstrom H, Khudairy HA: Synovectomy of the elbow in rheumatoid arthritis. *Acta Orthop Scand* 1975; 46:744.
4. Bryan RS, Morrey BF: Extensive posterior exposure of the elbow: A triceps-sparing approach. *Clin Orthop* 1982; 166:188.
5. Bryan RS, Morrey BF: Rheumatoid arthritis of the elbow, in Evarts CM (ed): *Surgery of the Musculoskeletal System.* London, Churchill Livingstone Ltd, 1983, pp 62–73.
6. Coonrad RW: Seven year follow-up of Coonrad total elbow replacement, in Inglis AE (ed): *Symposium on Total Joint Replacement of the Upper Extremity.* St Louis, Mosby–Year Book, Inc, 1982.
7. Copeland SA, Taylor JG: Synovectomy of the elbow in rheumatoid arthritis: The place of excision of

the head of the radius. *J Bone Joint Surg [Br]* 1979; 61:69.
8. Dee R: Total replacement of the elbow joint. *Orthop Clin North Am* 1973; 4:415.
9. Eichenblat M, Haas A, Kessler I: Synovectomy of the elbow joint in rheumatoid arthritis. *J Bone Joint Surg [Am]* 1982; 64:1074.
10. Geens S: Synovectomy and debridement of the knee in rheumatoid arthritis. Part I. Historical review. *J Bone Joint Surg [Am]* 1969; 51:617.
11. Gelman MI, Ward RJ: Septic arthritis: A complication of rheumatoid arthritis. *Radiology* 1977; 122:P17.
12. Inglis AE: Triaxial total elbow replacement: Indications, surgical technique, and results, in Inglis AE (ed): *Symposium on Total Joint Replacement of the Upper Extremity*. St Louis, Mosby–Year Book, Inc, 1982, pp 100–110.
13. Inglis AE: Revision surgery following a total elbow arthroplasty. *Clin Orthop* 1982; 170:213.
14. Inglis AE, Pellicci PM: Total elbow replacement. *J Bone Joint Surg [Am]* 1980; 62:1252.
15. Inglis AE, Ranawat CS, Straub LR: Synovectomy and debridement of the elbow in rheumatoid arthritis. *J Bone Joint Surg [Am]* 1971; 53:652.
16. Last RJ: *Anatomy, Regional and Applied,* ed 6. Boston, Little Brown & Co, Inc, 1966, p 111.
17. Marmor L: Surgery of the rheumatoid elbow. Follow-Up study on synovectomy combined with radial head excision. *J Bone Joint Surg [Am]* 1972; 54:573.
18. McCarthy D: *Arthritis and Allied Conditions.* Philadelphia, Lea & Febiger, 1985; pp 742–750.
19. Morrey BF: *The Elbow and Its Disorders.* Philadelphia, WB Saunders Co, 1985.
20. Morrey BF, An KN: Articular ligamentous contributions to the stability of the elbow joint. *Am J Sports Med* 1983; 11:315.
21. Morrey BF, Askew L, An KN, et al: A biomechanical study of normal functional elbow motion. *J Bone Joint Surg [Am]* 1981; 63:872.
22. Porter DB, Park N, Richardson C, et al: Rheumatoid arthritis of the elbow. The results of synovectomy. *J Bone Joint Surg [Br]* 1974; 56:427.
23. Souter WA: Arthroplasty of the elbow with particular reference to metallic hinge arthroplasty in rheumatoid patients. *Orthop Clin North Am* 1973; 4:395.
24. Swanson AB: *Flexible Implant Resection Arthroplasty in the Hand and Extremities.* St Louis, Mosby–Year Book, Inc, 1973.

CHAPTER 10

The Wrist

Michelle Gerwin, M.D.

Chitranjan S. Ranawat, M.D.

Roberta Brockman, M.D.

INTRODUCTION

In the management of the patient with rheumatoid arthritis, the involvement of the wrist is often initially overlooked while attending to the weightbearing joints. In fact, there is little in the literature about rheumatoid wrist involvement before the mid-1960s. The wrist is not only important in positioning the hand but is integral to the strength and dexterity of the entire upper extremity. Thus, wrist stability without pain is necessary for proper function and normal strength of the hand.

Fifty percent to 80% of patients with rheumatoid arthritis will eventually have wrist involvement. In 30% of patients, involvement is initially unilateral, with 95% of patients progressing to bilateral wrist involvement.[38] In a large series of patients with rheumatoid arthritis, the wrist was the first site of involvement in 2.7%.[38]

This chapter discusses the pathomechanics of rheumatoid arthritis of the wrist as well as its clinical and radiographic presentation. Indications, contraindications, and the results of surgical and conservative treatments are also discussed.

ANATOMY

The wrist is a complex joint consisting of the articulation of the eight carpal bones with the radius and ulna proximally, and the metacarpals distally. The carpal bones are divided into two rows with the scaphoid forming the link between them. Motion occurs across the radiocarpal and intercarpal joints.

Ligaments

The ligaments of the wrist consist of an extrinsic and an intrinsic group. The extrinsic ligaments course between the carpal bones and the radius, ulna, or metacarpal, while the intrinsic ligaments originate and insert within the carpal bones. There are three strong deep volar radiocarpal ligaments within the extrinsic system (the superficial ligaments are weaker): the radiocapitate, radiolunate, and radioscapholunate ligaments. The other components of the extrinsic system are the radiocollateral ligament and the ulnocarpal complex (triangular fibrocartilage, meniscus, ulnolunate ligament, and ulnar collateral ligament) (Fig 10–1). The dorsal radiocarpal ligaments are weaker than their volar counterparts.[45]

The intrinsic ligaments of the wrist are divided into three groups: the short (volar, dorsal, interosseous), intermediate (lunate-triquetral, scaphoid-lunate, scaphoid-trapezium), and long (volar intercarpal, dorsal intercarpal).[45]

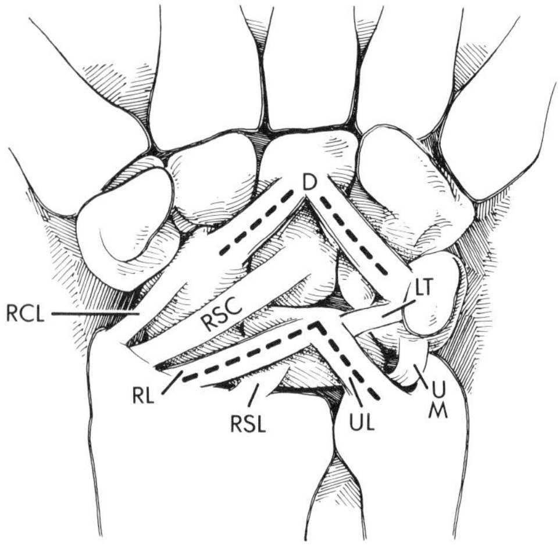

FIG 10–1.
Schematic drawing of volar wrist ligaments. *RSL* = radial collateral ligament; *RSC* = radioscaphocapitate ligament; *RL* = radioulnate ligament; *RCL* = radioscapholunate ligament; *LT* = lunate-triquetral ligament; *UL* = ulnolunate ligament; *UM* = ulnocarpal meniscus homologue; *D* = deltoid or V ligament. (From Jennings JF, Peimer CA: Ligamentous injuries of the wrist in athletes, in Nicholas JA, Hirshman EB (eds): *The Upper Extremity in Sports Medicine.* St Louis, Mosby–Year Book, Inc, 1990, p 459. Used by permission.)

Dorsal Compartments

There are six dorsal compartments containing extensor tendons, created by the extensor retinaculum and the distal radius. The first contains the abductor pollicis longus and extensor pollicis brevis; the second, the extensor carpi radialis longus and brevis; the third, the extensor pollicis longus; the fourth, the extensor digitorum communis and extensor indicis proprius; the fifth, the extensor diqiti quinti; and the sixth, the extensor carpi ulnaris (Fig 10–2). The dorsum of compartments 1 through 5 is the extensor retinaculum and the compartments are divided by septa between the retinaculum and distal radius. The sixth compartment is unique in that it has its own fibro-osseous tunnel which is not connected to the extensor retinaculum. The extensor retinaculum swings over the distal ulna to attach to the triquetrum and pisiform through the sheath of the flexor carpi ulnaris. It has no attachments to the distal ulna and so does not form any compartments over the distal ulna. Thus, even with removal of the extensor retinaculum, the extensor carpi ulnaris is maintained in its position over the distal ulna by its fibro-osseous tunnel. In this way the ex-

FIG 10–2.
A, extensor retinaculum to illustrate septa and compartments after tendons have been removed. Note first compartment has a septum dividing it in half. **B,** cross section through distal radioulnar joint to illustrate extensor compartments with tendons in situ. *APL* = abductor pollicis longus; *ECRB* = extensor carpi radialis brevis; *ECRL* = extensor carpi radialis longus; *ECU* = extensor carpi ulnaris; *EDC* = extensor digitorum communis; *EDM* = extensor digiti minimi; *EIP* = extensor indicis proprius; *EPB* = extensor pollicis brevis; *EPL* = extensor pollicis longus. (From Bogumill G: Anatomy of the forearm, wrist and hand, in Nicholas JA, Hirshman EB (eds): *The Upper Extremity in Sports Medicine.* St Louis, Mosby–Year Book, Inc, 1990, p 388. Used by permission.)

A

B

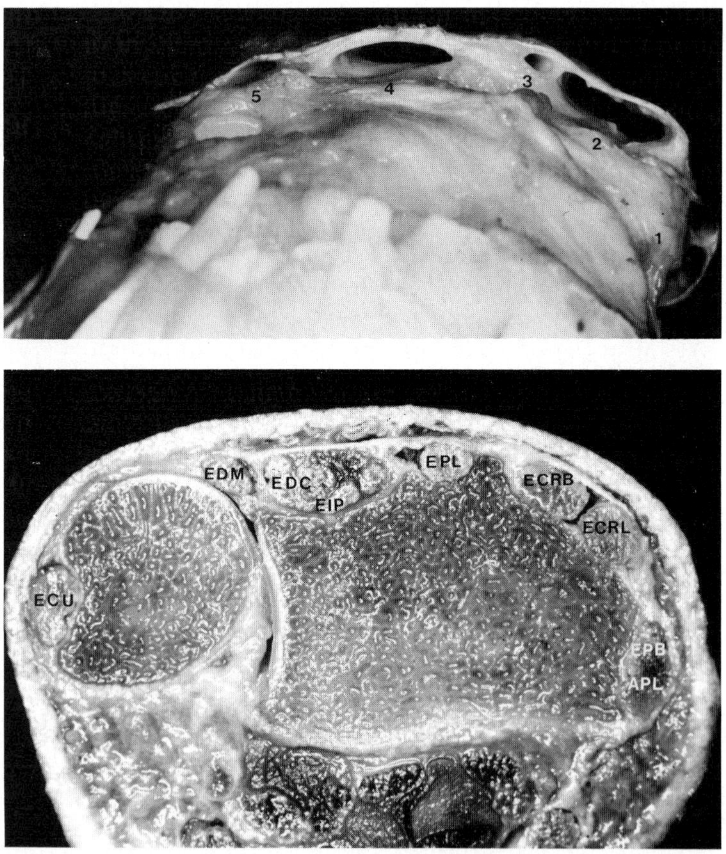

tensor retinaculum does not block forearm rotation.[41]

BIOMECHANICS

The need for motion in the wrist is especially important when other joints in the body are affected. Normal motion at the wrist is approximately 70 degrees each of dorsal and volar flexion. Radial and ulnar deviation is 15 and 40 degrees, respectively, limited by the radial styloid and triangular fibrocartilage. Pronation and supination yield 160 degrees of rotation with motion at both the proximal and distal radioulnar joints.[21] While extremes of motion are helpful in performing certain tasks, they are not necessary for normal function in day-to-day life. Activities of daily living require a more limited range of motion: approximately 30 degrees of extension, 5 degrees of flexion, and 10 degrees of radial and 15 degrees of ulnar deviation[33] (Fig 10–3).

The center of rotation of the wrist varies with the extremes of flexion-extension or radioulnar deviation. In a functional range of motion, it lies within the proximal pole of the capitate. The wrist extensors and flexors exert more of a radial and ulnar force on the wrist than the finger motors because of their increased distance from the center of rotation.[21]

PATHOPHYSIOLOGY

Alteration in the synovium is the basic lesion in rheumatoid arthritis, occurring in either the synovium of joints or of tendon sheaths. The diseased synovium expands and stretches the ligaments of joints and penetrates tendons. The enzymatic activity of the inflammatory cells in the synovium may erode cartilage and bone, create ligamentous laxity, and lead to tendon ruptures.[42] Rheumatoid synovitis of the wrist involves the radiocarpal joint, distal radioulnar joint, and the extensor and flexor tendons. At any given time, one or all of these entities may be involved.

Radiocarpal Collapse

The extent of diseased synovium in the wrist joint complex may go relatively unnoticed initially. The disease process works in two ways, destroying the interosseous ligaments as well as the articular cartilage. Thus carpal collapse may occur rapidly.[42] Because synovium is concentrated around ligaments, and there are relatively few ligaments in the midcarpal joint,[45] the midcarpal joint may be relatively spared.

The carpus is suspended from the radius by a

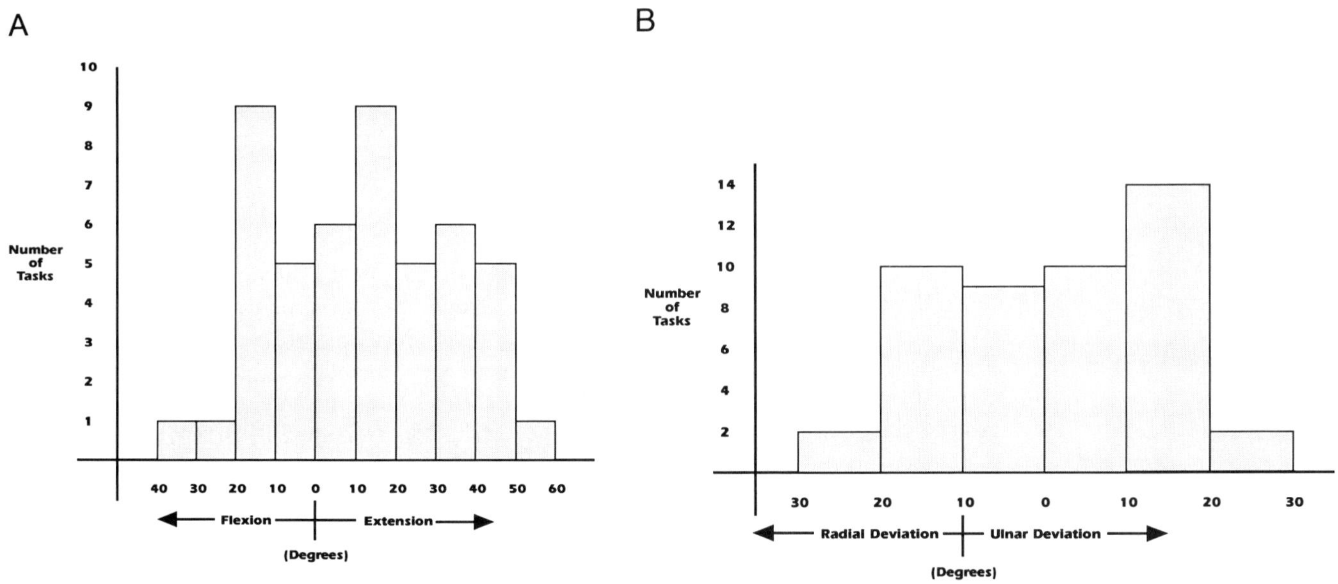

FIG 10–3.
A,B, histograms demonstrating average flexion-extension and radioulnar deviation used by normal subjects performing standard activities of daily living. (From Palmer AK, Werner FW, Eng MM, et al: *J Hand Surg [Am]* 1985; 10:39. Used by permission.)

ligamentous sling that originates from the volar radial and dorsal ulnar borders of the distal radius. Destruction of the deep radioscapholunate and radiocapitate ligaments destabilizes the proximal pole of the scaphoid and allows it to slip into palmar flexion.[34] Loss of the dorsal ulnar support of the radiocarpal joint allows the ulnar carpus to gradually slip into a palmar position.[47] This combination—shortening of the radial carpus, volar subluxation of the ulnar carpus, and dorsal displacement of the distal ulna—creates a relative supination deformity of the carpus.[21]

Even before subluxation, the proximal carpal row may become displaced in the ulnar direction on the radius.[42] An increase in the slope angle of the lunate fossa of the radius relative to the long axis of the radius, as well as ulnar minus variance, may predispose the carpus to ulnar translation.[22]

At this point, the volar position of the extensor carpi ulnaris tendon (carried palmarward by the drop of the ulnar carpus)[48] and the relatively unopposed force of the extensors carpi radialis longus and brevis pull the wrist into radial deviation. The metacarpophalangeal joints as a result are pulled into ulnar deviation by finger flexors and extensors. This plays a role in the ulnar deviation of the metacarpophalangeal joints.[32] It is known that the loss of extensor carpi ulnaris function alone from other causes does not produce this deformity, and thus the internal derangement of the ligamentous support to these joints by the rheumatoid synovitis is an important factor.[48]

Although this schema represents a likely scenario, cause and effect have not been established. For instance, radial deviation of the wrist may occur secondary to either rupture of the extensor carpi ulnaris tendon, collapse of the carpal scaphoid, or ulnar deviation of the fingers.[31] This must be kept in mind when evaluating the complex disorder of rheumatoid involvement of the wrist.

When destruction of the articular surface is rapid, and motion is limited, spontaneous panarthrodesis may occur. This is characteristic of juvenile rheumatoid arthritis, and if the fusion occurs in a functional position, the patient is asymptomatic.[31] In the adult rheumatoid patient, radiolunate ankylosis usually occurs first, with some patients progressing to degeneration of the articular surface of the scaphoid and radioscapholunate ankylosis.[21] Wrist motion may be preserved depending on the degree of articular cartilage damage.[32]

Distal Radioulnar Joint

The distal radioulnar joint is stabilized by the triangular fibrocartilage complex, the radioulnar ligaments, the sigmoid notch of the radius, and the extensor carpi ulnaris. The extensor retinaculum and ulnar collateral ligament do not play a role in stabilization of the distal radioulnar joint.[41] Attenuation of the dorsal carpal ligament, however, may play a role in instability of the distal radioulnar joint. This ligament courses over the distal ulna and ends in the pisiform and pisohamate ligament. It is separated from the distal radioulnar joint by areolar tissue, allowing for pronation and supination. Synovitis in the sixth compartment may stretch this ligament and allow for dorsal subluxation of the ulna.[22] As the extensor carpi ulnaris tendon slips volar to the distal ulna, it allows for more dorsal displacement of the ulna. This, together with the bony erosions of the distal ulna, puts the extensor tendons at risk of rupture.

Tendon Rupture

Extensor tendon rupture was initially described by Vaughan-Jackson in 1948 in patients with distal radioulnar joint arthritis, but not rheumatoid arthritis[49] (Fig 10–4). It was later described by Straub and Wilson in 1956 in seven patients with rheumatoid arthritis in whom end-to-side repairs were performed.[43]

The three basic factors responsible for tendon rupture at the wrist are rheumatoid synovitis, erosion by osseous structures, and pressure of the dorsal retinaculum, all of which cause tendon avascularity and attrition. Proliferation of the tenosynovium around the dorsal tendons has a deleterious effect on their nutrition in addition to directly penetrating the tendon. The dorsally displaced distal ulna, which is deformed early in the rheumatoid process, and the constricting condensed portion of the extensor retinaculum contribute to the combination of factors leading to rupture of the extensor digiti minimi and extensor digitorum communis tendons. The extensor pollicis tendon may undergo a similar process as it turns around Lister's tubercle.[42] The tenosynovitis may involve the second dorsal compartment,

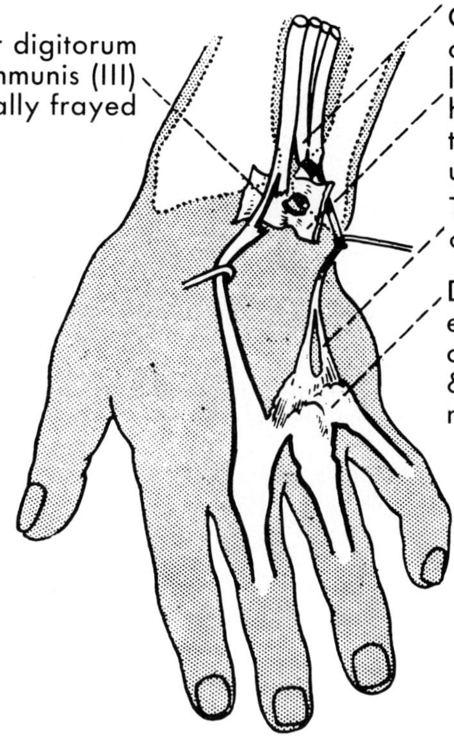

FIG 10–4.
Attrition rupture of the extensor tendon due to distal radioulnar joint arthritis as originally described by Vaughan-Jackson in 1948. (From Vaughan-Jackson DJ: *J Bone Joint Surg [Br]* 1948; 30:528. Used by permission.)

where it may weaken the extensors carpi radialis longus and brevis, but it rarely causes tendon ruptures. When the tenosynovitis involves the first dorsal compartment, it presents like deQuervain's syndrome.[21]

Flexor tendon rupture may be caused by synovial invasion or attrition secondary to bony spicules resulting from erosion of the carpus on the floor of the carpal canal.[21, 23, 36] With erosion of the scapholunate ligament by rheumatoid synovial proliferation, and palmar flexion of the scaphoid, its now irregular surface erodes through the volar radiocarpal ligament and can lead to attrition of the flexor pollicis longus and profundus to the index finger. Loss of active flexion of the fingers with weakness may be associated with adhesions between the flexor digitorum profundus and superficialis tendons within the carpal canal.[42]

CLINICAL PRESENTATION

Wrist pain may not be the primary complaint of patients with rheumatoid arthritis and multiple joint involvement. However, any complaint relative to the wrist should not be overlooked. Early attention to disease may prevent later radiocarpal collapse or tendon rupture.

Patients will usually present with complaints relating to the dorsal or volar aspect of the wrist. It is important at this time to evaluate the ipsilateral shoulder and elbow. A patient with severe shoulder and elbow involvement who is able to feed himself due to a wrist flexion contracture, will not benefit from a wrist arthrodesis in a neutral position. Knowledge of the natural history of the disease process, and careful physical examination of the patient will lead to accurate diagnosis and appropriate treatment.

Dorsal Synovitis

The disease process on the dorsal aspect of the wrist usually follows a distinct pattern. Initially, there is thickening at the ulnar aspect of the wrist joint caused by synovitis of the extensor carpi ulnaris tendon sheath and of the radioulnar articulation. Synovitis of the distal radioulnar joint leads to destruction of the ligamentous support of the distal ulna and triangular fibrocartilage. The distal ulna then subluxates dorsally to form a prominence beneath the common extensor tendons.[42] The syndrome of subluxation of the distal ulna, radial deformity of the wrist, and dropped fingers from extensor tendon rupture was described by Backdahl as the caput ulnae syndrome.[2] It also includes pain and weakness of the wrist in pronation and supination.[2] The "piano keyboard sign" is produced when the ulnar head is depressed and reduced, and springs back up with release. This does not occur in a stable distal radioulnar joint.[2, 16]

Synovitis may then appear in the other tendon sheaths as well as in the wrist joint. On the dorsum of the wrist, the synovitis of the extensor tendon sheaths is very obvious as swelling proximal and distal to the extensor retinaculum, and will usually produce pain on movement of the digits[32, 42] (Fig 10–5). The extensor tendon swelling halts abruptly at the midcarpal level, which marks the end of the tendon sheath, although swelling may extend distally on the extensor pollicis longus tendon. Rarely, tenosynovitis involves the first dorsal compartment.[42]

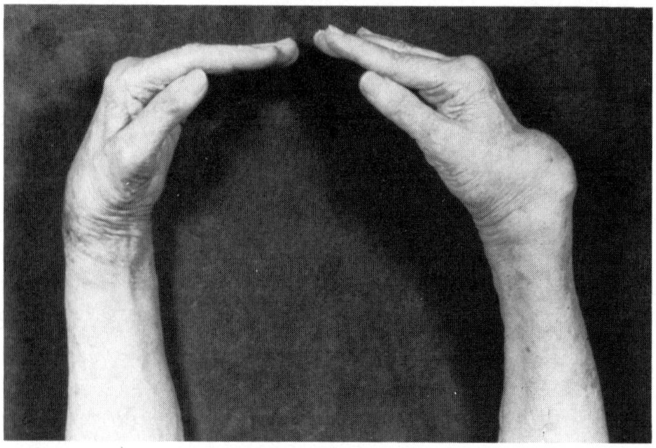

FIG 10–5.
A patient with significant dorsal tenosynovitis of the right wrist producing a dumbbell swelling proximal and distal to the extensor retinaculum. This can be compared with the less severely involved left wrist.

Rupture of the digital extensor tendons usually presents as painless and sudden loss of extension of the digit, usually the little finger which may be followed by the long and ring fingers.[48] Impending rupture must be suspected when extension against resistance elicits pain referred to the distal margin of the extensor retinaculum.[40, 48] Extensor tendon rupture must be differentiated from other clinical entities which can mimic rupture, namely volar subluxation of the extensor tendon and posterior interosseous nerve compression.

If a patient lacks digital extension and the tendon can be palpated on top of the metacarpophalangeal joint, then that tendon is most likely ruptured. Loss of extension due to metacarpophalangeal joint synovitis usually results in the tendon slipping into an ulnarly subluxed position into the intermetacarpal valley.[42] If the patient has some extension of the digit present, the extensor digitorum communis should be palpated moving across the dorsum of the wrist. The presence of the "scallop sign" on the radiograph (synovial erosion of the sigmoid notch of the radius) is associated with distal ulnar erosion of the extensor tendons, and should increase suspicion that an extensor tendon rupture is present. Obviously, absence of the scallop sign does not rule out extensor tendon rupture.

Extensor tendon ruptures must also be differentiated from the clinical presentation of posterior interosseous nerve compression.[24, 29] Posterior interosseous nerve compression in rheumatoid patients is secondary to compression of the nerve in the supinator muscle due to elbow synovitis and anterior capsular swelling. Clinically, these entities can be differentiated because with extensor tendon ruptures there is an absence of a "tenodesis effect," as finger extension does not occur with passive wrist flexion.[29] Diagnosis can be made definitively by electromyogram (EMG).

Volar Synovitis

Early recognition of volar synovitis is difficult because the transverse carpal ligament and palmar fascia tend to delay the clinical evidence until significant changes have occurred.[36, 42] Localizing symptoms of pain in the distribution of the median nerve are often overlooked because of the generalized painful nature of the disease. Careful sensory examination of the distribution of the median and ulnar nerves is imperative.[42] Patients may present with one or more of the following: carpal tunnel syndrome, pain and swelling over the volar aspect of the wrist, and progressive loss of active flexion of the fingers (with greater passive than active flexion).[36, 42, 48] The swelling accentuates the palmar slope of the wrist and obliterates the forearm slope[36] (Fig 10–6).

Penetration of tendons in the volar compartment of the wrist may occur, with the profundus tendons more frequently involved. The flexor digitorum profundus to the index finger and the flexor pollicis longus are the tendons most frequently ruptured, although tendon rupture occurs much less frequently in the volar compartment than it does in the dorsal compartment.[36] A provocative test for flexor tenosynovitis is the "sublimis test" in which a single digit's proximal interphalangeal joint flexion is tested with the other digits held in extension, thus anchoring the profundus tendons. This elicits pain in patients with flexor tenosynovitis by forcing the tendons to glide on one another.[6] Loss of flexion of the flexor pollicis longus and flexor digitorum profundus tendon to the index finger can mimic anterior interosseous nerve compression.[28]

Tenosynovitis in the carpal tunnel may less often extend medially and involve the canal of Guyon, causing ulnar nerve symptoms.[42]

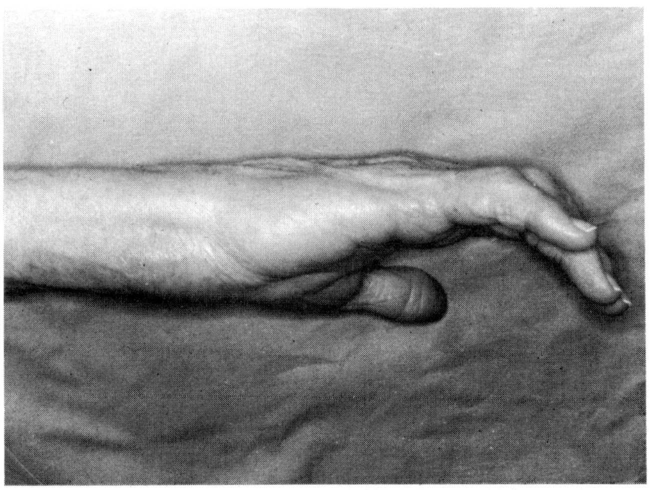

FIG 10–6.
Hypertrophic synovitis at the wrist level may cause carpal tunnel syndrome. (From Milford L: Arthritic hand, in Crenshaw AH (ed): *Campbell's Operative Orthopaedics*, ed 7. St Louis, Mosby–Year Book, Inc, 1987, p 401. Used by permission.)

RADIOGRAPHIC FINDINGS

Normal Radiographic Anatomy

The normal radiographic anatomy of the wrist is essential knowledge for interpretation of the pathologic anatomy of the rheumatoid wrist. The normal volar tilt of the radius is 11 degrees with an inclination of 22 degrees and an articular length of 9 mm (from the ulnar cartilage to the height of the radial styloid). Carpal height, as described by Youm et al.,[52] is the ratio of the height of the carpus (from the base of the third metacarpal to the articular surface of the radius) to the length of the third metacarpal and is usually 0.54 ± 0.03. The carpal-ulnar distance is the ratio of the distance from the midcapitate to the extended line of the ulna, to the length of the third metacarpal and is usually 0.3 ± 0.03 (Fig 10–7). On lateral radiograph, the normal radioscaphoid angle is 58 degrees; the normal radiolunate angle is less than 15 degrees. The average scapholunate angle is 47 degrees; greater than 70 degrees in-

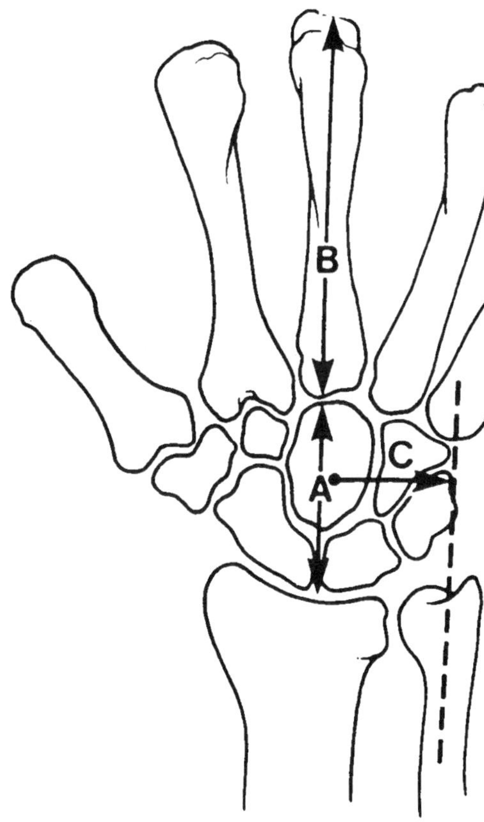

FIG 10–7.
Measurement of carpal height and carpal ulnar distance. (From Youm Y, McMurty RY, Flatt AE, et al: *J Bone Joint Surg [Am]* 1978; 60:423–431. Used by permission.)

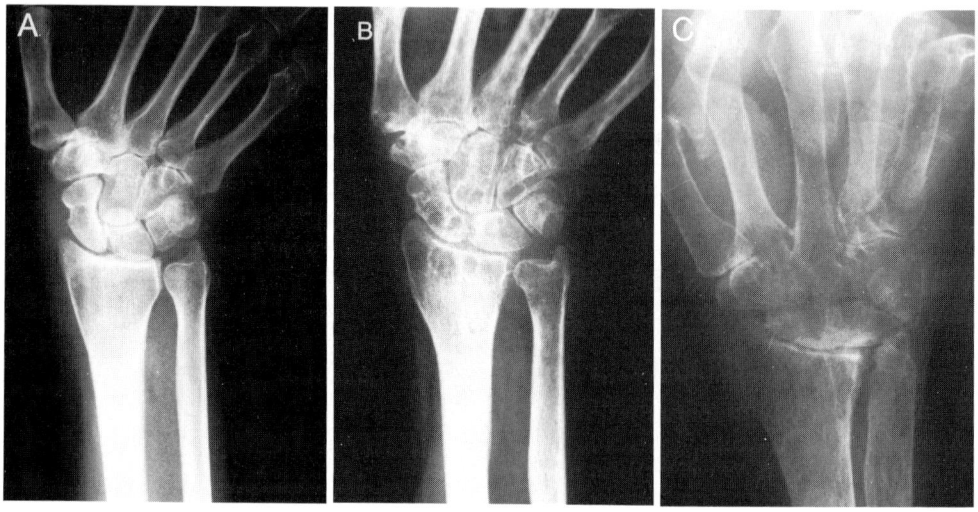

FIG 10–8.
Progressive radiographic changes in rheumatoid arthritis. **A,** a cyst is present in the scaphoid and there are erosive changes in the adjacent margin of the scaphoid and lunate. **B,** there are marginal erosions in the radial and ulnar styloid processes and lunate. **C,** advanced changes are present with joint space narrowing, subchondral sclerosis, and destruction of the head of the ulna. (From Ranawat CS, Frieberger RH, Jordan LR, et al: *J Bone Joint Surg [Am]* 1969; 51:1269–1281. Used by permission.)

dicates dorsal intercalated segment instability (DISI); less than 30 degrees indicates volar segment intercalated instability (VISI). A capitolunate angle of greater than 20 degrees, signifies midcarpal instability.

Pathologic Changes

Radiograph

The first findings on plain films of the rheumatoid wrist are osteoporosis and soft tissue swelling. The earliest bone lesions are marginal erosions at the sites of ligamentous attachments: the ulnar styloid process, the scaphoid and lunate, and the radial styloid process (Fig 10–8). Also frequently seen is erosion of the radius at the sigmoid notch by the roughened distal ulna—the "scallop sign" (Fig 10–9). Less frequently seen are minor erosive lesions on the volar margin of the lower end of the radius and the head of the ulna, and the other carpal bones. Pseudocysts are also seen on the volar aspect of the radius, and when large are usually associated with eventual volar carpal dislocation.[35] Other changes, such as destruction and dorsal dislocation of the distal ulna, narrowing of the joint spaces of the radiocarpal and midcarpal joints, and volar subluxation of the carpus with radial deviation are found late in the disease process[35] (Fig 10–10).

Once bony lesions are present, microfocal radiographic techniques can be used to evaluate progression of disease. High magnification and resolution

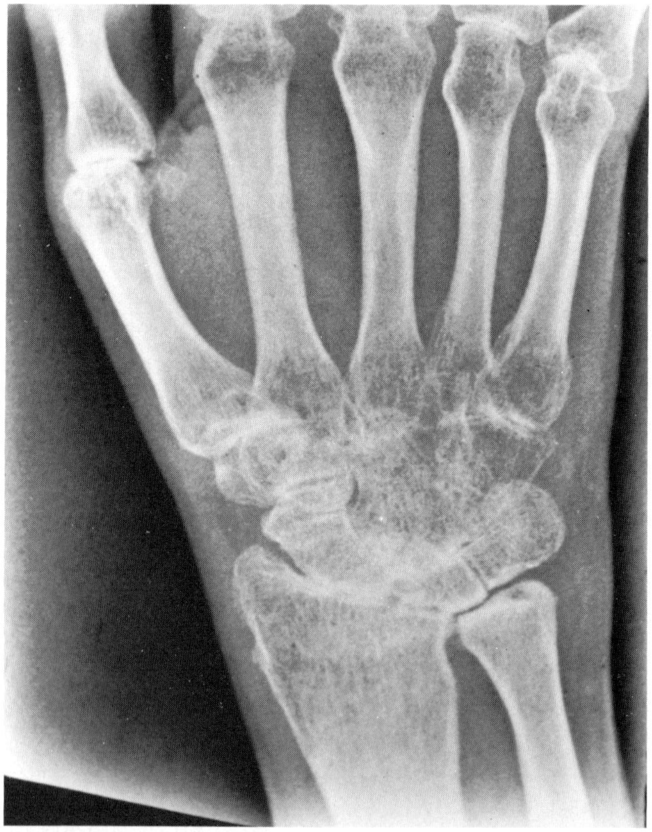

FIG 10–9.
Anteroposterior radiograph demonstrating synovitic erosion of the radius at the sigmoid notch termed the "scallop sign."

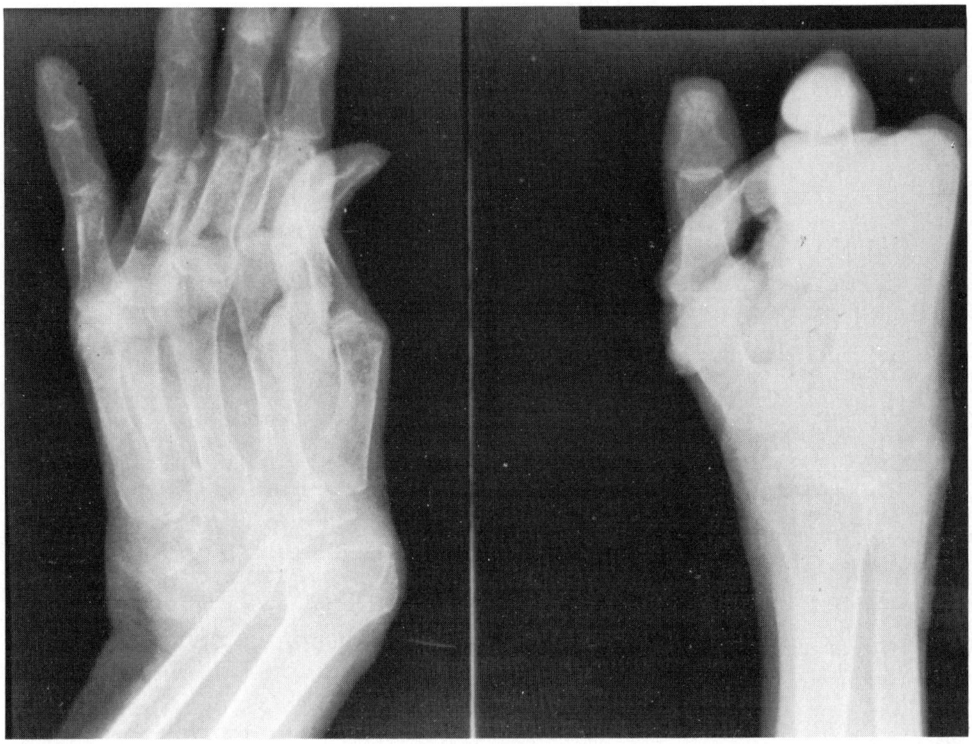

FIG 10–10.
Late destruction of the wrist by rheumatoid arthritis, with radiocarpal dislocation.

allow measurements of structures as small as 35 μm and allow accurate measurement of the number and size of lesions in the rheumatoid hand. Over time, the number of erosions increases until it approaches a constant value. Mean erosion area is a more sensitive indicator of disease progression than erosion number and continues to increase as the disease progresses.[8]

In order to allow for comparison of populations of patients with rheumatoid arthritis, a grading system of radiographic changes has been developed. The most widely used system assigns a number from 0 to 4 based on the overall appraisal of change.[17] More recently, a system has been developed that grades radiographic severity of disease as a function of two scores: one for joint space narrowing and sclerosis, and one for defects and destruction. This allows for measurement of the two major pathologic features of the disease: destruction of cartilage, and chronic inflammatory erosion in the bone.[37] This system, while more accurate, is complex and cumbersome.

Arthrogram

The arthrogram can be used to detect early evidence of disease even before bony lesions are present. A corrugated pattern of the synovial cavity represents villous proliferation of the synovium and is the earliest radiographic evidence of rheumatoid arthritis.[35] On arthrogram, communication is also frequently seen between the radiocarpal and radioulnar joints, and the radiocarpal and midcarpal joints, representing ligamentous destruction.[35] In addition, the extensor tendon sheaths are noted at times to communicate with the radiocarpal joint, indicating erosion into the tendon sheaths by the hypertrophic synovium. Pseudocysts always communicate with the radiocarpal joint.[35] Synovial proliferation can be seen as the presence of an abnormally large synovial pouch between the radius and the radiocarpal ligament, and the presence of abnormal synovial pouches between the radial collateral ligament and the scaphoid and the triquetrum and pisiform.[35]

The characteristic abnormality of a rheumatoid wrist is a corrugated synovial profile and one or more of the abnormalities described above. The knowledge gained by arthrography has contributed to the usefulness of early synovectomy[35] (Fig 10–11).

Magnetic Resonance Imaging and Computed Tomography

With the advent of magnetic resonance imaging (MRI) and computed tomography (CT), more careful evaluation of the soft tissue and bony architecture of the wrist can be done. Evaluation of the bony structure of the radiocarpal joint is important when planning arthrodesis or arthroplasty in the face of significant bone loss.

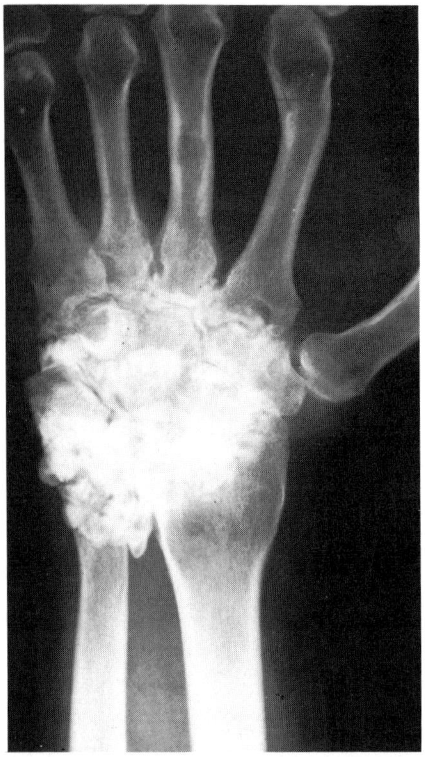

FIG 10–11.
Arthrography in rheumatoid arthritis, demonstrating the corrugated pattern of the synovial cavity of the wrist. (From Ranawat CS, Frieberger RH, Jordan LR, et al: *J Bone Joint Surg [Am]* 1969; 51:1269–1281. Used by permission.)

TREATMENT

CONSERVATIVE TREATMENT

It is important to stress that physical therapy in patients with rheumatoid arthritis should be begun early to prevent joint contractures and deformity, and maintain function. Physical therapy must be continued between episodes of inflammation and remission.

Splints

The goals of splinting are to relieve pain, decrease synovitis through rest, immobilize the wrist in a functional position, and prevent contractures. Splints should be removed frequently to allow for range-of-motion exercises. Prolonged immobilization in casts should be discouraged because it will result in stiffness. When inflammation subsides, isometric strengthening exercises should be begun.[3] Ideally, the splint should resist the ulnar force on the carpus, the radial force on the hand, and the dorsal force on the distal ulna.[21] In addition to daytime use of splints, cockup wrist splints can be used at night for treatment of carpal tunnel syndrome.

Occupational Therapy
Patients are referred to an occupational therapist for splinting and assistive devices at home to help with activities of daily living. They are also instructed in a home exercise program to retain joint mobility and improve functional strength.

Injections

Some have advocated control of rheumatoid synovitis by injections of antimetabolites, such as thiotepa and nitrogen mustard, or of radioactive material in the diseased joint.[39] Cortisone can also be used to decrease the synovial inflammation.[30]

SURGICAL TREATMENT

Goals

The decision to operate is made after careful consideration of the patient's functional, psychological, and social requirements in addition to assessment of the actual anatomic damage. Indications for surgery are persistence of synovitis after several months of nonoperative management, or progressive radiographic changes. Surgery may either be prophylactic or therapeutic. The aims of surgery of the rheumatoid wrist are: (1) to remove diseased synovium via synovectomy, (2) to prevent or repair tendon ruptures, and (3) to provide a painless, stable wrist joint in a functional position.[42]

With any procedure, it needs to be stressed that the skin of rheumatoid patients is delicate and of poor quality. It should be handled with care, and incisions should be of ample length to keep the skin tension free. Skin sutures should be placed with a "no touch" technique, and should be of nonabsorbable monofilament that can be left in place for 2 to 3 weeks if necessary.

Volar Tenosynovectomy

Goals
The object of tenosynovectomy is to remove the diseased synovium before the tendon damage occurs.[30]

Indications

Indications for volar tenosynovectomy are painful progressive synovitis for several months without relief from conservative therapy. Other indications are loss of flexion of the fingers, tendon rupture, and carpal tunnel syndrome.[36]

Contraindications

Pain in the wrist is frequently improved by tenosynovectomy, though most synovectomies are performed too late.[15, 30]

Technique

The palm and wrist are approached through a curving incision (Fig 10–12). This allows exposure of the median nerve and of the superficialis and profundus tendons, as well as the flexor pollicis longus. The incision avoids injury to the superficial branch of the median nerve and allows exposure of the canal of Guyon. The transverse carpal ligament, is exposed and divided. The nerve is carefully freed and the recurrent branch is identified and traced through the fibers of the carpal ligament into the muscles at the

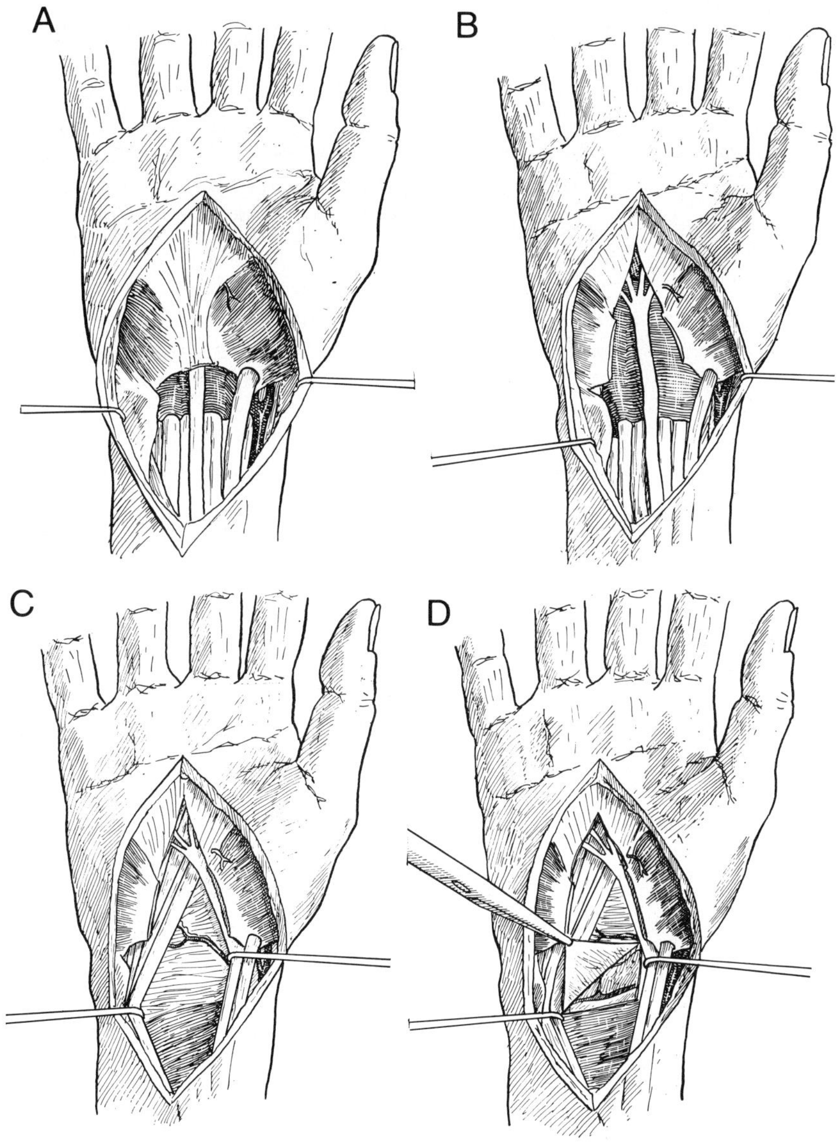

FIG 10–12.
Volar tenosynovectomy as described by Straub and Ranawat. **A,** flexor retinaculum exposed. **B,** flexor retinaculum sectioned, median nerve and tendons exposed. **C,** tenosynovium removed and tendons retracted to expose capsule. **D,** joint inspected for bony spicules protruding into the carpal canal. (From Straub LR, Ranawat CS: *J Bone Joint Surg [Am]* 1969; 51A:1–20. Used by permission.)

base of the thumb. It is important that the exposure extend proximally as far as the muscle substance of the flexor digitorum superficialis. The tendons are gently separated and the tenosynovectomy is performed, with special attention to the profundus tendons since these are usually more severely involved. If necessary, the tendons can then be retracted and a volar synovectomy of the wrist joint can be performed after reflecting the anterior radiocarpal ligament as a flap. Any bony spicules in the carpal canal should be removed. The wound is closed without repair of the transverse carpal ligament, and the wrist is kept in a gentle compressive dressing for 2 weeks.

Results

Results of surgery are considered successful if the patient is relieved of pain, if the preoperative range of finger motion is restored with improvement of strength of grasp, and if there is no recurrence of the synovitis.[42]

Distal Ulna Resection

Goals

Arthritis of the distal radioulnar joint is detrimental to wrist function. The inflamed radioulnar joint causes pain in pronation and supination and thus limits function. In addition, the diseased ulna, roughened by the erosive effect of inflammatory synovium, displaces dorsally as its ligamentous reins loosen, and erodes the extensor tendons above it. The goal of distal ulnar resection is to remove this noxious force while maintaining stability of the distal ulna.

The Darrach procedure is probably the easiest way of accomplishing a distal ulnar resection.[12] The distal ulna can then be stabilized by a slip of extensor carpi ulnaris to prevent dorsal translation. This helps to correct both the radial deviation and supination deformity seen in wrists in rheumatoid arthritis.[20, 21]

Bowers designed a modification of the Darrach procedure for patients who still have a functionally adequate or reconstructible triangular fibrocartilage, in which only the radial aspect of the distal ulna is resected.[4] The ulnar ligament complex is left intact, ulnar support to the wrist is preserved, the distal ulna is stabilized, and yet radioulnar impingement is eliminated. The gap left between the radius and ulna may be filled with either dorsal capsule or a tendon interposition[4] (Fig 10–13). Watson designed a similar technique: a 270-degree matched hemiresection of the distal ulna is performed to conform to the concave radial metaphysis, and no interposition is needed[51] (Fig 10–14).

Indications

Patients with involvement of the distal radioulnar joint with rheumatoid arthritis with pain on pronation and supination, or extensor tendon rupture, benefit from resection of the distal ulna.

Contraindications

Patients with preoperative evidence of ulnar translocation with displacement of the lunate from the lu-

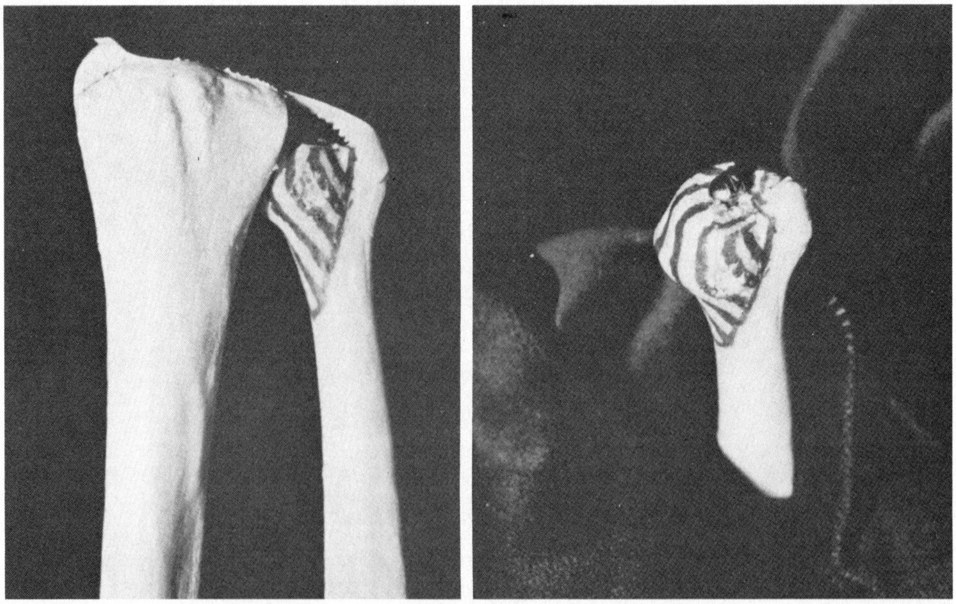

FIG 10–13.
Skeletal specimen demonstrating the resection of the distal ulna as described by Bowers. This space is then filled with a capsule or tendon "anchovy." (From Bowers WH: *J Hand Surg [Am]* 1985; 10:169–178. Used by permission.)

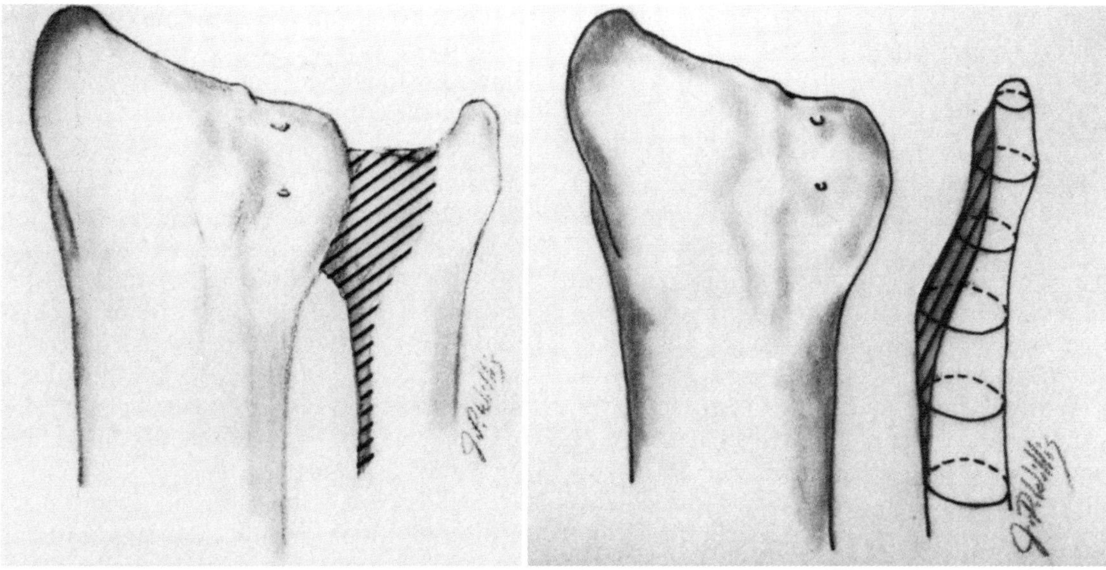

FIG 10–14.
Hemiresection of the distal ulna in a convex curve to conform to the concave distal radius as described by Watson et al. Ideally, no interposition is necessary here. (From Watson HK, Ryu JY, Burgess RC: *J Hand Surg [Am]* 1986; 11:812–817. Used by permission.)

nate fossa may have an increase in their ulnar translocation after a Darrach procedure (Fig 10–15). If the lunate is within the lunate fossa preoperatively, then the chance for ulnar translation is small. Without an adequate or reconstructible triangular fibrocartilage, the Bowers modification offers no advantage over a simple Darrach procedure.

If the patient has positive ulnar variance greater than 2 mm, or an unusually long ulnar styloid, then the styloid may impinge on the triquetrum if a hemiresection of the distal ulna is performed, and ulnar shortening should also be done. Extensor carpi ulnaris stabilization is done if there is volar displacement or instability in its compartment[4].

Patients who have high demands on their wrist will not do well after hemiresection of the distal ulna, because the tendency for the radius and ulna to impinge is increased in power grip when the ul-

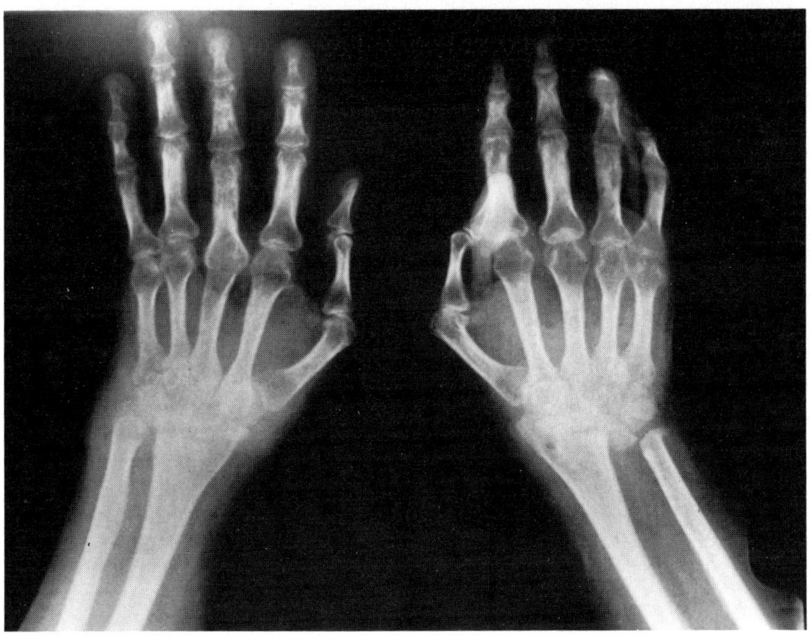

FIG 10–15.
The Darrach procedure. The radiograph demonstrates the appearance of the wrist after resection of the distal ulna. It is evident that ulnar translocation of the carpus has taken place or the right.

nar head can no longer counter the pull of the pronator quadratus.[4]

Technique

The distal ulna is approached through a standard dorsal incision. The extensor retinaculum is incised between the fifth and sixth dorsal compartments. The capsule of the distal radioulnar joint is then reflected in a sleeve fashion off of the radius to expose the distal ulna. Care is taken in this dissection to avoid the dorsal cutaneous branch of the ulnar nerve. The periosteum is reflected from the distal ulna and an osteotomy is made 1 cm proximal to the ulnar styloid (at the level of the proximal extent of the sigmoid notch). The ulnar styloid can be osteotomized at its base and left in situ, or it can be dissected free and removed with the remainder of the distal ulna. The remaining distal ulna is rounded to a bullet-nose configuration, and the periosteum and radioulnar capsule are closed securely to provide firm attachment for the ulnar styloid and aid in stabilization of the distal ulna.

Modifications

The distal ulna may be additionally stabilized with extensor carpi ulnaris tendon. The extensor carpi ulnaris is split longitudinally and the ulnar half is transected proximally. This slip of extensor carpi ulnaris with its distal insertion left intact is then woven through a dorsal drill hole in the distal ulna and sutured to itself with the wrist held in pronation and ulnar deviation. This prevents dorsal displacement of the distal ulna (Fig 10–16).

The Bowers modification involves resection of only the ulnar articular surface and subchondral bone. The remaining shaft and styloid are left intact

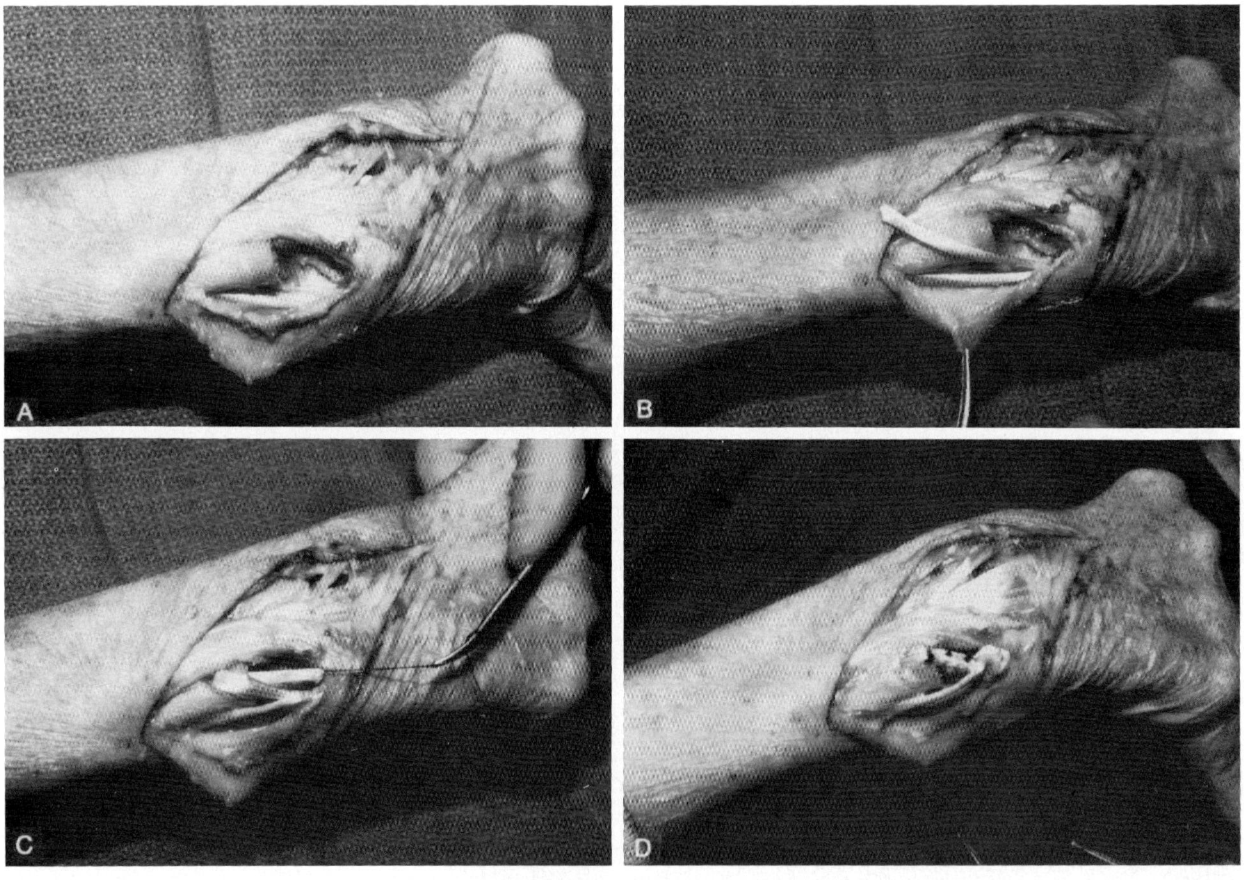

FIG 10–16.
Stabilization of the distal ulna with the extensor carpi ulnaris. **A,** after distal ulnar resection, the extensor carpi ulnaris can be seen in the direction of the ulna and volar to the remaining segment. **B,** the tendon is divided longitudinally and one slip is transected proximally, thus creating a distally based slip. **C,** the distally based slip is then passed through a drill hole made in the dorsal cortex of the distal ulna and out through the medullary canal. **D,** the slip of extensor carpi ulnaris is then sutured to itself while holding the distal ulna reduced. (From Leslie BM, Carlson G, Ruby L: *J Hand Surg [Am]* 1990; 15:547–551. Used by permission.)

and should be round in cross section and resemble a tapering dowel. The radioulnar space is then maintained using an "anchovy" of tendon or muscle about the size of the resected head.[4]

The Watson modification involves resection of the distal ulna in a 270-degree arc, matching the defect to the sigmoid notch. This obviates the need for an "anchovy," but is technically more difficult.[51] Whichever procedure is chosen, early postoperative motion enables a speedy functional recovery of range of motion.

Complications
The distal radioulnar joint is stabilized by the radioulnar ligaments, the triangular fibrocartilage complex, and the extensor carpi ulnaris. The Darrach procedure removes these stabilizers, and the stability of the distal ulna depends on the periosteal sleeve, the interosseous membrane, and the pronator quadratus. Postoperatively, patients may have dorsal subluxation of the distal ulna associated with pain and a snapping sensation[20, 21] unless a distal ulna stabilizing procedure is performed. Ulnar translocation of the carpus postoperatively has been attributed to the Darrach procedure, but this has not been confirmed. More likely it represents progression of the disease process.

Dorsal Stabilization

Goals
The goal of dorsal stabilization surgery is to stabilize the progressive volar and ulnar displacement of the radiocarpal joint, and remove all diseased synovium from the extensor tendons as well as the radiocarpal and midcarpal joints. A dorsal approach is used to allow repositioning of half of the extensor retinaculum to create a smooth gliding surface for the extensor tendons. A successful outcome of dorsal stabilization surgery should provide a painless stable wrist with an arc of motion of 15 to 30 degrees.

Indications
Indications for dorsal stabilization are painful synovitis with or without bone destruction even in the presence of a good range of motion, or painful minor subluxation with weakness of grasp.

Contraindications
Range of motion of the wrist preoperatively should be at least 30 degrees. Wrists that have less than a 30-degree arc of motion preoperatively will go on to fusion. It is important to note that this procedure should only be performed before significant radiocarpal subluxation or dislocation has occurred with either a fixed deformity or a flail wrist.[42]

Technique
A straight dorsal incision is made with care taken to preserve the dorsal venous system, and to protect the superficial branch of the radial nerve and the dorsal branch of the ulnar nerve. The extensor retinaculum in incised longitudinally over the second dorsal extensor compartment, and dissected in a radial and ulnar direction to expose the first through sixth dorsal compartments. A complete synovectomy is then performed of all compartments. After tenosynovectomy, the tendons are retracted and the dorsal ligament of the wrist joint is preserved and reflected in the opposite direction to the retinaculum. Care must be taken during synovectomy of the carpal joints, since the blood supply and stability of these bones may be compromised. After complete synovectomy of the wrist joint, the dorsal ligament is replaced. If the articular cartilage is entirely gone and the joint is unstable, it is reduced and fixed with crossed Kirschner wires. The distal ulna is then resected by one of the methods described previously (usually a Darrach procedure), and synovectomy of the distal radioulnar joint is performed. The extensor retinaculum is then divided in half and the distal half is sutured to itself deep to the extensor tendons. The proximal half is sutured to itself superficial to the extensor tendons to help prevent bowstringing of the tendons (Fig 10–17).

The wrist is immobilized in plaster cast fixation for 4 to 6 weeks and the Kirschner wires are removed at 2 to 3 weeks.

Results
Eighty-three percent of patients have good pain relief, although 30% of patients may require a secondary procedure owing to increasing synovitis (20%), tendon ruptures, instability, and increasing radiographic evidence of intraarticular wrist destruction.[7] Average loss of range of motion postoperatively is 30 degrees with 10% of wrists going on to spontaneous ankylosis.[42]

Dorsal Tenosynovectomy With or Without Distal Ulna Resection

Goals
This procedure is performed in patients with extensor tenosynovitis without involvement of the radiocarpal joint. In addition, strengthening or reposi-

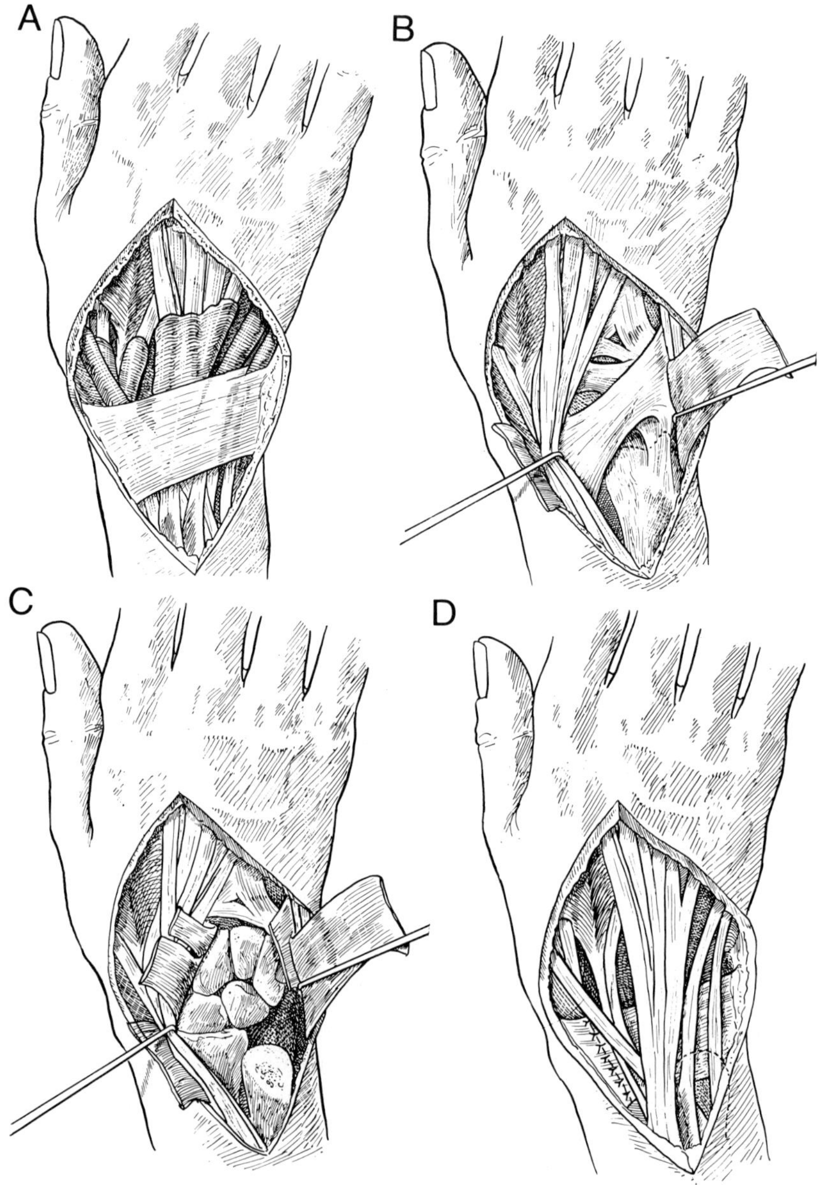

FIG 10–17.
Dorsal stabilization of the wrist. **A,** the extensor retinaculum and tenosynovium have been exposed. **B,** the extensor retinaculum here has been divided over the second dorsal extensor compartment and reflected radially and ulnarly to expose all extensor compartments. **C,** the wrist joint has been opened by reflecting the radiocarpal ligaments. Synovectomy can then be performed along with distal ulnar resection. **D,** the radiocarpal ligaments can then be sutured back in place. Here the extensor retinaculum is sutured under the extensor tendons, but more commonly this is divided transversely, and half is sutured deep and half superficial the tendons to prevent bowstringing. (From Straub LR, Ranawat CS: *J Bone Joint Surg [Am]* 1969; 51:1–20. Used by permission.)

tioning of the extensor carpi ulnaris can be performed at this time to reduce the radial deviation of the carpus and ulnar deviation of the digits.

Indications

The indications for this procedure are tenosynovitis that has not responded to adequate conservative treatment, or tendon rupture. If the distal radioulnar joint is painful, then a distal ulna resection should be performed.[42]

Technique

The procedure is similar to that performed for a dorsal stabilization except that a wrist synovectomy is not done. If an extensor carpi ulnaris repositioning is to be performed, a sling can be created from the dorsal extensor retinaculum with its base on the ulnar side of the sheath of the extensor digiti quinti. The free end of the flap is then passed around the extensor carpi ulnaris and sutured to itself, thus reconstructing the fibro-osseous tunnel and the dorsal position of the extensor carpi ulnaris.[41] The extensor carpi radialis longus is transferred to the extensor carpi ulnaris, which not only strengthens the ulnar extensors but keeps it in a dorsal position.[43] Postoperatively, the wrist should be splinted in a neutral position since the usual position of dorsiflexion may allow for bowstringing of the extensor tendons.[10]

Results
The average loss of range of motion after this procedure is 20 degrees, slightly more when a distal ulna resection is performed.[42] Improvement in supination and pronation is noted in all patients.[42]

Treatment of Tendon Ruptures

Goals
The primary goal of tendon surgery should be prevention of rupture with early synovectomy. Once rupture has occurred, treatment should be aimed at restoring function as completely as possible. The extensor tendons most commonly involved are the extensor digitorum communis of the ring and little fingers and the extensor digiti minimi. The next most common is the extensor pollicis longus tendon. Complete rupture of all the tendons of the extensor digitorum communis occurs infrequently.

Indications
Any ruptured digital extensor tendon should be repaired by the end-to-side technique to the adjacent digital extensor tendon, if possible. Attempts at end-to-end repair have been unsuccessful. The proximal musculotendinous unit usually retracts after rupture and is fibrotic so that it cannot be stretched to reach the distal tendon without a significant amount of tension.[21]

Volar flexor tendon ruptures are usually treated by free tendon grafts or transfer from an adjacent superficialis tendon. End-to-end repair, as in extensor tendons, is not possible.

Contraindications
Tendon repair is contraindicated when severe metacarpophalangeal disease is present with contracture of the joint and loss of motion.

Technique
Rupture of extensor digitorum communis tendons is treated by suture to the adjacent tendon in an end-to-side fashion.[43] Rupture of the tendons to the ring and little fingers can be treated by end-to-side transfer to the extensor digitorum communis to the long finger and extensor digiti quinti, respectively.[30] Complete rupture of the extensor digitorum communis tendons can be treated with an extensor carpi radialis longus or flexor digitorum superficialis transfer.[30, 43] The flexor digitorum superficialis is brought up to the dorsal aspect of the wrist either through the interosseous membrane or around the radial aspect of the forearm.[30] Extensor pollicis longus rupture is treated with transfer of the extensor indicis proprius. In a patient with severe involvement of the wrist, wrist fusion will allow for the wrist motors to be used in transfer to the ruptured extensor tendon.

Results
Poor results of tendon reconstruction are related to extensive involvement of tendon substance by diseased synovium, associated metacarpophalangeal synovitis and volar subluxation, and giving way of the tendon repair.[43]

Arthrodesis

When a significant wrist deformity is present with cartilage destruction, only arthrodesis will correct the deformity and restore alignment without a total wrist replacement. A partial fusion may allow for retention of some motion in addition to correction of alignment. Partial radiocarpal arthrodeses were suggested by spontaneous radiolunate fusions resulting in painless wrists with good function. These patients had good range of motion as well as halting of the progressive deterioration of the wrist with ulnar translation of the carpus.

Radiolunate and Radioscapholunate Arthrodesis
Goals.—The goals of radiolunate and radioscapholunate arthrodesis are to relocate the lunate in the lunate fossa, correct radial deviation of the wrist and midcarpal malalignment, and maintain carpal height. This should allow the wrist to function in an optimal position.[22]

Indications.—Indications for a radiolunate arthrodesis are radiolunate joint space narrowing with preservation of capitolunate articular surface and a midcarpal space of at least 1 mm. Additional indications for limited arthrodesis are ulnar translation of the carpus, and carpal collapse (dorsal or volar intercalated segment instability).[22, 31]

When the midcarpal joint is in good condition, but there is deterioration of the scaphoid articular surface, a radioscapholunate fusion and midcarpal synovectomy is an acceptable procedure. The midcarpal joint usually remains aligned even in severe rheumatoid arthritis, with a functional range of motion.

If the midcarpal articular surfaces are not in good condition, then a lunocapitate arthroplasty can be performed by replacement of the head of the capitate with a silicone prosthesis.

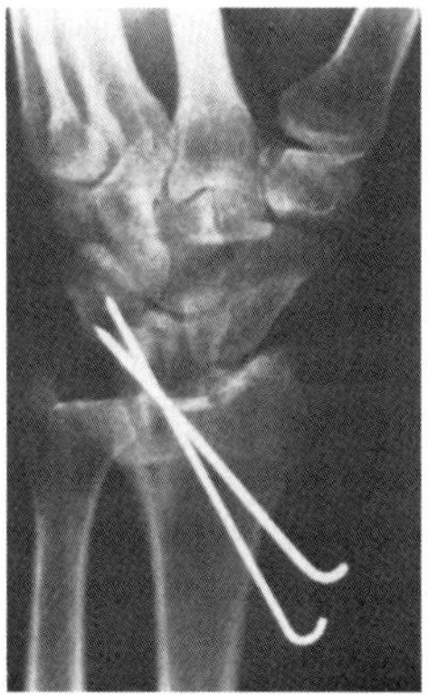

FIG 10–18.
Radiolunate fusion. Intraoperative radiography demonstrates the lunate reduced into the lunate fossa, keyed bone graft, and fixation with Kirschner wires. (From Linscheid RL, Dobyns JH: *J Hand Surg* 1985; 10:821–829. Used by permission.)

Contraindications.—Contraindications to the procedure are extensive midcarpal osseous destruction or ankylosis, or scaphoid or lunate resorption decreasing the chance of obtaining fusion.[46]

Technique.—Through a dorsal approach the lunate is fixed back in the lunate fossa with a 0.0625-in. Kirschner wire. A slot is then made in the dorsal aspect of both the lunate and radius with a sagittal saw. A corticocancellous graft obtained from the iliac crest is laid into this slot, with the cortical side dorsal. The graft should be cut long so that a slight amount of distraction is possible. Extra Kirschner wires are then used to stabilize the radiolunate joint and the wrist is placed in a short arm cast for 12 weeks. The Kirschner wires are removed at 6 weeks (Fig 10–18).

The radiocarpal arthrodesis is performed similar to the radiolunate arthrodesis with transfixing Kirschner wires across the radioscapholunate articulation and local bone graft.[46] If the articular surface of the head of the capitate is destroyed, the damaged head can be replaced with a small silicone implant (Fig 10–19).

Results.—Early results of radiolunate arthrodesis are promising, showing no wrists deteriorating to total spontaneous fusion. Most patients have pain relief with retention of functional range of motion of the wrist. This procedure, because it alters the normal kinematics of the wrist, probably only represents a temporizing measure because forces around the lunate are increased.[22] Although radioscapholunate and radiolunate arthrodeses may be a temporizing measure, they can easily be salvaged by a panarthrodesis[45].

Panarthrodesis

Goals.—In fusion, a neutral wrist position is most functional for personal hygiene and activities of daily living without compromising grip strength.[18] Position can be tailored to individual needs. Five to 10 degrees of ulnar deviation is necessary to counterbalance the ulnar pull at the metacarpophalangeal joints caused by the zigzag pattern of collapse.[21, 26] In patients requiring bilateral arthrodeses, both wrists should be fused in a neutral position.[18] Most patients can compensate for their lack of wrist motion with shoulder and elbow movement.

Indications.—It is the procedure of choice in patients with advanced, fixed volar carpal dislocation, wrist instability caused by severe bony deformity, or wrist extensor rupture.[27] Other indicators are poor bone stock, prior infection, or high demand (including dependence on ambulatory aids).[9, 18]

In patients with bilateral wrist disease, the dominant wrist should be considered for arthroplasty, while the nondominant wrist should receive arthrodesis.[18]

Contraindications.—Any patient considered a candidate for wrist arthrodesis should have the ipsilateral shoulder and elbow examined, as arthrodesis with severe shoulder and elbow involvement may compromise upper extremity function.

Technique.—The approach to total wrist arthrodesis is similar to that of dorsal stabilization. Resection of the distal ulna is mandatory to allow for rotation of the forearm. The articular surfaces of the carpal bones and distal radius are roughened and the largest Steinmann's pin possible is passed anterograde through the carpus and out the soft tissue between the second and third metacarpal. The wrist is then held in neutral flexion and 5 degrees of ulnar deviation as the pin is passed in a retrograde fashion up the canal of the distal radius with the tip of the pin buried in the intermetacarpal soft tissue, or within the third metacarpal. Bone graft obtained from resection of the distal ulna is placed in the radiocarpal and midcarpal joints. If there is severe bone loss, an autologous iliac cancellous bone graft may be necessary. A plaster cast is used for external immobilization for 6 to 8 weeks. Total wrist arthrodesis leaves the wrist in a neutral position (Fig 10–20).

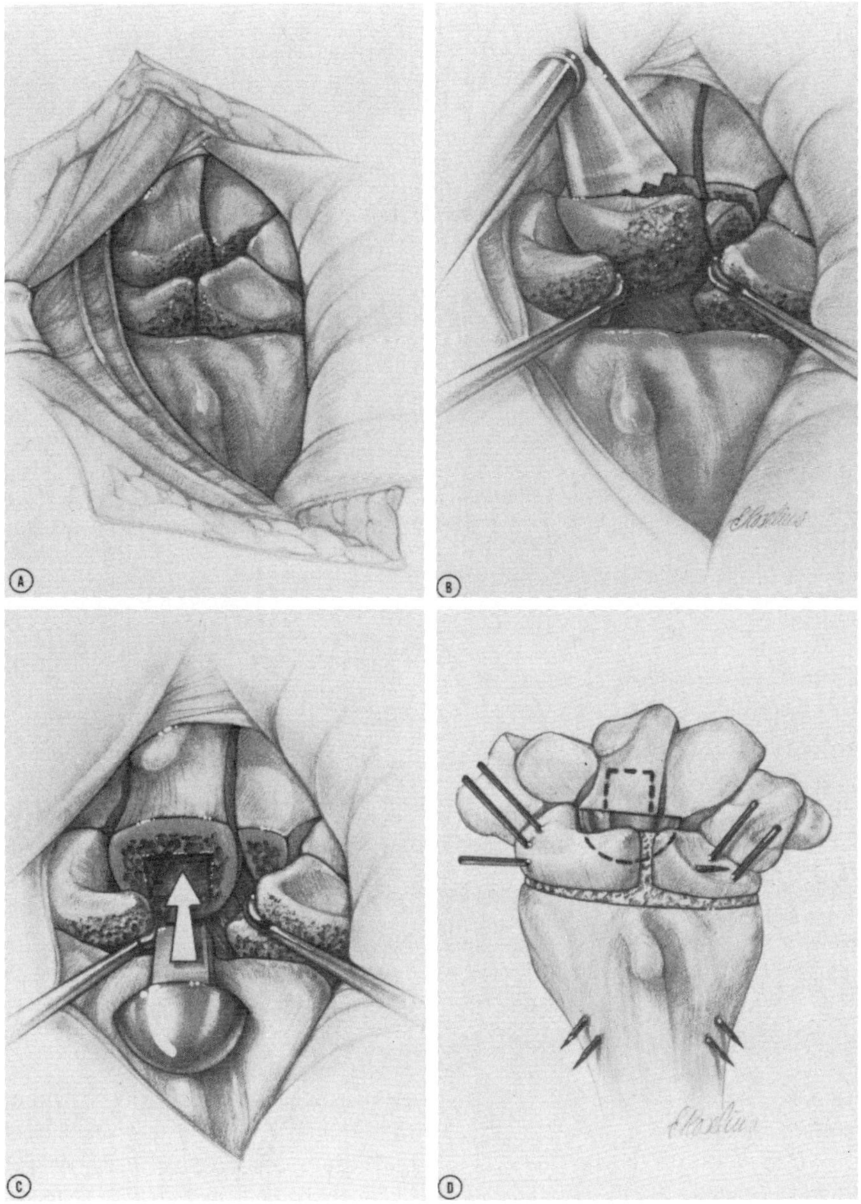

FIG 10–19.
Radioscapholunate fusion. **A,** after exposure of the radiocarpal and midcarpal joints, the articular surfaces are inspected. **B,** if there is degeneration of the radiocarpal and midcarpal joints, the head of the capitate may be resected. **C,** the head of the capitate is then replaced with a condylar implant. **D,** appearance of the wrist after radioscapholunate arthrodesis and capitate arthroplasty. (From Taleisnik J: *J Hand Surg [Am]* 1987; 12:1–8. Used by permission.)

Complications.—The most common complications of this procedure are radiographically demonstrable failure of arthrodesis and symptomatic hardware.[18]

Results.—Wrist arthrodesis is a universally successful procedure with 97% excellent results reported.[18] Most patients feel that the absence of pain and increased strength far outweigh the loss of motion.[26] When fusion is performed on the dominant side, the patient may have difficulty with fine motor activities such as handwriting or the use of eating utensils. The few patients that are not satisfied are those that miss the motion afforded by an arthroplasty on the contralateral side.

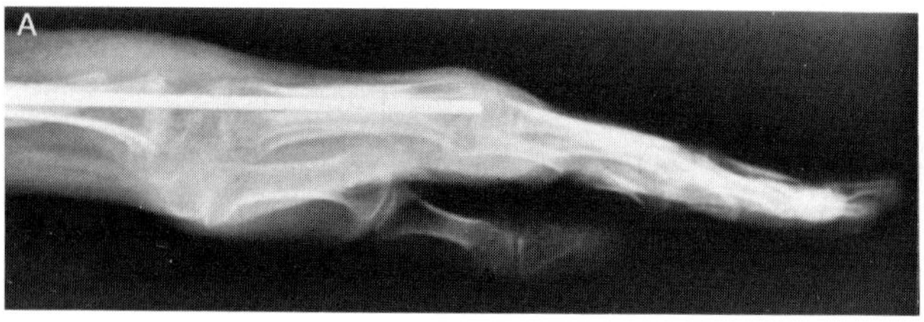

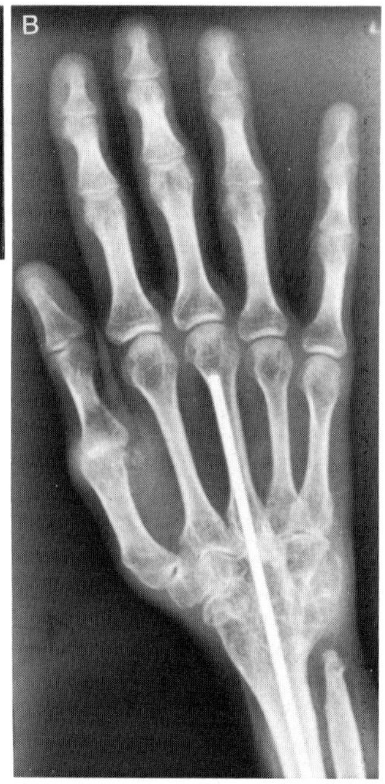

FIG 10–20.
A,B, wrist arthrodesis with internal fixation by a Steinman pin through the third metacarpal and distal radius.

Arthroplasty

Arthroplasty is performed to improve alignment and retain motion in the radiocarpal articulation. Palmar shelf arthroplasty may provide short-term relief of symptoms. Good long-term results are obtained with total wrist replacement arthroplasty.

Palmar Shelf Arthroplasty

Indications.—This procedure was designed for wrists that are severely subluxated or dislocated, to provide a stable painless joint while retaining motion (Fig 10–21).

Technique.—After synovectomy and excision of the distal ulna, the distal radius is shortened to allow reduction of the dislocated carpus, and the radial styloid is removed completely. A distally projecting shelf of bone is then fashioned from the anterior radial cortex. It should extend the entire width of the radius but not project more than 3 mm or else it will interfere with flexion. The articular surface of the carpal bones should not be disturbed to prevent fusion. A Steinmann's pin is placed across the radiocarpal joint for stability, and removed 6 weeks later.[1]

Results.—Early results were promising,[1] but longer-term results demonstrated a high rate of recurrent pain (84%) and spontaneous fusion (68%) although the pain was less severe.[15]

Total Wrist Arthroplasty

There are several prostheses available for wrist arthroplasty. Important considerations in implant arthroplasty are centering of the prosthesis, fixation of the prosthesis, and soft tissue balance.[11] Soft tissue contractures that result from rheumatoid arthritis can make centering the prosthesis difficult. Tendons are malpositioned or ruptured and muscle forces ex-

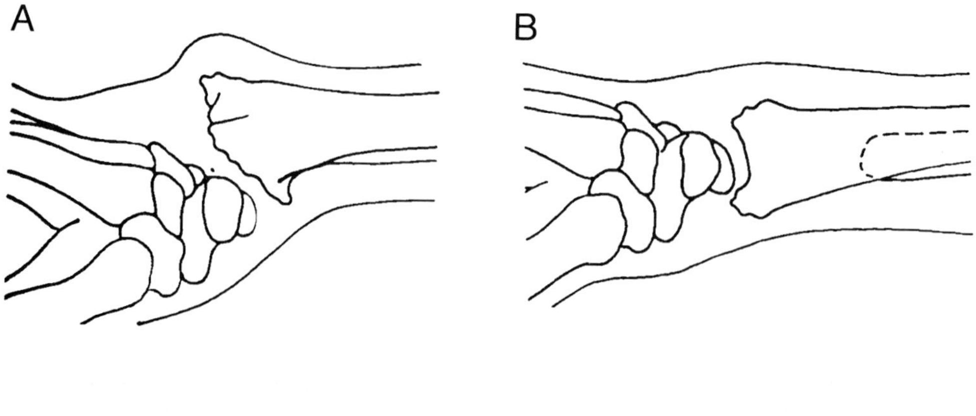

FIG 10–21.
Palmar shelf arthroplasty. **A,** the preoperative deformity with volar erosion of the distal radius. **B,** the reconstructed radiocarpal joint. A volar lip is created extending the full width of the radius and projecting 2 to 3 mm. (From Albright JA, Chase RA: *J Bone Joint Surg [Am]* 1990; 52:896–906. Used by permission.)

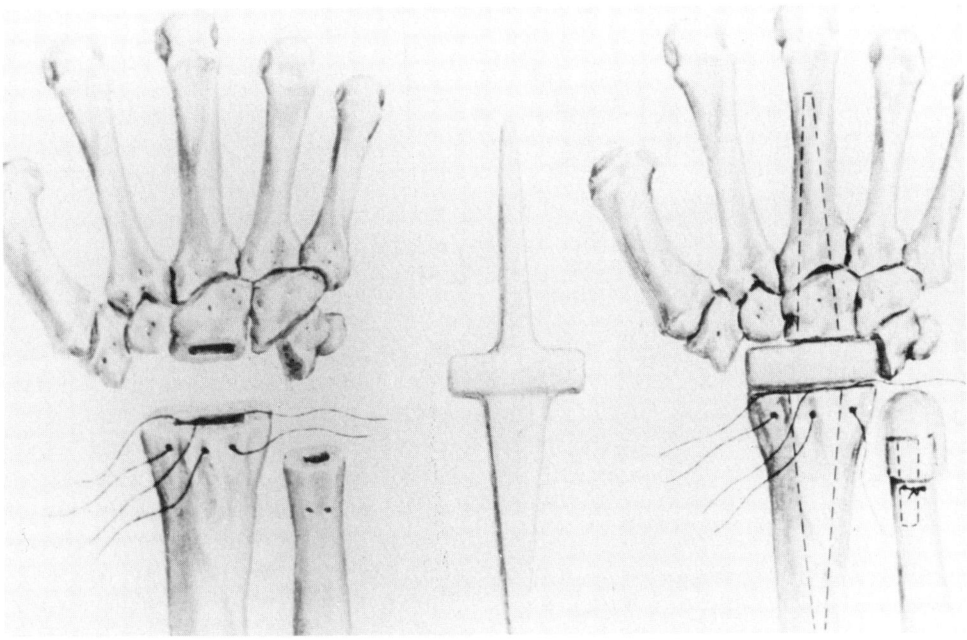

FIG 10–22.
The Swanson prosthesis *(center)*. The usual area of resection of the radiocarpal joint is depicted on the *left*. The prosthesis is inserted into the intramedullary canal of the radius and through the capitate into the intramedullary canal of the third metacarpal. The ulnar head implant is shown in place *(right)*.

erted through them are altered.[11, 14] Prostheses available for implantation include the Swanson, the Meuli, the Volz, and the spherical triaxial prostheses.

The Swanson prosthesis has been in use since the early 1970s. It has a flexible hinge and intramedullary stems which are not fixed[44] (Fig 10–22). For this reason, this prosthesis should be considered an implant spacer rather than a replacement, and used as an adjunct to resection arthroplasty. The purpose of the implant is to maintain joint space while allowing for development of a new capsular-ligament system.[11, 44] Unfortunately, this implant has a 25% rate of fracture or silicone synovitis requiring revision (Fig 10–23). This problem is probably related to the

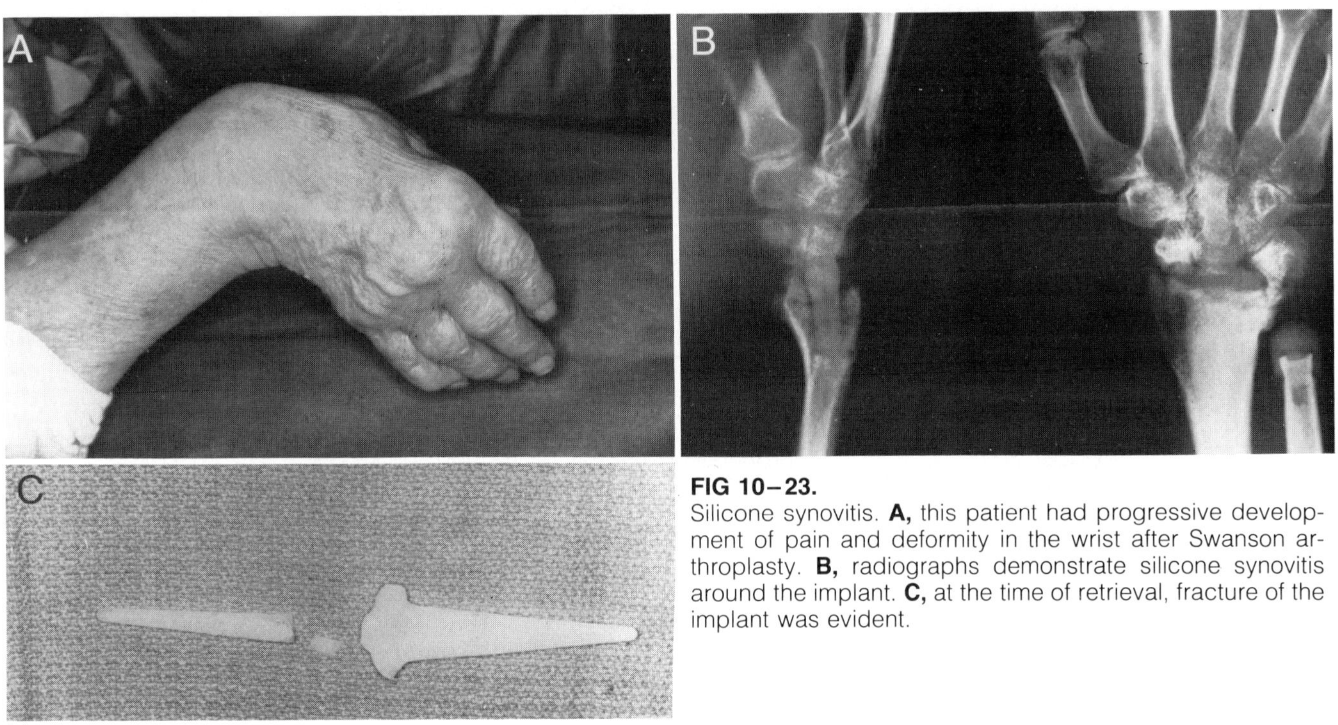

FIG 10–23.
Silicone synovitis. **A,** this patient had progressive development of pain and deformity in the wrist after Swanson arthroplasty. **B,** radiographs demonstrate silicone synovitis around the implant. **C,** at the time of retrieval, fracture of the implant was evident.

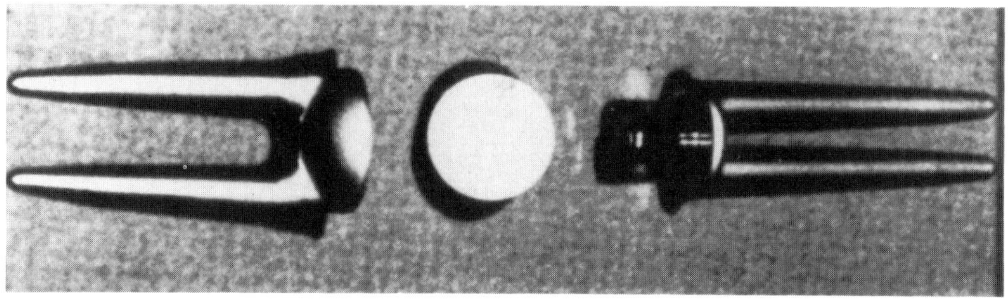

FIG 10–24.
The Meuli prosthesis consists of a polyester ball seated on the trunion end of the radial component, and a shallow, cupped distal metacarpal component.

amount of flexion accomplished and length of follow-up. Patients with a greater range of motion had an increased chance of fracturing their prosthesis.[5]

The Meuli prosthesis, designed in 1972, was the first true prosthesis.[25] It consisted of a polyester ball seated on the trunion end of a metal radial component, and a shallow, cupped distal metacarpal component (Fig 10–24). Intramedullary fixation is accomplished through cementation of the double-pronged components. This prosthesis had a high rate of tendon imbalance, a reoperation rate of 33% for major complications, and a 9% dislocation rate[11] (Fig 10–25).

The Volz prosthesis, designed in 1974, had a single-stemmed radial component with a polyethylene articular surface, and a distal carpometacarpal articulation with a double-pronged stem for intramedullary fixation. Extension, flexion, and radioulnar deviation were limited by prosthesis design.[50] This is a nonlinked prosthesis and has had a high rate of tendon imbalance and dislocation.[19]

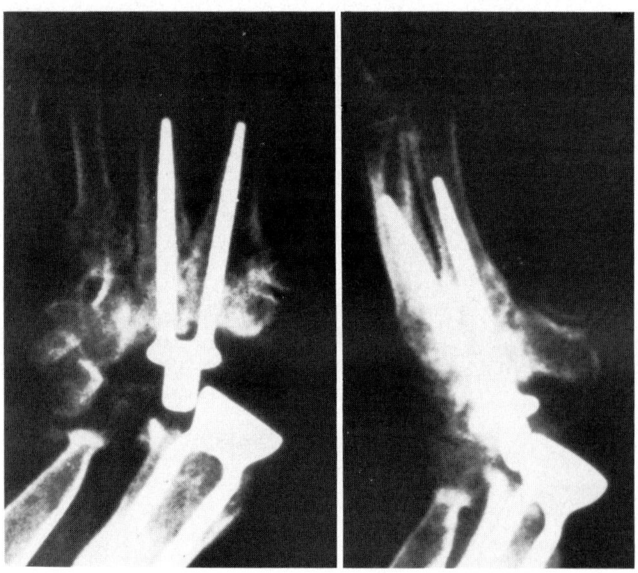

FIG 10–25.
The Meuli prosthesis had a high incidence of complications requiring reoperation, including a 9% dislocation rate.

The Spherical Triaxial prosthesis is a semiconstrained prosthesis. Metacarpal and radial components articulate with a polyethylene bearing and an axle restraint to prevent dislocation. The radial component has a stem for the radius and an ulnar offset of the articulation to allow the center of motion of the wrist to approximate the position of the capitate in both planes. The radial component also has a 12-degree palmar tilt (Fig 10–26). The metacarpal component has a stem for the third metacarpal and an offset short stem for the second metacarpal and scaphoid to prevent rotation. The metacarpal and radial components fit together by means of a polyethylene bushing, and all components are locked together with a central axle (Fig 10–27).

Goals.—The Spherical Triaxial prosthesis is designed to provide 90 degrees of flexion, 80 degrees of extension, and 15 degrees of radial and ulnar deviation (Fig 10–28). The axle is not loaded during normal range of motion.[14] Alignment is very important in positioning the prosthesis. The center of rotation should be 2 mm volar to the radial canal axis, and the carpal height should be restored to 40% to 60% of the length of the third metacarpal.

The advantage of the Spherical Triaxial prosthesis is that it properly restores the center of motion of the wrist, the carpal height, and tendon tension. The semiconstrained design allows for shifts in the center of motion with flexion, extension, and radial and ulnar deviation. The other older prostheses did not accurately restore the center of motion, which led to tendon imbalance and eventual ulnar deviation.

Indications.—Total wrist arthroplasty is an alternative to arthrodesis when there are intact wrist extensor tendons with severe joint destruction (usually class III or IV radiographic disease). This is especially important in the patient with complete upper extremity involvement in which maintenance of wrist motion is important.

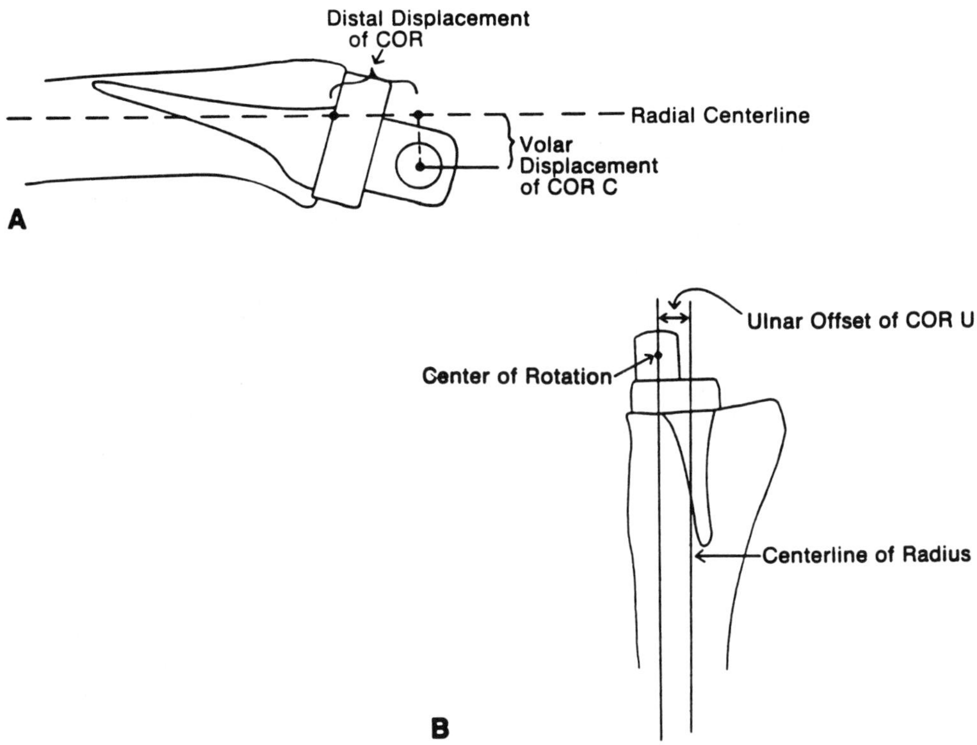

FIG 10–26.
The offset of the center of rotation *(COR)* is measured relative to the long axis of the medullary canal of the radius. **A,** volar offset. **B,** ulnar offset. (From Figgie HE, Inglis AE, Straub LR, et al: *J Arthroplasty* 1986; 1:149. Used by permission.)

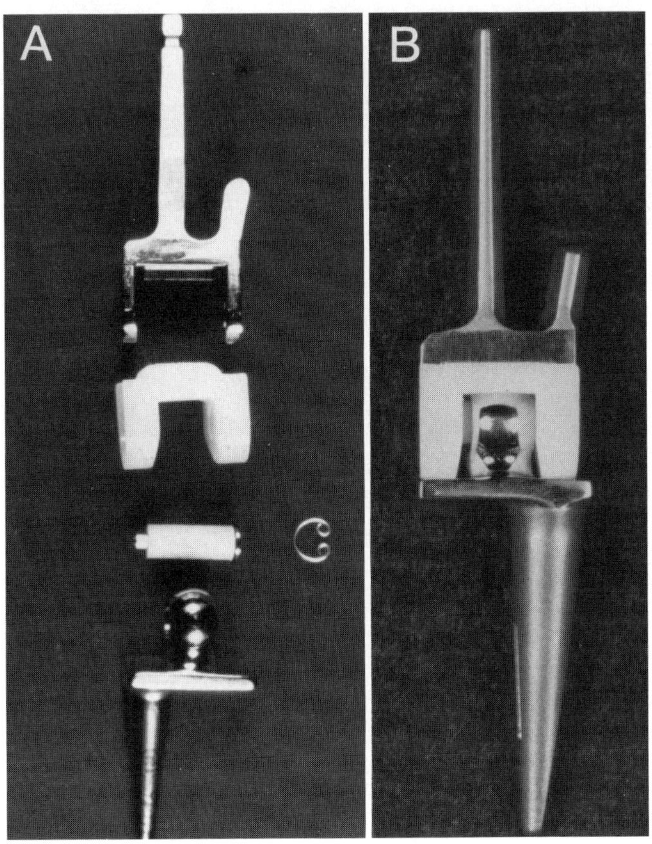

FIG 10–27.
The Spherical Triaxial prosthesis. **A,** an exploded view demonstrates how radial and metacarpal components fit together with the polyethylene bushing and central axle. **B,** assembled view.

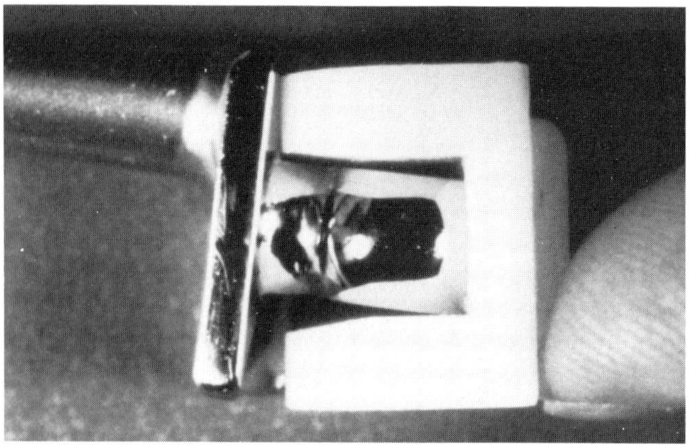

FIG 10–28.
The semiconstrained design of the Spherical Triaxial prosthesis allows for 15 degrees of radial and ulnar deviation.

Contraindications.—Patients with absent wrist extensor power, severe flexion contracture, or a dislocated wrist are probably better treated with arthrodesis. Additionally, as with any implant arthroplasty, previous infection is a contraindication. A relative contraindication is the need for heavy loading, as with the use of an ambulatory aid.

Technique.—The approach to the wrist is similar to that used for arthrodesis (Fig 10–29,A–D). After exposure of the radiocarpal and radioulnar joints, a distal ulnar resection is performed. The appropriately sized radial cutting block is used to perform the distal radial osteotomy and insure that the proper amount of radius is resected. The carpal osteotomy is then performed with axial tension to remove the desired amount of the carpus. Excess carpal bones or capsule should be resected since they

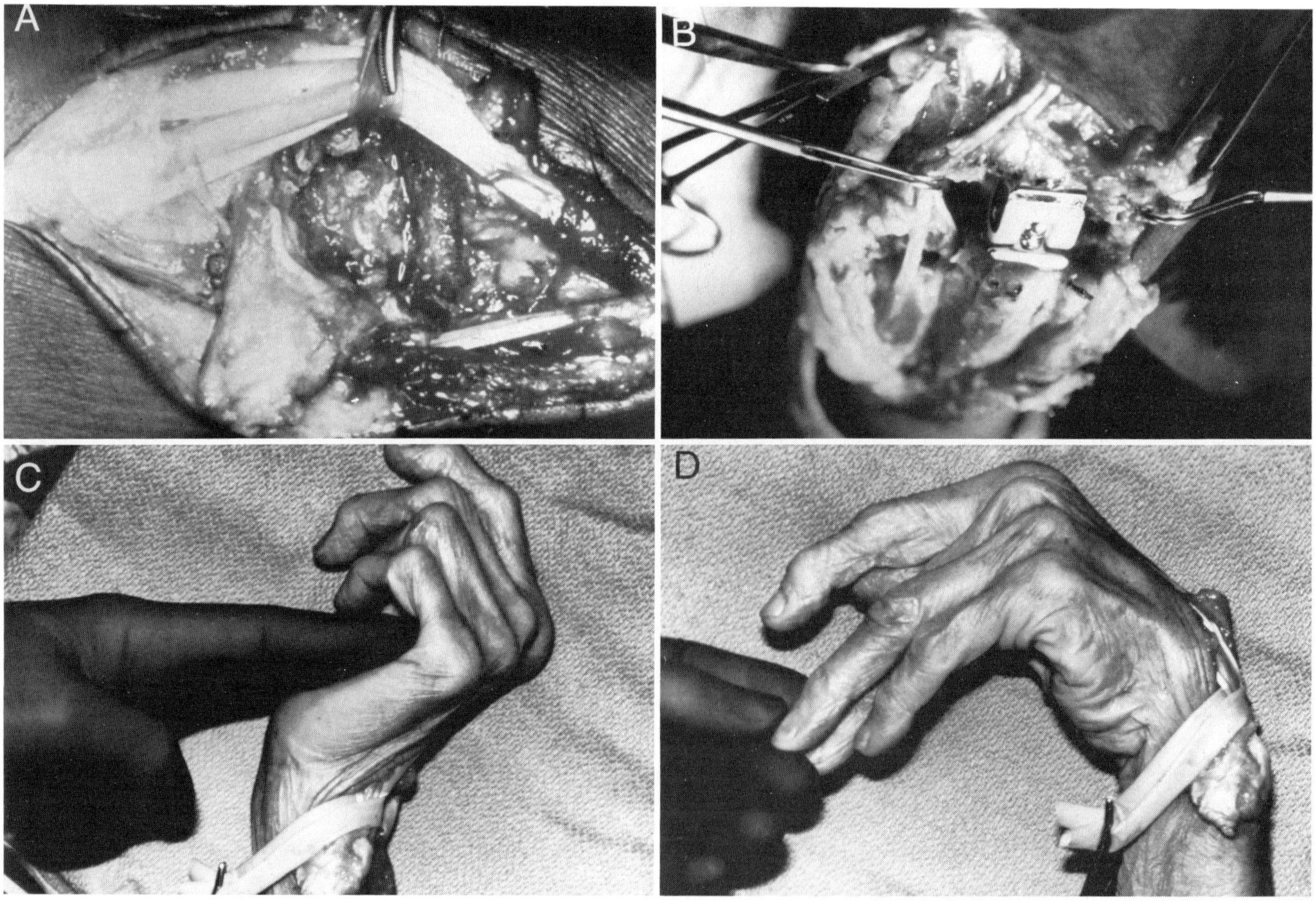

FIG 10–29.
Technique for Spherical Triaxial total wrist arthroplasty. **A,** through a standard longitudinal dorsal incision, extensor tenosynovectomy is performed, and the wrist joint is exposed. **B,** after appropriate bony resections, a trial reduction is performed with the prosthetic components. **C,D,** intraoperative range of motion is performed to insure there are no bony or soft tissue blocks to motion.

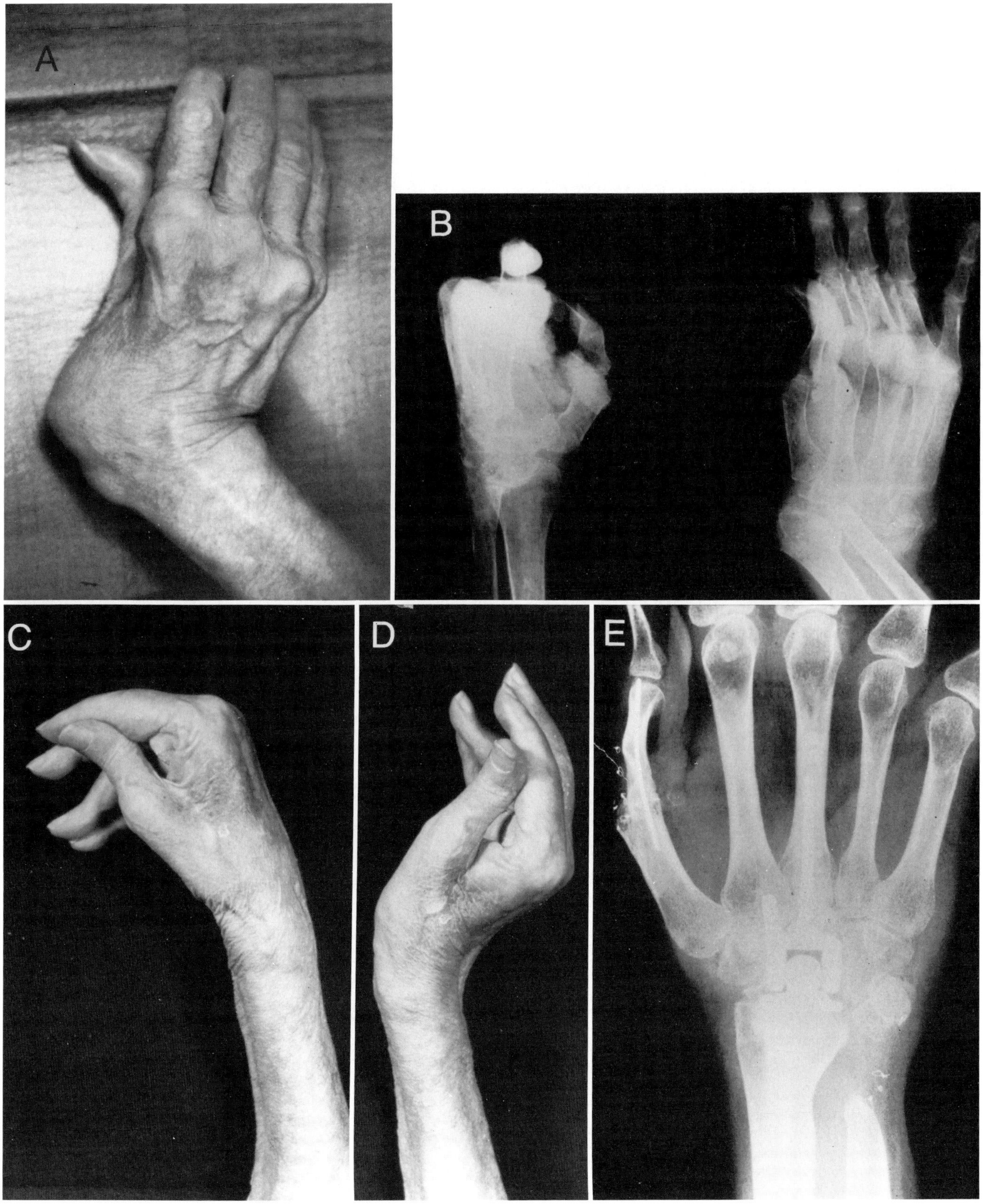

FIG 10–30.
Spherical triaxial total wrist arthroplasty. **A,** preoperative appearance of a wrist with severe rheumatoid arthritis changes. **B,** preoperative radiographs demonstrate radiocarpal subluxation. **C,D,** postoperative range of motion. **E,** postoperative radiograph demonstrates spherical triaxial total wrist arthroplasty in good position.

can block flexion.[13] An awl is used to find the shaft of the radius, and the canal of the second and third metacarpal. Rasps are used to enlarge the canal of the second and third metacarpals. A trial reduction is performed with the true prosthesis without the axle, before cementation, to assess fit. After cementation, the components are reduced with the axle in place, and the capsule and dorsal retinaculum are closed in the usual fashion.

Complications.—Loosening causing failure is the most important complication and occurs in 3% of Spherical Triaxial wrist arthroplasties.[14] Infection is always a possibility. The salvage procedure after failed arthroplasty is arthrodesis. When arthrodesis is performed after removal of an arthroplasty, supplemental bone graft should be used, either from the iliac crest or from metacarpal heads salvaged from the concomitant metacarpophalangeal joint replacement.[18]

Results.—Long-term follow-up has shown that 80% of patients have good or excellent results, with an average improvement in range of motion of 15 de-

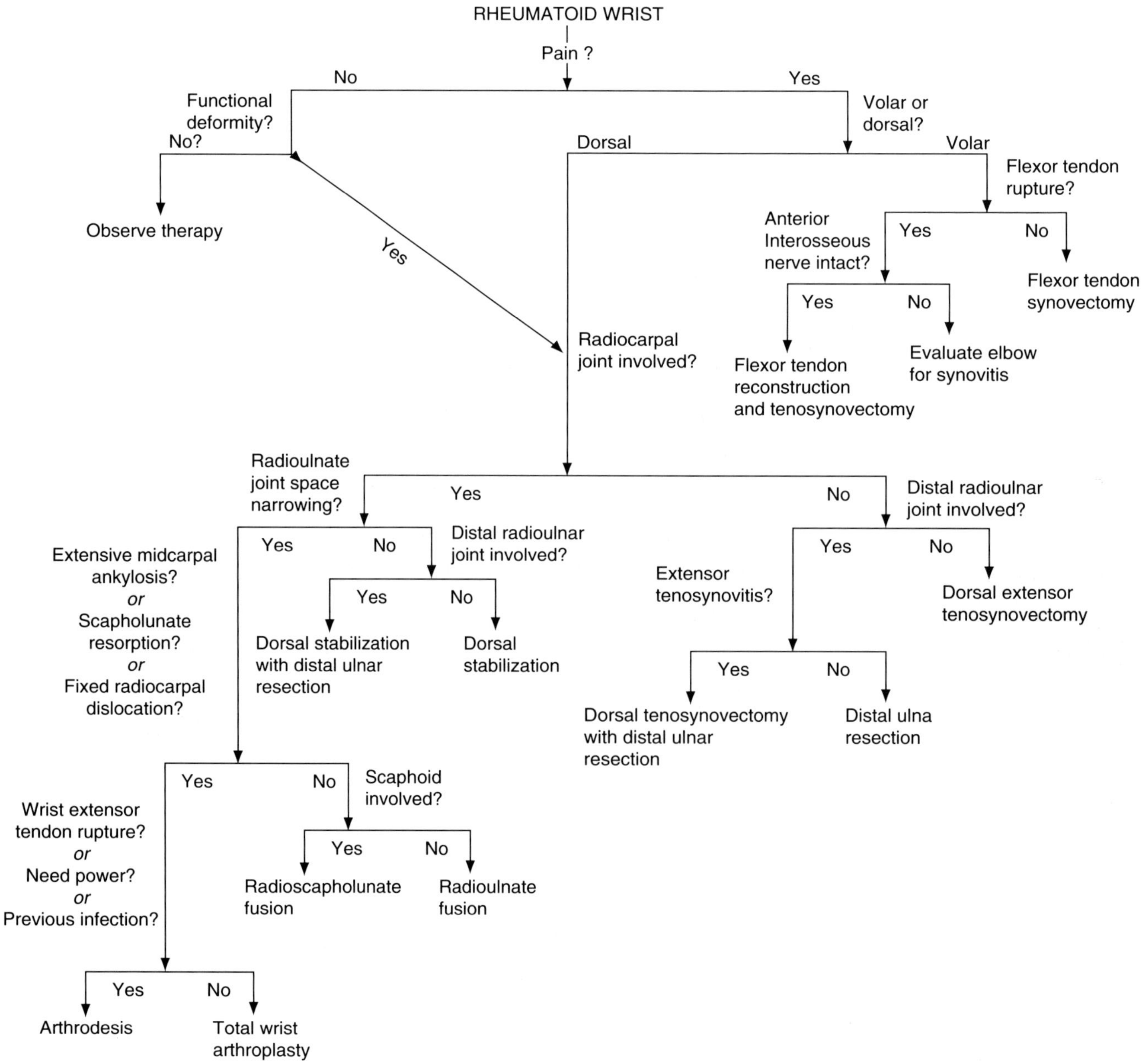

FIG 10–31.
Algorithm for surgical treatment of the rheumatoid wrist.

grees (range 35–50 degrees). The preoperative appearance of a wrist with severe rheumatoid arthritis, and the postoperative results of Spherical Triaxial total wrist arthroplasty are shown in Figure 10–30,A–E. Patients that developed postoperative tendon attrition had preoperative ruptures which were repaired. The position of the center of motion in the dorsal or volar plane and the restoration of carpal height correlated best with the eventual range of motion, functional score, and component shift.[13]

Patients with contralateral wrist fusions prefer arthroplasty because the retained motion allows them to perform activities requiring precision and dexterity.[14]

CONCLUSIONS

The primary goal of surgery is always relief of pain and promotion of a stable functional wrist. When conservative therapy fails, the only option available is surgical intervention (Fig 10–31). The most important prophylactic procedure is prevention of tendon rupture. Thus, during frequent follow-up examination, close scrutiny most be paid to synovitic involvement of the extensor tendons. If this occurs and it is not responsive to conservative therapy, an extensor tendon synovectomy must be performed. At this time the distal radioulnar and radiocarpal joints are evaluated and, if involved, the appropriate procedures are performed. At our institution, we favor dorsal stabilization, wrist panarthrodesis, and total wrist arthroplasty over other varieties of limited procedures. The dorsal stabilization is performed for wrist synovitis with cartilage destruction and no fixed deformities or significant subluxation. In our hands, the Darrach procedure (occasionally with stabilization with a slip of extensor carpi ulnaris tendon) is the simplest procedure for distal ulnar resection, and meets our goals. If bony destruction is severe and deformities are fixed, an arthrodesis or arthroplasty is necessary. The choice depends on the quality of the bone, the quality of the wrist extensors, and the needs of the patient.

Good treatment of the rheumatoid wrist involves complete assessment of the rheumatoid patient including the extent of involvement of other joints and the patient's needs for activities of daily living. Once these are assessed, close evaluation of the patient for progression of disease, and prompt intervention when necessary, assures a satisfactory outcome for both patient and surgeon.

REFERENCES

1. Albright JA, Chase RA: Palmar shelf arthroplasty of the wrist in rheumatoid arthritis. *J Bone Joint Surg [Am]* 1990; 52:896–906.
2. Backdahl M: The caput ulnae syndrome in rheumatoid arthritis. A study of morphology, abnormal anatomy, and clinical picture. *Acta Rheum Scand* 1963; 5(suppl):1–75.
3. Biundo JJ, Hughes GM: Rheumatoid arthritis rehabilitation: Practical guidelines. Part I. *J Musculoskeletal Med* 1991; 8:85–96.
4. Bowers WH: Distal radioulnar joint arthroplasty: The hemiresection interposition technique. *J Hand Surg [Am]* 1985; 10:169–178.
5. Brase DW, Millender LH: Failure of silicone rubber wrist arthroplasty in rheumatoid arthritis. *J Hand Surg [Am]* 1986; 11:175–183.
6. Brewerton DA: The rheumatoid hand. President's address. *Proc R Soc Med* 1966; 59:225.
7. Brumfeld R Jr, Kuschner SH, Gellman H, et al: Results of dorsal wrist synovectomies in the rheumatoid hand. *J Hand Surg [Am]* 1990; 15:733–735.
8. Buckland-Wright JC, Clarke GS, Walker SR: Erosion number and area progression in the wrists and hands of rheumatoid patients: A quantitative microfocal radiographic study. *Ann Rheum Dis* 1989; 48:25–29.
9. Carroll RE, Dick HM: Arthrodesis of the wrist for rheumatoid arthritis. *J Bone Joint Surg [Am]* 1971; 53:1365–1369.
10. Clayton ML: Surgical treatment at the wrist in rheumatoid arthritis. *J Bone Joint Surg [Am]* 1965; 47:741–750.
11. Cooney WP III, Beckenbaugh RD, Linscheid RL: Total wrist arthroplasty problems with implant failure. *Clin Orthop* 1984; 187:121–128.
12. Darrach W, Dwight K: Derangements of the inferior radioulnar articulation. *Proc N Y Acad Med Med Rec* 1915; 87:708.
13. Figgie HE, Inglis AE, Straub LR, et al.: A critical analysis of alignment factors influencing functional results following tripsherical total wrist arthroplasty. *J Arthroplasty* 1986; 1:149.
14. Figgie MP, Ranawat CS, Inglis AE, et al: Trispherical total wrist arthroplasty in rheumatoid arthritis. *J Hand Surg [Am]* 1990; 15:217–223.
15. Gellman H, Rankin G, Brumfield R Jr, et al: Palmar shelf arthroplasty in the rheumatoid wrist. *J Bone Joint Surg [Am]* 1989; 71:223–227.
16. Jackson IT, Milwand TM, Lee P, et al: Ulnar head resection in rheumatoid arthritis. *Hand* 1979; 4:252.
17. Kellgren JH, Lawrence JS: Radiologic assessment of rheumatoid arthritis. *Ann Rheum Dis* 1957; 16:485–493.
18. Kobus RJ, Turner RH: Wrist arthrodesis for treatment of rheumatoid arthritis. *J Hand Surg [Am]* 1990; 15:541–546.
19. Lamberta FJ, Ferlic DC, Clayton MC: Volz total wrist arthroplasty in rheumatoid arthritis: A preliminary report. *J Hand Surg [Am]* 1980; 5:245–252.

20. Leslie BM, Carlson G, Ruby L: Results of extensor carpi ulnaris tenodesis in the rheumatoid wrist undergoing distal ulnar excision. *J Hand Surg [Am]* 1990; 15:547–551.
21. Linscheid RL, Dobyns JH: Rheumatoid arthritis of the wrist. *Orthop Clin North [Am]* 1971; 2:649.
22. Linscheid RL, Dobyns JH: Radiolunate arthrodesis. *J Hand Surg [Am]* 1985; 10:821–829.
23. Mannerfelt L, Norman O: Attrition ruptures of flexor tendons in rheumatoid arthritis caused by bony spurs in the carpal canal. *J Bone Joint Surg [Am]* 1969; 51:270.
24. Marmor L, Lawrence JF, Dubois EL: Posterior interosseous nerve palsy due to rheumatoid arthritis. *J Bone Joint Surg [Am]* 1967; 49:381.
25. Meuli HC: Reconstructive surgery of the wrist joint. *Hand* 1972; 4:88.
26. Millender LH, Nalebuff EA: Arthrodesis of the rheumatoid wrist. *J Bone Joint Surg [Am]* 1973; 55:1026–1034.
27. Millender LH, Nalebuff EA: Reconstructive surgery in the rheumatoid hand. *Orthop Clin North Am* 1975; 6:709–732.
28. Millender LH, Nalebuff EA, Feldon PG: Rheumatoid arthritis, in Green DP (ed): *Operative Hand Surgery.* New York, Churchill Livingstone Inc, 1982.
29. Millender LH, Nalebuff EA, Holdsmith DE: Posterior interosseous nerve syndrome secondary to rheumatoid arthritis. *J Bone Joint Surg [Am]* 1973; 55:753.
30. Nalebuff EA: Rheumatoid hand surgery—Update. *J Hand Surg [Am]* 1983; 8:678–682.
31. Nalebuff EA, Garrod KJ: Present approach to the severely involve rheumatoid wrist. *Orthop Clin North Am* 1984; 15:369–380.
32. Norris SH: Surgery for the rheumatoid wrist and hand. *Ann Rheum Dis* 1990; 49(suppl 2):863–870.
33. Palmer AK, Werner FW, Eng MM, et al: Functional wrist motion: A biomechanical study. *J Hand Surg [Am]* 1985; 10:39.
34. Pekin TJ Jr, Zugiflen NJ: Navicular displacement in rheumatoid arthritis. Its recognition and significance (abstract). *Arthritis Rheum* 1965; 6:292.
35. Ranawat CS, Frieberger RH, Jordan LR, et al.: Arthrography of the rheumatoid wrist joint. *J Bone Joint Surg [Am]* 1969; 51:1269–1281.
36. Ranawat CS, Straub LR: Volar tenosynovitis of the wrist in rheumatoid arthritis. *Arthritis Rheum* 1970; 13:112–117.
37. Sharp JT, Lidsky M, Collins LC, et al: Methods of scoring the progression of radiological changes in rheumatoid arthritis. *Arthritis Rheum* 1971; 14:706–720.
38. Short CL, Bauer W, Reynolds WE: *Rheumatoid Arthritis. A Definition of the Disease and Clinical Description Based on a Numerical Study of 293 Patients and Controls.* Cambridge, Mass, Harvard University Press, 1957.
39. Sledge CB, Atcher RW, Shortkroff S, et al: Intraarticular radiation synovectomy. *Clin Orthop* 1984; 182:37–40.
40. Souter WA: The hand in rheumatic disease, in Lamb DW, Kuczynski K (eds): *The Practice of Hand Surgery.* Boston, Blackwell Scientific Publishers, 1981.
41. Spinner M, Kaplan EB: Extensor carpi ulnaris: Its relationship to the stability of the distal radial ulnar joint. *Clin Orthop* 1970; 68:124–129.
42. Straub LR, Ranawat CS: The wrist in rheumatoid arthritis. *J Bone Joint Surg Am* 1969; 51:1–20.
43. Straub LR, Wilson EH Jr: Spontaneous rupture of extensor tendons in the hand associated with rheumatoid arthritis. *J Bone Joint Surg [Am]* 1956; 38:1208–1217.
44. Swanson AB: Flexible implant arthroplasty for arthritic disabilities of the radiocarpal joint: A silicone rubber intramedullary stemmed flexible hinge implant for the wrist joint. *Orthop Clin North Am* 1973; 4:383.
45. Taleisnik J: The ligaments of the wrist. *J Hand Surg [Am]* 1976; 1:110.
46. Taleisnik J: Combined radiocarpal arthrodesis and midcarpal (lunocapitate) arthroplasty for treatment of rheumatoid arthritis. *J Hand Surg [Am]* 1987; 12:1–8.
47. Taleisnik J: *The Wrist.* New York, Churchill Livingstone Inc, 1985.
48. Taleisnik J: Rheumatoid arthritis of the wrist. *Hand Clin* 1989; 1:251–278.
49. Vaughan-Jackson OJ: Rupture of extensor tendons by attrition at the inferior radioulnar joint. Report of two cases. *J Bone Joint Surg [Br]* 1948; 30:528–530.
50. Volz RG: The development of a total wrist arthroplasty. *Clin Orthop* 1976; 116:209.
51. Watson HK, Ryu JY, Burgess RC: Matched distal ulnar resection. *J Hand Surg [Am]* 1986; 11:812–817.
52. Youm Y, McMurty RY, Flatt AE, et al.: Kinematics of the wrist. I. An experimental study of radioulnar deviation and flexion-extension. *J Bone Joint Surg [Am]* 1978; 60:423–431.

CHAPTER 11

The Hand

Allan E. Inglis, M.D.

INTRODUCTION

Rheumatoid arthritis of the hand is extremely disabling to the patient with rheumatoid disease because even minor deformities or alterations in hand function result in reduced function of the upper extremity. The hand serves the individual in two ways. First, it is the individual's major tactile contact with the environment. Second, it is the major structure of prehension. The full sensory modality of the finger tips is remarkable. One must recall that a person can easily hold the two ends of a pin or edges of a razor blade between the finger tips without discomfort and yet with full awareness of the nature of the edges and points. Normal two-point discrimination is 5 mm. However, blind people easily read braille in which the elevated dots are 2 mm apart or less. Rheumatoid or inflammatory arthritis may destroy these two hand functions through compression neuropathies, vasculitis neuropathies, muscle atrophy, tendon ruptures, osteopenia, and joint destruction. Indeed, the hand is vulnerable to the pathologic destructive effects of rheumatoid disease because of its anatomic complexity (Fig 11–1).

Neural damage from rheumatoid arthritis may occur in a variety of ways. The median nerve may be compressed from volar tenosynovitis of the ulnar bursa. Similarly, the ulnar nerve may be involved just before, or within the canal of Guyon. Vasculitic brachial plexus neuropathy may produce sensory and motor changes in the entire upper extremity. Indeed, rheumatoid vasculitis may be of sufficient severity that the ischemia may result in digital gangrene (Fig 11–2).

Tendon damage may also occur. Rheumatoid nodules may develop on the tendon surfaces, thereby restricting their excursion or at times leading to tendon rupture. Proliferative rheumatoid tenosynovitis may cause locking of the flexor tendons as they glide beneath the digital flexor pulleys.[14] Additionally, flexor tenosynovitis may be of sufficient severity that the tendons become adherent to one another or rupture (see Fig 11–20,D). This is of particular importance within the carpal canal where nine tendons are confined to a narrow space. Tendon ruptures, particularly the insertions of the flexors digitorum superficialis and profundis, are common. At times, the tendons may become attenuated due to rheumatoid involvement.[26] This is particularly common with attenuation of the central slip of the extensor digitorum communis into the base of the middle phalanx producing a boutonnière deformity[17] (see Fig 11–14,A). Attenuation or thinning of the insertion of the extensor pollicis brevis into the base of the proximal phalanx of the thumb will lead to flexion deformities of the thumb.[9]

Deformities of the metacarpophalangeal (MP) joints are also common in more advanced cases of rheumatoid arthritis.[20] Tendon imbalance and attenuation is an important cause of ulnar drift of the lesser fingers.[6, 21] Inflammatory synovitis of the joints of the hand may cause disabling instability due to ligament attenuation. Although these liga-

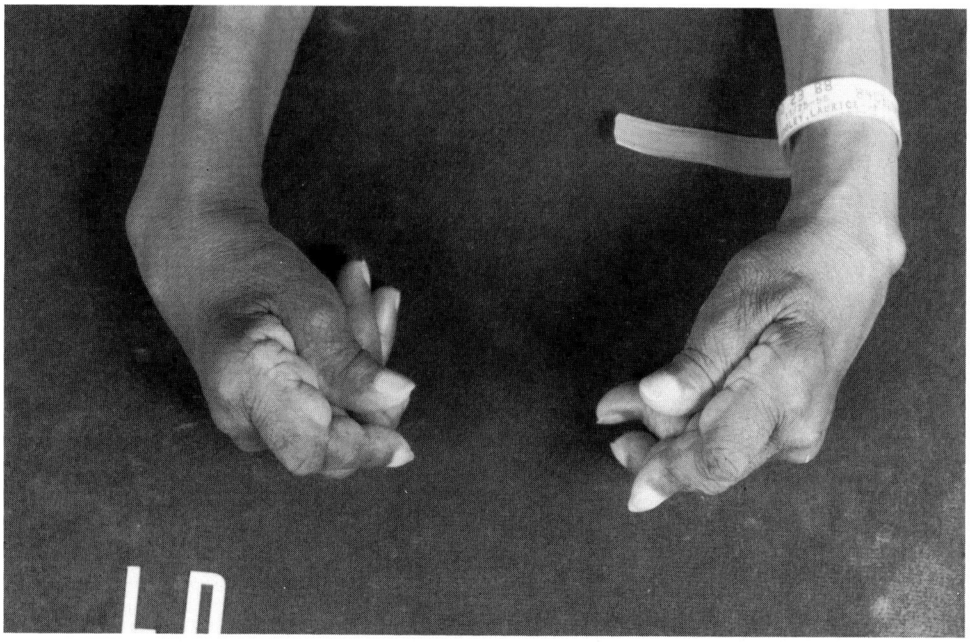

FIG 11–1.
Advanced hand deformities due to rheumatoid arthritis.

ments are normally quite sturdy, they are also small. Therefore, when rheumatoid synovium gets beneath the bony attachments of these ligaments, the ligaments may stretch or give way.

As with other joints, the rheumatoid synovium and pannus may destroy the articular surfaces and produce subchondral cysts.[8] These erosions and cysts cause a loss of joint surface integrity, producing bony collapse. Malalignment of the joint occurs as these surfaces collapse. The combination of ligamentous attenuation, muscle imbalance, and loss of articular integrity all contribute to joint dislocations, contractures, and rotatory subluxations. Indeed, rheumatoid arthritis or inflammatory arthritis affects virtually every structure in the hand.

RHEUMATOID THUMB INVOLVEMENT

Rheumatoid nodules are common along the pressure surfaces of the distal phalanx and the interpha-

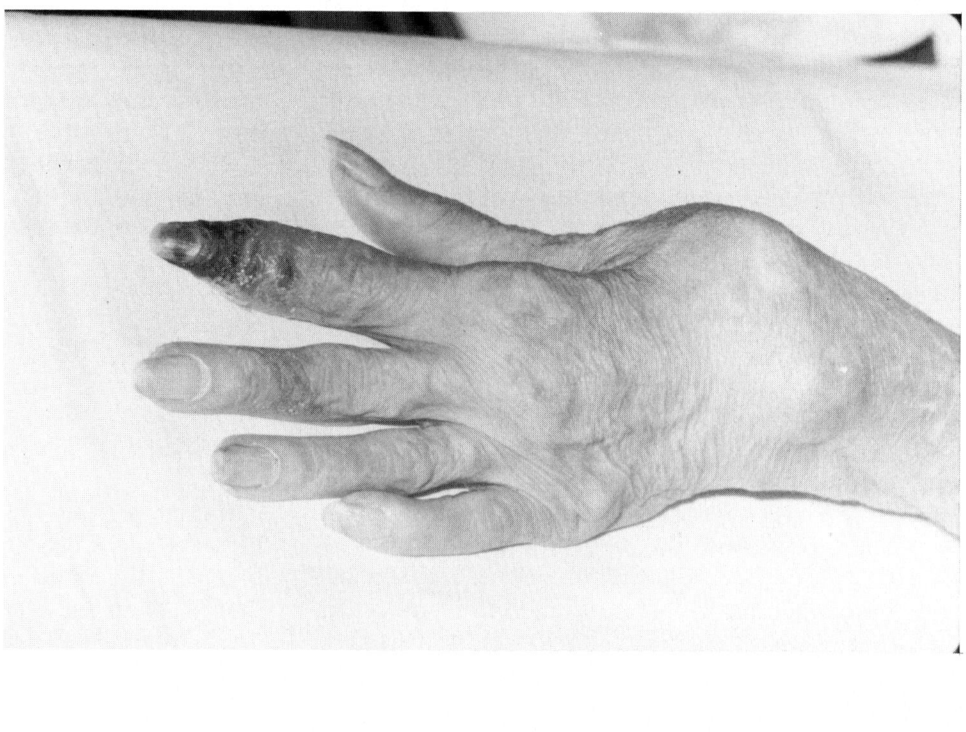

FIG 11–2.
Rheumatoid vasculitis involving the distal phalanx of the index finger. The patient had undergone corrective surgery on the contralateral wrist.

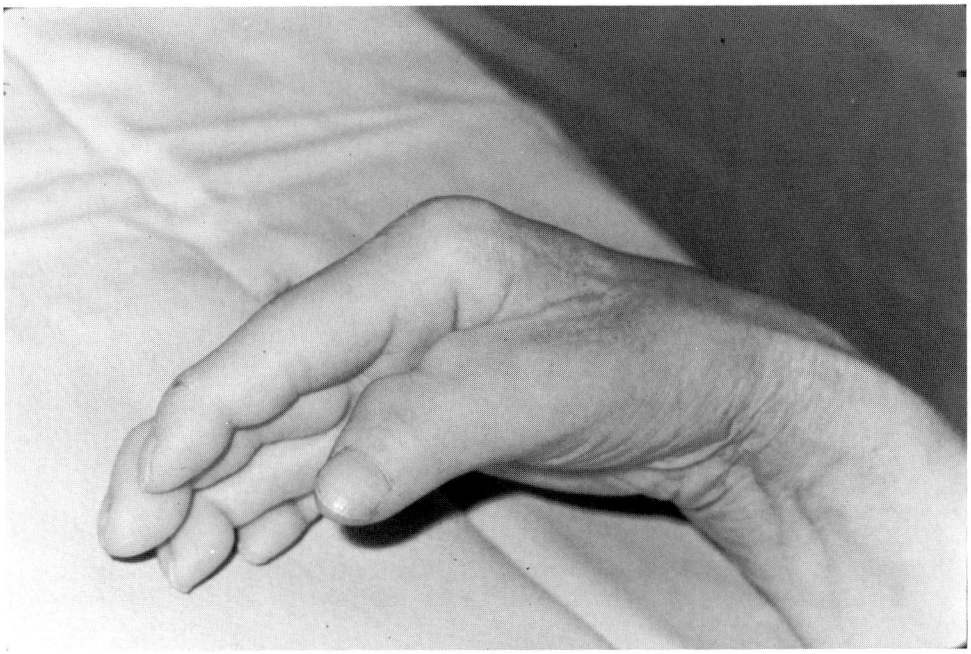

FIG 11–3.
Rheumatoid nodules along the ulnar border of the thumb. These usually occur along the pressure areas of the thumb.

langeal joint of the thumb (Fig 11–3). These nodules frequently accompany instability and hyperextension deformities of the interphalangeal joint. These large, rheumatoid nodules frequently are unsightly (Fig 11–4) and interfere with side-to-side pinch. Surgically, these nodules may be tedious and time-consuming to remove as they often involve the neurovascular bundle on the ulnar border of the thumb. The recurrence level is low and the patients are grateful for the removal of these unsightly and disabling masses.

Rupture of the flexor pollicis longus usually occurs in the palm at the level of the carpometacarpal joint, or less commonly, at the MP joint.[3, 26] This is the result of either a bony excrescence or bony projection from the basal joint or a nodule just proximal to the MP joint pulley. Ruptures should not be treated with primary repair because the tendon ends have been abraded or damaged and therefore are not in a condition for repair. They are treated with a tendon transfer, usually a superficialis tendon from the ring finger. These superficialis tendons are usu-

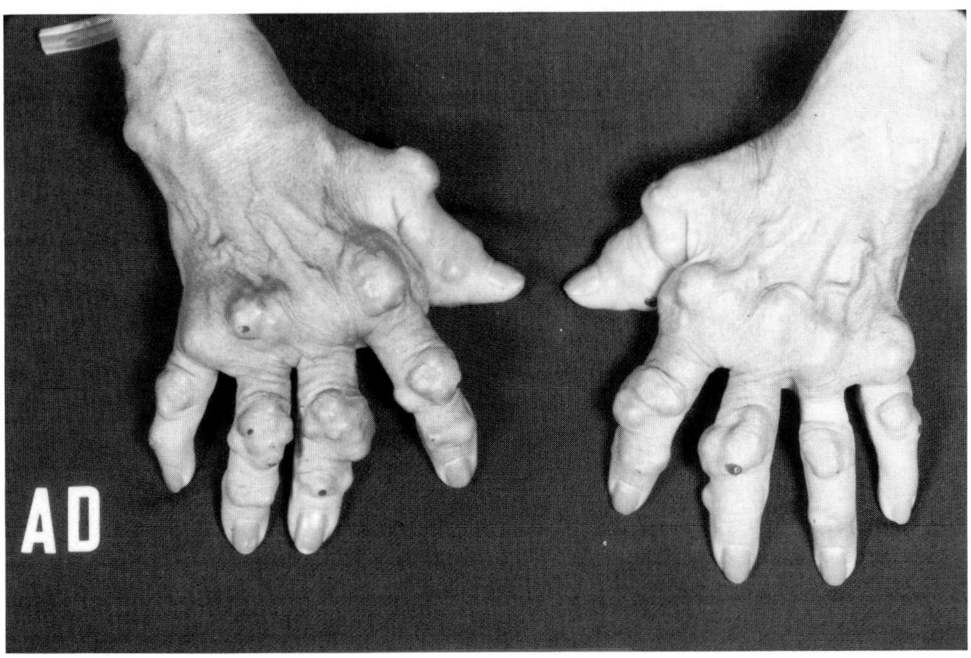

FIG 11–4.
Rheumatoid nodules. These are unsightly and interfere with thumb function.

ally healthy and will hold the repair sutures. Additionally, the superficialis tendon has sufficient excursion to provide good functional MP and interphalangeal joint flexion.

Involvement of the trapeziometacarpal joint is disabling because the stability and strength of the entire thumb is diminished. Initially, treatment is conservative with splints and steroid injections. If this does not provide lasting relief, then surgical therapy is required.[9] Two basic therapeutic approaches may be considered in inflammatory arthritis: resection arthroplasty and implant arthroplasty. Resection arthroplasty of the trapezium with or without fascial or tendon transposition into position has produced good results.[1, 7, 8] Excision of the trapezium is carried out through a curving incision beginning on the dorsum of the first metacarpal and extending in a curving manner to the volar aspect of the wrist overlying the scaphoid bone. The superficial branches of the radial nerve are carefully protected, including those of the dorsal and volar branches of the superficial branch of the radial nerve. The subcutaneous tissue about the extensor pollicis brevis and abductor pollicis longus and around the basal joint is carefully elevated and retracted to provide exposure of the radial artery as it passes around the trapezium and distal to its course between the origin of the first dorsal interosseous muscle and the first and second metacarpal bones. The artery is carefully retracted proximally.

A capsulotomy is then performed about the basal joint. It is important to leave a thick, substantial capsular cuff for subsequent repair following removal of the trapezium bone. Removal of the trapezium is facilitated by the use of a Knowles pin drilled through its substance (Fig 11–5). A suture is placed about the threads of the pin to prevent it from being drilled too deeply or into the flexor carpi radialis tendon. This pin will allow the trapezium to be moved from side to side allowing for sharp ligament detachment. The pin should not be used to pry out the trapezium. Gentle pressure on the pin, much as with a "joy stick" on a computer keyboard, will allow exposure and excision of the trapezium. The tendon of the abductor pollicis longus is then identified and released from where it inserts into the base of the first metacarpal bone. It should be transferred into a drill hole at the junction of the lower and middle thirds of the first metacarpal. This transfer will provide active abduction and will tend to stabilize and hold the base of the first metacarpal into the defect left by the removed trapezium. The capsule is carefully and securely closed. The thumb is then placed in an appropriate bulky dressing which is exchanged in 3 to 4 days for a well-molded plaster "thumb spica" that holds the thumb in abduction. An alternative to this procedure has been a fascial arthroplasty recommended by Carroll in which a strip of tendon from the flexor carpi radialis or palmaris longus is used to fill the defect left by the excised trapezium. The basic technique is the same as the resection arthroplasty, except that the abductor pollicis longus is not transferred distally. The fascial or tendinous slip must be sutured into the base of the cavity to prevent unintended displacement of the fascial mass.

Implant arthroplasty is an alternative therapeutic measure that is particularly useful when the periarticular structures are only moderately damaged. There are, however, no firm data suggesting that implant arthroplasty is superior to resection arthroplasty.[9] If implant arthroplasty is elected, then the same surgical approach is used with the exception that the incision is carried 1½ in. proximally along the tendon of the flexor carpi radialis.[11] Again, the trapezium is removed with the aid of the Knowles pin (see Fig 11–5). We have used both the Eaton[4] and the Swanson[25] implant with success. The Eaton implant has a central hole through which the tendon of the flexor carpi radialis can be passed to secure the implant tightly into place. The stems of these implants are shaped differently and therefore the hole

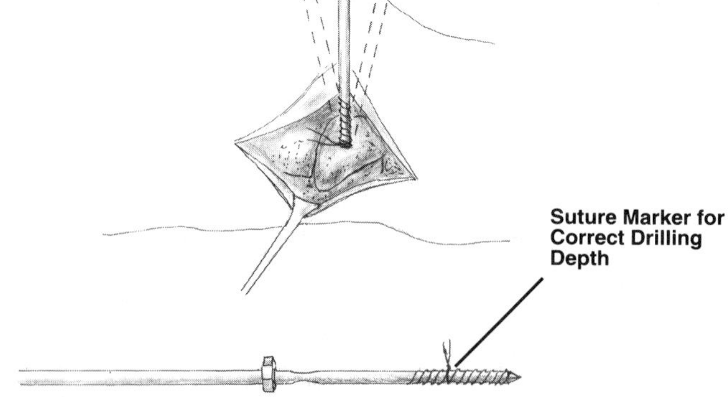

FIG 11–5.
A Knowles pin or other threaded pin can be drilled into the center of the trapezium bone.

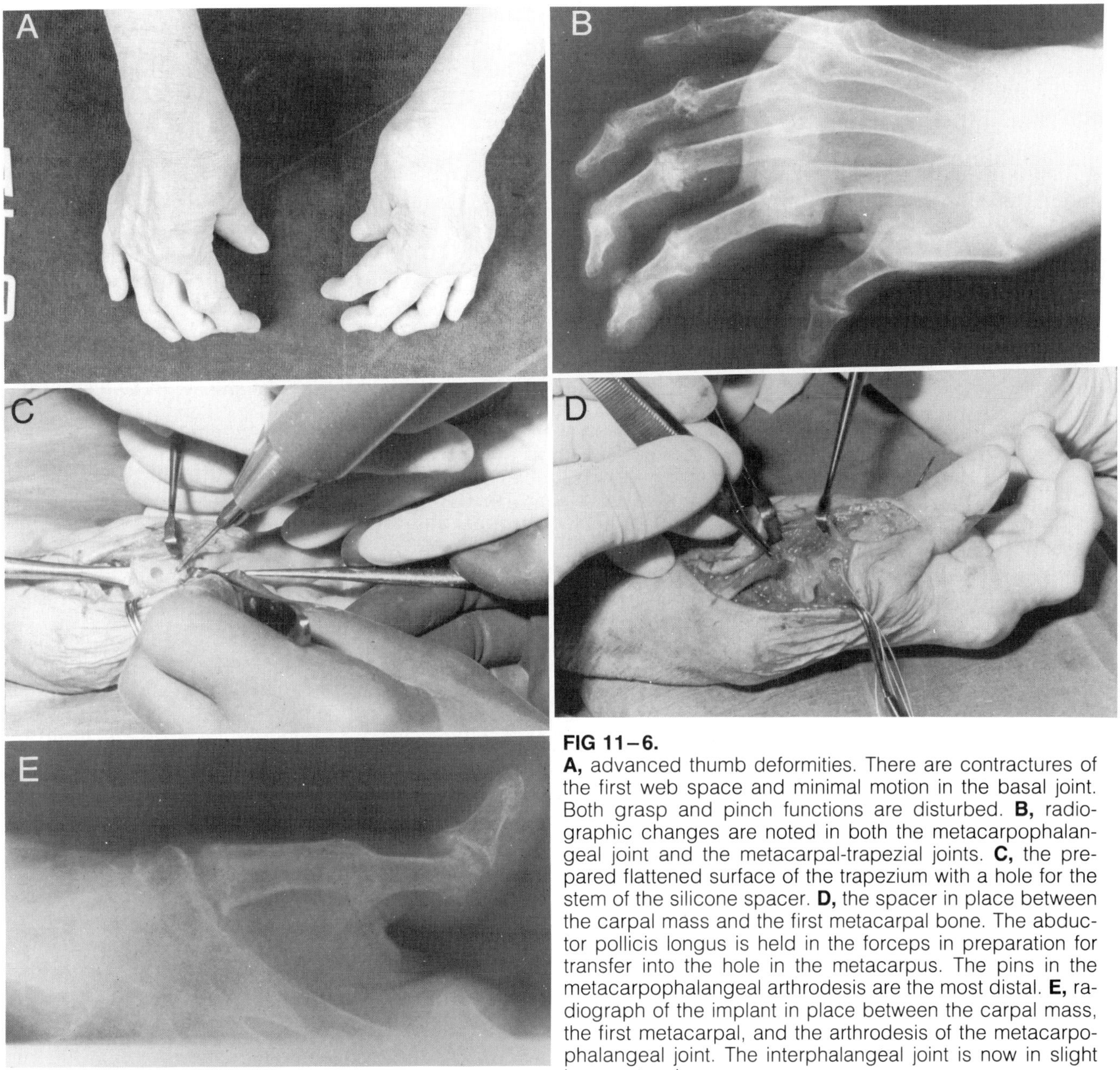

FIG 11–6.
A, advanced thumb deformities. There are contractures of the first web space and minimal motion in the basal joint. Both grasp and pinch functions are disturbed. **B,** radiographic changes are noted in both the metacarpophalangeal joint and the metacarpal-trapezial joints. **C,** the prepared flattened surface of the trapezium with a hole for the stem of the silicone spacer. **D,** the spacer in place between the carpal mass and the first metacarpal bone. The abductor pollicis longus is held in the forceps in preparation for transfer into the hole in the metacarpus. The pins in the metacarpophalangeal arthrodesis are the most distal. **E,** radiograph of the implant in place between the carpal mass, the first metacarpal, and the arthrodesis of the metacarpophalangeal joint. The interphalangeal joint is now in slight hyperextension.

in the base of the first metacarpal must be prepared differently. It will be noted that these implants usually do not fit squarely and properly on the scaphoid bone and will dislocate when the thumb is abducted. Therefore, a portion of the deeper trapezoid bone must be burred away to allow additional space for seating of the implant. If the Eaton implant is used, a portion of the tendon of the flexor carpi radialis must be harvested from the distal forearm. The flexor carpi radialis tendon is split longitudinally and passed through the defect in the deep capsule where the trapezium has been resected. The free tendon is then passed through the aperture in the implant. The implant will become firmly seated. This tendon is then passed through the capsule and woven back and forth through the capsule during the capsular closure. The technique for the Swanson implant arthroplasty is the same except that the tendon of the flexor carpi radialis is not used to secure the implant. Final implant stability is achieved by a secure capsular closure and reinforced, if needed, by a portion of the abductor pollicis longus tendon. The hand is treated the same way postoperatively as in the resection arthroplasty. Exercises are initiated 5 weeks after surgery. As a precaution we recommend a removable molded splint for an additional 4 weeks to be worn when the patient is not exercising the thumb.

When there is gross destruction of the carpometacarpal joint with ankylosis of the carpal bones (Fig 11–6,B), i.e., the trapezium, scaphoid, and trapezoid, an alternative procedure is recommended. In these situations, there is usually a contracture of the first web space, and very little motion at the basal joint, with painful thumb function (Fig 11–6,A). The incision in this instance begins more distally and continues around the base of the carpometacarpal joint, stopping at the point where the flexor carpi radialis enters the carpus. The superficial branches of the radial nerve, including the palmar branch, are carefully protected. The basal joint is identified and the capsular structures incised. The tendon of the abductor pollicis longus is then released and prepared for subsequent transfer. Approximately 3 mm of bone is removed with an oscillating saw from the base of the first metacarpal. This provides exposure of the remaining trapezium. This surface is then flattened and prepared for a Swanson implant. Using a burr, a hole is prepared in the trapezium and in the first metacarpal (Fig 11–6,C). A Swanson implant is selected of sufficient size that the two hubs fit against the cortical shell of the first metacarpal. The two stems of the Swanson implant are then trimmed leaving approximately 1 cm of the stem on each side of the hub. The implant is inserted into the bone, thereby providing a *stable*, interpositional arthroplasty. The tendon of the abductor pollicis longus is transferred into a drill hole distally into the shaft of the first metacarpal bone (Fig 11–6,D). At times, it may be necessary to carefully elevate the muscle fibers of the first dorsal interosseous muscle from the first metacarpal to obtain additional abduction. The thumb is abducted and the hand is placed in a bulky dressing. When the swelling has subsided the hand is placed in a lightweight thumb spica for 6 weeks. This procedure has proved particularly useful in those cases with severe basal joint disease (Fig 11–6,E).

THE METACARPOPHALANGEAL JOINT OF THE THUMB

Rheumatoid arthritis of the MP joint of the thumb produces disability and pain. There may be only painful synovitis or there may be joint destruction with instability and joint dislocation. If the synovitis persists for any period of time there will be attenuation of the extensor pollicis brevis muscle as it passes over the joint. As the tendon becomes attenuated there will be a gradual loss of the ability to fully extend the MP joint. As the attenuation proceeds, there will be further loss of the capsule and the extensor hood of the joint. As the hood is weakened, the extensor pollicis longus will become displaced in the direction of the ulna. In extreme cases, this displacement may allow the tendon to drop below the center of rotation. This produces flexion of the MP joint and hyperextension of the interphalangeal joint of the thumb. As the synovitis continues, there is also displacement of the abductor pollicis brevis and the adductor pollicis such that they no longer assist in extension and stabilization of the MP joint. The synovitis may disrupt the ligamentous support and the volar plate with resultant instability of the MP joint. Any or all of these deficiencies may result in reduced grasp and poor pinch function of the thumb.

Inflammatory arthritis of the MP joint can be managed initially with intraarticular steroids and resting splints. If these are not sufficient, then surgical therapy can be recommended.[8]

Synovectomy of the MP joint of the thumb is performed through a dorsal, darted incision. The subcutaneous tissues are undermined to expose the adductor pollicis and the abductor pollicis brevis as well as the extensors pollicis longus and brevis. The joint is entered through the interval between the extensor pollicis longus and the extensor pollicis brevis. The capsule and the synovium are then removed. The rheumatoid synovium beneath the collateral ligaments and palmarward are removed with the joint in flexion. Following removal of these tissues, the retinaculum is closed with nonabsorbable sutures. Nonabsorbable sutures are used so that early flexion can be initiated. A dorsal splint is worn for 7 days to allow the soft tissues to heal. Exercises are then initiated emphasizing flexion and extension. A night splint is worn for 1 month to prevent a flexion contracture.

When the rheumatoid synovitis has proceeded to the point where there has been rupture or attenuation of the extensor pollicis brevis, an alternative procedure must be used. The same surgical approach is employed. However, the attenuated or ruptured remnant of the tendon is detached from the base of the proximal phalanx. The tendon of the abductor pollicis brevis and the adductor pollicis are isolated for subsequent extensor hood reconstruc-

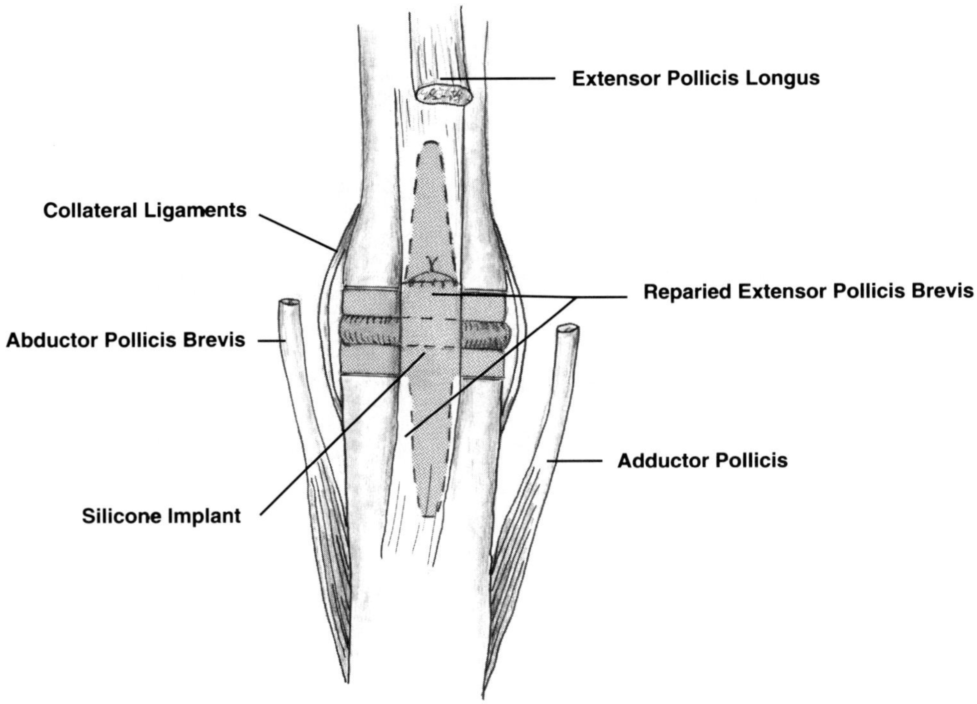

FIG 11–7.
The thumb metacarpophalangeal (MP) implant arthroplasty. The collateral ligaments have been retained for stability. The tendon of the extensor pollicis brevis has been repaired back to the base of the proximal phalanx. The extensor pollicis longus is restored to the dorsum of the MP joint and supported by the tendons of the adductor pollicis longus and the abductor pollicis brevis.

tion. A synovectomy is then carried out. The tendon of the extensor pollicis brevis is restored to its normal position at the base of the proximal phalanx with a suture into bone. The extensor pollicis longus is centralized and stabilized with sutures from the abductor pollicis brevis and the adductor pollicis. This reconstructed hood is then stabilized with a small wire across the joint. The wire is removed in 3 weeks and, as with simple synovectomy, a night splint is used as the exercise program is started.

In those cases in which the rheumatoid disease has destroyed the MP joint of the thumb and yet there are intact collateral ligaments, an implant arthroplasty can be recommended. When implant arthroplasty is considered, it is essential that the collateral ligaments be retained. Frequently there is a subluxation or even a dislocation of the MP joint, yet the collateral ligaments are still intact and functional.[24] The operative procedure is similar to that used for synovectomy and dorsal hood reconstruction previously described. However, the head of the first metacarpal is osteotomized just distal to the insertions of the collateral ligaments. The base of the proximal phalanx is debrided and flattened. The intermedullary cavities are then carefully reamed and broached for the appropriate silicone spacer. At times it may be necessary to shorten the stem going into the proximal phalanx, particularly when arthrodesis of the interphalangeal joint is planned. The implant is then inserted. The extensor pollicis brevis is brought forward and attached to its normal position in the base of the proximal phalanx with nonabsorbable sutures. It is important that this tendon be sutured into the bone itself. The extensor pollicis longus is restored to the midline and the abductor pollicis brevis and the adductor pollicis are used in the hood reconstruction (Fig 11–7). We follow Swanson's suggestion and stabilize the joint in extension with a pin in the tendon sheath of the flexor pollicis longus. This pin is kept in place for 3 weeks at which time a removable dorsal splint is used to stabilize the extensor hood reconstruction. Active flexion and extension exercises are begun at that time (Fig 11–8,A and B).

Arthrodesis of the MP joint is indicated when there has been destruction of the joint and its ligamentous support. It is also an alternative in patients in whom great strength is required in an otherwise normal hand. Arthrodesis is carried out, again through a darted, dorsal incision. The extensor pollicis longus is carefully protected and the entire hood system is restored so that extension of the interphalangeal joint will be as normal as possible. The position for arthrodesis follows the "rule of 15's."[8] In this position the thumb is abducted 15 degrees, flexed 15 degrees, and rotated inward 15 degrees. This position allows for an optimal grasp span and retains good position for pinch or opposition to the little finger. This position also optimizes the forces to the basal thumb and to the interphalangeal joint during pinch and grasp.

Deformities of the interphalangeal joint have

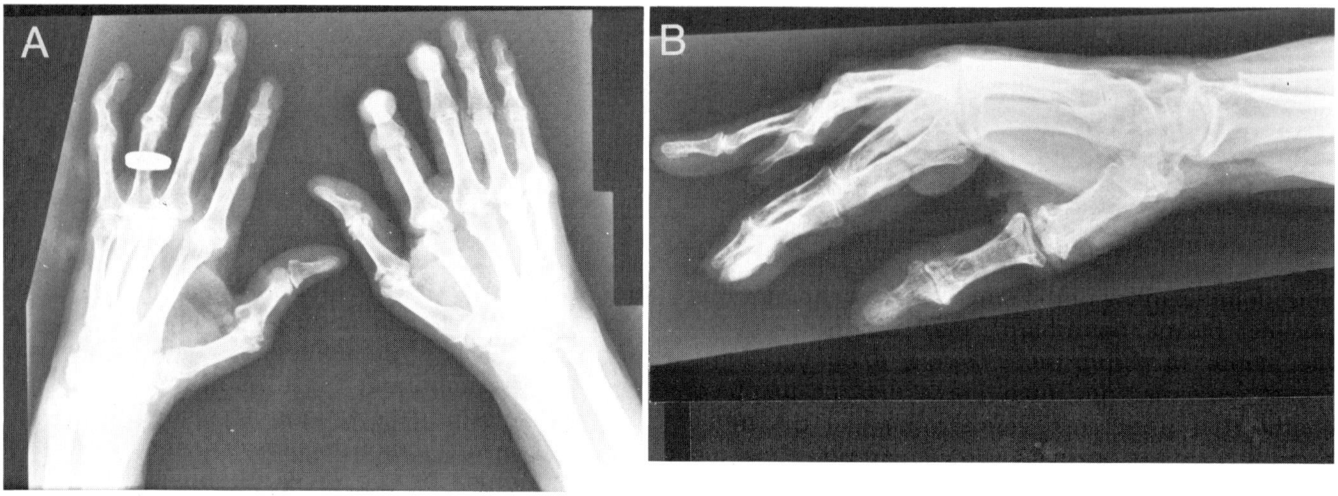

FIG 11–8.
A, radiographs of rheumatoid arthritis involving the metacarpophalangeal joints of the thumb. The head of the first metacarpal has been destroyed and instability and palmar dislocation has occurred despite retention of the collateral ligaments. **B,** following arthroplasty, the thumb is now in good alignment for pinch and grasp.

been described and categorized according to joint destruction and position.[16] When the interphalangeal joint of the thumb becomes unstable, then arthrodesis in the position of function is the procedure of choice. The position must be carefully ascertained taking into consideration the condition of the index finger and the functional requirements of the patient. Some patients prefer tip pinch, whereas others prefer pulp pinch. In general, pulp pinch is preferred with a broader pinch area and somewhat higher allowable pinch forces. Frequently, arthrodesis of the interphalangeal joint is combined with implant arthroplasty of the MP joint.

THE METACARPOPHALANGEAL JOINTS OF THE LESSER FINGERS

The major deformities and loss of function in inflammatory arthritis of the MP joints of the lesser fingers are similar to those observed in the thumb. Two basic processes produce these deformities: active and passive forces. The passive forces are those in which the rheumatoid disease damages the soft tissue structures about the MP joints.[6, 19, 21] Damage to the collateral ligaments produces medial-lateral instability of the MP joint. Damage to the capsule and surrounding hood structures allows the extensor mechanism to rotate and the fingers to migrate in an ulnar direction.[22] The articular surfaces may also be damaged with loss of joint surface integrity and stability. Further damage may result from proliferative synovitis causing capsular distention and distortion. The active forces leading to deformity include displacement and malposition of the tendons including the flexors digitorum superficialis and profundis as well as the six extensor tendons. Additionally, the intrinsic muscles, including the abductor digiti minimi, with their attachments to the base of the proximal phalanges may produce palmar subluxation and rotational deformities. The combination of these active and passive deformities tends to produce intrinsic contractures, volar subluxation of the MP joints, and ulnar drift of the entire phalanges.

Conservative treatment includes intraarticular steroids and splinting, and gentle exercises. When the synovitis of the MP joint becomes severe, arthrocentesis with instillation of 5 to 10 mg of methylprednisolone (Depo-Medrol) is useful. There are few intraarticular injections of steroids that are as immediately beneficial and long-lasting as those in the MP joints. Technically, the instillation is best accomplished with the joint flexed 90 degrees. A ball-point pen with the point *retracted* is then pressed gently lateral or medial to the extensor tendon directly over the flexed joint for 10 seconds. This will leave a small indentation for 10 minutes or more in the skin which serves as a guide for the subsequent arthrocentesis (Fig 11–9,A). Frequently, it is necessary to inject all four MP joints using the marked area of indented skin (Fig 11–9,B).

Resting splints may be recommended for patients with ulnar drift involving the MP joints. These resting splints are most beneficial when used at night. Experience has shown that resting splints do

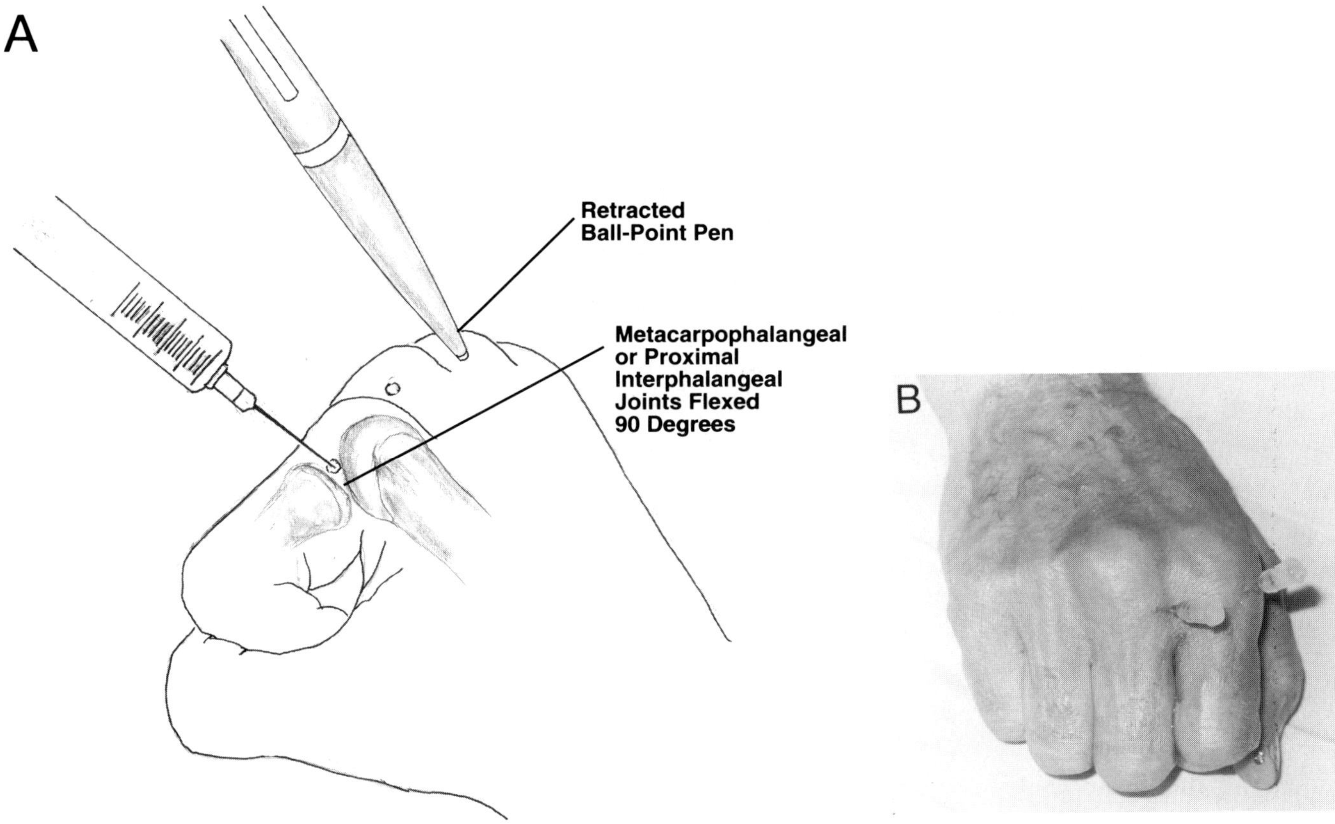

FIG 11–9.
A, steroid instillation into the metacarpophalangeal joints. Pressing the retracted ball-point pen for 5 to 10 seconds over the exact spot for the injection will facilitate locating the injection site after the antiseptic has been applied. These marks will last for several minutes. **B,** the needles are in place with the joints flexed 90 degrees.

not correct or prevent further ulnar drift but will relieve or reduce pain in the MP joints. These splints are also helpful in reducing wrist pain. Patients should be advised that the splints are used to relieve pain and discomfort, not to prevent further deformity. This explanation will avoid disappointment and ultimately further compliance with other therapeutic measures. The resting splints should be fabricated by occupational therapists during a comprehensive occupational therapy program. These programs should include an assessment of overall hand function and deficiency. The therapist will then be able to devise special handles for knives, forks, combs, and other tools that are used in the activities of daily living. Should surgical therapy be required, a baseline of function will have been established and the patient will have an acquaintance with the therapist and a knowledge of what can be accomplished through the therapeutic program.

The major disabling deformities within the MP joints of the lesser fingers are subluxation and ulnar drift. Both of these deformities are caused by the inflammatory tissue.[6] This tissue will have damaged the joints with secondary destruction of the supporting capsular structures and ligaments and, ultimately, damage to the articular surfaces and the subchondral bone. In the early phases of this inflammatory reaction there may be merely distention of the capsule and stretching of the ligaments by the hyperplastic inflamed synovium. As this tissue proliferates beneath the collateral ligaments, there is progressive loss of ligamentous and capsular substance and attenuation of the collateral ligaments. The capsule hood and extensor tendon will become displaced into the adjacent ulnar "valleys" (Fig 11–10,A and B). As the synovitis continues, there will be loss of articular cartilage and damage to the underlying bony structures. This loss of ligamentous, capsular, and bony support allows the proximal phalanges of the fingers to move both ulnarward and in a palmar direction.

These deformities of volar subluxation and ulnar drift are accelerated by the tensions developed by the muscles of the hand. The interosseous muscles,

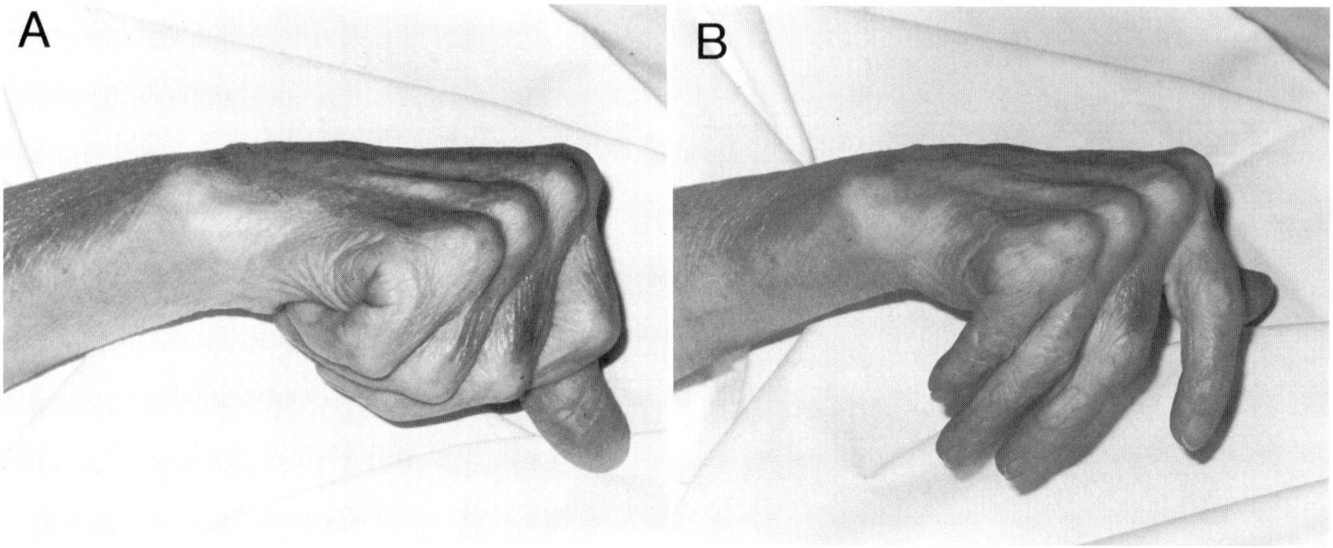

FIG 11–10.
A, rheumatoid arthritis involving the metacarpophalangeal (MP) joints. This patient has retained excellent grasp owing to the uninvolved interphalangeal joints of the fingers. **B,** the patient attempting to extend the MP joints. There has been complete dislocation of the extensor mechanism into the adjacent ulnar valleys such that any attempt to extend the MP joints results in flexion. The abductor digiti minimi can be noted to rotate the little finger as well.

being primary flexors of the MP joints, will actively pull the proximal phalanges into a palmar subluxated position. The ulnar drift deformity is accelerated when the ligaments and capsular structures and bony supporting structures are damaged by the pull or tension of the six digital extensor muscles, i.e., the extensors communis and indicis proprius and digiti minimi. Since the capsules and extensor hoods are damaged, these extensor muscles will migrate into the adjacent ulnar valleys, thereby producing an ulnar-directed force on the individual fingers. The extensor digiti minimi functioning as an abductor will also tend to deform the little finger in an ulnar direction. Rheumatoid wrist deformities in which the carpus rotates or deviates radially on the radius producing the "Z" deformity further accentuate the digital ulnar deformity.[16] With a normal MP joint, the finger moves laterally in full extension. This is allowed by the surface geometry of the head of the metacarpal bone and the base of the proximal phalanx.[27] The movement is guided by the collateral ligaments and the volar plate and the active forces provided by the surrounding muscles. If any of these constituents of normal motion, i.e., joint surfaces, ligamentous support, or muscle force, are injured or malaligned, abnormal motion will occur.

If pain and disability continue, conservative measures such as splinting, arthrocentesis with steroid instillation, or rheumatoid medications having failed, then surgery must be considered. In general, there are three categories of surgical treatment. The first is synovectomy of the MP joint; synovectomy involves realignment of the extensor mechanism. The second is realignment of the extensor mechanism without synovectomy. The third is implant arthroplasty with realignment of the extensor mechanism.[15, 23, 24] Each of these procedures has different indications. Again, it must be emphasized that these procedures are only indicated when conservative measures have failed.

Synovectomy of the MP joint of the lesser fingers is indicated when there is minimal or no damage to collateral ligaments and the articular surfaces of the joint (Fig 11–11,A). The extensor hood, sagittal bands, and collateral ligaments should be preserved (Fig 11–11,B). The capsule should be excised with the synovium. Removal of the synovium without excising the capsule will cause postoperative joint stiffness. There usually is early ulnar drift of the joint (Fig 11–11,C). The ulnar drift is corrected by centralization of the extensor mechanism. A longitudinal incision over the MP joint is used when the synovitis involves only one finger. The extensor tendon is incised longitudinally. This exposes the capsule of the MP joint. The capsule is excised over the dorsum of the head of the metacarpal along with the underlying synovium. The collateral ligaments are preserved as the capsule and synovium are removed. The entire joint surface should be visualized. The posterior synovectomy is carried out between the volar plate and the head and neck of the metacarpal. Using very small rongeurs, all of the synovium must be removed beneath the collateral ligaments. If there has been no ulnar drift, then the extensor tendon is sutured in the midline with fine, nonabsorbable sutures. If there has been ulnar drift with ulnar displacement of the extensor tendon, the incision is made along the *radial* border of the extensor tendon. Following synovectomy, the juncturae tendinum are released and the extensor tendon is realigned and imbricated with the sagittal band or hood structure centralized over the MP joint. An active flexion-extension exercise program is initiated on the third postoperative day, including both active-resistive and active-assistive exercises. If there is any question about digital alignment, dynamic splints are used to promote flexion and extension of the MP joint. The nonabsorbable sutures will allow the active exercise program to proceed without fear of suture failure during the first 3 weeks following surgery.

Recentralization of the extensor mechanism without synovectomy is an uncommon surgical procedure. It is used particularly in patients with systemic lupus erythematosus in whom the initial synovitis has subsided and there is only residual ulnar drift with migration of the extensor mechanisms into the adjacent ulnar valleys. There is usually no articular damage. Typically, the patient is able to maintain the MP joints in full extension if the fingers are placed in full extension and is able to flex the joints normally. However, as the patient flexes the MP joints, the extensor mechanisms become displaced into the adjacent ulnar valleys. Once in the fully flexed position, it is not possible for the patient to *actively* extend the MP joints as the extensor tendons have slipped below the center of rotation of the joint. The surgical procedure in this situation is recentralization of the extensor mechanisms, release of the juncturae tendinum (Fig 11–12) and release of the abductor digiti minimi.

The skin incision is transverse across the metacarpal heads. The extensor hood is incised along the *radial* border of the extensor tendon. The extensor

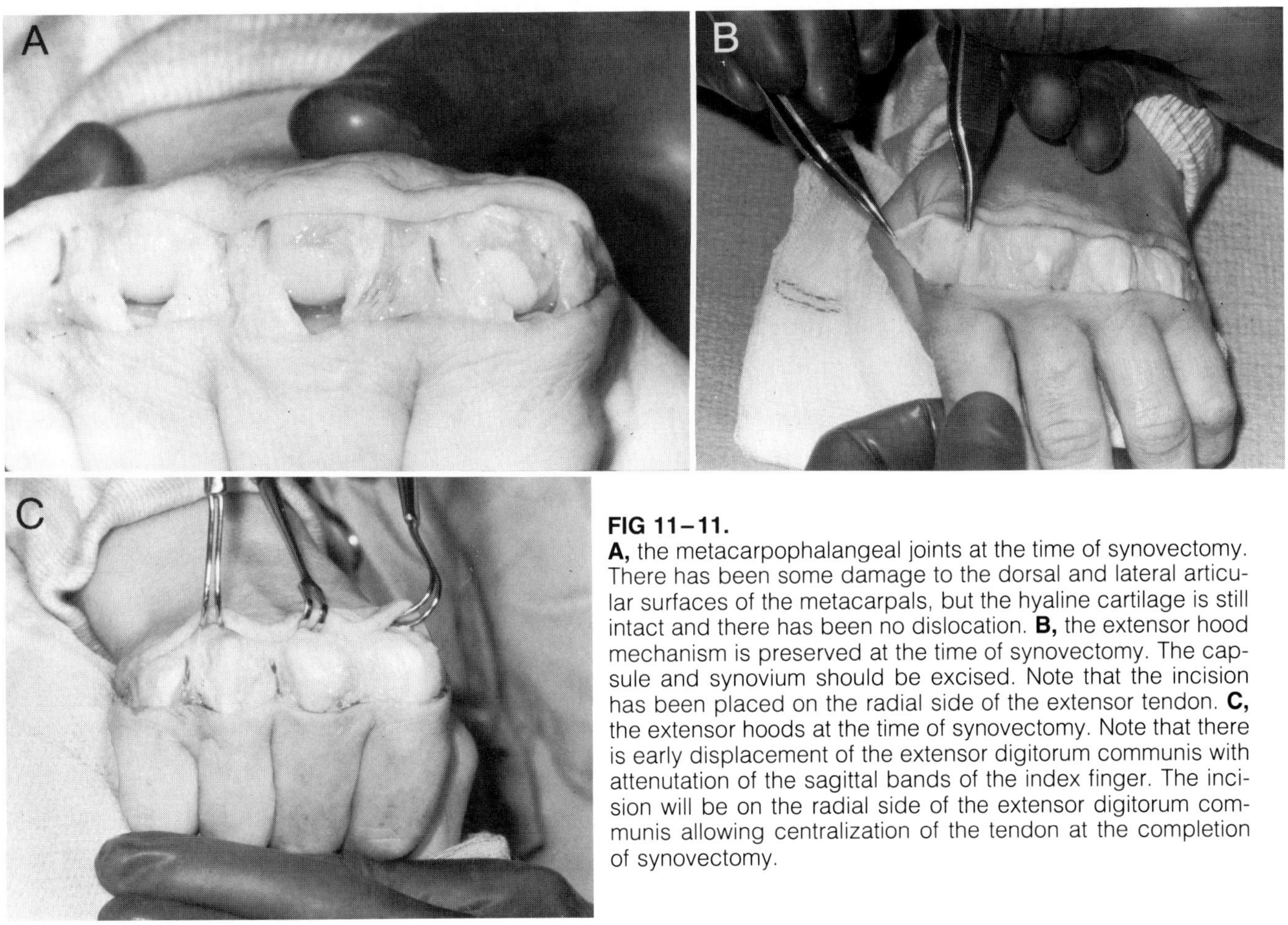

FIG 11–11.
A, the metacarpophalangeal joints at the time of synovectomy. There has been some damage to the dorsal and lateral articular surfaces of the metacarpals, but the hyaline cartilage is still intact and there has been no dislocation. **B,** the extensor hood mechanism is preserved at the time of synovectomy. The capsule and synovium should be excised. Note that the incision has been placed on the radial side of the extensor tendon. **C,** the extensor hoods at the time of synovectomy. Note that there is early displacement of the extensor digitorum communis with attenutation of the sagittal bands of the index finger. The incision will be on the radial side of the extensor digitorum communis allowing centralization of the tendon at the completion of synovectomy.

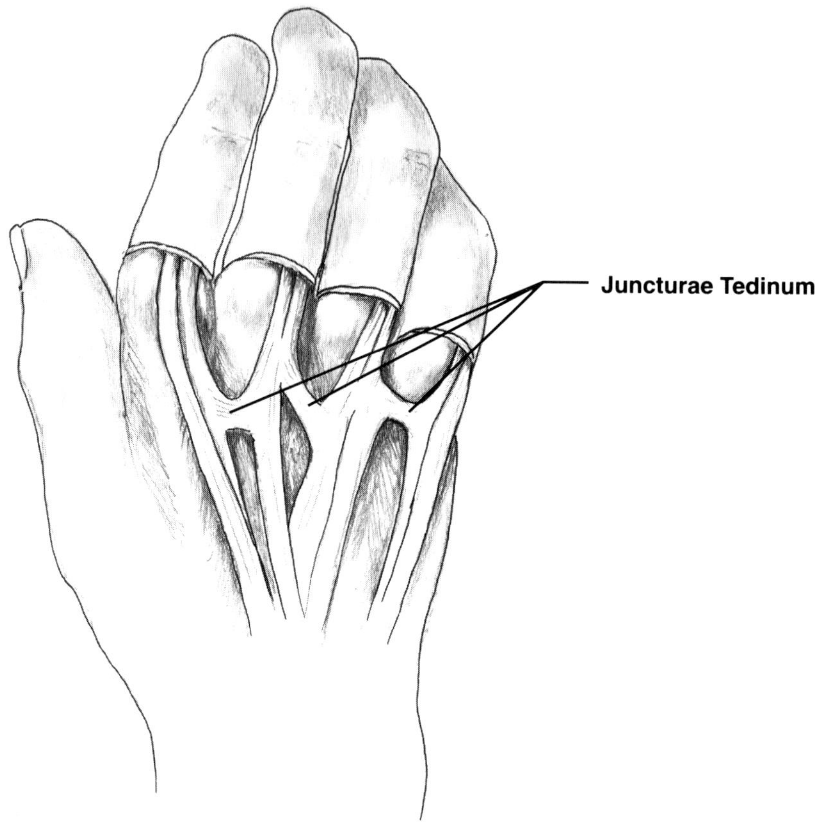

FIG 11–12.
Illustration of the juncturae tendinum and their tethering effect on the adjacent extensor tendons.

tendon with the sagittal band is released within the web space. There are frequently small adhesions between the sagittal bands of the adjacent MP joints. Following this, the extensor hood is easily centralized over the MP joint. An imbricating, horizontal mattress suture is used to hold the tendon in place. The suture is passed through the center of the extensor digitorum communis tendon (Fig 11–13). The attenuated and stretched radial sagittal band is held tightly over the top of the MP joint. The needle and suture is passed in a horizontal mattress fashion through this structure over the center of the MP joint and brought again through the center of the tendon of the extensor digitorum communis. The extensor digitorum communis tendon will move up and over and on top of the MP joint as the suture is drawn tight. Three or four of these sutures are placed in a similar manner thereby securing the extensor mechanism in a normal position. This will of course tighten the ulnar sagittal band structures. This newly imbricated structure resembles the normal extensor hood system. The adjacent juncturae are incised, thereby reducing cross-tension between the extensor tendons. This procedure is carried out for each of the involved MP joints. The tendon of the abductor digiti minimi is released from its insertion into the base of the ulnar border of the proximal phalanx of the little finger.

It is frequently necessary to release the sagittal band along the ulnar border of the little finger to insure proper alignment of the extensor tendon of the little finger. The hand is then placed in a bulky bandage with the fingers in the fully corrected position. On the third day following surgery, the patient is placed in a dynamic extension splint that holds the fingers in normal alignment. Because nonabsorbable sutures have been used, early motion is allowed. The patient will use the dynamic flexion-extension splint for 5 weeks, which allows full healing of the realigned extensor mechanism. This procedure is contraindicated when the MP joints cannot be passively extended preoperatively. If the MP joints cannot be fully extended, then resection arthroplasty with implant arthroplasty is needed.

Implant arthroplasty of the MP joints is required when there is pain or poor function in the joints. Implant arthroplasty is used when there has been joint damage or destruction with volar subluxation and ulnar drift of the fingers. It should be noted that there is *no* indication for surgery if there is normal interphalangeal joint flexion and extension with functional grasp and release, yet there is ulnar drift of the lesser fingers. The hand may appear unattractive because of ulnar drift and yet have strong grasp and release. Surgery on such a functional hand will result in an improved appearance. However, the power and the overall function of the hand will not be improved.

The original operation for such damaged and deformed joints was simple resection arthroplasty. Since then, the results have been improved significantly with the use of a silicone spacer between the resected metacarpal head and the proximal phalanx rather than disorganized scar tissue. The spacer tends to maintain longitudinal, transverse, and rotational alignment. The amount of bone resected from the metacarpal head, and when necessary the proximal phalanx, must be sufficient to allow for proper realignment and balancing of the extensor mechanism. For optimal results, the ligamentous and tendon balancing must be precise.

Surgical Technique

A transverse incision over the top of the MP joints is used (Fig 11–14,A). The subcutaneous tissues are undermined such that the extensor hoods of each of the MP joints can be visualized without tension on the skin. A longitudinal incision is made along the *radial* border of the extensor tendon. The capsule and the synovium are dissected away from the extensor hood. Keeping the synovium and capsule in one piece aids in the removal. When the synovectomy has been completed, a mark is placed on the head of the metacarpal to indicate the amount of metacarpal head to be removed that will allow insertion of the implant. The metacarpal head is then excised. It is dissected free of the collateral ligaments which are preserved, if possible. The synovectomy is then completed beneath the resected head and shaft of the metacarpal and the volar plate. The base of the proximal phalanx must be debrided and flattened if there has been erosion or osteophyte formation. The oscillating saw is used to flatten this surface and prevent distortion of the implant. The insertions of the interossei into the bases of the proximal phalanges are preserved. Using an awl, reamers, and broaches, the canal is opened to accept the stem of the implant. The edges of the implant that is selected should rest on the edges of the cortical bone. The subchondral bone of the proximal phalanx is then penetrated with an awl and the contents of the proximal phalanx are reamed to accept the stem of the implant. Each metacarpal joint is treated in a similar manner. The juncturae tendinum are released. The insertion of the abductor digiti minimi is released along with the sagittal band from the base of the proximal phalanx of the little finger. The individual joints are then irrigated and the implants are inserted (Fig 11–14,B).

The radial collateral ligament may be reattached. The extensor hoods are realigned and closed using a horizontal mattress suture technique (see Fig 11–13). The needle is passed through the center of the extensor tendon and then longitudinally into the adjacent hood as it is pulled directly over the middle of the MP joint using a horizontal mattress technique. The needle is then passed out through the ex-

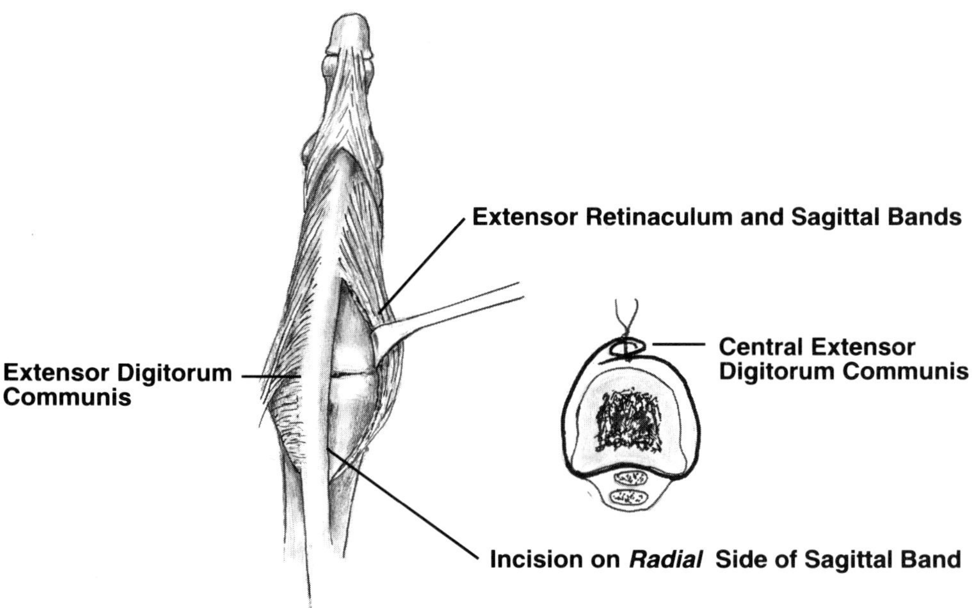

FIG 11–13.
The extensor hood incision and reconstruction. The incision is made through the sagittal band, the retinaculum, the capsule and the synovium, and the *radial* side of the extensor digitorum communis (EDC). Following implant insertion, the sutures are passed through the EDC through the middle of the tightened and otherwise redundant radial sagittal band and then back through the EDC.

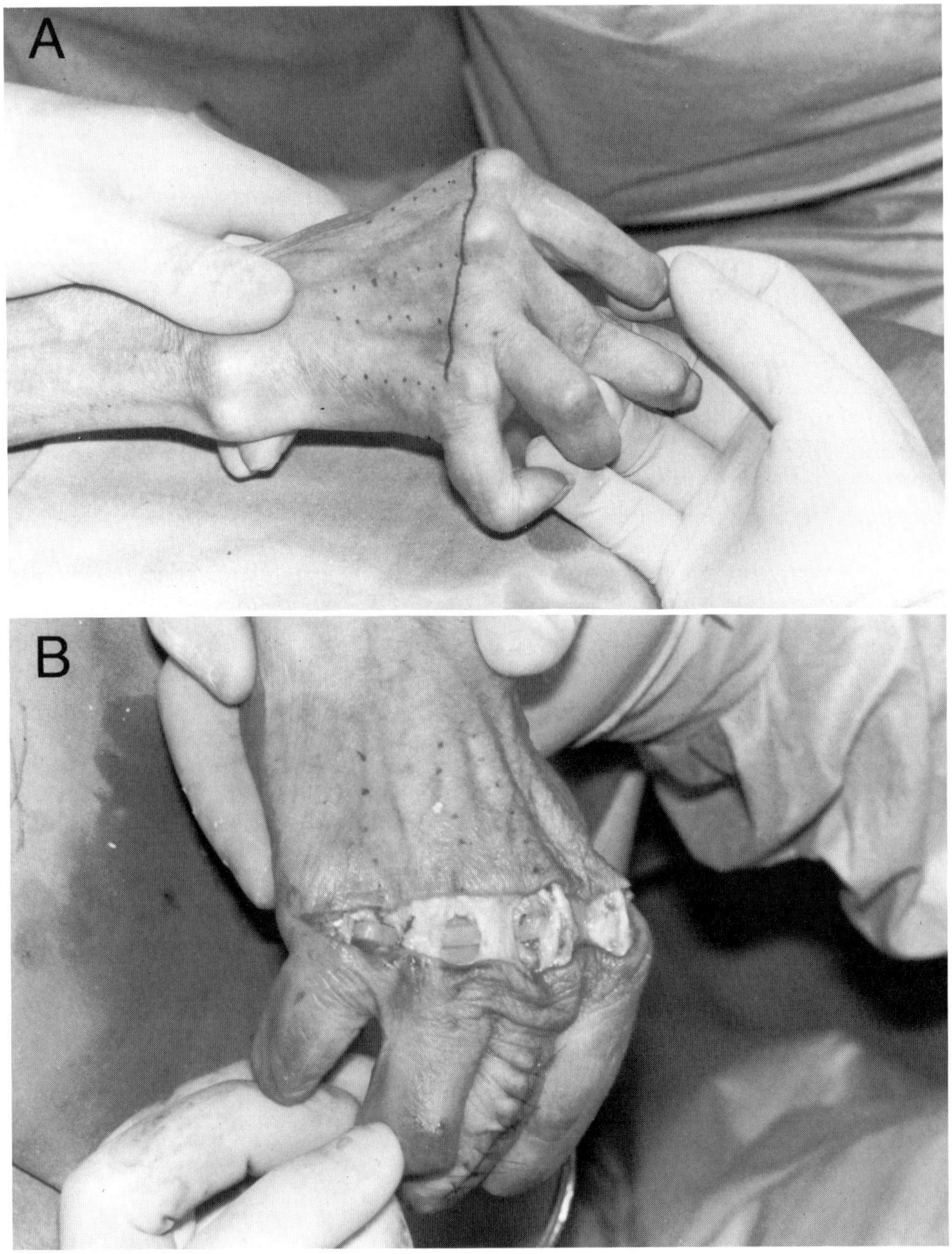

FIG 11–14.
A, incision for metacarpophalangeal implant arthroplasty. Note that the incision is directly over the proposed metacarpal head resection site. The small *dotted lines* indicate the alignment of the individual metacarpal bones allowing for a more precise, transverse, metacarpal neck osteotomy. There is a fixed proximal interphalangeal (PIP) joint swan-neck deformity that will require arthrodesis. There is also a boutonnière deformity of the ring finger that is rigid and in the position of function. **B,** the implants in place. The overall alignment of the fingers has been restored. The extensor tendons can be accurately centralized as in the index finger. The PIP joint of the index finger has been fixed in 40 degrees of flexion. The juncturae have been released.

tensor hood again. As the two suture limbs are tightened, the extensor hood will become realigned with the extensor digitorum communis directly over the center of the MP joint. Two or three or more of these sutures are placed in the hood structure to assure its continuity during the rehabilitation process. The skin margins only are closed with fine, nonabsorbable sutures. The hand is then placed in a large, bulky dressing with the finger in the newly aligned position. On the third day following surgery, a dynamic extension splint is fabricated and on the following day a dynamic flexion splint is prepared for nighttime use. The extension splint is used in the daytime to provide maximum extension and use of the hand in the usual activities of daily living. These splints are continued for 4 or 5 weeks. The extension splint is used a little longer than the flexion splint.

This same operative procedure and rehabilitation program can be combined with arthrodeses, realignment manipulations, or osteotomies of the proximal interphalangeal (PIP) joints. All of these procedures will improve the overall alignment of the

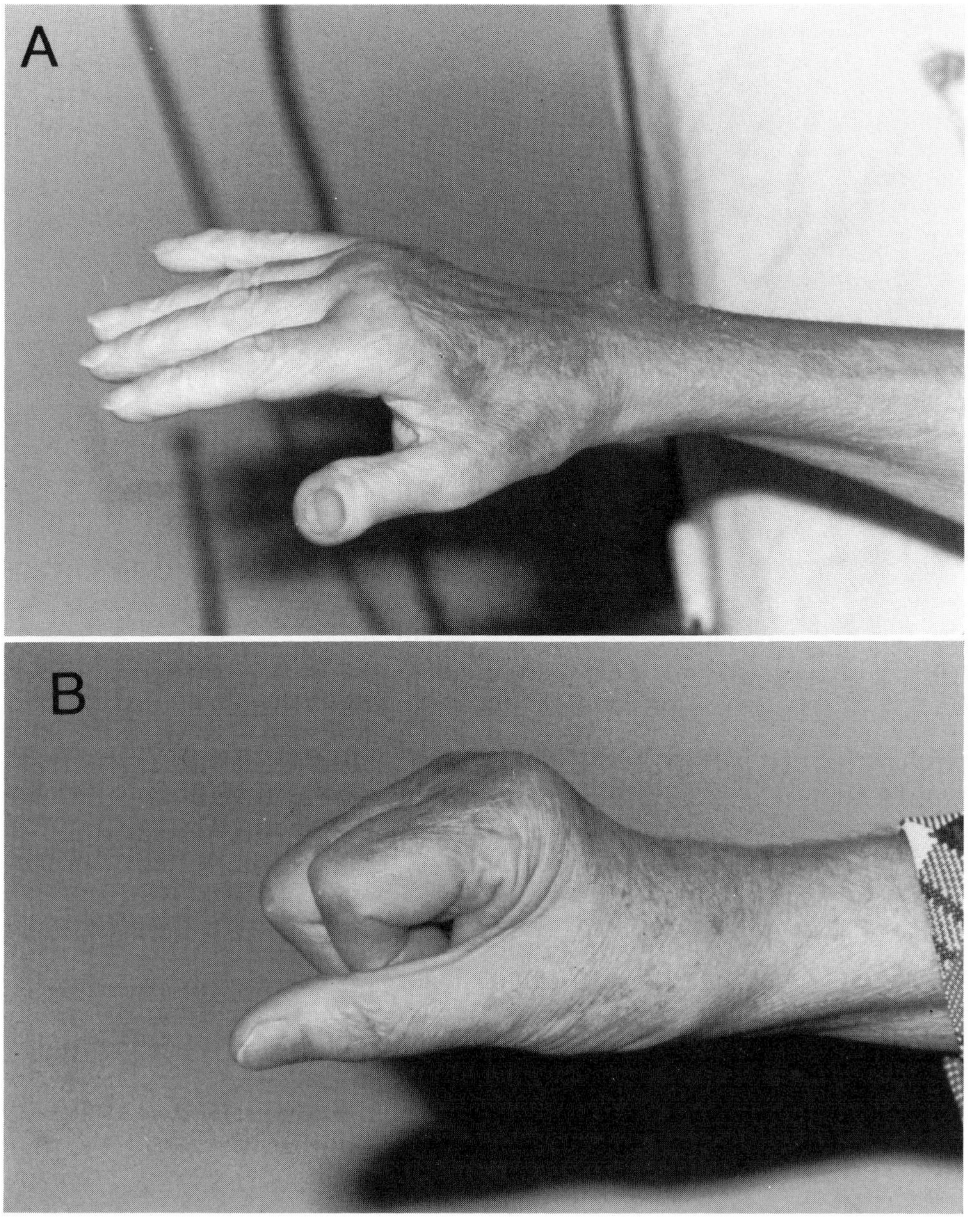

FIG 11–15.
A, metacarpophalangeal (MP) implant arthroplasty 6 months following surgery. Note that the longitudinal alignment is excellent. It should be noted also that the hand is not normal and that the MP joints lack some degree of extension. This should improve with time, and not at the expense of flexion. The result was reported as good. **B,** MP joint flexion. Flexion of the individual joints was 70 degrees. However, with good interphalangeal joint flexion, the patient was able to bring the fingers to the palm. The hand is still not normal. This hand was also rated as good.

fingers and the overall function of the hand. It is not expected that the hand will have greater power to grasp. However, the appearance and performance of the hand will be improved (Fig 11–15,A and B).

THE INTERPHALANGEAL JOINTS

The PIP joints, like the other joints of the hand, may have deformities secondary to muscle or ligamentous imbalance or damage due to joint surface destruction. The deformities therefore may be either actively or passively derived through joint destruction. The interphalangeal joint deformity may be simply an ankylosis in malposition or an angular deformity due to joint destruction. Alternatively, the patient may develop a swan-neck or hyperextension deformity or a boutonnière or flexion deformity of the PIP joint. Both are due primarily to muscle or ligamentous disease or injury.

The boutonnière deformity is caused principally by underlying joint synovitis which produces an attenuation and lengthening of the central slip of the extensor digitorum communis tendon[17] (Fig 11–16). The fine medial tendons of the lateral interosseus

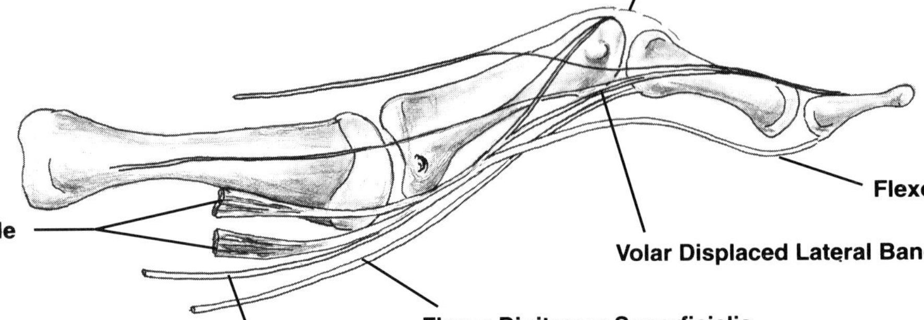

FIG 11–16.
A boutonnière deformity. The lateral bands have been displaced volarward so that they cannot assist in extension of the proximal interphalangeal (PIP) joint. Additionally, the extensor digitorum communis, having become attenuated and retracted proximally, now "overcontributes" to the lateral bands and in fact flexes the PIP joint.

bands become attenuated and lengthened as a part of the extensor mechanism of the PIP joint. The extensor digitorum communis then begins to "overcontribute" to the lateral interosseous bands through so-called lateral tendons, thereby contributing to a flexion deformity of the PIP joint. This deformity develops when, in attempting to extend the PIP joint, the joint in fact begins to flex. The lateral bands gradually migrate in a palmar direction producing an even greater flexor force across the joint. With this increased power there is an overpull of the extensor slip to the *distal interphalangeal joint.* This tends to produce a hyperextension deformity of that joint. The increase in relative strength of the lateral bands produces an imbalance between this structure and the tethering effect of the longitudinal retinacular (Landsmeer) ligament.[12] The distal interphalangeal joint begins to lose its capacity to fully flex as the longitudinal retinacular ligament becomes contracted.

The swan-neck or hyperextension deformity of the PIP joint is also caused by soft tissue contractures and secondary muscle imbalance. The hyperextension deformity is produced and maintained by an abnormal displacement of the lateral interosseous bands above the center of rotation of the joint (Fig 11–17). The transverse retinacular ligaments become foreshortened. Normally the lateral bands are held just above the center of rotation of the joint when the joint is extended. Early in the development of this deformity, the lateral bands are still able to move back below the center of rotation as the PIP and distal interphalangeal joints move into flexion. Once the lateral bands are below the center of rotation, normal interphalangeal joint flexion may occur. As the disease process continues, the volar plate of the PIP joint may stretch. In combination with permanent shortening of the transverse retinacular ligaments, the PIP joint may not be able to flex fully or may become permanently hyperextended. The inflammatory process involving the joint may, in addition to producing a contracture of the transverse retinacular ligaments, cause damage to the joint itself, further impeding normal flexion of the joint. Fixed swan-neck deformities greatly diminish the overall function of the hand, interfering with pinch and particularly with normal grasp.

Angular and rotational deformities of the PIP joint may occur when the inflammatory arthritis damages the condyles of the distal proximal phalanx. In time, the joint may rotate during pinch due to lateral pressure from the thumb or from the torque forces involved in power grasp. Angular or rotational deformities occur as a result of simple collapse of the condyles allowing the articular surfaces of the proximal middle phalanx to fall into the defects. This is particularly apparent in arthritis mutilans. The damaged articular surfaces may either ankylose or become unstable. Instability is also a problem in the distal interphalangeal joint with the same etiology as in the PIP joint.

Surgical therapy for the boutonnière deformity can be considered after conservative measures have failed and there is continuing pain and disability. Conservative measures should include a resting splint and arthrocentesis. Steroid injections into the PIP joint frequently have a long-lasting salutary effect. Again, the joint is located with the finger in full

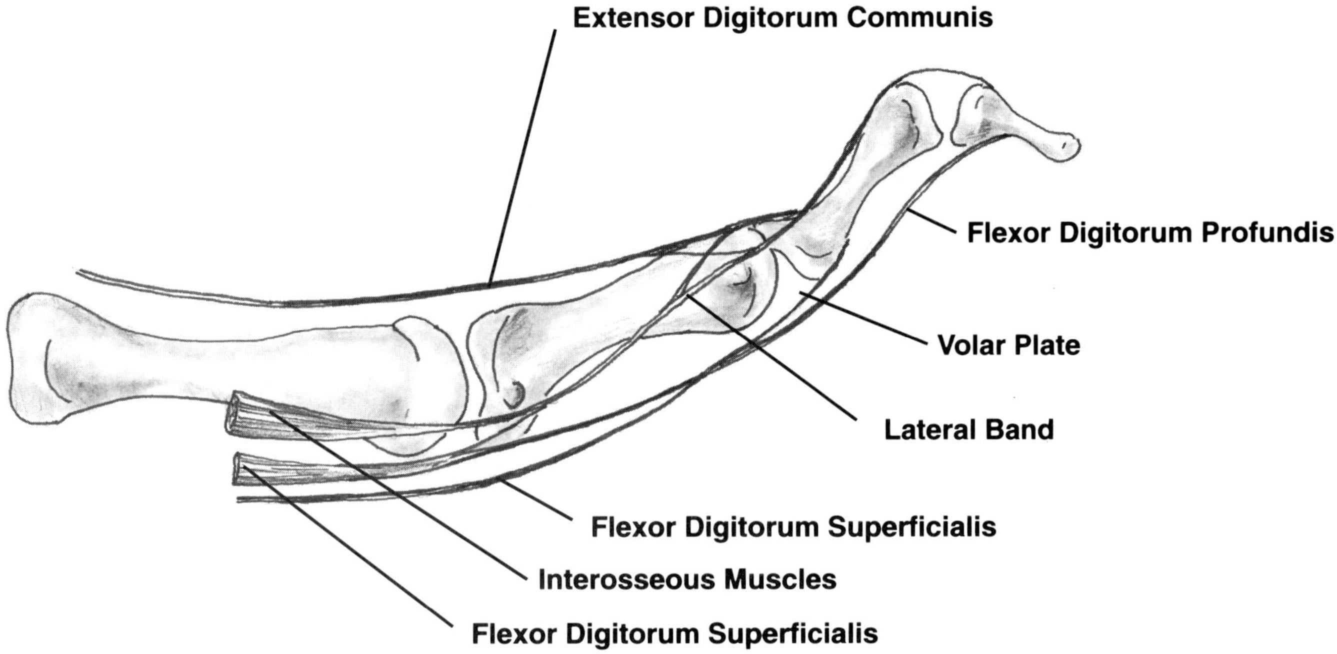

FIG 11–17.
A swan-neck deformity. The lateral interosseous bands have been displaced dorsally above the center of rotation of the proximal interphalangeal (PIP) joint preventing normal flexion of the PIP joint.

flexion. A small dimple can be palpated and then marked with a blunt retracted ball-point pen. Usually, only a small amount of local anesthetic and steroid can be injected (Fig 11–18,A and B). The conservative surgical treatment of a disabling flexion deformity usually is arthrodesis. Soft tissue correction with tendon transfers are difficult and unpredictable. The major problem with a soft tissue reconstruction is in reestablishing the normal soft tissue balance and tension so that at the end of the proce-

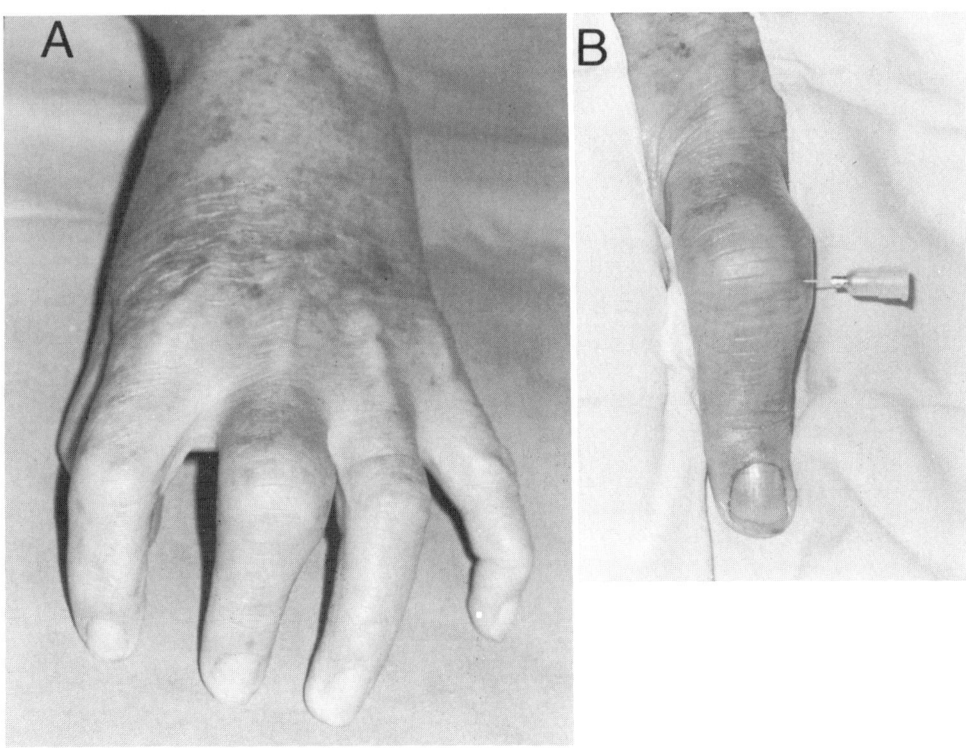

FIG 11–18.
A, isolated proximal interphalangeal (PIP) joint synovitis. The finger is assuming a flexion posture of an early boutonnière deformity. **B,** the PIP joint steroid injection is made just to one side of the extensor slip and above the collateral ligament. The joint is always more distal than anticipated.

dure the joint can extend fully and flex normally.

The position selected for arthrodesis must be carefully determined preoperatively and should allow functional grasp and pinch while at the same time placing the finger in enough extension to permit the hand to be inserted into a glove, pocket, or purse. Slightly more flexion is needed ulnarward in each of the PIP joints. Alternatively, implant arthroplasties may be recommended in the long and ring fingers if the extensor mechanism can be restored to the joint. This procedure provides greater flexibility in grasp while retaining functional power. The collateral ligaments must be preserved to prevent angular instability. The index and little fingers, however, are not candidates for implant arthroplasty. The index finger is a major apposing digit for the thumb in pinch. The torque forces generated during normal pinch are sufficiently great that the implant, even with the collateral ligaments retained, is unable to provide satisfactory lateral resistance for this function. A stable PIP joint is necessary for satisfactory pinch. Similarly, the little finger is important in normal power grasp. An implant in the PIP joint does not provide sufficient stability in the grasp mode. Therefore, arthrodesis is recommended.[2]

Surgical correction of the flexible swan-neck deformity is best accomplished through one of three procedures. Each provides a tendinous tether holding the PIP joint in slight flexion and thereby preventing the lateral interosseous bands from moving above the center of rotation of the joint. The first procedure is the lateral retinacular ligament reconstruction.[13] In this procedure, a small limb of the lateral interosseous band is developed (Fig 11–19, A–C) and passed beneath Grayson's ligament into the area of the flexor tendon sheaths. The small tendon is then passed through a small incision in the A-2 pulley. The tendon is tightened so that the PIP joint is maintained in 20 degrees of flexion. The tendon is then sutured to itself, producing a permanent tether. This device will allow normal flexion but will limit PIP joint flexion to no more than 20 degrees.

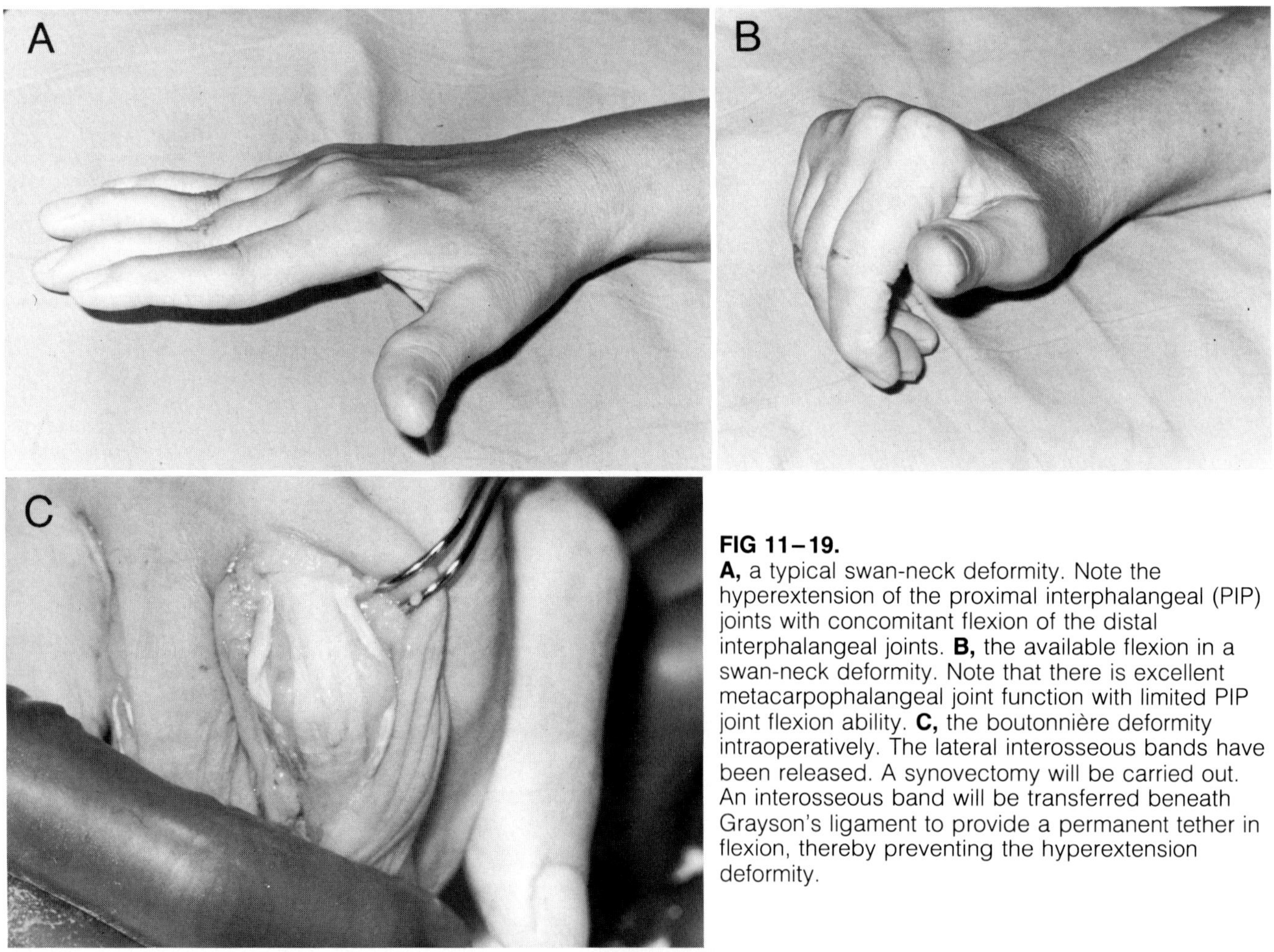

FIG 11–19.
A, a typical swan-neck deformity. Note the hyperextension of the proximal interphalangeal (PIP) joints with concomitant flexion of the distal interphalangeal joints. **B,** the available flexion in a swan-neck deformity. Note that there is excellent metacarpophalangeal joint function with limited PIP joint flexion ability. **C,** the boutonnière deformity intraoperatively. The lateral interosseous bands have been released. A synovectomy will be carried out. An interosseous band will be transferred beneath Grayson's ligament to provide a permanent tether in flexion, thereby preventing the hyperextension deformity.

The joint then is pinned in the correct position for 4 weeks. The pin prevents accidental extension of the joint which would disrupt the sutures in the tether.

Another method of swan-neck correction involves transfer of one of the two tendinous insertions of the flexor digitorum superficialis. A direct volar approach is used. The neurovascular bundles are carefully protected and the two slips of the flexor digitorum superficialis insertion are identified. One of the slips is divided proximally, approximately 1 in. or more from its normal insertion into the base of the proximal phalanx. It is then sutured into the A-2 flexor tendon pulley. The tendon is passed through a substantial portion of the pulley and sutured back onto itself with the finger held in approximately 20 degrees of flexion. A pin is placed across the PIP joint to prevent inadvertent extension of the digit and disruption of the tendon repair. These methods of swan-neck deformity correction have produced lasting correction with good retained flexor power and digital flexibility.

A third method of correction is unusual and effective. Frequently, following MP joint implant surgery, there will be residual stiffened swan-neck deformities or deficiencies in PIP joint flexion. In this situation, the joint may be carefully manipulated into 40 degrees of flexion and then longitudinally pinned from the dorsum of the proximal phalanx to the middle phalanx. The ligaments will stretch. The condyles may undergo a compression fracture that allows improved flexion. The collateral ligaments will maintain the normal alignment of the PIP joint. The pin is removed at 3 weeks and active flexion exercises are initiated. This regimen results in improved grasp, especially when combined with implant arthroplasty of the MP joint.

If the PIP joint is ankylosed in hyperextension, corrective osteotomy is the procedure of choice.[2] The precise angle or position for arthrodesis, as with the boutonnière deformity, must be carefully determined. It will depend on the overall size of the digit as well as the motion available at the MP and distal interphalangeal joints. A functional grasp and alignment for pinch are the goals. The fingers must be able to be flexed to bring the finger tips to within 4 cm of the palm.

VOLAR AND DIGITAL SYNOVITIS

Synovitis of the radial and ulnar bursae and the synovium within the fingers produces substantial hand disabilities.[5] These may be in the form of reduced median nerve function but are more commonly manifested by a reduction in digital flexion and extension. The radial and ulnar bursae and digital synovium allow for efficient gliding of the nine flexor tendons within hand. Rheumatoid or inflammatory arthritis may involve the synovium directly or may produce nodules within the synovium. The synovitis usually involves the palmar bursae; alternatively, the flexor tendons within the fingers may be affected. The synovitis may obstruct normal motion beneath the digital pulleys. At times, nodules will form that become trapped on one side or the other of the digital pulleys.

The initial therapeutic measures include steroid instillations into the ulnar and radial bursae and into the tendon sheaths of the fingers. Caution must always be taken to avoid the median nerve. A chemical neuritis may arise if the perineurium of the median nerve is violated. Should the needle penetrate the nerve the patient will complain of immediate paresthesias and the needle can be withdrawn. Should surgical therapy be required, it is important to determine the precise location of the obstructing proliferative synovitis. Digital synovitis can easily be ascertained by palpating the tendon sheath and then passively flexing and extending the finger. The synovial mass can be felt beneath the finger tip, in the palm, and in the finger itself.

It may be necessary to carry out a digital synovectomy in conjunction with an MP implant arthroplasty. Certainly, the MP implant cannot be expected to function properly if synovium is trapping the flexor tendons of the fingers. In this situation the palmar synovectomy is carried out with a transverse incision just proximal to the A-1 pulleys. The neurovascular structures are identified and a proximal digital synovectomy is performed. The finger should passively flex and extend smoothly at the completion of the procedure. The MP implant arthroplasty can then be carried out.

Volar synovectomy must be complete if it is to be effective (Fig 11–20,A). The entire ulnar and radial bursae must be excised with minimal trauma to the accompanying flexor tendons (Fig 11–20,B). The median nerve must be decompressed (Fig 11–20,D). Not only must the synovium be removed from the tendon but the parietal synovia throughout the carpal tunnel must be removed (Fig 11–20,C and D). If necessary, an additional incision must be made to remove synovium from the digital tendon sheaths. Nodules must be excised and tendon ruptures repaired (Fig 11–20,D). The entire visceral and parietal

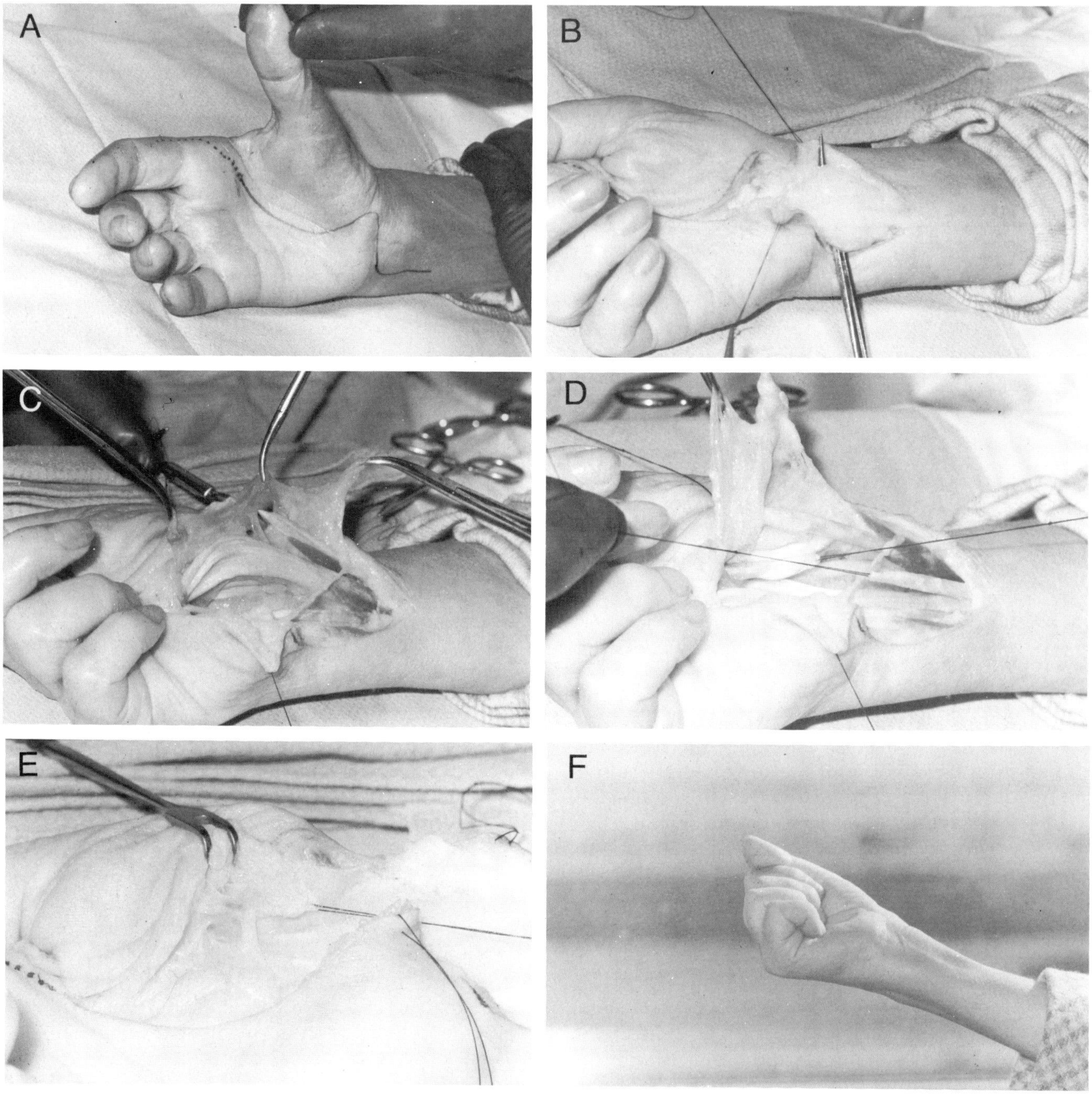

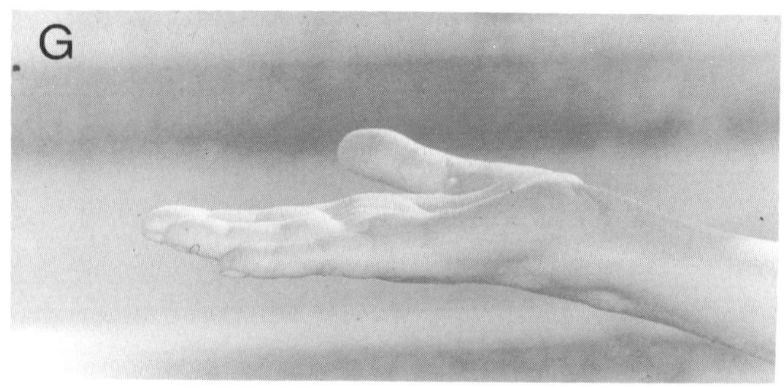

FIG 11–20.
A, the incision for palmar synovectomy. Note that the proximal midincision does not pass over the palmar cutaneous branch of the median nerve. The incision also can be carried out along the midlateral border of the index finger if this is the only digital sheath involved. When the other digital sheaths are involved, a transverse incision just distal to the midpalmar crease and over the A-1 pulleys is recommended. **B,** the large synovial mass surrounding and engulfing the flexor tendons. The median nerve and flexor tendons must be carefully dissected away from this inflammatory synovial mass. **C,** the flexor tendons. Note the flexor pollicis longus in the background. **D,** a ruptured flexor digitorum superficialis tendon. Owing to the good condition of the tendon, it could be repaired. **E,** the recurrent branch of the median nerve as it passes around the flexor retinaculum. A proliferative synovitis surrounds the nerve as well as the nearby flexor tendons. Careful synovectomy of the tendons and nerve was required. **F,** flexion following synovectomy and tendon repair. Early motion is essential to allow individual tendon function following surgery. **G,** extension following volar synovectomy.

synovium must be removed from the carpal canal.

Of considerable importance in volar synovectomy is the postoperative dressing. It is recommended that the fingers be placed in nearly full flexion rather than in their functional position. In this position, the flexor tendons will have retracted maximally into the forearm. On the fourth postoperative day the fingers are brought passively into full extension. At this point, the immature adhesions will be disrupted and the tendons may move freely. There is usually enough postoperative edema to provide some lubrication. The patient is allowed to fully extend and fully flex the fingers. Usually, this is done with the aid of an occupational therapist. Dynamic flexion-extension splints may be helpful. The early results of volar and digital synovectomy were disappointing because the hands were splinted in the position of function and intertendinous adhesions developed. The technique of early manipulation and active motion has resulted in excellent results with little recurrence (Fig 11–20,E,F).

CAVEATS IN SURGERY OF THE RHEUMATOID HAND

It must be recalled that rheumatoid arthritis involving the hand is a global physiologic problem. The hand is a visible structure and often the patient will seek a more cosmetically acceptable hand rather than a more functional hand. Certainly, cosmesis is important to these disabled patients. However, if they are expecting dramatic increases in overall function with restoration to full function, they will be disappointed. Surgery on a musician's hand is always problematic. In this case it is necessary to see the patient use his or her instrument to determine precisely what can be accomplished through surgical therapy. Expectations can be discussed and revised at the same time. Whereas removal of rheumatoid nodules is always appreciated, stiff fingers resulting from arthrodesis may be disturbing to the patient, even though power and function are improved.

It is also essential to have a full assessment of the entire upper extremity before hand surgery is recommended. Frequently, the hand operation will precede elbow and shoulder surgery. In most instances, corrective wrist surgery precedes hand surgery. This can be complicated, particularly when the wrist is painless, yet deformed and contributing to digital deformities. In general, the painful or most disabling problems should be given priority.

CONCLUSIONS

Careful study and planning is required in the management of rheumatoid disease in the hand. It is desirable to obtain as much information through rheumatological and occupational therapeutic consultations as possible. Alterations in drug therapy programs along with steroid instillation may be all that is required to reduce pain and disability. Hand therapists, after a comprehensive functional study, may have suggestions about splints and asssistive devices for use in the activities of daily living. A formulated plan of needs and priorities should be developed and discussed with the patient if surgical therapy is required. Goals should be modest to avoid disappointment. Rarely is strength increased, while grasp, release, and pinch are the rule. Although the patient rarely requests an improvement in appearance, the usual improved cosmetic result is graciously appreciated. The availability or regional anesthesia and infection control, even in immuniocompremised patients, allows the surgeon some latitude in the planning of surgical procedures unless there is the potential of vascular compromise. Medical technology has made available improved hand function in patients with disabling inflammatory arthritis.

REFERENCES

1. Burton RI: Basal joint arthrosis of the thumb. *Orthop Clin North Am* 1973; 4:331–348.
2. Carroll RE, Hill NA: Small joint arthrodesis in hand reconstruction. *J Bone Joint Surg [Am]* 1969; 51:1219.
3. Clayton ML: Surgery of the thumb in rheumatoid arthritis. *J Bone Joint Surg [Am]* 1962; 44A:1376–1386.
4. Eaton RG: Replacement of the trapezium for arthritis of the basal articulations. *J Bone Joint Surg [Am]* 1979; 61:76–82.
5. Ferlic DA, Clayton ML: Flexor tenosynovectomy in the rheumatoid finger. *J Hand Surg* 1978; 3:364–367.
6. Flatt AE: The pathomechanics of ulnar drift. Final report. Social and Rehabilitation Services Grant no. RD2226M, 1971.
7. Gerivs WH: A review of excision of the trapezium for osteoarthritis of the trapezio-metacarpal joint after twenty five years. *J Bone Joint Surg [Br]* 1973; 55B:56–57.
8. Goldner JL, Clippinger FW: Excision of the greater multiangular bone as an adjunct to mobilization of the thumb. *J Bone Joint Surg [Am]* 1959; 41:609.
9. Inglis AE, Hamlin C, Sengelmann RP, et al: Reconstruction of the metacarpophalangeal joint of the

thumb in rheumatoid arthritis. *J Bone Joint Surg [Am]* 1972; 54:704–712.

10. Jackson IT, Paton KC: The extended approach to flexor tendon synovitis in rheumatoid arthritis. *Br J Plast Surg* 1973; 26:122–131.
11. Kessler I: Silicone arthroplasty of the trapeziometacarpal joint. *J Bone Joint Surg [Br]* 1973; 55B:285–291.
12. Landsmeer JMF: Anatomical and functional investigations on the articulation of the human fingers. *Acta Anat (Basel)* 1955; 25(suppl 24):5–69.
13. Littler JW: Restoration of the oblique retinacular ligament for correction of hyperextension deformity of the proximal interphalangeal joint, in Fourniee A (ed): *La main rhumatismale.* Paris, Expansion Scientifique Française, 1966, p 471.
14. Millender LH, Nalebuff EA: Preventative surgery—tenosynovectomy and synovectomy. *Orthop Clin North Am* 1975; 6:765–792.
15. Millender LH, Nalebuff EA, Amadio P, et al: Interpositional arthroplasty for rheumatoid carpometacarpal joint disease. *J Hand Surg* 1978; 6:533–541.
16. Moberg E: Arthrodesis of finger joints. *Surg Clin North Am* 1960; 40:465–470.
17. Nalebuff EA, Millender LH: Surgical treatment of the boutonnière deformity in rheumatoid arthritis. *Orthop Clin North Am* 1975; 6:753.
18. Paul WD: Systemic manifestations of rheumatoid arthritis (rheumatoid disease) accentuated by steroid therapy. *J Iowa Med Soc* 1961; 51:205–216.
19. Smith RJ, Kaplan EB: Rheumatoid deformities at the metacarpophalangeal joints of the fingers. A correlative study of anatomy and pathology. *J Bone Joint Surg [Am]* 1967; 49:31.
20. Stack HG, Vaughan-Jackson OJ: The zig-zag deformity in the rheumatoid hand. *Hand* 1971; 3:62.
21. Straub LR: The etiology of finger deformities in the hand affected by rheumatoid arthritis. *Bull Hosp Joint Dis* 1960; 21:322–329.
22. Straub LR, Wilson EH: Spontaneous rupture of extensor tendons in the hand associated with rheumatoid arthritis. *J Bone Joint Surg [Am]* 1956; 38:1208.
23. Swanson AB: Silicone rubber implants for replacement for arthritis or destroyed joints in the hand. *Surg Clin North Am* 1968; 48:1113.
24. Swanson AB: Flexible implant arthroplasty for arthritic finger joints. Rationale, technique and results of treatment. *J Bone Joint Surg [Am]* 1972; 54:435.
25. Swanson AB, Herndon JH: Flexible (silicone) implant arthroplasty of the metacarpophalangeal joint of the thumb. *J Bone Joint Surg [Am]* 1977; 59:362–368.
26. Vaughan-Jackson OJ: Attrition ruptures of tendons as a factor in the production of deformities in the rheumatoid hand. *Proc R Soc Med* 1959; 52:132–134.
27. Zancolli E: *Structural and Dynamic Bases of Hand Surgery.* Philadelphia, JB Lippincott Co, 1968, p 139.

CHAPTER 12

The Hip

Michael J. Maynard, M.D.

Chitranjan S. Ranawat, M.D.

William F. Flynn, Jr., M.D.

INTRODUCTION

Since the introduction of the "low friction arthroplasty" by Sir John Charnley in the early 1960s,[11] the surgical treatment of inflammatory arthritis has advanced rapidly. The widespread adoption, investigation, and adaptation of Charnley's low friction principles have fostered rapid advancement of bioengineering technology and vastly improved our understanding of the biomechanical principles germane to joint reconstruction. Patients with rheumatoid arthritis have gained particular benefit from this revolution in surgical therapy as its application has expanded to include the hip, knee, shoulder, elbow, wrist, and other joints. Total hip arthroplasty (THA) has improved over the course of myriad evolutionary changes to become a surgical procedure with relatively broad indications and highly predictable, durable success.

Severe coxarthrosis, of a degree sufficient to indicate surgical intervention, may derive from a wide range of etiologies summarized below.

I. Degenerative disease.
   A. Osteoarthritis.
   B. Posttraumatic arthritis.
   C. Avascular necrosis (AVN).
   D. Structural derangement, e.g., congenital dysplasia of the hip (CDH), Legg-Calvé-Perthes disease (LCP), Charcot's joint, and slipped capital femoral epiphysis (SCFE).

II. Inflammatory arthritis.
   A. Rheumatoid arthritis (RA).
   B. Juvenile rheumatoid arthritis (JRA, Still's disease).
   C. Seronegative spondyloarthropathy, e.g., ankylosing spondylitis, psoriatic arthropathy.
   D. Crystalline arthropathy (gout, calcium pyrophosphate deposition [CPPD]).
   E. Infectious arthritis.

III. Connective tissue disease.
   A. Systemic lupus erythematosus (SLE).
   B. Mixed connective tissue disease.

IV. Endocrine, metabolic, miscellaneous.
   A. Ochronosis.
   B. Hemochromatosis.
   C. Pigmented villonodular synovitis (PVNS).
   D. Acromegaly.

The discussion that follows focuses primarily on issues related to the surgical treatment of *rheumatoid arthritis* as it relates to involvement of the hip joint. The clincial and radiographic presentation, indications for surgery, medical and surgical planning considerations, and surgical techniques are discussed. Rehabilitation, complications, long-term results, and future directions are also discussed.

RHEUMATOID ARTHRITIS

Symptomatic involvement of one or both hips requiring surgical therapy has been reported to occur in 10% to 20% of patients with an established diagnosis of RA.[26, 32, 46] However, a direct correlation between clinical findings and radiographic evidence of hip abnormalities has been universally lacking. Irrefutable evidence of arthritic involvement may appear on hip radiographs of RA patients whose clinical examination remains normal. The converse of this situation also often appears early in the course of the rheumatoid disease process when synovitis may cause severe hip pain and functional disability in the complete absence of any demonstrable radiographic changes. This variability of the presentation and clinical course of the disease observed among patients underscores an important point to remember—that destruction of the hip eventually requiring surgical relief should not be viewed as an inevitable event in the natural history of RA. Appropriate management of anti-inflammatory medicines, physical therapy, activity level, ambulatory aids, and nutrition can, in fact, successfully avoid or delay the need for hip surgery in many patients.

JUVENILE RHEUMATOID ARTHRITIS

The term *juvenile rheumatoid arthritis* or *JRA* encompasses several different disease entities, or subtypes, which vary considerably in their initial presentation, clinical course, and ultimate prognosis. Overall, up to 10% of children diagnosed as having JRA will develop significant functional disability related to the hip.[57] However, in those patients presenting with the polyarthritis subtype of the disease, approximately 50% will develop hip involvement that results in destruction of the joint.[10]

Early identification of those JRA patients with a pathologic condition of the hip is crucial. The majority of these patients are skeletally immature and, left untreated, may rapidly develop severe soft tissue contractures. If diagnosed early, physical therapy, occasionally augmented by surgical soft tissue release, can successfully delay or avoid THA. However, if significant contractures go untreated and are allowed to exert a persistent effect on an immature skeleton, severe bony deformity or ankylosis, or both, inevitably result (Fig 12–1). Increasing bony deformity correlates directly with increasing surgical technical difficulty and may, in and of itself, mandate surgical intervention at an extremely young age in the interest of preserving some chance of surgical success. This worst-cast scenario—when joint implant arthroplasty becomes the only option for maintaining or regaining ambulatory capability in a young child—represents a clinical catastrophe since the prospects for growth disturbance and eventual failure of an arthroplasty implanted in a child are significant.

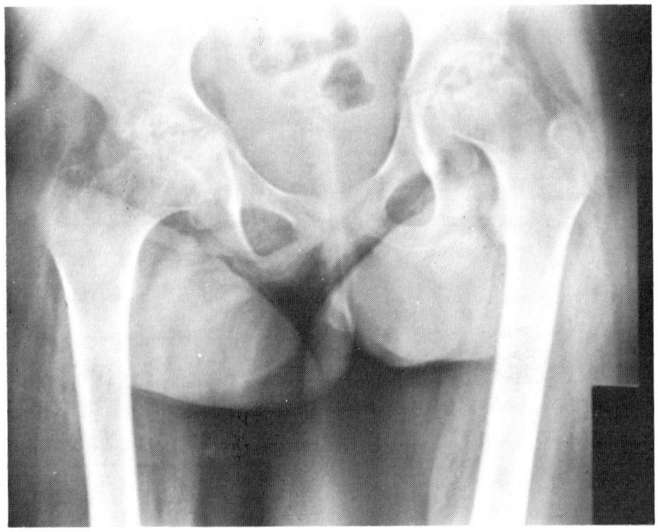

FIG 12–1.
Severe hip involvement in a patient with juvenile rheumatoid arthritis. The triradiate cartilages and capital femoral epiphyses are still open.

There are several considerations, unique to the treatment of arthritic children, which the treating surgeon must take into account. In particular, motivation and related psychosocial issues are important with respect to the ultimate functional outcome of young arthritis patients and must be considered in any therapeutic plan.[57] In addition, hip reconstruction in these patients nearly always presents significant surgical technical difficulties.

OTHER INFLAMMATORY ARTHRITIDES

Patients with a diagnosis of ankylosing spondylitis can demonstrate a 50% prevalence of clinically significant hip arthritis.[8] Greater than 50% of those affected have bilateral involvement.[29, 66] Bony deformities commonly seen radiographically in association with ankylosing spondylitis include protrusion deformities and complete ankylosis. Heterotopic ossification of the soft tissues about the hip occurs frequently after surgery and prophylaxis is therefore indicated in these patients.[8, 42, 52]

Psoriasis gives rise in 10% of patients to hip arthritis. This has been reported to be as high as 40% in patients with juvenile onset.[33, 58] THA should be considered for these patients if pain and functional disability become severe despite appropriate medical management. Patients suffering from Reiter's disease, Crohn's disease, and ulcerative colitis also occasionally present with associated hip arthritis. Hip involvement of a severity requiring arthroplasty is uncommon but not unknown.

Gout and CPPD, (pseudogout) may cause hip arthritis. Joint space narrowing and subchondral cysts are seen radiographically and, in severe cases, joint arthroplasty may be indicated. The metabolic stress of surgery has been known to precipitate an acute flare-up in patients with gout or pseudogout.

SLE and mixed connective tissue disease may rarely present with direct involvement of the hip joint. More commonly, the hip changes seen in association with these disorders are secondary to the use of high-dose corticosteroids in the control of the primary disease. In some patients, this leads to osteonecrosis of the femoral head, subsequent femoral head collapse, and consequent painful arthritis of the hip joint. Osteoporosis, and osteoarthritic changes, including joint space narrowing and osteophyte formation, are seen radiographically late in the disease process.

Ochronosis, hemochromatosis, PVNS, and acromegaly can cause destruction of the hip joint. Though the discussion of these diseases is often grouped—as it is here—with a discussion of the inflammatory arthritides, the radiographic presentation of the hip changes in these diseases is often more similar to that seen in osteoarthritis. In ochronosis, a metabolic defect causes homogentisic acid to accumulate in the synovium and cartilage. Destruction of joint surfaces and a characteristic black staining are seen clinically. Hemochromatosis, another genetically determined metabolic disease, occasionally leads to deposition of iron in the synovium accompanied by deposition of calcium pyrophosphate in the articular cartilage—eventually causing destruction of the joint surfaces. The pathologic process seen in PVNS involves synovial pigmentation and hypertrophy of unknown cause. Cartilage destruction, joint space narrowing, and cyst formation can be detected radiographically. Acromegaly, an endocrine disorder characterized by an excess of growth hormone, involves the joints through hypertrophy, degeneration, and regeneration of cartilage and bone. Osteophytic changes are usually prominent and the large size of the bones may require the fabrication of custom oversized tools and implants for an appropriate prosthetic reconstruction.

CLINICAL AND RADIOGRAPHIC FEATURES OF RHEUMATOID ARTHRITIS

Significant rheumatoid involvement of the hip may present with a variety of symptoms including pain, tenderness, gait disturbance, decreased range of motion (soft tissue contractures), synovitis, and bursitis. Leg length discrepancy may be present secondary to asymmetric soft tissue contractures or asymmetric migration of the femoral heads during the formation of pelvic protrusion deformities. Adult patients usually present with pain that is aggravated by walking and weightbearing, typically in the groin, as their chief complaint. The pain may persist at rest and may be present at night. Decreasing functional range of motion is commonly only a secondary complaint.

By contrast, JRA patients seldom complain of hip pain, but rather control their pain, over time, by decreasing voluntary motion.[57] As a result, they often develop a pronounced limp and advanced hip flexion and adduction contractures. Compensatory lumbar hyperlordosis and even scoliosis may appear. A resultant course of progressively diminishing ambulation is the late symptom which often precipitates referral to the orthopaedic surgeon.

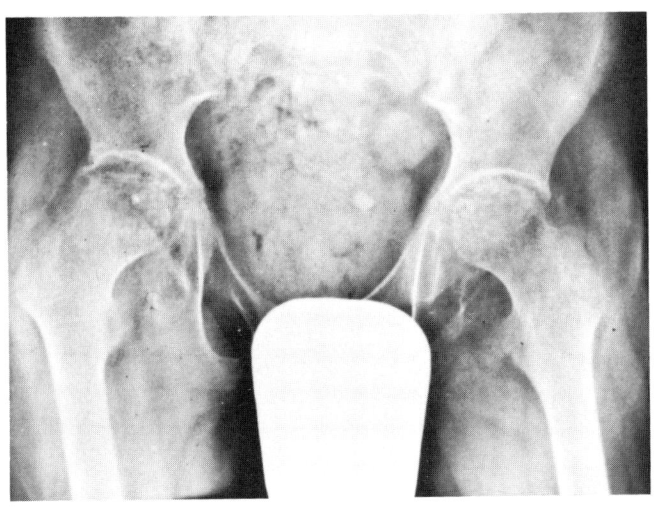

FIG 12–2.
A 25-year-old woman with juvenile rheumatoid arthritis. Note marked periarticular osteopenia and erosive joint disease.

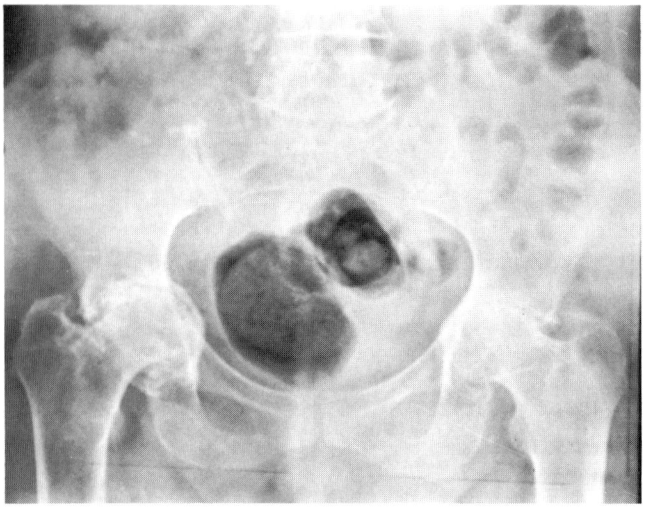

FIG 12–3.
The hip on the left has developed a severe protrusion deformity secondary to rheumatoid arthritis.

Radiographs of hips affected by RA reveal osteopenic bone in the majority of patients (Fig 12–2). Loss of joint space due to destruction of the articular cartilage is common. Osteophyte formation is uncommon. Protrusion deformity may be present in up to 30% of patients. The appearance of this deformity represents significant bone loss in the pelvis and presents difficult technical problems to the operating surgeon (Figs 12–3 and 12–4). Cyst formation, also signifying bone destruction, may also be apparent. As alluded to previously, patients who have received corticosteroid therapy may demonstrate signs consistent with AVN and consequent collapse of the femoral head[46] (Fig 12–5,A and B).

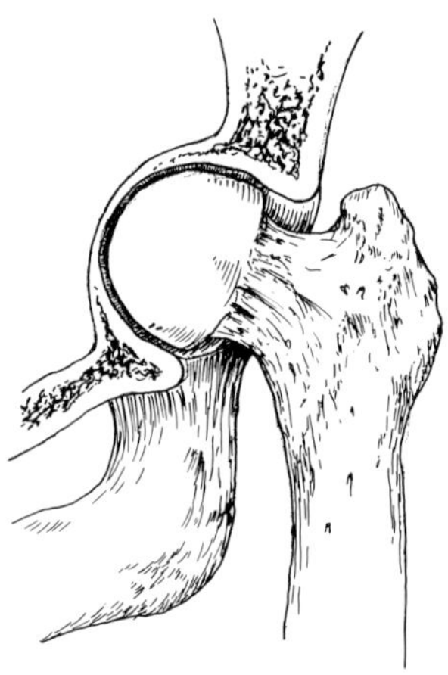

FIG 12–4.
Migration of the femoral head during protrusion deformity. The mechanism underlying the progressive deformity is thought to be a weakening of the bone of the acetabular wall secondary to osteoporosis caused by the inflammatory process active in rheumatoid arthritis.

SURGICAL INDICATIONS

Over the years, various surgical techniques have been advocated in the treatment of the rheumatoid hip. Some of the most commonly performed operative procedures are:

I. Synovectomy.
II. Soft tissue release.
III. Fusion.
IV. Girdlestone resection.
V. Arthroplasties.
  A. Cup.
  B. Femoral endoprosthesis.
    1. Unipolar.
    2. Bipolar.
  C. Surface replacement.
  D. Total hip replacement.
VI. Revision surgery.

Synovectomy

Open hip synovectomy has narrow indications and significant risks. Control of fulminant synovitis that is unresponsive to medical therapy, in the setting of absent or minimal damage to the articular cartilage, is the only indication for which synovectomy of the hip might reasonably be considered.[57, 63] The procedure requires extensive surgical exposure of the hip and carries with it the danger of disruption of the blood supply to the femoral head—causing AVN—especially if the hip is dislocated as part of the procedure. Theoretically, arthroscopic synovectomy might be an attractive alternative to open synovectomy, but the effectiveness of this approach has yet to be fully evaluated. Reported results of open synovectomy have been discouraging[1] and the juxtaposed encouraging results of arthroplasty have caused synovectomy to be largely abandoned in the recent past.

Soft Tissue Release

Classically, the natural history of the untreated RA hip, in both the juvenile and adult forms, inexorably leads to the development of soft tissue contractures in flexion and adduction. Lumbar hyperlordosis,

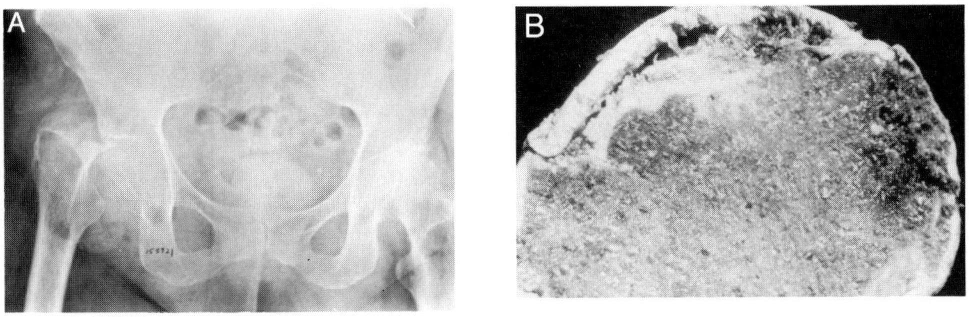

FIG 12–5.
A, marked osteonecrosis with dissolution of the femoral head and hip fracture-dislocation. **B,** gross specimen of subchondral collapse in an osteonecrotic femoral head in a patient with rheumatoid arthritis treated with corticosteroids.

scoliosis, knee flexion contracture, pelvic tilt, and apparent limb-length inequality may also appear as direct clinical sequelae. In the juvenile, these contractures may develop long before any significant intraarticular damage to the involved hip has occurred. In the adult, however, the vast majority will have preexisting associated articular pathologic changes.

In the absence of intraarticular damage, soft tissue release as an isolated surgical procedure may be indicated. This situation most often presents itself in the JRA patient where it may be used as an adjunct to an aggressive physical therapy program aimed at preserving joint motion and postponing or avoiding total joint arthroplasty. Absolute prerequisites are: (1) the absence of intraarticular abnormalities on clinical and radiographic examination, and (2) the absence of acute synovitis. The presence of either of these will severely compromise the postoperative rehabilitation and effectively negate the benefits of the surgery.

Adduction contracture release can often be performed percutaneously by selective tenotomy of the adductors near their pelvic origins—as is commonly performed in the treatment of patients with cerebral palsy. Hip flexion contracture release often requires a more extensive open procedure to achieve an adequate result. A course of aggressive postoperative physical therapy to maintain the motion gained at surgery is indispensable if this treatment is to succeed.

The performance of soft tissue release is most often required in the achievement of appropriate joint motion and limb length during THA. Familiarity with the performance of soft tissue release appropriate to the correction of each type of contracture is essential if the procedure is to be successful.

Osteotomy

Osteotomy has a limited role in the treatment of joints with early changes due to RA and is most often applicable to the JRA population. It can be considered as an option in a patient who develops excessive femoral anteversion, valgus, or subluxation and secondary hip dysplasia. In order for osteotomy to achieve a successful outcome, active hip synovitis must be absent and there must be preservation of the articular surfaces which are to be loaded after the mechanical rearrangement effected by the osteotomy. Unfortunately, healthy articular cartilage is rarely available since rheumatoid involvement of the hip is usually global. A drawback of osteotomy is the requirement for postoperative immobilization while the osteotomy heals—which may result in significant loss of joint motion. In the setting of active synovitis, this could even cause joint ankylosis. However, in appropriately selected and managed patients, osteotomy usually achieves excellent pain relief and may achieve excellent long-term functional results.[37]

Occasionally, a patient may present with an ankylosed hip where the limb position compromises function and personal hygiene. A simple repositioning osteotomy of the proximal femur may be of benefit to these patients.

Hip Fusion

This procedure has a place in the treatment of young, heavy, active laborers whose occupation requires them to be on their feet a significant proportion of the time. It is also an attractive option in the treatment of a primarily infected hip.

However, the polyarticular nature of RA presents a relative contraindication to the performance of a surgical hip fusion. This is because, even if not already present, one can expect a high associated incidence of eventual contralateral hip, lumbar or ipsilateral knee involvement. Any of these problems, alone or in combination, with an existing hip fusion would result in severe functional disability and would degrade the rehabilitation and long-term durability of contralateral or ipsilateral joint arthroplasty.

Girdlestone Resection

This procedure was originally described by Girdlestone[25] for the treatment of the chronically infected hip joint. The surprisingly good functional results obtained by this operation, which called for excision of the femoral head and neck and a portion of the acetabular margins followed by a period of traction and slowly progressive weightbearing, caused its use to flourish as a treatment for all types of hip arthritis—prior to the advent of modern hip arthroplasty.[63] The evolution of THA has contracted the relatively expanded indications enjoyed by the Girdlestone resection pseudarthrosis operation while, ironically, reestablishing it as a primary option for its original indication: the treatment of the chronically infected hip *(arthroplasty)*.

In the surgical management of patients with RA, a Girdlestone resection arthroplasty is most often indicated as a final salvage procedure after recurrent infections in a hip that has received multiple implantations, removals, and reimplantations of THAs. Occasionally, it may be used as a temporary measure for several months or years—during a period of observation and surveillance for infection—after removal and antibiotic treatment of an infected THA. Even in the absence of infection, a Girdlestone pseudarthrosis may be an attractive alternative if bone loss secondary to aseptic loosening of a THA makes reconstruction unlikely to succeed.

Arthroplasty

The earliest significant work in hip arthroplasty is generally credited to Smith-Petersen[61] who introduced his cup or mold arthroplasty in the 1920s. The next step in the evolution of hip arthroplasty, introduced by Moore[36] and others, consisted of unipolar and eventually bipolar femoral endoprosthesis designs—some of which are still in use. Sir John Charnley's low friction arthroplasty, consisting of a metallic femoral stem and polyethylene acetabular socket each fixed to bone with acrylic cement, provided the final major advance in the development of THA. Unipolar and bipolar femoral endoprostheses continue to be used by many surgeons in the treatment of hip fractures in elderly or sedentary patients who have an intact acetabular articular surface.

The introduction of surface replacement arthroplasty, a modification of THA that minimizes the amount of required bone resection while attempting to simply "resurface" the femoral head and acetabulum, enjoyed early popular support. However, long-term results have revealed that, compared to the performance of cemented total hip replacement arthroplasties in similar patients, its durability has been disappointing.[38, 53]

It is our opinion and experience that, of all available primary reconstructive procedures using an implanted prosthesis, cemented THA is currently the surgical alternative with the most predictably satisfactory long-term performance in hips afflicted with inflammatory arthritis.

The fundamental indication for THA in rheumatoid patients is severe pain or functional disability despite optimal medical management. This assumes that all other potential causes of hip pain, such as spine or other joint involvement, tumor, synovitis, and other soft tissue inflammation have been ruled out or are not amenable or responsive to nonsurgical therapy. In addition, there should be objective radiographic evidence of hip abnormalities.

Absolute contraindications include acute or chronic infection at any site and any medical condition which contraindicates anesthesia and surgery. Poor condition of the skin or vasculature of the involved extremity and previous sepsis in the involved joint are relative contraindications. Massive obesity and occupation requiring heavy labor are also relative contraindications but usually do not apply to the RA patient population.

Finally, the summary condition of the patient, including other joint involvement, motivation, personal expectations, and overall ability to comply with postoperative rehabilitation, should be taken into account. Patient, rheumatologist, and surgeon should all realize that the polyarticular nature of the disease may require the surgical treatment of several joints before any significant functional benefit is obtained. Furthermore, while pain relief is a consistently predictable outcome of joint replacement arthroplasty in RA, range of motion and overall functional improvement are much less so. Postoperative rehabilitation can be made difficult and may not achieve optimal results if met by an uncooperative patient. Therefore, it is important to enlist the help of nurses, psychologists, social workers, and physical and occupational therapists prior to any surgical intervention. This team approach, while particularly applicable to young patients, is beneficial for all patients with inflammatory arthritis. In cases where the patient's toleration of multiple planned procedures is in doubt, it may be prudent to perform a relatively simple procedure first, i.e., assess the patient's ability to comply with the required postoperative protocol, before proceeding with surgery, which entails more painful and arduous rehabilitation.[60]

MEDICAL CONSIDERATIONS

The patient with inflammatory arthritis poses unique problems to the physician coordinating perioperative management. For this reason every patient with any form of inflammatory arthritis should be managed perioperatively by a medical consultant familiar with these considerations.

The possibility of inflammatory involvement of chest, common in RA and ankylosing spondylitis, makes thorough preoperative assessment of each patient's cardiopulmonary status particularly crucial. This testing should be aimed at defining the preparatory and precautionary measures that may be warranted during anesthesia and recovery. Many of these patients present for surgery while on chronic corticosteroid therapy. These patients are therefore often adrenally suppressed and must receive appropriate additional doses of corticosteroids to meet the requirements imposed by the metabolic stress of surgery.

A thorough preoperative search for potential sources of bacteremia and infection is critically important. This must include, as a minimum, evaluation of the lungs, heart, skin, teeth and gums, and urinary tract. Patients with a history of gastrointestinal problems should be examined further for possible occult infection (e.g., gallbladder disease or diverticular abscess). Any preexisting source of infection must, of course, be eradicated prior to surgery. After surgical implantation of a prosthetic joint, periodic surveillance of potential sources of bacteremia should become part of routine medical management. Prophylactic antibiotics are mandatory prior to dental work and any invasive medical instrumentation (e.g., cystoscopy or colonoscopy) performed on these patients for the rest of their lives.

GENERAL SURGICAL CONSIDERATIONS

Surgical technical difficulties most often arise secondary to osteoporosis and bony deformity, especially protrusion, which lead to a decrease in the amount of good-quality bone available for the support of an implanted prosthesis. Significant osteoporosis is present in most hips affected by RA. Up to 40% of RA patients presenting for THA may demonstrate protrusion of the femoral head and medial wall of the acetabulum into the pelvis.[44] Some patients, those with JRA in particular, present with subluxation and acetabular dysplasia—clinically quite similar to the presentation of CDH. Coupled with severe deformity, the small bones seen in JRA patients often require the fabrication of custom implants and surgical tools.[7, 56] All of these considerations affect the choice of fixation and prosthetic implant, may lengthen the operative time, and may indicate the use of bone grafting or special prosthetic devices.[31, 35, 49, 51]

Soft tissue contractures are frequently present in the rheumatoid hip and usually require the performance of extensive soft tissue releases as mentioned earlier. If contractures are particularly severe, limb shortening may be necessary to achieve proper joint stability and motion.

Surgical Planning Considerations in Multiple Joint Involvement

Significant involvement of the cervical spine occurs in 30% to 40% of patients with RA.[45] Therefore, radiographic evaluation of the cervical spine for possible instability is mandatory prior to surgery. If cervical spine instability exists, it should be given first priority for surgical intervention. In addition to instability, deformity or loss of flexibility of the cervical spine is also commonly associated with RA, JRA, and ankylosing spondylitis. Additionally, patients with JRA may have temporomandibular joint involvement and micrognathia. These problems often mandate the use of special techniques, such as bronchoscopy-guided intubation or tracheostomy, if general anesthesia is to be induced.[56] To avoid the problems associated with these techniques, regional anesthesia is often the method of choice for the performance of lower extremity surgery in patients with RA.[57]

Many patients have significant involvement of both upper and lower extremity joints. If practical, surgical intervention should first address the lower extremities to avoid the weightbearing demands of lower extremity rehabilitation upon upper extremity arthroplasties. However, this requires that the patient's upper extremities be functional enough to assist weightbearing during lower extremity rehabilitation using canes, crutches, or walkers. If this is not the case, upper extremity arthroplasty may be required prior to lower extremity arthroplasty in order to achieve the ability to use the ambulatory aids required for lower extremity rehabilitation.

Lower extremity operative planning must take the status of both hips, both knees, both ankles, and both feet into account (Fig 12–6). First priority should be given to insuring that the feet and ankles are stable and plantigrade and without areas of skin breakdown or impending breakdown which could present a potential source of infection. Once the feet and ankles are satisfactory, the hips and knees may be addressed.

In a patient with ipsilateral hip and knee involvement, the hip operation should be performed first unless there is such severe flexion deformity or instability of the knee that it would effectively preclude ambulation and adequate rehabilitation of the hip. This order of priority derives from the fact that hip rehabilitation generally requires less functional range of motion at the ipsilateral knee than knee rehabilitation requires at the ipsilateral hip. If both hips or both knees, or both hips and both knees, are involved, bilateral hip or knee arthroplasties can be carried out at a single operative setting if the patient's medical status allows this.[46]

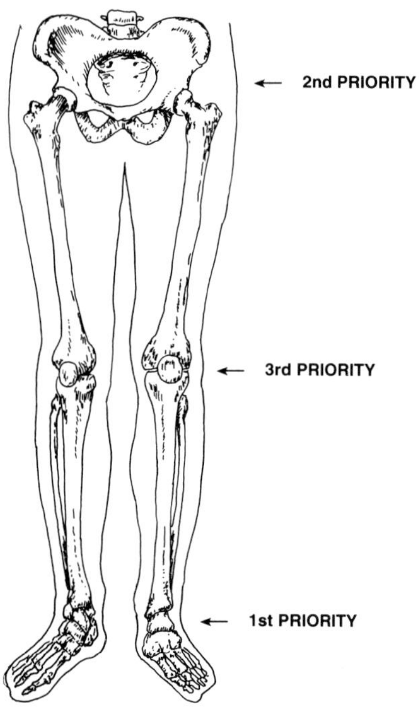

FIG 12–6.
Rheumatoid arthritis often involves multiple lower extremity joints. In a patient with multiple symptomatic joints in the ipsilateral limb, first priority should be given to achieving a stable, plantigrade foot and ankle. Second priority is given to the hip. Third priority is given to the knee.

SURGICAL PROCEDURE

Long-Range Preparation

Proper surgical technique begins with appropriate preparation. Good-quality radiographs, standardized to allow accurate estimation of magnification and templating, are the first necessity. Scrutiny of these films should seek to answer three questions:

1. Can reconstruction be performed using available off-the-shelf prostheses, or should ordering of a specially sized, modified, or custom-made implant and associated bone-working tools be considered?
2. Is there a significant superior or medial protrusion deformity, and will bone grafting be required to make up for bone loss in order to restore the hip center of motion to the proper position?
3. Is cemented or noncemented fixation likely to be the optimal choice for best long-term performance?

To answer the first question, templates of the intended implant system must be available for comparison with the radiographs (templating). JRA patients, with their small bone size and frequent anteversion, valgus, and protrusion deformities, and acromegaly patients, with their large bone size, are the most likely patient groups to require fabrication of custom implants, or modification of existing implants, in order to achieve proper prosthetic fit. If a custom implant is indicated, computed tomography (CT) scanning of the hip joints and proximal half of the femora is required to provide the detailed anatomic information.

Several reports have described methods for the radiographic evaluation of protrusion.[28, 35, 49, 51, 62] The primary significance of the magnitude of a protrusion deformity is that it reflects the amount of bone loss in the direction of the protrusion. This bone loss must either be replaced with bone graft or effectively offset by the prosthetic implants in order to achieve a successful reconstruction. The movement of the center of rotation of the joint off of the proper anatomic position, as takes place in progressive protrusion, also disrupts the balance of the muscle forces across the hip joint by changing their directions of pull and the lengths of their arms. Over time, this leads to the development of soft tissue contractures. These contractures must be ameliorated during joint reconstruction in order to achieve restoration of the center of rotation to the proper position and restore muscle balance.

Our preferred method of locating the proper anatomic position of the acetabulum has been described in detail elsewhere[49] (Fig 12–7). It can be summarized as follows: On an anteroposterior (AP) radiograph of the pelvis one starts by drawing two parallel, horizontal lines—the upper one crossing the tops of the iliac crests and the lower one crossing the bottoms of the ischial tuberosities. Next, a vertical line is drawn, crossing perpendicular to the first two lines, and passing through a point designated *A* located 5 mm lateral to the intersection of Köhler's and Shenton's lines. Next, a point designated *B* is also located on the vertical line, superior to point *A* at a distance equal to one fifth of the overall length of the vertical line between the two horizontal lines. Now a third horizontal line, of length equal to the distance *AB*, is erected laterally and perpendicularly from point *B*. The lateral end of this line is designated point *C*. The true acetabulum lies within the isosceles triangle defined by points *A, B,* and *C*. Retrospective analysis of reconstructed protrusion deformities has demonstrated that reconstructions that placed the center of rotation within 5 mm of the anatomic position located in this manner had significantly better long-term durability compared with those placed 10 mm or more from this position.[49]

Once the surgeon has located the proper anatomic position of the acetabulum, its relationship to the actual bony acetabular limits will help define the technical requirements for acetabular reconstruction. If there is medial protrusion, a medial bone graft will likely be indicated in all but the mildest cases (Fig 12–8). Small to moderate amounts of superior bone loss can often be treated by surgically opening the mouth of the acetabulum and using a larger prosthesis. In cases where superior migration has enlarged the acetabulum by more than 15% to 20%, as estimated on the AP view, bone grafting will be required (Fig 12–9). The best sources of bone graft, if available, are the resected femoral head and neck, and the iliac crest. Otherwise, femoral head allografting may be necessary and should be anticipated. Depending on the shape of the defect, the type and shape of the graft, and the quality and quantity of the supporting pelvic bone, fixation of the graft may be by interference fit, or with screws. In some cases, the use of a protrusion ring may also be beneficial. The surgeon treating a large protrusion deformity should be familiar with the preparation and fixation of bone grafts and the use of protrusion rings and should have these devices available in the operating suite.

The question of whether to use cemented or noncemented fixation involves the assessment of several variables including the patient's age and remaining life expectancy, activity level, bony defor-

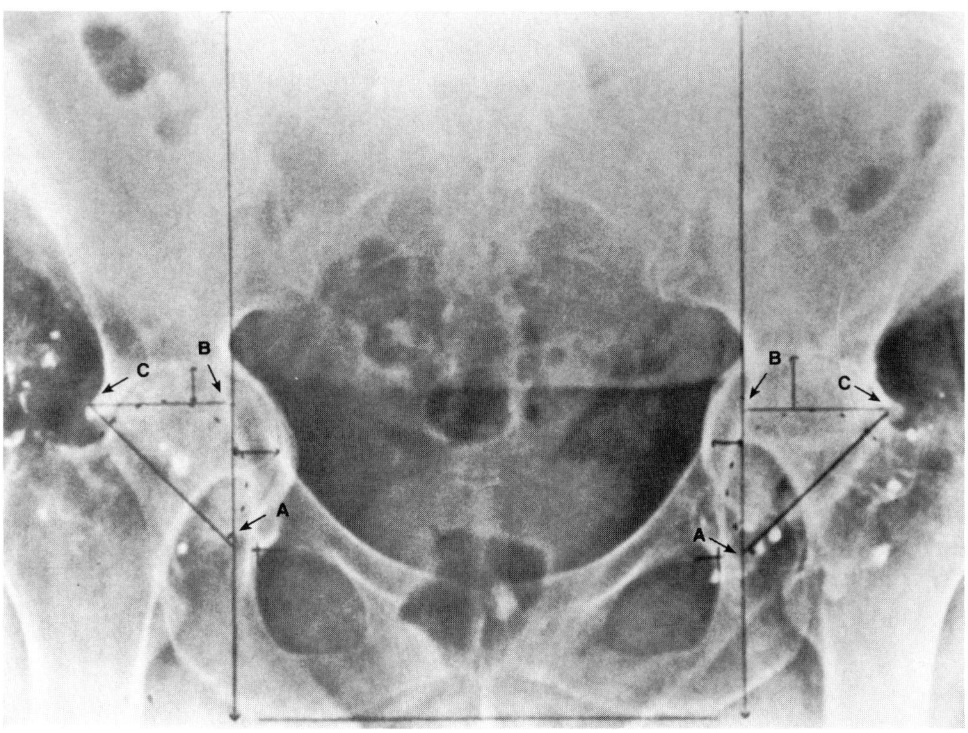

FIG 12–7.
Graphic representation of Ranawat's method for radiographically determining the proper location of the acetabulum. A detailed description is given in the text. (From Ranawat CS, Zahn MG: *J Arthroplasty* 1986; 1:131–137. Used by permission.)

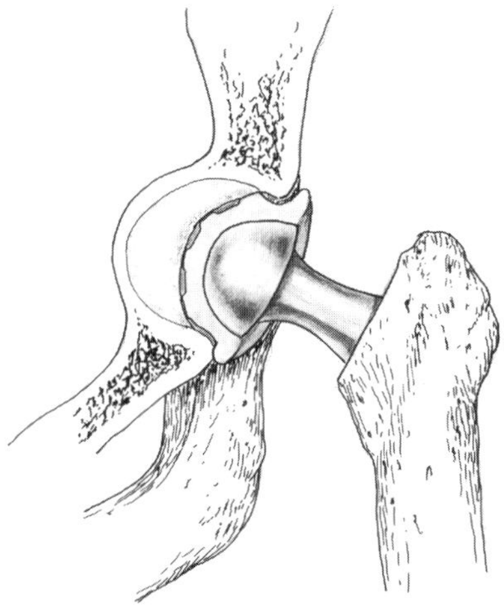

FIG 12–8.
Artist's conception of acetabular reconstruction using a femoral head autograft to fill a medial protrusion defect.

mity, and bone quality. Improvements in cementing technique have rendered cemented fixation extremely reliable and durable for both femoral stem fixation and socket fixation in the presence or absence of bone grafting. Therefore, the advantages of using noncemented fixation in a particular rheumatoid patient should be clear-cut if cement fixation is ruled out.

Thus far, noncemented fixation of acetabular sockets has produced encouraging results in the treatment of all arthritides where none, or minimal, bone grafting has been done.[23] The durability of this technique, when used with bone grafting of the weightbearing portions of the acetabulum, is questionable and has not been extensively reported. We recommend cemented socket fixation in most cases where structural (i.e., weight bearing) bone grafting has been utilized. Noncemented socket placement is recommended in young patients, in whom no structural bone grafting has been performed, and whose bone is of sufficient quality to provide adequate purchase for initial screw fixation.

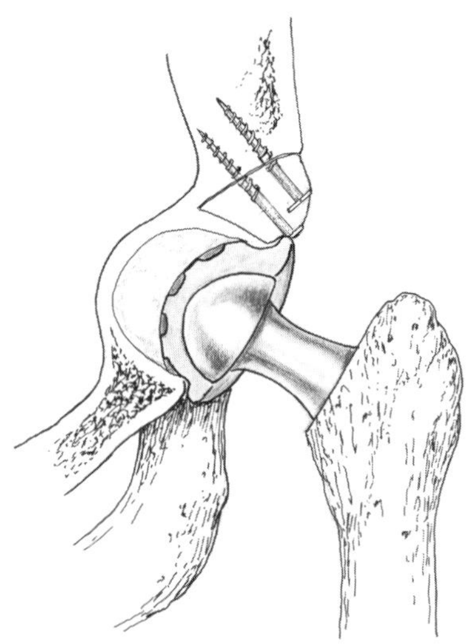

FIG 12–9.
Medial and superior bone grafting for bone loss created by protrusion.

In youthful patients consideration for implantation of a noncemented femoral implant should be given. Experience with noncemented femoral implants in osteoarthritic patients has demonstrated that success of noncemented stem fixation is related to the correctness of the implant fit to the patient's anatomic geometry and the patient's ability to form a bony bond to the implant. In our opinion, the quality of the patient's bone—with respect to its ability to successfully achieve bone ingrowth—can be judged radiographically by measuring the "cortical index" of the femoral shaft. The index is the percentage of the diameter of the diaphyseal shaft, just distal to the metaphysis, which is made up by cortical bone (Fig 12–10). In our experience, a cortical index of 48% or greater seems to correlate with a high rate of success for noncemented femoral implants. However, even in the presence of an acceptable femoral cortical index, a mismatch between implant geometry and patient anatomy will usually lead to failure of fixation and subsidence of the implant. When noncemented fixation is intended, inspection at surgery should (1) verify acceptable bone quality, as determined by the consistency and appearance of the cancellous bone in the metaphysis, and (2) insure a proper match between implant geometry and patient anatomy. If either are found to be questionable, cemented fixation remains the procedure of choice. Therefore, we usually recommend cemented stem fixation in all but the youngest of RA patients for whom precise custom-fit implants have been made.

As a final aspect of long-term preparation, the surgeon should consider alternative courses of action if intraoperative technical complications, such as femoral fracture or perforation of the medial wall of the acetabulum, occur, as can easily happen when dealing with osteoporotic bone. The knowledgeable surgeon will prepare solutions to these problems in the form of additional bone graft, wire mesh, long-stem implants, cerclage wires, and other devices.

Immediate Preoperative Preparation

Total hip arthroplasty patients, especially those with inflammatory arthritis, should be admitted to the

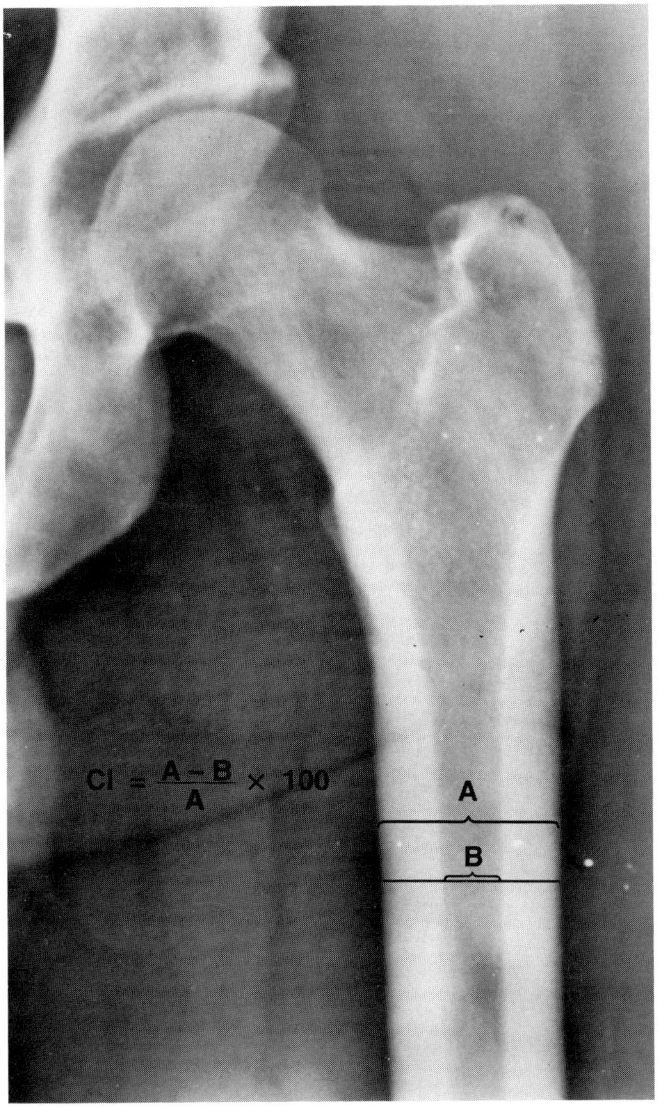

FIG 12–10.
The cortical index (CI) is measured radiographically on the femoral shaft just distal to the metaphyseal-diaphyseal junction. It is the percentage of total shaft diameter occupied by cortical bone at this point and appears to be related clinically to the quality of bone with respect to strength, degree of mineralization, and ability to achieve a successful bond with a bone-ingrowth implant.

hospital no later than the night before surgery. This allows time for adequate last-minute patient instruction and physical preparation, and the assembly of all essential preoperative evaluations. Most standard protocols include a patient shower with pHisoHex or povidone-iodine (Betadine), and a bowel-cleaning enema on the night before surgery. In addition, most anesthesia protocols require that the patient ingest nothing by mouth after midnight of the night before surgery as a precaution against aspiration of stomach contents during anesthesia. Hospital admission on the day before surgery facilitates the accomplishment of these precautions.

We believe that epidural anesthesia, with controlled hypotension if possible, is the anesthesia method of choice for the performance of THA. This method has several advantages, all related to lowering of the blood pressure in the operative field. Firstly, there is reduced bleeding from all sources, which leads to significantly shorter operative time by reducing the time the surgeon is occupied with hemostasis. Secondly, cemented fixation of implants appears to be improved by weakening of the hydraulic barrier formed by the blood in bone. This effectively decreases the resistance to cement intrusion into the bone and has been demonstrated to foster statistically significant improvement of the radiographic appearance of the acetabular cement-bone interface achieved at surgery.[47]

Intravenous antibiotic prophylaxis is started just prior to surgery, with completion of infusion of the first dose just prior to the incision. It is continued for 48 hours post operation. Our drug of choice is cefazolin. Vancomycin is administered to patients with known or suspected allergy to penicillin and its analogues.

Surgical Approach

The performance of a proper hip arthroplasty requires a wide exposure. We prefer in most cases to place the patient in the lateral position and use a posterolateral approach to the hip joint, without trochanteric osteotomy (Fig 12–11). However, when

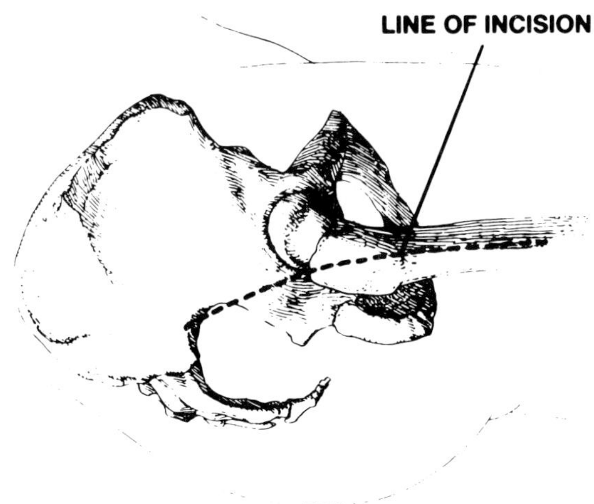

FIG 12–11.
Dashed line indicates the approximate line of incision with respect to the bony anatomy. (From Ranawat CS, Maynard MJ: *Techniques Orthop* 1991; 6:17–25. Used by permission.)

there is a severe distortion of the femoral or acetabular anatomy, as is often the case in RA and JRA, the surgeon should be prepared to perform a trochanteric osteotomy for exposure, or for trochanteric advancement, if necessary.

At the time of the skin incision, the subcutaneous tissues are also sharply divided to expose the fascia. Then, palpation of the greater trochanter will aid the surgeon in choosing the proper position for the fascial incision. An appropriately placed fascial incision will course approximately 1 cm anterior to the insertion of the gluteus maximus onto the femoral shaft. The fascia lata and fascia of the gluteus maximus are divided sharply and the fibers of the gluteus maximus are separated bluntly or with electrocautery, in line with the muscle bundles. The tendinous insertion of the gluteus maximus onto the shaft of the femur is divided with electrocautery. At this point, attention is given to hemostasis and installation of protective moist sponges and a Charnley retractor at the wound edges. The short external rotators of the hip are now detached from their insertions on the posterior edge of the greater trochanter and are allowed to retract posteriorly. The hip capsule is opened at its insertion onto the posterior femoral neck and a trapezoid capsular flap is formed by cutting the capsule radially at the upper border of the piriformis superiorly and at the lower border of the inferior gemmellus inferiorly. The capsular flap and the short external rotators will later be repaired to the greater trochanter (Fig 12–12). A narrow bent Hohmann retractor is placed under the gluteus minimus and the capsulotomy is extended superiorly and anteriorly. An Aufranc retractor is placed inferior to the femoral neck. The quadratus femoris is detached all along its femoral insertion down to the level of the lesser trochanter and then the inferior part of the hip capsule is released as far inferiorly as can be easily viewed.

The hip can then usually be dislocated posteriorly with gentle adduction, flexion, and internal rotation of the femur. This may not be the case, however, if significant protrusion is present. Under these circumstances, two options exist. The surgeon may, at this point, decide to proceed with trochanteric osteotomy, thus "unroofing" the hip joint to allow easier dislocation. The other option is to osteotomize the femoral neck in situ and proceed with mobilization of the femoral shaft to allow further exposure of the acetabulum and eventual removal of the femoral head and neck fragment from the socket.

If possible after dislocation, the center of rotation of the femoral head should be estimated and marked prior to femoral neck osteotomy. Measurements are made and recorded from this point to the tip of the greater trochanter and the top of the lesser trochanter. The femoral neck cut is then performed at a 45-degree angle to the shaft of the femur at the level where the lateral end of the cut lies at the intersection of the superior cortex of the femoral neck and the greater trochanter (Fig 12–13). The cut neck is sealed with bone wax to reduce bleeding during acetabular preparation and fixation.

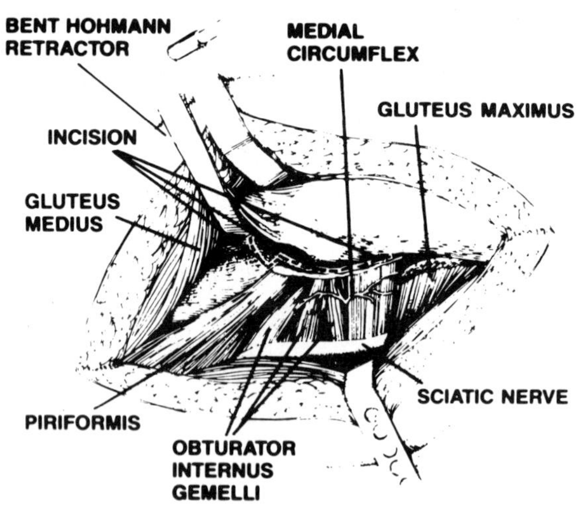

FIG 12–12.
Course of posterior capsulotomy. (From Ranawat CS, Maynard MJ: *Techniques Orthop* 1991; 6:17–25. Used by permission.)

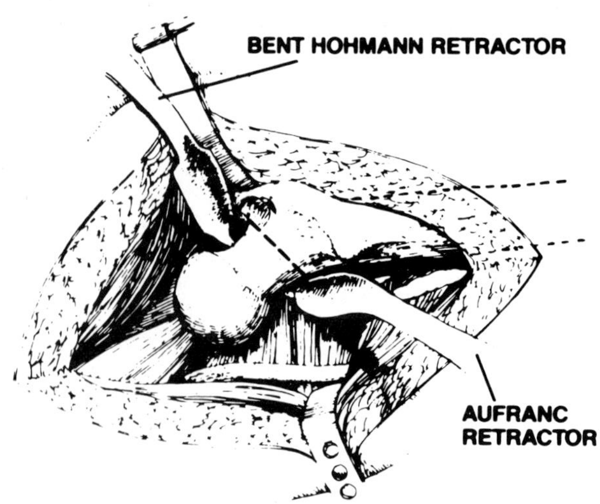

FIG 12–13.
Dotted lines indicate the approximate position for femoral neck osteotomy. (From Ranawat CS, Maynard MJ: *Techniques Orthop* 1991; 6:17–25. Used by permission.)

Acetabular Reconstruction

After removal of the femoral head from the acetabulum, a Charnley retractor is placed over the anterior lip of the acetabulum in front of the cut femoral neck. An Aufranc retractor is placed beneath the transverse acetabular ligament. The ligament is left intact, if possible, to act as a cement dam. A broad bent Hohmann retractor is placed into the bone just above the midpoint of the posterior wall. A Steinmann's pin is placed superiorly to retract the gluteus medius and minimus. If trochanteric osteotomy has been avoided, the femur is mobilized anteriorly by releasing the reflected head of the rectus femoris muscle and the anterior hip capsule at the superomedial quadrant of the acetabular margin (Fig 12–14). The synovium and labral tissue obscuring the mouth of the acetabulum are sharply dissected away. Any soft tissue in the acetabular fossa is removed to allow a view of the true medial wall of the acetabulum, if possible.

In primary arthroplasty, the most constant landmarks for determining proper acetabular placement are the anterior and posterior attachment points of the transverse acetabular ligament and the rounded curve of the ischial bone as it passes beneath this ligament. The surgeon should identify these structures early and later attempt to place the inferior edge of the prosthetic socket in close proximity to them. A dummy prosthesis can then be held in this position at the start of, and frequently during, acetabular reconstruction to aid in the selection of the appropriate size and type of implant and the planning of any required bone grafting or protrusion ring placement.

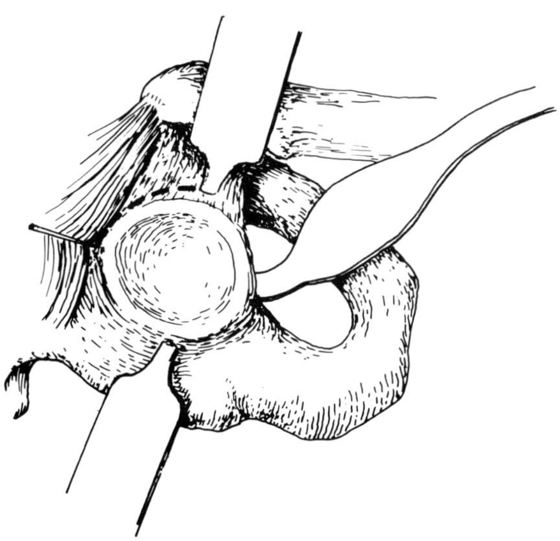

FIG 12–14.
Placement of retractors for exposure of the acetabulum. *Dashed line* indicates where the anterior capsule and rectus femoris muscle are released for proper anterior mobilization of the femur. (From Ranawat CS, Maynard MJ: *Techniques Orthop* 1991; 6:17–25. Used by permission.)

Preparation of the acetabulum proceeds with thorough debridement of all soft tissue, including cartilage, until a bed of bleeding bone is achieved. Care should be taken during this debridement to recognize and avoid violation of any preexisting medial wall defects and avoid making any new perforations.

Next, preparation and placement of any required bone grafting should be performed. In cases of mild to moderate medial protrusion, a wafer of bone can often be fashioned from the removed femoral head and placed to fill the defect. If severe protrusion deformity exists, femoral head autograft or allografts may be required. A fundamental requirement of bone graft preparation is the removal of all soft tissue and cartilage from the graft. Once this has been achieved, the intended use of the graft determines further preparation. If the graft is to be placed in a position where it will bear a load, the structural integrity of the graft should be preserved as much as possible. This is done by removing as little cortical and hard subchondral bone as possible during sculpting of the graft to fit the defect. This is also important to avoid splitting the graft if screws are to be placed through it for fixation. Graft shaping is often facilitated by first shaping one part of the graft to allow it to be wedged into a defect and then using the acetabular reamers to trim it down into the appropriate exterior contour. If the graft is intended as a grouting material or as a filler for smaller, cystic defects, it can be ground up in a bone mill to form a sort of mash. When using allograft bone, we remove most of the fat from this type of preparation, to avoid its potentially antigenic effects, by mixing the bone mash with water and then straining it through a cloth surgical sponge several times. If large, structural (or loadbearing) grafting has been placed, cement fixation of the prosthetic socket is employed. Cement fixation holes should be fashioned. If possible, place two relatively large (5–8 mm diameter, 8–10 mm depth) holes, one each in the ischium and pubis, and several smaller holes in the superior aspect of the prepared bed, in the ilium or bone graft, or in both. The position for placement of the large inferior holes is usually obvious because after removal of the articular cartilage, bleeding cancellous bone reveals the medullary portion of the ischial and pubic bones where the holes should be placed (Fig 12–15). Locations where impaction of the cement at

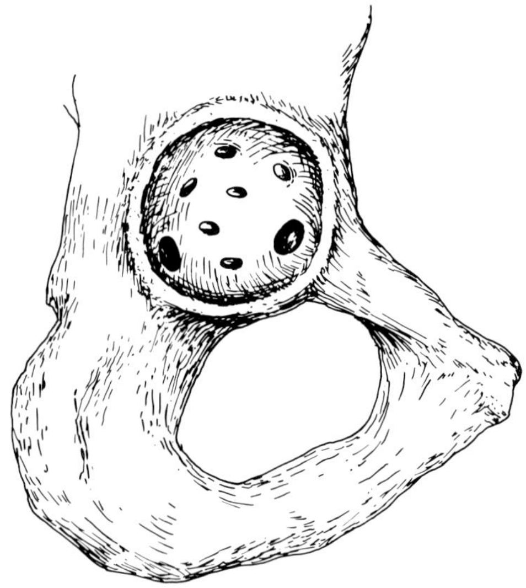

FIG 12–15.
Large cement fixation holes are placed in the ischium and pubis, and several smaller holes are placed in the ilium. (From Ranawat CS, Maynard MJ: *Techniques Orthop* 1991; 6:17–25. Used by permission.)

implantation might lead to interposition of cement between host bone and graft bone should be firmly sealed with cement or morselized bone graft, or both.

If a stable interference fit has been achieved between the graft and the bony defect, and adequate native bone is also available for cement fixation, implantation of a protrusion ring may not be necessary. However, if the graft fixation is unstable, or little purchase by the cement directly onto the pelvic bone can be expected, a protrusion ring should now be fixed in place.

As discussed previously, the guiding principle of socket positioning is the normalization of the center of rotation of the hip in terms of the superoinferior, AP, and medial-lateral directions. Once adequate bony reconstruction has been achieved to support this, the appropriate trial device may be used to assess the acetabulum and insure provision for a homogeneous cement mantle of adequate thickness. During this maneuver one should identify landmarks that can be used to insure proper position during actual implantation of the prosthetic socket.

The bone is then thoroughly cleaned by a pulsatile lavage. The bone is dried by packing the end of a clean, dry sponge individually into each of the large fixation holes and then pressing the rest of the roll into the acetabulum and holding it there for several seconds. The timing of this maneuver is crucial. The cement should already be mixed and within approximately 1 minute of the proper consistency for implantation at the time of final lavage and drying. In this way, as soon as drying is complete, the sponge can be removed and the cement immediately pressed into a bed of clean, dry bone.

Simplex acrylic cement is preferred because of its superior strength and handling characteristics. Some evidence suggests that mixing the cement under vacuum or centrifuging the cement after mixing removes trapped air bubbles and improves the strength properties of the cement.[19, 20] We prepare the cement as follows:

1. The cement reagents are heated in a blanket warmer prior to surgery. This speeds up the rate at which the cement cures after mixing. It also seems to aid in the release of air trapped in the cement during mixing, by causing it to bubble out.
2. The powdered and liquid forms of the cement are mixed in a bowl with minimal stirring (usually less than 30 seconds).
3. The cement is allowed to sit undisturbed in the bowl for several minutes, during which time most of the air trapped during mixing bubbles to the surface.

Simplex cement at 3 to 5 minutes of setting, when it is slightly firmer than toothpaste consistency, can be rolled into a doughy ball. At this consistency, part of the cement should be coated over the outer surface of the prosthesis while it is on the holder. The rest of the cement is placed into the acetabulum and swiftly pressed into each of the large fixation holes with the index finger (Fig 12–16). Then, the cement is uniformly pressed in using a

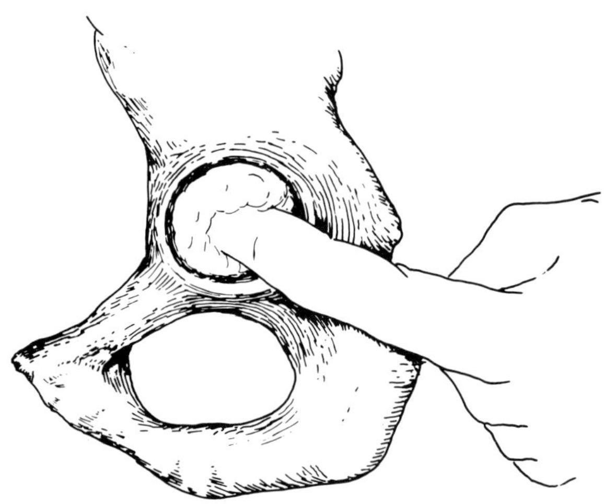

FIG 12–16.
Cement is pressed into the fixation holes with the index finger. (From Ranawat CS, Maynard MJ: *Techniques Orthop* 1991; 6:17–25. Used by permission.)

sturdy rubber impactor. With this tool, pressure is applied for 2 to 3 minutes (Fig 12–17).

Next, immediately prior to implantation of the socket, any blood that has collected on the cement is cleaned off with suction or a dry sponge. Then, using a curette, the cement is removed from the transverse acetabular ligament and nearby inferior margin of the acetabulum for a distance of about 5 mm, this to avoid pushing cement into the obturator foramen when the socket is placed (Fig 12–18). Excess cement is cleared from the periphery of the acetabulum. The prosthetic socket, using the appropriate holder, is inserted into the cement, positioned, and impacted down into the proper medial position. It is also positioned at approximately 40 degrees of lateral opening and 15 degrees of anteversion. Thus positioned, the prosthesis will completely occlude both of the large cement fixation holes placed in the ischial and pubic bones. If one or both are not completely occluded, recheck the socket position with respect to anteversion and lateral opening. Pressure is maintained on the prosthesis while the cement hardens. Very often a portion of the prosthesis is left uncovered by bone superiorly. During the cement-curing process digital pressure should be maintained on any part of the superior and posterior cement mantle that is left uncovered by bone. Once the cement has hardened, palpate the edges of the acetabulum searching for excess cement, which is removed using osteotomes and a rongeur.

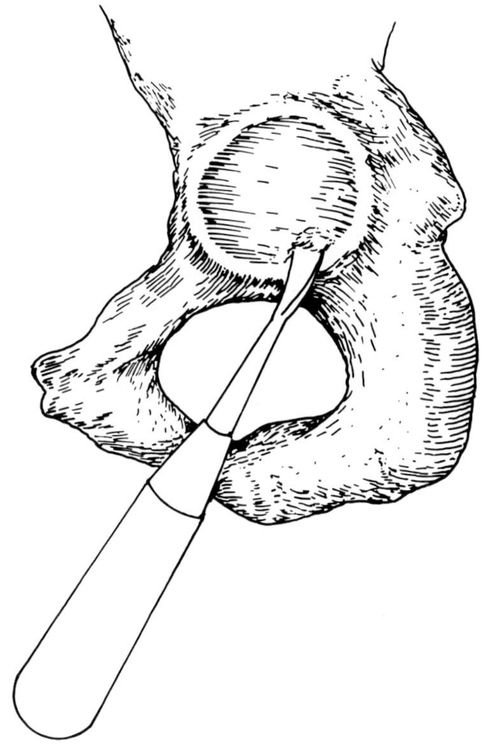

FIG 12–18.
Cement is cleaned away from the acetabular ligament prior to implantation of the prosthesis. (From Ranawat CS, Maynard MJ: *Techniques Orthop* 1991; 6:17–25. Used by permission.)

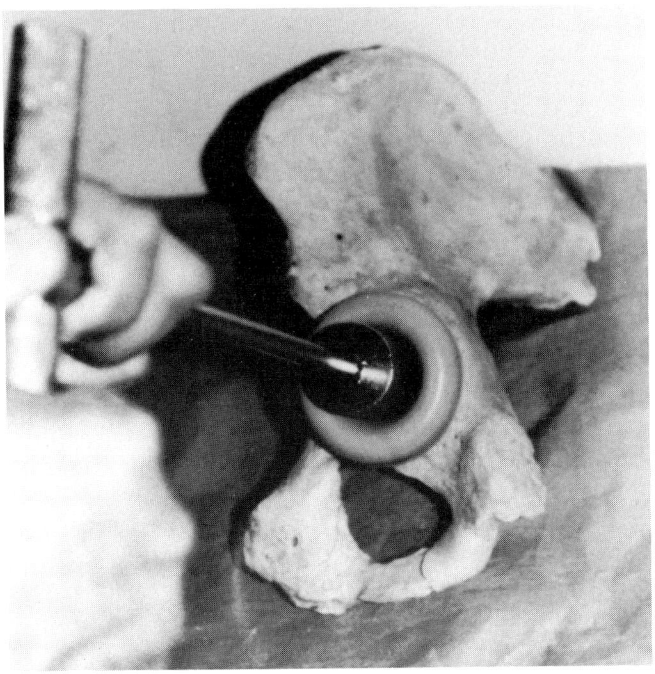

FIG 12–17.
A rubber balloon impactor is used to further press down the cement mass for several minutes. (From Ranawat CS, Maynard MJ: *Techniques Orthop* 1991; 6:17–25. Used by permission.)

Implantation of a noncemented socket may be practical if the amount and quality of available pelvic bone stock provides reasonable expectation of bone ingrowth and durable long-term fixation. It may also be desirable where there is inadequate cancellous bone available for microinterlock with cement, as is often the case in revision arthroplasty. The principles of noncemented socket postioning are completely analogous to those for cemented sockets. The size of the metal shell should be chosen to achieve a "wedge" or "press" fit in the prepared acetabular bed, if possible. Fixation may then be secured by placement of screws through the shell into the iliac bone overlying the superior acetabular dome. Screws should be directed to avoid intrapelvic penetration and should obtain purchase in the patient's native iliac bone. Reliance upon screws anchored in grafted bone should be avoided.

Femoral Reconstruction

The acetabular retractors are removed and a moist sponge is placed to protect the socket. A large posterior femoral neck retractor is placed under the proximal femur and the leg is flexed and internally rotated, when no trochanteric osteotomy has been performed, to allow easy access to the femoral canal. (If an osteotomy has been performed, the leg is covered in a sterile bag, and placed in external rotation and flexion, with the foot supported on a low stool off the anterior side of the table.) An Aufranc retractor is placed to retract the soft tissues at the inferior margin of the femoral neck and a narrow-angled Hohmann retractor is placed between the gluteus medius and minimus superiorly to gain further exposure of the femoral canal and greater trochanter (Fig 12–19).

A "canal finder," or a straight intramedullary reamer with a pointed leading end, is used to locate the medullary canal of the femur. The optimal starting point for this maneuver is at the piriformis fossa—located at the posterior corner of the intersection of the femoral neck and the greater trochanter (Fig 12–20). The first reamer should be passed to a distance of approximately 150 mm. The medullary canal should then be prepared with progressively larger reamers. Excessive reaming is not advisable, however, since this may remove the cancellous bone required for adequate cement interdigitation. Preoperative planning using appropriate radiographs and templates can give the surgeon an estimate of the size required. The proximal femur is then broached up to the appropriate size using the broaches provided by the manufacturer of the prosthesis intended for implantation. During broaching, the desired amount of femoral anteversion should be maintained with each broach. The appropriate amount of femoral anteversion is determined by the patient's anatomy and gender, and the position of the just-implanted socket. In general, this falls into the range of 0 to 15 degrees. The objective is a total anteversion of 25 to 45 degrees when the anteversion of the socket and stem are considered together. Females fare better with combined anteversion closer to 45 degrees while males require only around 20 to 30 degrees for satisfactory function. If a custom implant and tools have been provided, the procedure is modified accordingly.

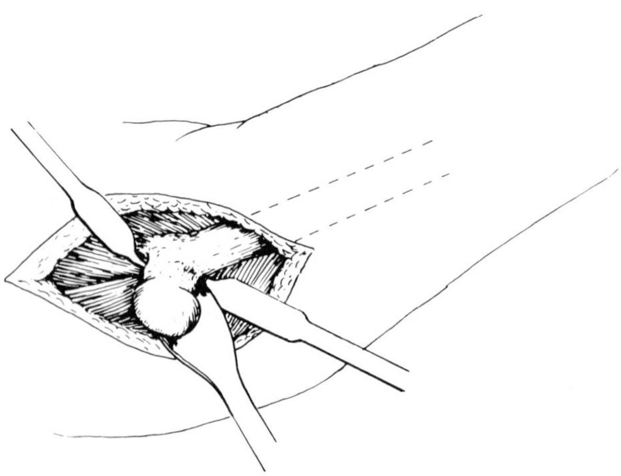

FIG 12–19.
Placement of retractors for exposure of the femur. (From Ranawat CS, Maynard MJ: *Techniques Orthop* 1991; 6:17–25. Used by permission.)

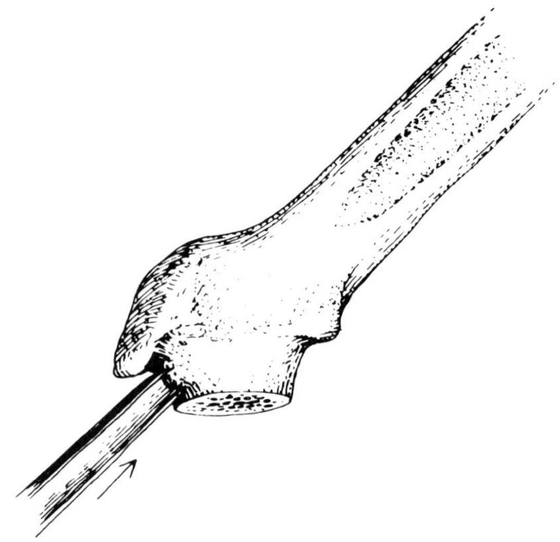

FIG 12–20.
The medullary canal is approached starting at the piriformis fossa. (From Ranawat CS, Maynard MJ: *Techniques Orthop* 1991; 6:17–25. Used by permission.)

A trial implant of the appropriate size should now be placed into the medullary canal and impacted to the position desired for the actual implant. If using a modular system, the appropriate neck and head trials should be attached and a trial reduction performed. Prior to trial reduction, the distances from the center of rotation of this reconstruction to the greater trochanter and the top of the lesser trochanter should be measured. Comparison of these figures with those obtained prior to femoral neck osteotomy will aid the surgeon in the critical assessment of the trial reduction with respect to offset and leg length. During trial reduction, the surgeon should assess the total anteversion, anterior capsule tension, leg length, and position required to dislocate the hip. The total anteversion is judged by rotating the hip, while at neutral flexion-extension, to the position where the prosthetic neck is perpendicular to the face of the socket. At this position, the total anteversion is the amount of internal rotation of the hip. Two factors may confound this determination.

First, the use of an elevated posterior rim on

the socket (which *is* recommended) may make the perpendicular position a little more difficult to judge. Secondly, if the patient or operating table have been tilted during the procedure it may be difficult to determine the frontal plane of the patient—the plane of reference for internal rotation—unless the tilt is corrected. Anterior capsule tension should be assessed by palpation with the hip in neutral flexion-extension, adduction-abduction, and rotation. With a finger palpating the anterior capsule, the surgeon should use the other hand to rotate the femur externally. A small amount of external rotation should produce a palpable tightening of the capsule. If the capsule does not develop tension, consideration should be given to increasing the femoral neck length, or performing a trochanteric advancement, in order to lessen the probability of dislocation. If, on the other hand, the capsule develops excessive tension, consideration should be given to either reducing the neck length or offset, or both, or to releasing the capsule. It is usually prudent to release the anterior capsule or adductor muscles in favor of preserving offset and neck length. Leg length is judged by assessment of soft tissue tension and the measurements previously described. The position of the hip at dislocation is seen by rotating the hip internally while at approximately 10 degrees of adduction and 30 degrees of flexion. The goal is a minimum of 65 degrees in males and 75 degrees in females. If the trochanter has been osteotomized, trial reduction should be used to determine the proper position for wire placement to effect an appropriately tensioned repair.

Often, when a severe protrusion deformity has been corrected, the effective bony limb lengthening is not accommodated by the soft tissues, including the neurovascular structures, which have shortened over time as the deformity progressed. If satisfactory trial reduction cannot be obtained, the surgeon should first attempt to remedy this by judicious soft tissue releases. Tissues which can be released entirely from the proximal femur without significant detriment include the anterior capsule, the gluteus maximus and minimus muscles, and the iliopsoas muscle. The adductors and rectus femoris can be tenotomized at their pelvic insertions. The gluteus medius can also be significantly released by isolation and elevation proceeding proximally up to its origin, with care to avoid injury to the superior gluteal nerve and artery.

If satisfactory reduction and joint motion are still unobtainable after all appropriate releases have been done, the proximal femur must be osteotomized to allow more distal placement of the prosthetic stem in the bone. Occasionally, simple revision of the femoral neck cut may achieve satisfactory results. If more bone shortening is required, however, the trochanter must be osteotomized, if this has not been done already. Then the level of the required femoral shaft osteotomy can be determined by reducing the trial femoral implant into the prosthetic socket and holding it alongside the femoral shaft while an assistant applies an appropriate amount of soft tissue tension by pulling the leg distally. The site for osteotomy is marked opposite to where the neck of the trial stem falls. The femur may now require further broaching to accept the intended implant at its new position.

After successful trial reduction, the trial implants are removed and the retractors are replaced in the previously described positions. A cement restrictor should now be placed in the femoral canal. The distance at which it is to be placed should be measured directly off of the actual prosthesis which should, by now, be available in the sterile field. It should be placed deep enough to allow approximately 2 cm of cement distal to the tip of the prosthesis when fully seated.

If trochanteric repair is required, two wires should be placed through a drill hole in the lateral cortex of the proximal femur, at a position determined during trial reduction. After these intramedullary wires are placed, trial placement of the femoral stem into the canal should again be done to insure the absence of significant obstruction. One or two additional wires should be placed around the femoral shaft through a drill hole in the lesser trochanter or femoral shaft.

Cement preparation is now done as previously described with the additional step of placement of the cement into a plastic cement gun. The cement is mixed in a bowl, allowed to sit uncovered for a time to allow the bubbles to rise and clear, and then placed into the gun.

After the cement restrictor is placed, the medullary canal is thoroughly lavaged with a water pick and suction. When the cement is within a minute of the proper consistency (toothpastelike), a final lavage is performed followed by a drying maneuver with a clean, dry sponge. The sponge is packed into the canal and removed immediately prior to cement implantation. As soon as the sponge is removed, a final quick suction of the bottom of the canal is performed and the cement is swiftly placed into the canal in a retrograde fashion, filling from distally to proximally (Fig 12–21). The cement is pressed down by placing the thumb of the distal hand to occlude the medial side of the top of the medullary canal

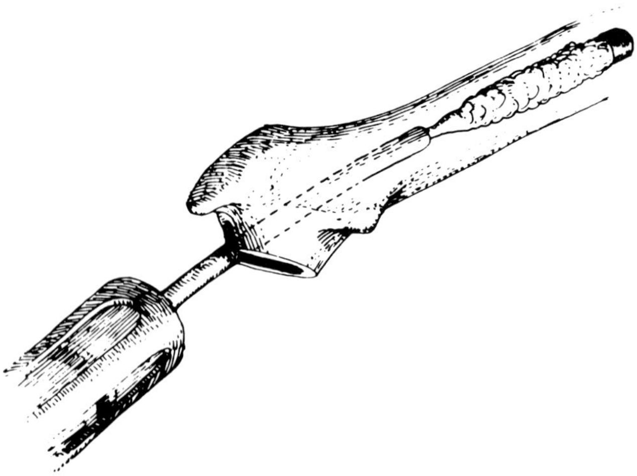

FIG 12–21.
Cement is delivered retrograde into the medullary canal using a cement gun. (From Ranawat CS, Maynard MJ: *Techniques Orthop* 1991; 6:17–25. Used by permission.)

while pushing a finger of the proximal hand (usually the index finger) into the cement (Fig 12–22). More cement is placed to fill the defect created by the pushing finger and the procedure is repeated two or three times. Sufficient impaction is usually signaled by the emergence of displaced fat and blood onto the surface of the proximal femur. A doughy consistency of cement optimizes the effectiveness of this technique.

The prosthesis is prepared for implantation by cleaning and drying, if necessary, and coating the proximal metaphyseal area circumferentially with cement. This eliminates the chance introduction of water, blood, or other material between the cement and the prosthesis during implantation. Along with the textured surface found in modern implants, it insures an improved mechanical bond of the cement to the prosthesis. After the cement column has been prepared, the prosthesis should be pressed down manually into the cement in a slow, steady fashion. This maneuver should be controlled to achieve a neutral or slight valgus position of the stem, the desired anteversion, and the proper proximal-distal position in one smooth movement. Occasionally, impaction of the prosthesis with a few blows from an impactor and mallet may be necessary to achieve the appropriately distal position. Gentle pressure should be used to maintain the position of the prosthesis while all excess cement is cleaned away and the cement is allowed to harden. During cement curing, the surgeon should compact any exposed cement using forceps and a moist sponge. Once the cement has hardened, the appropriate femoral head prosthesis, if not already attached, may be fitted to the trunion with standard technique.

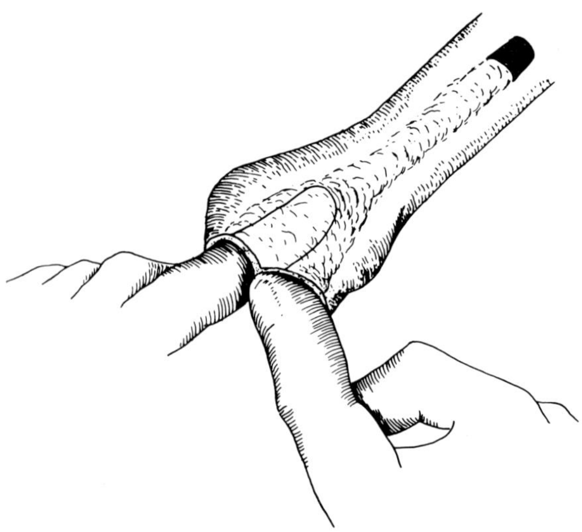

FIG 12–22.
Digital technique of pressing cement. (From Ranawat CS, Maynard MJ: *Techniques Orthop* 1991; 6:17–25. Used by permission.)

Placement of a noncemented femoral component may be desirable in younger patients that have good bone stock. The technical details will vary according to the implant system. In general, the procedure for femoral preparation differs from the technique for cemented implants in that broaching of the femoral canal is more precise and is aimed at achieving a stable interference fit between the prosthesis and the bone that will foster the achievement of bone ingrowth for long-term fixation.

Two drill holes are now made in the posterior edge of the greater trochanter for use in reattaching the posterior soft tissues. A loop of suture is placed through each hole, using a straight needle, for later use. The hip is now reduced. A last check of position and soft tissue tension is performed. The insertion of the gluteus maximus may be repaired. The short external rotators of the hip and the posterior capsular flap are secured to one another with two nonabsorbable sutures. These sutures are then drawn through the holes made in the greater trochanter using the suture loops previously installed for this purpose. Then, with the hip placed in an abducted and externally rotated position, the sutures are used to draw the posterior soft tissues up snugly against the posterior surface of the greater trochanter and are securely tied (Fig 12–23).

The entire wound is now thoroughly irrigated with an antibiotic-saline solution. Two large suction drains are placed in the joint and are brought out

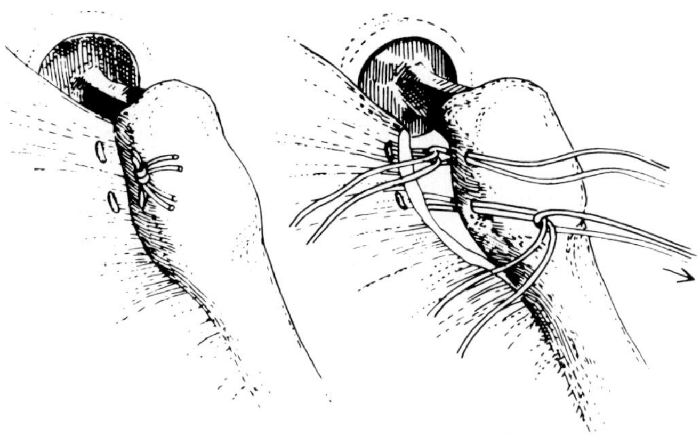

FIG 12–23.
Posterior capsular repair through drill holes in the greater trochanter. (From Ranawat CS, Maynard MJ: *Techniques Orthop* 1991; 6:17–25. Used by permission.)

through the fascia and skin anteriorly and distally. The fascia lata and fascia over the gluteus maximus are repaired with interrupted sutures. The subcutaneous tissues are also closed with a single layer of interrupted sutures and the skin is closed with a running nylon stitch. The wound is dressed with silk soaked in povidone-iodine, covered with sterile gauze, and held in place with an elastic bandage that surrounds the hip, upper thigh, and pelvis.

TYPICAL HOSPITAL COURSE AND REHABILITATION

Primary THA generally requires from 1 to 2 hours to complete. Surgical blood loss concomitant to a primary hip arthroplasty requires 1 to 3 units of blood during and after surgery. Autologous predeposit of blood by the patient for his or her own use is available at many centers and often avoids nonautologous transfusion.

The suction drains placed in the hip at surgery are usually removed after 24 to 48 hours. Abduction slings or an abduction pillow is applied for a few days after surgery to protect the hip from dislocating forces while the patient is convalescing from surgery. Prophylactic antibiotics, as previously mentioned, are begun before surgery and continued intravenously for 24 to 48 hours post operation. Anticoagulant therapy is usually started the night after surgery. The type of therapy will vary according to the patient's medical history. Our rehabilitation protocol calls for the patient to begin standing up at the bedside by the second postoperative day. Progressive ambulation usually begins by the third postoperative day. In cases where cement fixation has been used, full weightbearing is allowed immediately after surgery. If a trochanteric osteotomy has been performed, special precautions and limited weightbearing on the hip are in order. Where a noncemented device has been implanted, an extended period of minimal weightbearing is prescribed.

Ambulatory assistive devices for rehabilitation are tailored to the patient's needs. Patients with rheumatoid involvement of the upper extremities may require a special walker with platforms which avoids weightbearing on the hands and wrists. Most patients progress to discharge after a hospital stay of 7 to 10 days. Some patients with inflammatory arthritis may require further supervised rehabilitation and, based upon individual needs, these patients are transferred, if possible, to a rehabilitation facility that is able to accomodate their personal requirements. In most cases, an unsupervised program of ambulation at home is all that is necessary for a successful outcome after THA.

Our long-term THA rehabilitation protocol requires the use of an ambulatory aid for at least 2 months after surgery. A walker or two crutches is prescribed for the first month. This may progress to a single crutch for an additional month and then to a cane thereafter. Full benefit from the surgical intervention is usually realized by the end of 12 months.

Postoperatively, the performance of a THA requires the observance of special precautions to avoid dislocation of the prosthetic joint. These are aimed at avoiding extremes of motion at the hip while the soft tissues heal. After a posterior surgical approach, acute flexion and internal rotation of the hip must be avoided. In this regard, the patient is carefully instructed in proper leg and body positioning as part of the rehabilitation protocol. Patients should use an elevated toilet seat and avoid soft or low chairs for several months after surgery. They should not lean forward from a sitting position and should not bend over at the waist from a standing position. Special assistive reachers and other devices are provided and should be used for dressing and other activities of daily living. A pillow held between the legs while sleeping is also prescribed for the first few months.

INTRAOPERATIVE COMPLICATIONS

The overall intraoperative surgical complication rate in primary THA is less than 5%.[63] The prevalence of neurologic complications related to THA is approximately 1% to 3%[4, 15, 21, 59] and the majority of these resolve within 6 months after surgery.[50] Although the prevalence of vascular complications is not known, they probably occur in less than 1% of cases.[5, 39, 50] Significant malpositioning of the prosthetic components manifesting as postoperative joint instability and dislocation occurs in less than 3% of cases.[50, 63] Infection attributable to the surgical procedure after primary hip arthroplasty is less than 2% in the rheumatoid population.[63, 67] The osteoporosis commonly present in rheumatoid bone should make gentle manipulation of the limb and careful utilization of bone-working tools a constant priority of the surgeon in order to avoid occasional bony complications such as femoral perforation or fracture, and perforation of the medial wall of the acetabulum.

POSTOPERATIVE COMPLICATIONS

Deep Vein Thrombosis

Various reports in the literature have reported the rate of deep vein thrombosis (DVT) (all sites) following THA at 50% to 80%, although not all are symptomatic.[30, 40, 41] Based on clinical suspicion and ventilation-perfusion scan, the prevalence of related pulmonary embolism (PE) is estimated to be 6% to 19%. Fatal PE associated with THA has been reported to be as high as 1% to 3% in patients not receiving prophylaxis.[30, 41] Thus, because of the obvious potential for significant morbidity and mortality, prophylaxis and surveillance are important components of perioperative and postoperative management.

Epidural anesthesia during the operation and aspirin therapy in the immediate postoperative period are utilized for most patients according to our current DVT prophylaxis protocol. All patients receive venographic evaluation of the affected extremity on or about postoperative day 5. If thrombosis is demonstrated, warfarin therapy is started. All patients undergoing bilateral arthroplasty, and those with a prior history of PE, are begun on warfarin on the night after surgery, in lieu of aspirin therapy.

The incidence of DVT or PE may affect the function of the arthroplasty itself to the degree to which the event interferes with the course of postoperative rehabilitation. Otherwise, the long-term effects upon durability and function are neglible.

Infection

The incidence of early infection, defined as that appearing within 6 months of surgery, is similar for all diagnoses and is less than 1%.[50, 63] The overall long-term infection rate for THA performed using routine antibiotic prophylaxis and modern surgical technique is approximately 2%.[6] The long-term rate for various subgroups of patients varies significantly, however. The infection rate for osteoarthritic patients is approximately 0.3%, while RA patients have a risk of 1.2%.[67] The risk for psoriatic patients has been reported to be 5.5%, and for diabetic patients, 6.6%.[67] Patients in these groups also have a higher incidence of infection at other sites, such as lung, urinary tract, and skin, than do nonaffected patients. This is thought to be due to immunosuppression caused by the disease processes themselves and related medications which degrade the effectiveness of the immune response.

Established infection within a prosthetic joint is a devastating complication. The standard treatment of an established infection is removal of the implants and all associated fixation, and debridement of all locally infected soft tissue and bone. This is usually followed by a minimum of 6 weeks of appropriate intravenous antibiotic therapy.[50] Reimplantation of a new prosthesis may then be performed if the infectious source has been identified and removed and diagnostic testing demonstrates the eradication of the infectious organism. Occasionally, especially in cases of infection involving a particularly virulent pathogen, it may be wise to delay reimplantation until after a period of observation (sometimes up to a year or more), while off antibiotic therapy.

Reimplantation after infection is technically more demanding than primary arthroplasty and always requires an experienced surgeon with the necessary tools and implants. Occasionally, it may require the fabrication of custom tools and implants, and bone grafting.

Dislocation

Dislocation of the prosthetic femoral head from within the prosthetic acetabulum averages 0.5% to 3.0% in most reports[15, 50, 63] and may occur at any time after THA. It is most common during the first several postoperative weeks. During this period, soft tissue and muscle weakness about the hip are least able to resist any dislocating forces that may be applied.

Poor surgical technique may be a factor in dislocation. However, the vast majority of dislocations occur as a result of patient error—usually noncompliance in the observance of prescribed precautions. As mentioned previously, appropriate precautions usually involve the avoidance of certain body positions and activities. These will vary according to the details of the surgical technique as it relates to the weakening of various anatomic structures. Rehabilitation after THA should always include thorough instruction in these precautions and should provide, if possible, various aids such as long shoehorns, hand-extension devices for putting on hosiery, elevated toilet seats, and related devices which help the patient to avoid the extremes of hip motion in the early postoperative period.

If dislocation occurs, it should be considered a surgical emergency. Injury to neural and vascular structures may acutely accompany the dislocation or the relocation event.[6] A patient with suspected dislocation should be promptly transferred to a facility where radiographic evaluation and manipulative or operative treatment are available. The vast majority of dislocations are easily reducible with mild analgesics, muscle relaxants, and gentle manipulation by an experienced physician. Occasionally, closed reduction is not possible and operative open reduction under anesthesia may be required.[6]

Our treatment protocol after an acute dislocation includes hospital admission for observation, fitting of an abduction brace, and reinforcement of physical therapy and precautions. We insist that the patient wear the brace at all times, except when lying flat in bed, for a period of 6 weeks. The brace must be put on while lying flat prior to getting out of bed and must be removed while lying flat after returning to bed. After 6 weeks, some of the restrictions are removed, but brace usage is continued sometimes up to several months.

Trochanteric Complications

Trochanteric nonunion is reported to occur in 3.0% to 9.5% of cases in which a trochanteric osteotomy is performed as part of the surgical procedure.[9] The rate is increased in patients with repeat osteotomies and in those with osteoporosis or other conditions that are associated with poor bone healing. It has been reported to be as high as 24% in one series of patients with RA.[49] Nonunion may be painful but is rarely disabling because a fibrous union usually develops. Approximately 50% of patients with nonunion or fibrous union will demonstrate abductor weakness and a limp.[54] Complete nonunions have a higher rate of dislocation and limp and may require surgical repair.

Heterotopic Ossification

Heterotopic ossification (HO) is a complication which may appear clinically with redness, low-grade fever, and aching pain around the affected hip. The diagnosis can be made radiographically when a hazy appearance is seen in the soft tissue surrounding the hip. Males are affected two to three times more often than females, and the incidence in osteoarthritis is higher than in RA. Patients with ankylosing spondylitis, Paget's disease, and diffuse idiopathic skeletal hyperostosis (Forestier's disease) carry a higher risk.[42, 52] Though overall, heterotopic ossification of varying degree has been reported in up to 30% of all patients after THA,[6] the incidence of significant HO compromising function of the joint is probably less than 5%.[12]

For patients at particular risk, postoperative indomethacin has been shown to decrease the risk of HO.[2, 52] Low-dose postoperative irradiation, 1000 rad given in five fractions of 200 rad each, has also been shown to be very effective.[3] If severe HO does occur, it can significantly compromise joint function and may require surgical excision.

Leg Length Discrepancy

Leg length discrepancy is an occasional complication of hip reconstruction which may be quite annoying to the patient. Excessive lengthening is most often associated with a posterior surgical approach to the hip joint since lengthening may be required to achieve proper joint stability after this exposure.[50] On the other hand, limb shortening may be required to achieve joint stability in patients in whom severe soft tissue contractures are present. In most cases, leg length discrepancy that is deemed clinically significant postoperatively can be satisfactorily treated with the use of a shoe lift. Revision surgery is rarely indicated.

Metal Toxicity

Metal sensitization has not yet been shown to occur to any significant degree after implantation of cemented metal-on-plastic articulations.[6, 55] However, it is too early to assume that the same will be true of cementless components which, if they incorporate a metallic microstructured design for bone-ingrowth fixation, present a much larger surface area for the processes of local corrosion and ion leaching to take place.

Nickel and cobalt are two suspected human carcinogens routinely present in the most popular alloys used for implant fabrication.[6] Yet the observed incidence of primary malignant tumors arising in the vicinity of THAs has been vanishingly rare.[43, 64]

LONG-TERM RESULTS

General

Nearly 100% of RA patients experience dramatic, immediate, and complete relief of their hip pain after cemented THA.[44, 65] Functional improvement is also apparent in the vast majority of patients, but owing to the polyarticular nature of the disease, the degree of ultimate improvement seen over the long term is not as complete or predictable.

Cemented Fixation

The long-term performance of cemented THA in RA implanted prior to the advent of improved cementing techniques, which came into widespread use in the late 1970s, has been reported in the orthopaedic literature by many authors.* Review of a representative series of such patients treated at The Hospital for Special Surgery revealed greater than 80% survivorship of the arthroplasty longer than 12 years using the end point of revision surgery for actuarial analysis[65] (Fig 12–24). Aseptic loosening is uniformly reported in all series as the most frequent long-term complication associated with cemented THA for RA and it is the leading cause for revision arthroplasty (Fig 12–25,A and B). The main conclusion to be derived from the long-term experiences reported in the series cited above is that longevity of fixation of a cemented implant is directly related to the quality of the initial surgical technique, the quality and quantity of bone available to support the prosthesis, and patient-related variables such as age, activity level, and body weight.

Surgical technique is perhaps the single most important determinant. Current standards require thorough bone preparation and careful cement handling and pressurization to achieve satisfactory cement-bone microinterlock. Improvements in prosthetic design have made durable cement-prosthesis bonding relatively easy to achieve. Actuarial curves derived for a more recent series of patients treated using the improved cementing techniques described in detail above project significant improvement of long-term durability over the previous series. At

*References ferences 4, 7, 13–18, 21, 27, 31, 44, 46, 49, 51, 56, 63.

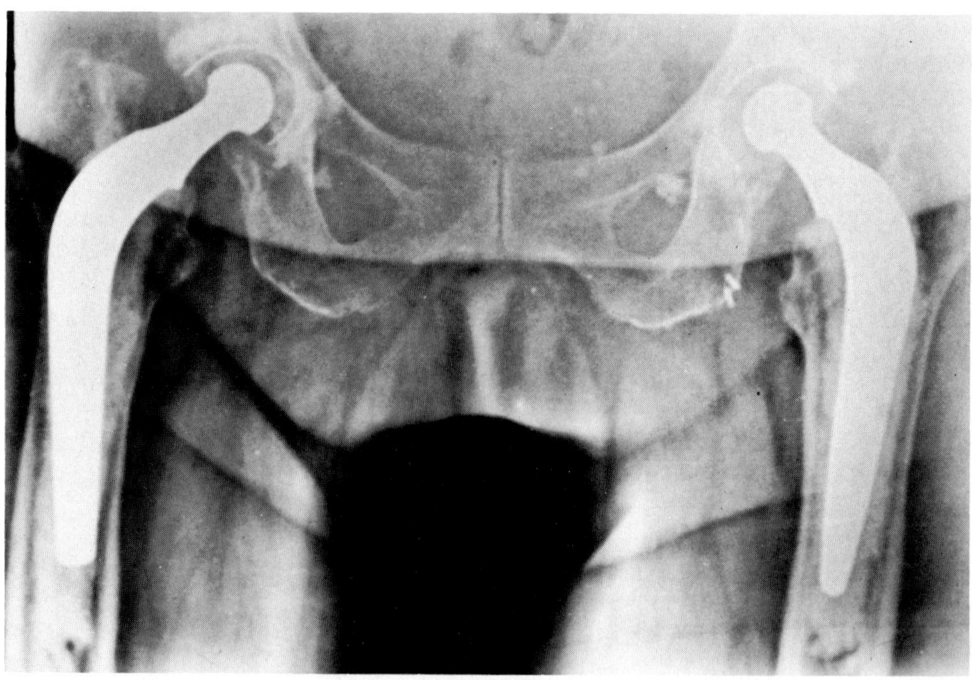

FIG 12–24.
A 73-year-old woman with rheumatoid arthritis. Radiographs demonstrate 14-year follow-up of Charnley low friction arthroplasties.

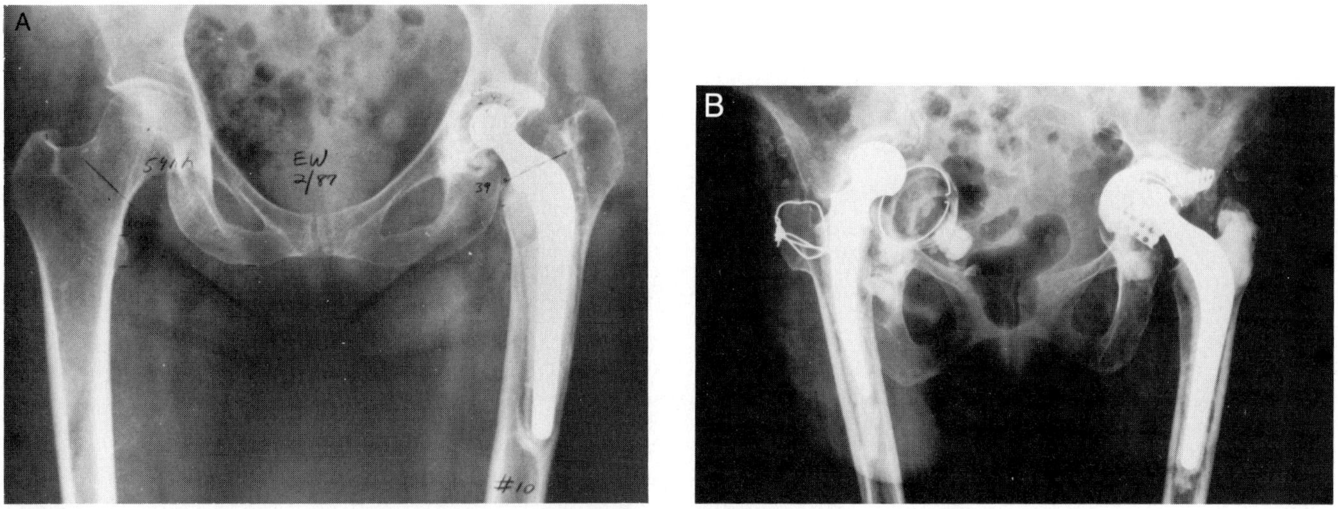

FIG 12–25.
A, femoral loosening with drift into a varus stem position. **B,** marked acetabular loosening with intrapelvic acetabular component.

present, a 90% success rate at 10 years can be predicted for the average patient receiving a cemented THA for RA.[48]

Alternatives to Cemented Fixation

Currently, much attention is focused on the development of suitable alternatives to cement fixation in an effort to provide a satisfactory solution to the problem of long-term implant fixation. The alternatives presently receiving the most scrutiny are "press-fit," "microstructured," and "hydroxyapatite osteoconductive" designs. The press-fit prostheses rely on intimate contact "interference" fit between prosthesis and bone for fixation. Microstructured prostheses have specially engineered surfaces designed to allow bone ingrowth into the pores of the surface for fixation by interdigitation of bone and implant. Hydroxyapatite osteoconduction prostheses are coated with hydroxyapatite ceramic on a microstructured surface. This substance is the main inorganic component of human bone matrix and is

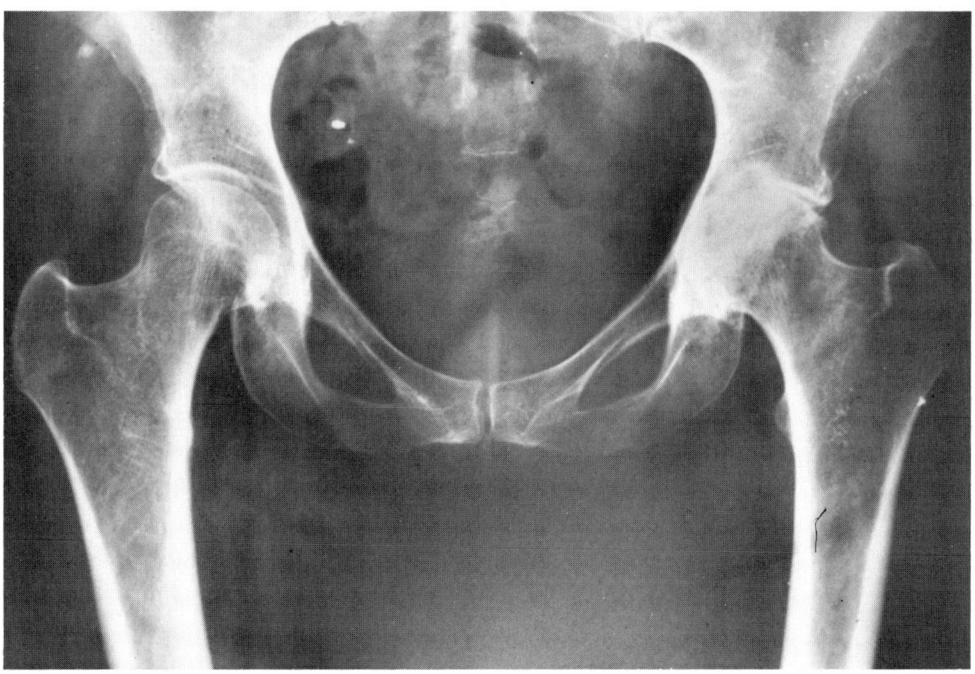

FIG 12–26.
A 73-year-old woman with rheumatoid arthritis affecting the left hip.

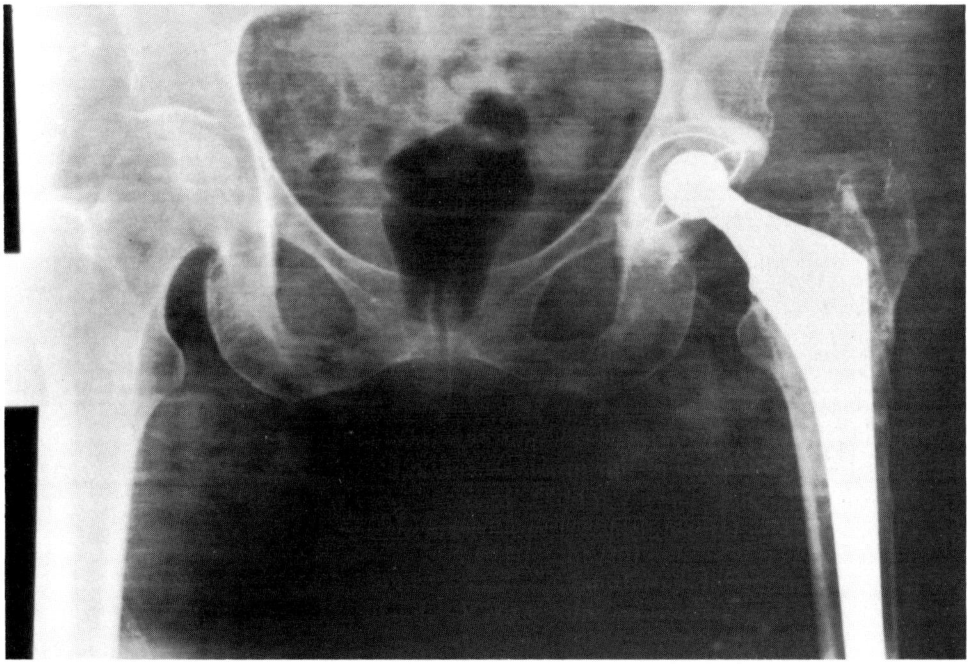

FIG 12–27.
Patient treated with a noncemented femoral component.

expected to facilitate the conduction of living bone ingrowth and interdigitation with the prosthesis.

Microstructured or porous-ingrowth prostheses have to date received the most extensive use. Controversy abounds concerning how much and what type of surface provides optimal fixation. Most surgeons agree, however, that good bone quality and proper prosthetic fit are prerequisites for success of these implants since the growth of bony interdigitation appears to require intimate contact without motion at the interface. Patients meeting indications for use of an uncemented implant include those at high risk for loosening of a cemented implant (i.e., young, active, heavy) who have good bone quality regardless of arthritic etiology.

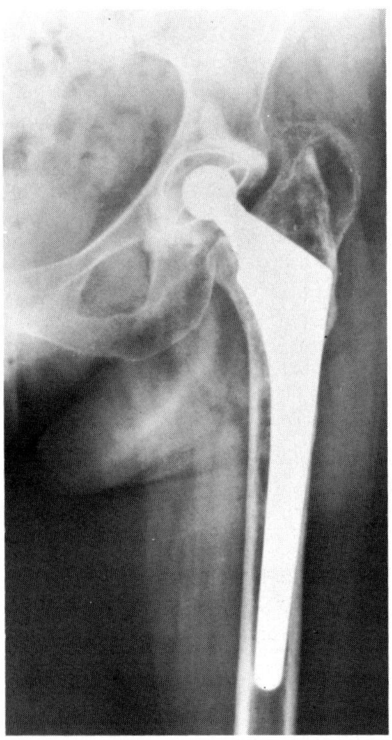

FIG 12–28.
Marked femoral component subsidence at 6-month postoperative examination.

The performance of uncemented acetabular fixation has thus far been excellent in a wide range of patients. Uncemented fixation of the femoral component has remained problematic, however, with persistent thigh pain presenting in up to 15% to 30% of patients[22, 24] (Figs 12–26, 12–27, and 12–28). Based on the assumption that the performance of uncemented sockets will remain good in the long term and the knowledge that modern cementing technique has significantly improved the durability of cemented stem fixation, the use of a "hybrid" arthroplasty consisting of an uncemented acetabular component and a cemented femoral component has become popular.[34]

REFERENCES

1. Albright JA, Albright JP, Ogden JA: Synovectomy of the hip in juvenile rheumatoid arthritis. *Clin Orthop* 1975; 106:48–55.
2. Almasbakk K, Rosyland P: Does indomethacin (IMC)

prevent postoperative ectopic ossification in total hip replacement? *Acta Orthop Scand* 1977; 48:556.
3. Ayers DC, Evarts C McC, Parkinson, JR: The prevention of heterotopic ossification in high risk patients by low dose radiation therapy following total hip arthroplasty. *J Bone Joint Surg [Am]* 1986; 68:1423–1430.
4. Beckenbaugh RD, Ilstrup DM: Total hip arthroplasty: A review of three hundred and thirty-three cases with long follow-up. *J Bone Joint Surg [Am]* 1978; 60:306–313.
5. Bergqvist D, Carlsson AS, Ericsson BF: Vascular complications after total hip arthroplasty. *Acta Orthop Scand* 1983; 54:157–163.
6. Bierbaum BE, Pomeroy DL, Berklacich FM: Late complications of total hip replacement, in Steinberg ME (ed): *The Hip and Its Disorders.* Philadelphia, WB Saunders Co, 1991, pp 1061–1096.
7. Bisla RS, Inglis AE, Ranawat CS: Joint replacement surgery in patients under thirty. *J Bone Joint Surg [Am]* 1976; 58:1098–1104.
8. Bisla RS, Ranawat CS, Inglis AE: Total hip replacement in ankylosing spondylitis with involvement of the hip. *J Bone Joint Surg [Am]* 1976; 58:233–238.
9. Boardman KP, Bocco F, Charnley J: An evaluation of methods of trochanteric fixation using 3 wires in the Charnley low friction arthroplasty. *Clin Orthop* 1978; 132:31–38.
10. Cassidy JT, Petty RE: *Textbook of Pediatric Rheumatology.* New York, Churchill Livingstone Inc, 1990.
11. Charnley J: Arthroplasty of the hip. A new operation. *Lancet* 1961; 1:1129.
12. Charnley J: The long term results of low-friction arthroplasty of the hip performed as a primary intervention. *J Bone Joint Surg [Br]* 1972; 54:61–76.
13. Charnley J: *Low Friction Arthroplasty of the Hip: Theory and Practice.* Berlin, Springer-Verlag, 1979.
14. Charnley J: Long term results of low friction arthroplasty, in Nelson JP (ed): *The Hip: Proceedings of the Tenth Open Scientific Meeting of the Hip Society, 1982.* St Louis, Mosby–Year Book, Inc, 1982, pp 42–49.
15. Charnley J, Cupic Z: 9 and 10 year results of low friction arthroplasty of the hip. *Clin Orthop* 1973; 95:9–25.
16. Collis DK: Long-term radiographic follow-up of total hip replacements. in Nelson JP (ed): *The Hip: Proceedings of the Tenth Open Scientific Meeting of the Hip Society, 1982.* St Louis, Mosby–Year Book, Inc, 1982, pp 1–26.
17. Colville J, Raunio P: Total hip replacement in juvenile rheumatoid arthritis. *Acta Orthop Scand* 1979; 50:197–203.
18. Coventry MB, Stauffer RN: Long-term results of total hip arthroplasty. in Nelson JP (ed): *The Hip: Proceedings of the Tenth Open Scientific Meeting of the Hip Society, 1982.* St Louis, Mosby–Year Book, Inc, 1982, pp 34–41.
19. Davies JP, Harris WH: Optimization and comparison of three vacuum mixing systems for porosity reduction of Simplex P cement. *Clin Orthop* 1990; 254:261–269.
20. Davies JP, O'Connor DO, Burke DW, et al: The effect of centrifugation on the fatigue life of bone cement in the presence of surface irregularities. *Clin Orthop* 1988; 229:156–161.
21. Eftekhar NS, Stinchfield FE: Experience with low friction arthroplasty: A statistical review of early results and complications. *Clin Orthop* 1973; 95:60–68.
22. Engh CA, Bobyn JD: Results of porous-coated hip replacement using the AML prosthesis, in Fitzgerald R Jr, (ed): *Non-Cemented Total Hip Arthroplasty.* New York, Raven Press, 1988, pp 393–406.
23. Fitzgerald RH Jr (ed): *Non-Cemented Total Hip Arthroplasty,* New York, Raven Press, 1988.
24. Galante JO: Clinical results with the HGP cementless total hip prosthesis, in Fitzgerald R Jr (ed): *Non-Cemented Total Hip Arthroplasty,* New York, Raven Press, 1988, pp 427–431.
25. Girdlestone GR: Acute pyogenic arthritis of the hip. An operation giving free access and effective drainage. *Lancet* 1943; 1:419.
26. Gschwend N: *Surgical Treatment of Rheumatoid Arthritis.* Philadelphia, WB Saunders Co, 1980.
27. Gustilo RB, Burnham WH: Long-term results of total hip arthroplasty in young patients, in Nelson JP (ed): *The Hip: Proceedings of the Tenth Open Scientific Meeting of the Hip Society, 1982.* St Louis, Mosby–Year Book, Inc, 1982, pp 27–33.
28. Hubbard MJS: The measurement of progression in protrusio acetabuli. *AJR* 1969; 106:506–508.
29. Julkunen H: Rheumatoid spondylitis. Clinical and laboratory study of 149 cases compared with 182 cases of rheumatoid arthritis. *Acta Rheum Scand Suppl* 1962; 4.
30. Kakkar VV, Fok PJ, Murray WJ, et al: Heparin and dihydroergotamine prophylaxis against thromboembolism after hip arthroplasty. *J Bone Joint Surg [Br]* 1985; 67:538–542.
31. Lachiewicz PF, McCaskill B, Inglis A, et al: Total hip arthroplasty in juvenile rheumatoid arthritis: Two- to eleven-year results. *J Bone Joint Surg [Am]* 1986; 68:502–508.
32. Lehtimäki MY, Kaarela K, Hämäläinen MMJ: Incidence of hip involvement and need for total hip replacement in rheumatoid arthritis. An eight-year follow-up study. *Scand J Rheumatol* 1986; 15:387–391.
33. Leonard DG, O'Duffy JD, Rogers RS III: A prospective evaluation of psoriatic arthritis in patients hospitalized for psoriasis. *Mayo Clin Proc* 1978; 53:511–518.
34. Maloney WJ, Harris WH: Comparison of a hybrid with an uncemented total hip replacement. *J Bone Joint Surg [Am]* 1990; 72:1349–1352.
35. McCollum DE, Nunley JA, Harrelson JM: Bone-grafting in total hip replacement for acetabular protrusion. *J Bone Joint Surg [Am]* 1980; 62:1065–1073.
36. Moore AT: Metal hip joint: A new self-locking Vitallium prosthesis. *South Med J* 1952; 45:1015.

37. Müller ME: Intertrochanteric osteotomy in the treatment of the arthritic hip joint, in Tronzo RG (ed): *Surgery of the Hip Joint.* Philadelphia, Lea & Febiger, 1973.
38. Murray WR, Van Meter JW: Surface replacement hip arthroplasty: Results of the first seventy-four consecutive cases at the University of California, San Francisco, in Nelson JP (ed): *The Hip: Proceedings of the Tenth Open Scientific Meeting of the Hip Society, 1982.* St Louis, Mosby–Year Book, Inc, 1982, pp 156–160.
39. Nachbur B, Meyer RP, Verkkala K, et al: The mechanisms of severe arterial injury in surgery of the hip joint. *Clin Orthop* 1979; 141:122–133.
40. Paiement G, Wessinger SJ, Waltman AC, et al: Low dose warfarin versus external pneumatic compression for prophylaxis against venous thromboembolism following total hip replacement. *J Arthroplasty* 1987; 2:22–26.
41. Paiement GD, Beisaw NE, Harris WH, et al: Advances in prevention of venous thrombembolic disease after hip and knee surgery. *Orthop Rev* 1989; 18(suppl):1–20.
42. Parkinson JB, Evarts C McC, Hubbard LF: Radiation therapy in the prevention of heterotopic ossification after total hip arthroplasty, in Nelson JP (ed): *The Hip: Proceedings of the Tenth Open Scientific Meeting of the Hip Society, 1982.* St Louis, Mosby–Year Book, Inc, 1982, pp 211–227.
43. Penman HG, Ring PA: Osteosarcoma in association with total hip replacement. *J Bone Joint Surg [Br]* 1984; 66:632–634.
44. Poss R, Maloney JP, Ewald FC, et al: Six to 11-year results of total hip arthroplasty in rheumatoid arthritis. *Clin Orthop* 1984; 182:109–116.
45. Ranawat CS: Rheumatoid arthritis of the cervical spine. *J Neurosurg* 1984; 3:3340–3343.
46. Ranawat CS: Surgery for rheumatoid arthritis: Lower limb, surgery of the hip. *Curr Orthop* 1989; 3:146–149.
47. Ranawat CS, Beaver WB, Sharrock NE, et al: Effect of hypotensive epidural anesthesia on acetabular cement-bone fixation in total hip arthroplasty. *J Bone Joint Surg [Br]* 1991; 73:779–782.
48. Ranawat CS, Cornell CN: The impact of modern cement techniques on acetabular fixation in cemented total hip replacement. *J Arthroplasty* 1986; 1:197–202.
49. Ranawat CS, Dorr LD, Inglis AE: Total hip arthroplasty in protrusio acetabuli of rheumatoid arthritis. *J Bone Joint Surg [Am]* 1980; 62:1059–1065.
50. Ranawat CS, Figgie MP: Early complications of total hip replacement, in Steinberg ME (ed): *The Hip and Its Disorders.* Philadelphia, WB Saunders Co, 1991. pp 1042–1060.
51. Ranawat CS, Zahn MG: Role of bone grafting in correction of protrusio acetabuli by total hip arthroplasty. *J Arthroplasty* 1986; 1:131–137.
52. Ritter MA, Gioe T: The effect of indomethacin on pararticular ossification following total hip arthroplasty. *Clin Orthop* 1982; 167:113–117.
53. Ritter MA, Gioe TJ: Conventional versus resurfacing total hip arthroplasty. A long-term prospective study of concomitant bilateral implantation of prostheses. *J Bone Joint Surg [Am]* 1986; 68:216–225.
54. Ritter MA, Gioe TJ, Stringer EA: Functional significance of non-union of the greater trochanter. *Clin Orthop* 1982; 159:177–182.
55. Rooker GD, Wilkinson JD: Metal sensitivity in patients undergoing hip replacement. *J Bone Joint Surg [Br]* 1980; 62:502–505.
56. Ruddlesdin C, Ansell BM, Arden GP, et al: Total hip replacement in children with juvenile chronic arthritis. *J Bone Joint Surg [Br]* 1986; 68:218–222.
57. Scott RD, Sledge CB: Juvenile rheumatoid arthritis, in Steinberg ME (ed): *The Hip and its Disorders.* Philadelphia, WB Saunders Co, 1991, pp 470–482.
58. Shore A, Ansell BM: Juvenile psoriatic arthritis: An analysis of 60 cases. *J Pediatr* 1982; 100:529–535.
59. Silski JM, Scott RD: Obturator nerve palsy resulting from intrapelvic extrusion of cement during total hip arthroplasty. *J Bone Joint Surg [Am]* 1985; 67:1225–1228.
60. Sledge CB: Surgery for rheumatoid arthritis. *Curr Orthop* 1989; 3:1–3.
61. Smith-Petersen MN: Arthroplasty of the hip. A new method. *J Bone Joint Surg [Am]* 1939; 21:268–288.
62. Sotelo-Garza A, Charnley J: The results of Charnley arthroplasty of the hip performed for protrusio acetabuli. *Clin Orthop* 1978; 132:12–18.
63. Steinberg M: Hip surgery, in Utsinger PD, et al, (eds): *Rheumatoid Arthritis.* Philadelphia, JB Lippincott Co, 1985.
64. Swann M: Malignant soft tissue tumor at the site of a total hip replacement. *J Bone Joint Surg [Br]* 1984; 66:629–631.
65. Unger AS, Inglis AE, Ranawat CS, et al: Total hip arthroplasty in rheumatoid arthritis: A long-term follow-up study. *J Arthroplasty* 1987; 2:191–197.
66. Wilkinson M, Bywaters EGL: Clinical features and the course of ankylosing spondylitis as seen in followup of 222 hospital referred cases. *Ann Rheum Dis* 1958; 17:209–228.
67. Wroblewski BM, Del Sel HJ: Urethral instrumentation and deep sepsis in total hip replacement. *Clin Orthop* 1980; 146:209–212.

CHAPTER 13

The Knee

Thomas P. Sculco, M.D.

INTRODUCTION

Rheumatoid arthritis, when longstanding, will affect the knee joint in 90% of patients.[15] When involvement of the knee joint is severe, ambulatory capacity is greatly impaired as a result of pain, joint stiffness, and angular deformity. The disease involvement tends to be symmetric. In more advanced cases with deformity, however, bone loss and soft tissue contracture may be quite severe. Conservative measures tend to be ineffective once cartilage loss becomes progressive. Arthroscopic synovectomy may be useful as an invasive procedure in the early disease presentation. Total joint arthroplasty remains the treatment of choice in patients with advanced knee joint destruction. Complications after joint replacement surgery, particularly infection, tend to be catastrophic and jeopardize the survival of the arthroplasty.

PATIENT PRESENTATION

As in other joint involvement in rheumatoid arthritis, a spectrum of disease severity exists. Early manifestations of knee joint involvement may be pain and swelling without evidence of cartilage damage. Although symmetry tends to be more common in rheumatoid patients, a monarticular initial presentation of rheumatoid arthritis in the knee joint can be encountered. The pattern of the disease varies considerably and in some patients the knee joint involvement may be mild with recurrent effusions and low-grade synovitis. In a more active disease state chronic synovitis advances to cartilage destruction and progressive pain with impaired ambulation.

In a subset of patients a proliferative synovitis with marked effusions may persist for extended periods and produce a mechanical dysfunction of the knee with chronic pain. Examination in these patients demonstrates a boggy swollen knee joint with limitation of knee flexion due to the bulk of the intraarticular fluid and synovium. A large popliteal cyst is frequently present which may extend into the proximal calf area. On occasion rupture of these popliteal cysts may occur and produce marked swelling and pain in the calf. Differential diagnosis in these patients may be unclear as calf pain is quite marked, as is calf swelling. Venograms will be negative for clot formation in the deep venous system and magnetic resonance imaging (MRI) will generally demonstrate soft tissue extension of synovial tissue from the posterior knee joint to the upper calf.

As knee joint destruction becomes more severe, deformity progresses and soft tissue contractures become more fixed. Range of motion becomes limited and painful and flexion contractures occur. Valgus deformity with or without a flexion contracture is common (Fig 13–1). External rotation both at the knee joint and hindfoot can be encountered in combination with valgus-flexion deformity. These biplane and triplane deformities, because of varying amounts of soft tissue contractures in different planes, are the most difficult to correct with knee arthroplasty. The technical aspects of these reconstructions are discussed later in this chapter.

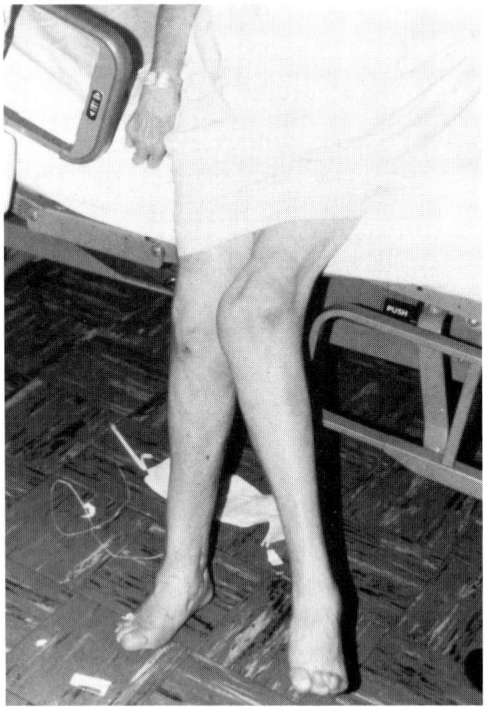

FIG 13–1.
Flexion-valgus deformity of the left knee is 65-year-old woman with rheumatoid arthritis.

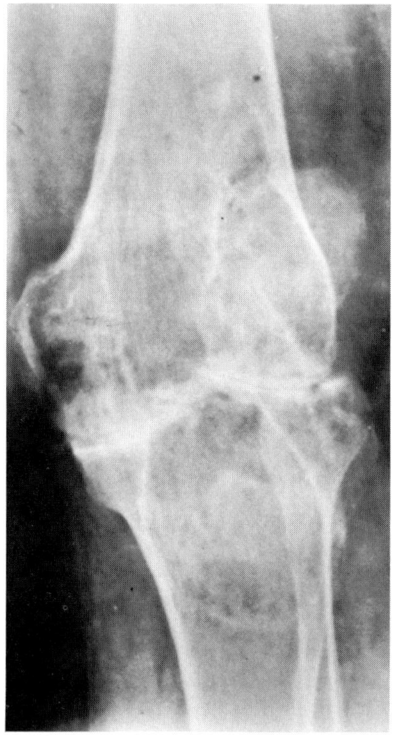

FIG 13–2.
Osteopenia and large tibial cyst in rheumatoid arthritis of the knee joint.

The rheumatoid patient presenting with knee involvement may also demonstrate local soft tissue problems which must be carefully evaluated preoperatively, particularly if surgery is contemplated. Garner et al.[17] demonstrated a twofold increase in wound healing in a controlled series of rheumatoid arthritis patients compared with nonrheumatoid patients.

Because many patients with rheumatoid arthritis are taking immunosuppressive and corticosteroid medication, and perhaps owing to the disease process itself, subcutaneous tissue about the knee joint will often become atrophic with associated changes of thinning and fragility to the epithelium. Vasculitis seen in these patients may further impair the blood flow to the extremities. The limbs may demonstrate ecchymoses beneath this deficient skin.

Aside from the knee joint abnormality, patients with rheumatoid arthritis presenting with knee joint disease will often have significant joint involvement elsewhere. This must be carefully evaluated to determine the order of surgical treatment for the patient with multiple diseased joints. Upper extremity disease will impair the patient's ability to use external devices after knee replacement surgery. Occupational therapy and physical therapy can be extremely helpful in suggesting assistive devices to improve the patient's prospects for rehabilitation after knee surgery. Other lower extremity involvement should be treated during the same hospital stay if significant disability and pain are directly related thereto. Complex lower extremity surgery will not be successful unless all dysfunctional joints are treated.

Most information concerning the extent of joint destruction can be obtained with plain knee radiographs, a standing anteroposterior, as well as lateral, and patellar views are recommended. Radiographic evaluation of the knee joint in rheumatoid arthritis varies depending upon the severity of the disease involvement. Early changes consist of periarticular osteopenia, subligamentous erosions, and global joint space narrowing. As the disease progresses the joint space narrowing becomes more marked, cystic changes are seen within bone, and osteopenia increases (Fig 13–2). Osteophyte formation, marked subchondral sclerosis, and loose bodies tend to be uncommon in the rheumatoid knee joint although these changes may be present in the patient with longstanding disease in whom there is an element of degenerative joint disease concomitant with their rheumatoid arthritis. Angular deformity, when present, is often associated with a bone deficit, most frequently on the tibial plateau on the concave side of the deformity.

CONSERVATIVE TREATMENT

The nonsurgical treatment of rheumatoid arthritis affecting the knee joint depends on the severity of the disease. In early cases nonsteroidal anti-inflammatory medication is the treatment of choice. In patients with more severe disease activity who are unresponsive to nonsteroidal anti-inflammatory medications, the rheumatologist may place the patient on disease-modifying drugs (e.g., gold salts) or immunosuppressive drugs. Intraarticular corticosteroid injections are also beneficial early in the disease when synovitis is marked. Braces do little to control angular deformity and generally are not particularly helpful in rheumatoid arthritic involvement of the knee.

Physical therapy can be of assistance when the degree of knee pain is mild. Quadriceps and hamstring exercises should be encouraged to maintain muscle function about the knee joint. Strengthening exercises to incorporate muscle groups of the entire lower extremity are not only useful when concentrated on the affected limb but also in exercising the contralateral limb. Range-of-motion exercises should be encouraged. The objectives of a physical therapy program are to maintain strength and mobility and this may become less possible as pain increases with joint motion and weightbearing. Local modalities such as ultrasound, cryotherapy, and diathermy are transiently helpful. With the rapid deterioration in function and general well-being that occurs in the rheumatoid patient once ambulatory ability is lost, the therapist should particularly stress gait training and assistive devices as necessary to maintain walking ability.

RADIATION SYNOVECTOMY

Radiation synovectomy, which qualifies as a nonsurgical measure although hardly conservative, may be utilized in patients with proliferative synovial disease and relatively preserved joint space. The indications are basically similar to those for a surgical synovectomy. Results of treatment have been mixed. Sledge et al.[60] reported 2-year follow-up results in 59 patients from an overall experience of 111 patients. Intraarticular dysprosium 165–ferric hydroxide macroaggregates were used to deliver a dose of 270 mCi. Dysprosium-165 has the advantage of having a 2.3-hour half-life and by combining it with a ferric macroaggregate, leakage of radiation from the joint is markedly reduced. When compared with gold-198 and yttrium-90 the half-life is 25 times shorter. Total body radiation was 0.3 rad with dysprosium-165 and liver levels were 3.2 rad compared to liver levels of 5.4 to 40 rad with gold-198 and yttrium-90.

Results were not dissimilar to those of surgical synovectomy with patients with early radiographic staging doing better than patients with more advanced radiographic destruction. Nineteen of 25 patients with stage I radiographic disease had good results whereas 20 of 34 patients with stage II radiographic disease had good results. Untoward local or systemic effects from the injection were not seen. No allergic reactions were reported. The main disadvantage of dysprosium-165 is that, owing to its short half-life, the hospital must be near the facility preparing the isotope.

SURGICAL TREATMENT

In the past a myriad of procedures were tried in the rheumatoid patient to maintain knee function. Osteotomy, which is useful in the treatment of knee osteoarthritis if limited to a single knee compartment, is not recommended in rheumatoid arthritis because of the diffuse nature of the joint involvement.

Open synovectomy was the traditional procedure of choice for patients with intractable synovitis despite medical treatment in whom synovial tissue was exuberant and the joint space was relatively spared. Open synovectomy requires a radical knee joint debridement and meniscal excision has also been performed as part of the procedure. Recovery tends to be slow with particularly prolonged knee stiffness and swelling. The procedure may be performed through two parapatellar incisions made in the midaxial plane of the knee joint to allow posterior compartment debridement. More commonly at this time, if open synovectomy is performed, a medial parapatellar or straight incision is used (Fig 13–3).

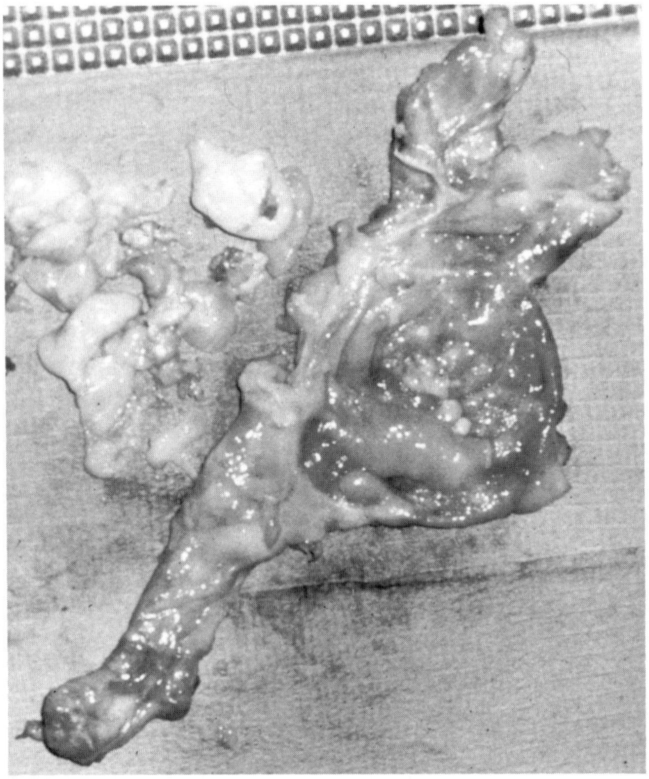

FIG 13–3.
Gross specimen of removed synovium by open synovectomy from the knee joint.

The literature is replete with reports of results of knee synovectomy in the rheumatoid patient, the consensus being that results in the short term are good but that results deteriorate as time passes and the disease process continues.[18, 27, 33, 46] In a recent long-term retrospective evaluation by Doets et al.,[10] results were quite disappointing. Eighty-three open knee synovectomies in 65 patients were followed for an average of 7 years. Most patients had stage II or stage III disease at the time of the synovectomy. In the stage II patients there were 18 good results, 14 fair, 8 poor, and 22 knees required reoperation. In the stage III patients there was only 1 good result in 16 knees and 11 of the 16 required total knee arthroplasty or double osteotomy.

Tillman[65] has argued that the beneficial results from synovectomy are related to the technique rather than the procedure itself. He has demonstrated only an 11% recurrence rate when subtotal (anterior and posterior incisions) synovectomy is performed compared with 25% recurrent synovitis when a partial synovectomy is performed, with a follow-up of about 7 years.

ARTHROSCOPIC SYNOVECTOMY

Arthroscopic knee synovectomy is the recommended method of removal of synovial tissue in the selected rheumatoid patient. The ideal patient for the procedure has active synovial disease which has remained unmitigated in the face of medical management. Loss of hyaline cartilage should be mild. Benefit from the procedure is multifold: (1) pain relief and improved range of motion results from the debulking of the overgrown synovium, (2) mechanical problems are removed by debriding of meniscal tags and other joint debris, and (3) the extensive lavage that occurs with the arthroscopic procedure may further remove debris and crystalline and immune complexes.

Arthroscopic synovectomy in the patient with significant synovial hypertrophy is tedious in that synovial tissue is present throughout the joint in copious amounts. This will interfere with arthroscopic visualization as the joint is initially entered. All compartments of the knee joint must be explored and debrided. A medial suprapatellar portal is used for the irrigation and the knee joint is distended. A medial and lateral portal is made to introduce the camera and instruments. Rotatory shavers tend to be most useful in the removal of synovial tissue and the camera and shaver portals may be switched so that all portals may be used to remove synovial tissue. If needed to more thoroughly remove synovial tissue, lateral suprapatellar and posterior medial or lateral portals may be used. Although all compartments should be debrided, most of the synovial tissue will extend into the suprapatellar pouch and care should be taken to fully decompress this area extensively.

Arthroscopic synovectomy is usually performed on an ambulatory basis. If the procedure is prolonged and multicompartmental, a suction drain should be used and the patient admitted to the hospital overnight. The procedure is performed without the use of a tourniquet and with epinephrine added to the irrigating saline solution. Epidural anesthesia is most commonly used. Portals are closed with subcuticular polyglycolic sutures and a Jones-type supportive dressing is applied. Protective weightbearing is begun with crutches and rapid progress to a cane is allowed pending the subsidence of pain and swelling. Because patients undergoing arthroscopic synovectomy will often have significant swelling, ice should be maintained on the knee for the first several days. The patient should be seen within a week of the arthroscopic synovectomy for reevaluation, and knee flexion is encouraged at this time. As knee joint swelling subsides, range-of-motion and strengthening exercises are started. Weightbearing progresses gradually as tolerated.

Results with knee joint arthroscopic synovectomy in rheumatoid arthritis have been encouraging in the short term. In a series of 16 synovectomies in ten rheumatoid patients whom I have followed for 2 years there has been one failure who will require total knee replacement and one patient with recurrent synovitis in one knee. Patients have been primarily stage I radiographically. Relief of pain has been excellent in the short term. There has been one significant hemarthrosis which resolved without further surgical treatment. Matsui et al.[37] have reported on a series of open and arthroscopic synovectomies. In the 41 arthroscopic procedures there were 83% good results at 3 years which deteriorated to 46% at 8-year follow-up. In the 26 patients undergoing open synovectomy there were 81% good results at 3 years and only 40% good results at 8 years. The authors support the use of arthroscopic synovectomy in patients with early radiographic disease and document the ease of recovery and reduced morbidity with the arthroscopic method. There is little postoperative pain, return to work is rapid, both knees can be operated upon at the same time, and range of motion rapidly returns.

The theoretical advantage of reducing lysozymal enzymes and collagenases by lessening the amount of inflammatory tissue in the joint is brought into question by the work of Myllyla et al.[40] They demonstrated only a minor reduction in lysosomal enzymes after synovectomy and no change in the amount of complement within the joint. Still, the main benefit from the procedure probably is relief of pain in the short term from the debulking of hypertrophic synovial tissue and the debridement of mechanically unsound meniscal and cartilage debris. As an arthroscopic procedure with reduced morbidity it is a useful intervention for intractable knee joint synovial disease which is its early yet active phase.

TOTAL KNEE ARTHROPLASTY

Total knee arthroplasty is the procedure of choice in patients that have significant joint destruction with or without angular deformity. The main clinical criteria for total knee arthroplasty are pain and difficulty in walking in patients in whom nonsurgical treatment or lesser surgical procedures have not been successful. In patients in whom there is advanced bilateral knee joint involvement, bilateral total knee arthroplasty is recommended. At The Hospital for Special Surgery in New York City, when both knees are to be replaced, the procedures are generally performed at one operative setting. Autologous blood is used in all patients although the rheumatoid patient is often anemic and may not be able to supply the 2 units of blood that are routinely collected preoperatively. At this time we are prospectively evaluating the use of recombinant erythropoietin as a bone marrow stimulant in patients who are unable to give their own blood. A 10-day course of erythropoietin is being administered.

Epidural anesthesia is used routinely for unilateral or bilateral knee replacement surgery. This is particularly useful in the patient with rheumatoid arthritis in that manipulation of the cervical spine is not necessary as it is in general anesthesia when intubation is required. The epidural catheter is commonly left in place postoperatively and further anesthetic or analgesics may be administered through the catheter to relieve pain during the first several days postoperatively. In patients in whom analgesics are administered, patient-controlled systems are used to allow the patient to administer his or her own medication. Additionally, reduction in the incidence of deep venous thrombosis has been demonstrated in patients undergoing epidural anesthesia.[42, 58]

Patients with rheumatoid arthritis may have multiple associated medical problems related to or distinct from their systemic disease and therefore rheumatologic-medical consultation is routinely obtained preoperatively. As discussed in Chapter 4, it is useful and extremely beneficial to the overall care and rehabilitation of rheumatoid patients if physical and occupational therapists, as well as nursing and social services, are able to examine and interview the patient preoperatively. This tends to allay anxiety and better inform the patient of the postoperative recovery and rehabilitation that will follow his or her surgery.

ORTHOPAEDIC EVALUATION

After medical clearance to proceed with knee replacement surgery has been obtained, orthopaedic evaluation should be directed at the entire musculoskeletal system, not just the affected knee joint. A careful examination of all upper extremity and lower extremity joints should be performed and special attention given to the cervical spine.

The neurovascular status of the lower extremities should be assessed and if abnormality is noted in circulatory function, vascular consultation should be obtained. If hyperreflexia is noted or other features of long tract dysfunction, further radiographic evaluation of the cervical spine including flexion-extension films and MRI, if indicated, should be obtained. Additionally, neurologic consultation is indicated if a question remains as to whether a possible cervical myelopathy exists.

THE KNEE JOINT

The degree of angular deformity must be considered preoperatively as this may influence the selection of the implant to be used during the replacement procedure (Fig 13–4,A and B). Specifically, if there is a severe biplane or triplane fixed deformity, the need for augmented implants may be necessary to produce a stable and corrected knee in all planes. The quality of the soft tissues about the knee should also be closely examined. If the skin is fragile and easily bruised, the surgeon may have difficulty with wound healing, which remains a major problem in the rheumatoid patient. The range of motion should also be noted, particularly if the knee joint is stiff in extension. In many of these patients it will be necessary to perform a quadricepsplasty to allow mobilization of the knee postoperatively.

External rotation deformities in association with valgus-flexion deformity are seen in patients with advanced rheumatoid arthritis. It is important preoperatively to note the degree of external rotation that will be correctable as part of the knee replacement surgery and the degree that is being contributed by the hip joint or (far more commonly) by the hindfoot. In patients with severe external rotation of the hindfoot it must be remembered that full correction at the knee joint should not be attempted. This will lead to excessive internal rotation of the knee implant, and major problems of the patellofemoral joint and its tracking may result. It is better to preserve the degree of external rotation at the hindfoot and correct this at a later date, either at the ankle or the associated hindfoot joint, or both.

OPERATIVE TECHNIQUE

Exposure

Exposure is not dissimilar to the standard approach to knee arthroplasty. A gentle medial parapatellar approach is preferred rather than a midline approach, as the amount of subcutaneous tissue tends to be greater when the incision is not placed in a straight line directly across the patella. There is also evidence that stresses on the incision are less when the incision is of the parapatellar type and this is of great importance in the rheumatoid patient in whom wounds and tissues are apt to delay in healing.[28] Care must be exercised throughout the procedure to prevent excess retraction or tension on skin edges and soft tissues (Fig 13–5). Skiving or the creation of multiple planes when cutting through subcutaneous tissue must be avoided. There should be no undermining of the subcutaneous tissue to create flaps for exposure. The line of incision should be directly to the joint without devascularizing the skin by unnecessary dissection.

In patients with severe contractures of the extensor mechanism and stiffness of the knee joint in the extended position, it may be impossible to mobilize the knee joint into flexion without avulsing the patellar tendon from its insertion into the tibia. This is a major problem as the fixation of the tendon back to its bony bed will require the use of metal staples, wire, or heavy nonabsorbable sutures. All present a problem as they are just beneath the skin and are an easy source of skin ulceration with contamination of the joint. Additionally, since the bone quality is poor in many of these patients, further avulsion may occur in the postoperative period with resultant weakness of the extensor mechanism and a lag on active extension. Therefore, a proximal V-Y quadricepsplasty[1, 7, 41, 57] should be performed (Fig 13–6,A–C). The quadriceps tendon can then be turned down distally for exposure and at the conclusion of the procedure a lengthening can be performed depending upon what is necessary to allow knee flexion. In my experience repairing the quadriceps with the knee in 30 to 40 degrees of flexion will allow knee

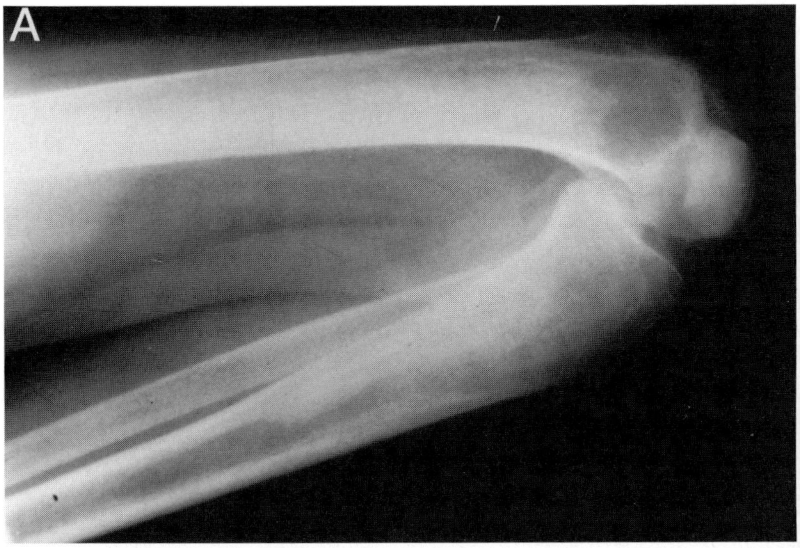

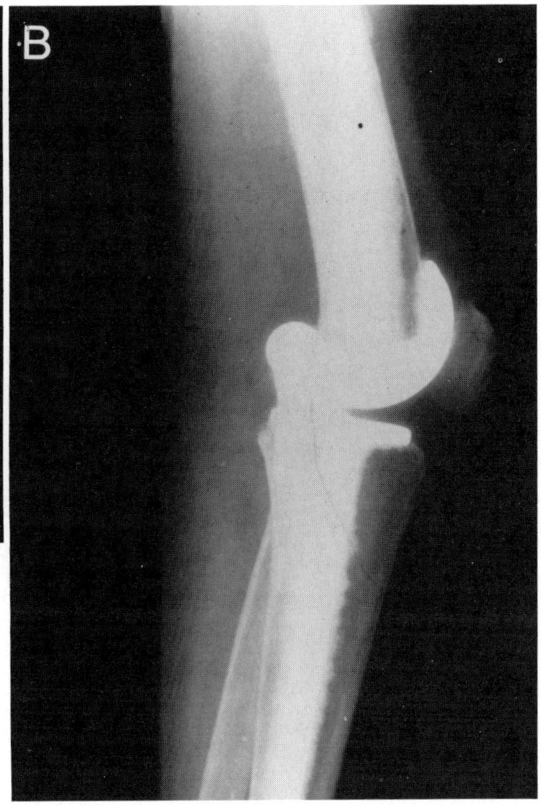

FIG 13–4.
A, a 26-year-old woman with 150-degree fixed flexion deformity. **B,** postoperative radiograph 8 years after GUEPAR replacement. Index procedure performed 1979. GUEPAR was used because of the marked bone resection required and the loss of collateral ligament support.

motion to approximate 75 to 80 degrees and an extensor lag, which may be present in the immediate postoperative period, will be gone at 3 to 6 months postoperatively. Postoperative rehabilitation is altered in these patients and a constant passive motion (CPM) machine is used, but only to allow 45 degrees of flexion for the first 7 to 10 days. At this point, further flexion is allowed, increasing by 5 degrees per day.

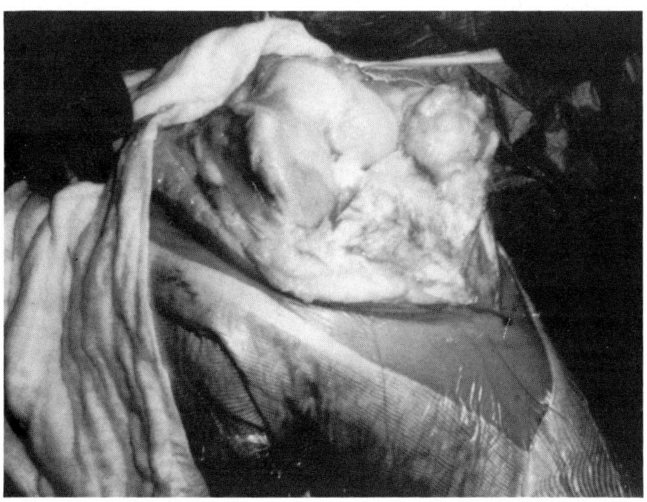

FIG 13–5.
Adequate knee joint exposure without undue tension on the skin incision.

Soft Tissue Balancing

The concepts of soft tissue balancing in the rheumatoid knee are the same as for knee joint deformity in the osteoarthritic patient. Since deformity may be quite severe in rheumatoid arthritis, especially the biplane and triplane deformity of valgus-flexion, and valgus-flexion with external rotation, it is important to review the management of these severely damaged knees.

The valgus knee deformity generally presents more complex soft tissue problems than the varus knee. In most of these deformities there exists a rotational component to the deformity and the patella often tracks laterally or is subluxed laterally because of the contracted lateral peripatellar soft tissues and the severely contracted patellofemoral ligament.

Initial exposure of the knee is similar to the varus knee with forward subluxation of the tibia being facilitated by periarticular soft tissue elevation around the proximal tibia. In the valgus knee the contracted soft tissues are on the concave side of the deformity, the lateral side. Therefore, the soft tissue release directed at the valgus deformity is performed

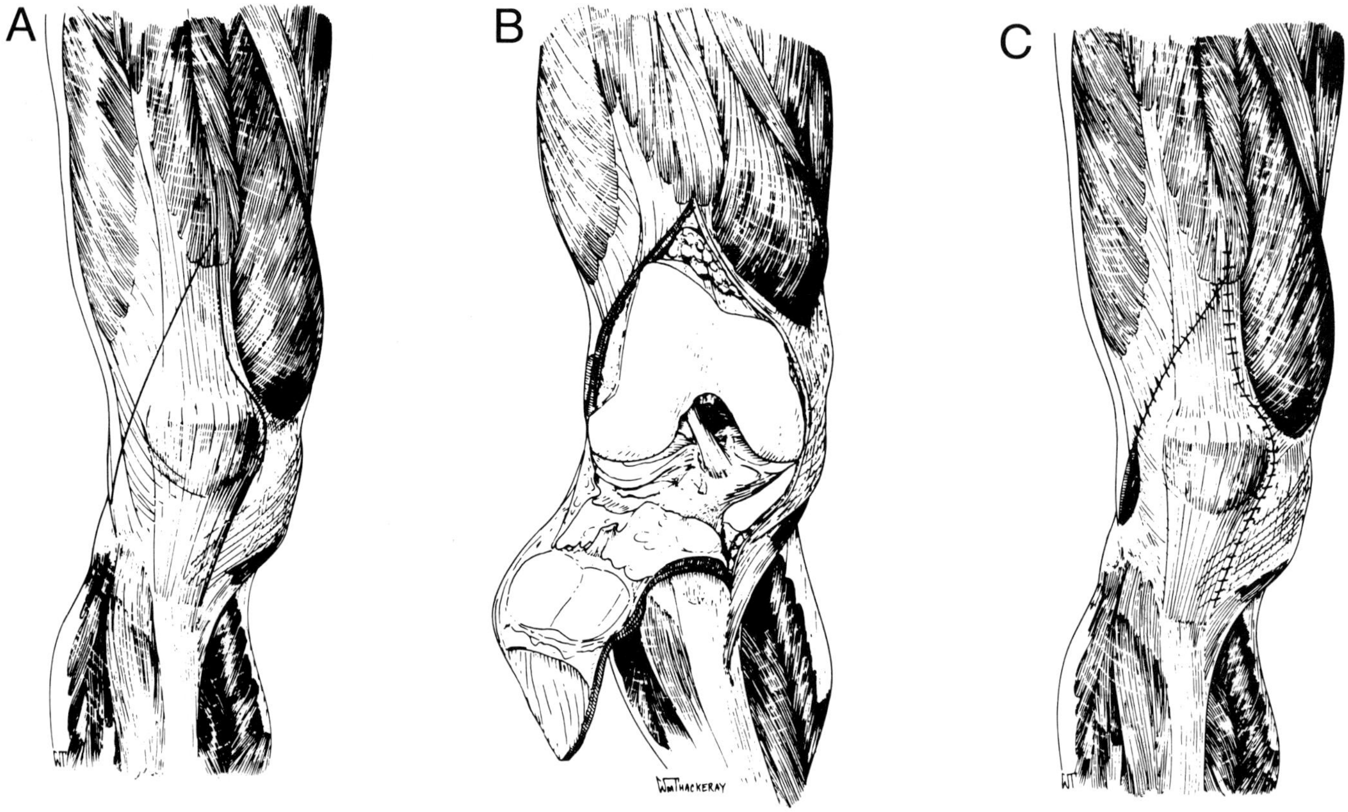

FIG 13–6.
A–C, the technique of V-Y quadricepsplasty for knee joint replacement in the knee that is stiff in an extended position with extensor mechanism contracture. (From Sculco TP: *Techn Orthop* 1986; 3:5–9. Used by permission.)

along the proximal tibial surface extending distally. All contracted soft tissues must be released from the upper tibia. The insertion of the patellar tendon may be elevated partially from its insertion into the tibia to allow better proximal exposure. As part of the valgus soft tissue release the insertion of the iliotibial band is released at its insertion into the tibia. More extensive dissection posterior along the tibial surface will be prevented by the presence of the fibular head.[56] In valgus deformity of less than 15 to 20 degrees, release along the tibial surface is adequate to achieve soft tissue symmetry across the joint.

In more severe valgus deformity, particularly when there are flexion and rotational components, soft tissue elevation and release must be extended to the lateral femur (Fig 13–7). This includes release of the origin of the lateral collateral ligament which may be dissected with a cautery and allowed to slide as a soft tissue sleeve. It is important to emphasize that these lateral soft tissues are not transected but are elevated in a subperiosteal manner from the bony origins. Essentially, they are then lengthened from their contracted state to more equally balance the lax soft tissues on the medial (convex) side of the

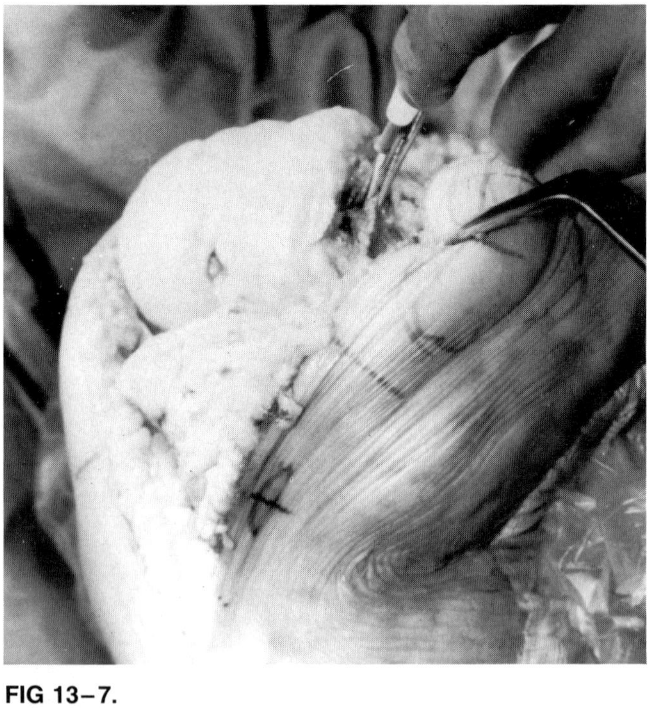

FIG 13–7.
Lateral collateral ligament subperiosteal release from femoral attachment in severe valgus deformity.

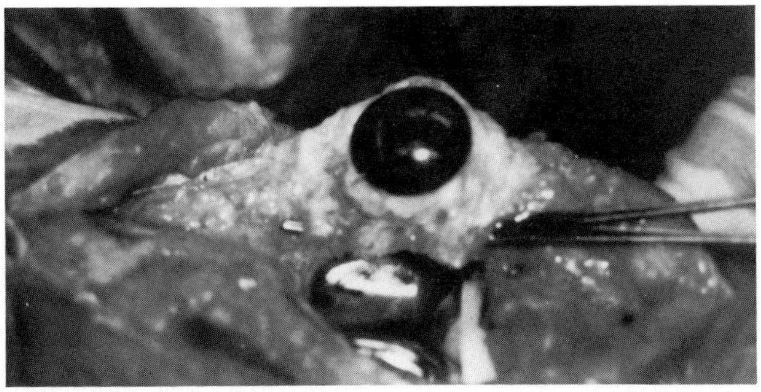

FIG 13–8.
Lateral retinacular release performed from inside the joint if patella tracks laterally or subluxes after replacement.

joint. If soft tissues remain contracted after tibial and femoral release, the iliotibial band should be released in a horizontal manner about 1 in. above the joint surface. The band can be palpated proximal to the knee joint by placing a varus stress on the knee. It is released sharply until the knee becomes more lax laterally to effect symmetry with the medial side of the joint. Release of the iliotibial band is generally the final component in the radical lateral release for the severely affected valgus knee.

In the valgus knee there is marked lateral retinacular contracture and shortening of the patellofemoral ligament. This tends to produce a lateral tilting or frank subluxation of the patella. This should be anticipated and a liberal lateral retinacular release of the patella should be performed as part of the initial exposure of the knee. This will facilitate eversion of the patella and improve patellar tracking. After trial implants have been inserted, a more extensive lateral release may be needed (Fig 13–8).

BIPLANE AND TRIPLANE DEFORMITY

The biplane and triplane deformities, i.e., those with angular and fixed deformities in more than one plane, are probably the most severe deformities confronted by the orthopaedic surgeon. Those most commonly encountered are the biplanar severe valgus-flexion deformity or the triplane deformity seen in juvenile rheumatoid arthritis and hemophilia of valgus-flexion–external rotation. Since these deformities exist in more than a single plane, asymmetry in soft tissue contracture and laxity exist in flexion-extension, in medial-lateral movement and rotation, and an attempt at release may lead to imbalances in various planes (Fig 13–9,A and B).

The basic surgical concept, as with less complex soft tissue contractures, is to balance the knee joint in all planes so that there is symmetric soft tissue tension across the joint. Because of the multiple nature of the contractures, the flexion or rotational de-

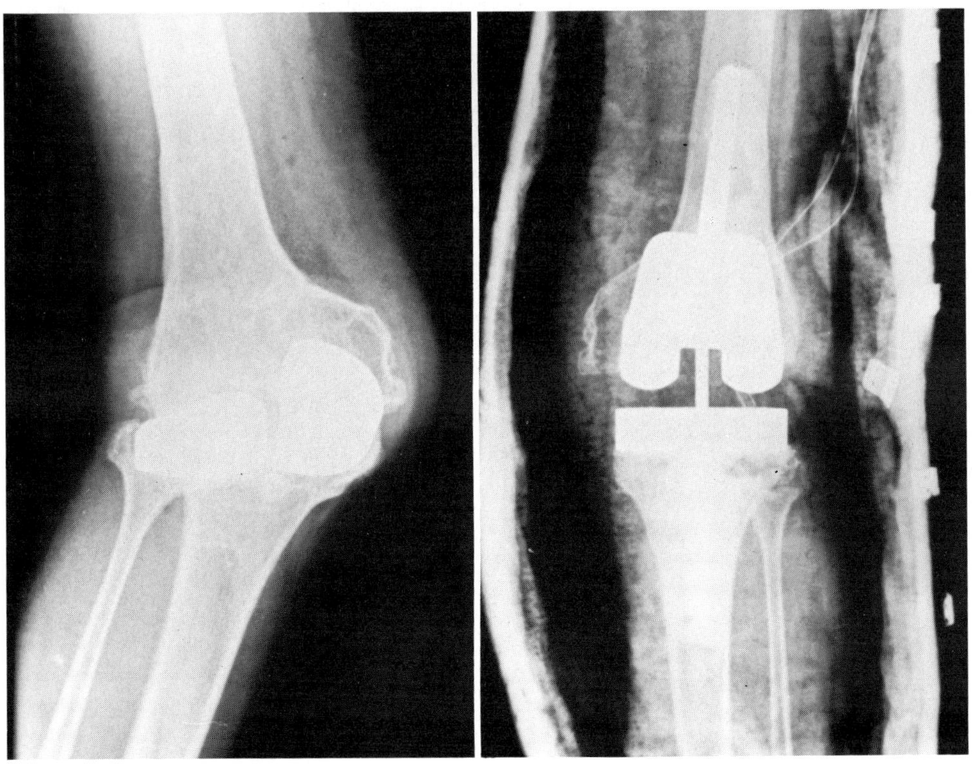

FIG 13–9.
A, a 53-year-old woman with failed McIntosh prostheses and valgus-flexion–external rotational deformity. **B,** postoperative radiograph of a total condylar III prosthesis used after radical soft tissue release.

formity may be greater than the angular deformity. The selection of implant must also be modified in these asymmetric knees. If the knee remains more unstable in flexion or extension after release, then an implant must be selected that has additional constraint or that augments areas of continued instability. An example of this is the knee that remains unstable in flexion but is well balanced in extension when a trial tibial implant of a particular size is used. Selecting a thicker tibial component to improve stability in flexion will prevent the knee from extending and leave the patient with a persistent flexion contracture. Therefore, in such a patient a posteriorly augmented femoral component, which may be of custom or modular design, must be available to allow stability of the knee in flexion without altering the extension gap (Fig 13–10,A–C).

Conversely, if the knee is stable in flexion with a particular tibial component but remains unstable in extension with a tendency to recurvatum, augmentation of the femoral implant must be performed to the distal femoral condylar surface. This will stabilize the knee in extension without altering the fit in flexion with the selected tibial implant (Fig 13–11,A–C).

In these more complex deformities there is often the need to be aggressive in effecting soft tissue symmetry. Instability may persist in one or another plane despite the use of a modular or custom implant and therefore more constrained devices may be necessary. The latter have an elevated tibial post which articulates with a deepened femoral box and provides additional medial-lateral and anteroposterior stability. Because of increased constraint in the implant there is a theoretical disadvantage that there will be increased shear and rotational stresses at the bone-cement interface and resultant early mechanical failure. Despite this, results with the total condylar III implant (Fig 13–12) for severe deformity and revision surgery has yielded good to excellent results in 77% of patients.[11, 55]

MANAGEMENT OF BONE DEFICITS

In patients with rheumatoid arthritis bone quality tends to be poor[30] and deformity may be severe. For this reason bone deficits may occur as angular deformity increases. Although there may be a bony deficit on the femoral condylar side of the joint, as a rule deficits are far more common on the tibial side. Bone

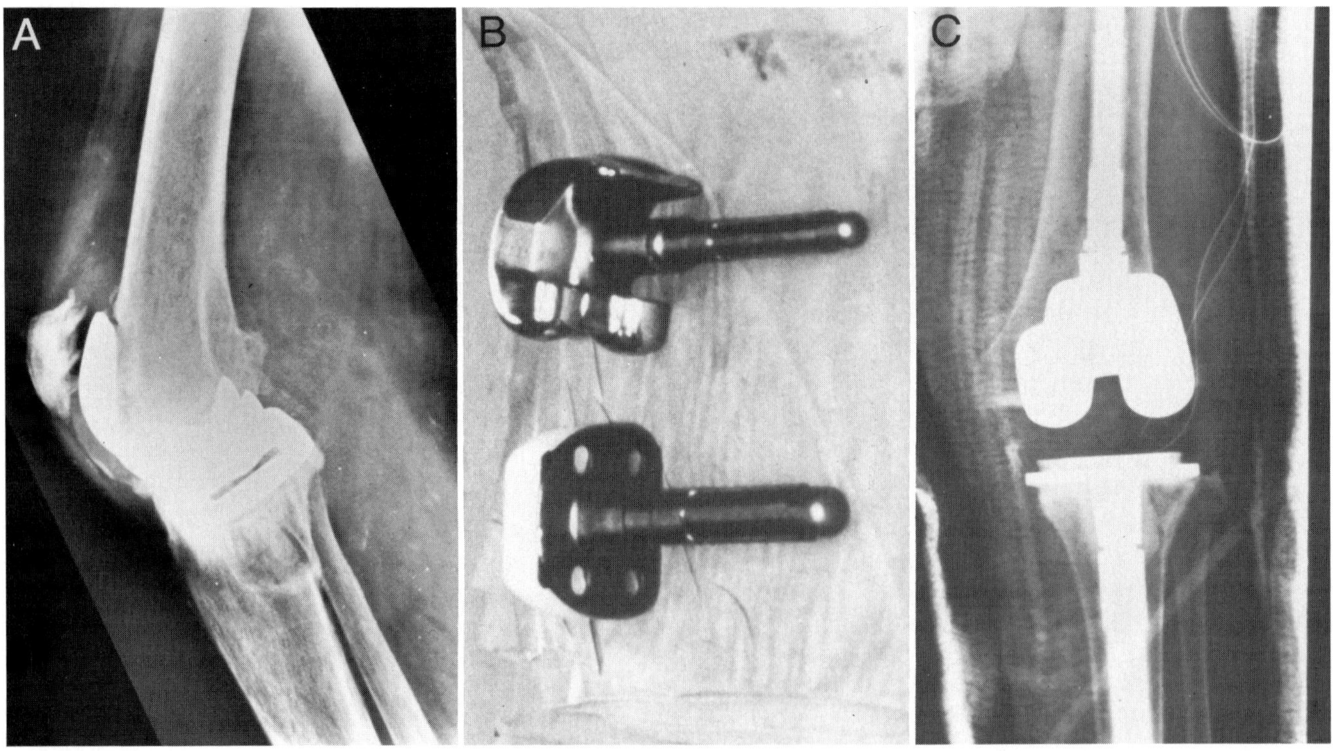

FIG 13–10.
A, failed knee replacement due to component loosening. **B,** custom posterior augmented femoral implant. **C,** postoperative radiograph. Proximal tibial bone grafting has also been utilized.

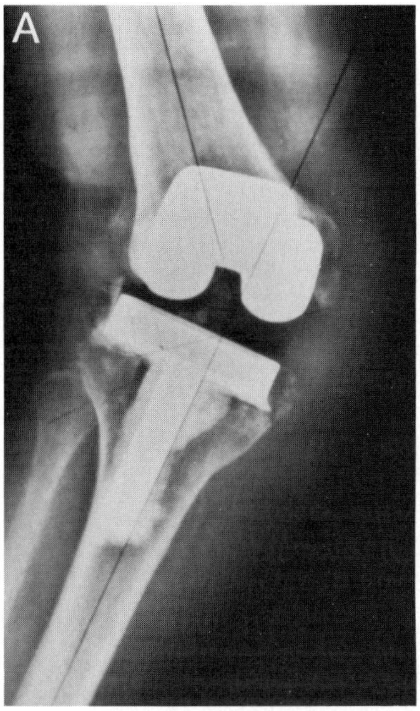

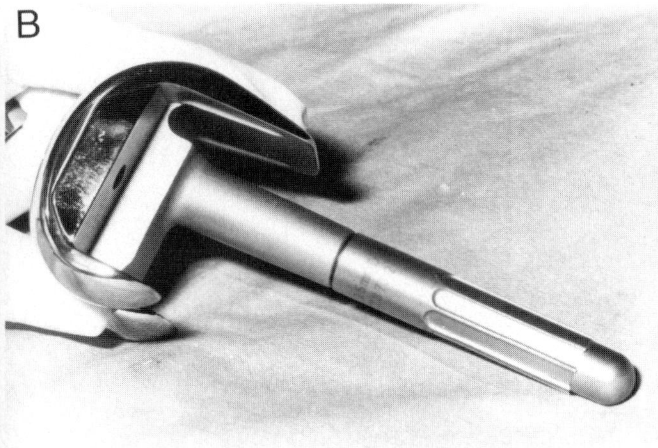

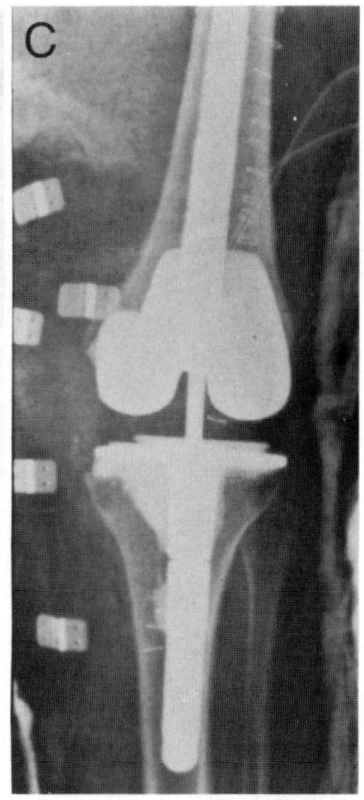

FIG 13–11.
A, marked valgus deformity with distal lateral femoral bone loss. **B,** modular femoral component with distal lateral augmentation to replace deficient femoral bone. **C,** postoperative radiograph demonstrating correction of the deformity and knee joint stability.

loss on the tibial side also occurs most frequently on the posterior surface of the tibial plateau, especially when there is a flexion contracture in combination with the angular deformity. The floor of the tibial defect is generally flattened, sclerotic, and devoid of cartilage. The tibia usually tends to sublux in these more severe deformities and therefore the bony rim of the tibial plateau tends to be damaged and often absent.

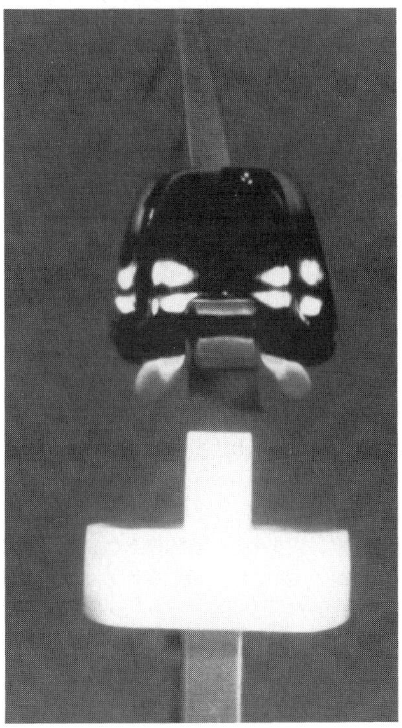

FIG 13–12.
Total condylar III prosthesis with stemmed femoral and tibial components and an augmented intercondylar eminence.

The management of bone loss in total knee replacement will vary depending on the location and the amount of bone loss. There are a number of methods available to augment and fill areas of bone deficiency and these include (1) the use of methylmethacrylate alone,[34] (2) methylmethacrylate reinforced with screws or mesh[44] (Fig 13–13), (3) bone grafting,[12, 58] and (4) custom or modular-augmented total knee systems. When confronted with a bone deficit the operating surgeon must not submit to the temptation of resecting proximal tibial bone to the base of the bone deficit except when the bone deficit is slight, i.e., less than 8 mm. This is approximately the amount of bone routinely resected from the tibial surface in a standard total knee arthroplasty. Resection of tibial bone will further complicate the technique of the arthroplasty should revision be necessary because valuable bone has been removed. Whenever possible in total knee surgery, bone stock should be spared. Additionally, when tibial bone is removed to the floor of a large defect, an increased gap is created in flexion that will require a thicker tibial implant to fill. This need for a thicker tibial implant will alter the patellofemoral tracking because the patella is fixed distally by the patellar tendon and therefore may come in contact with the thick implant when the knee is flexed. Also, excessive tibial resection will necessitate that the tibial implant

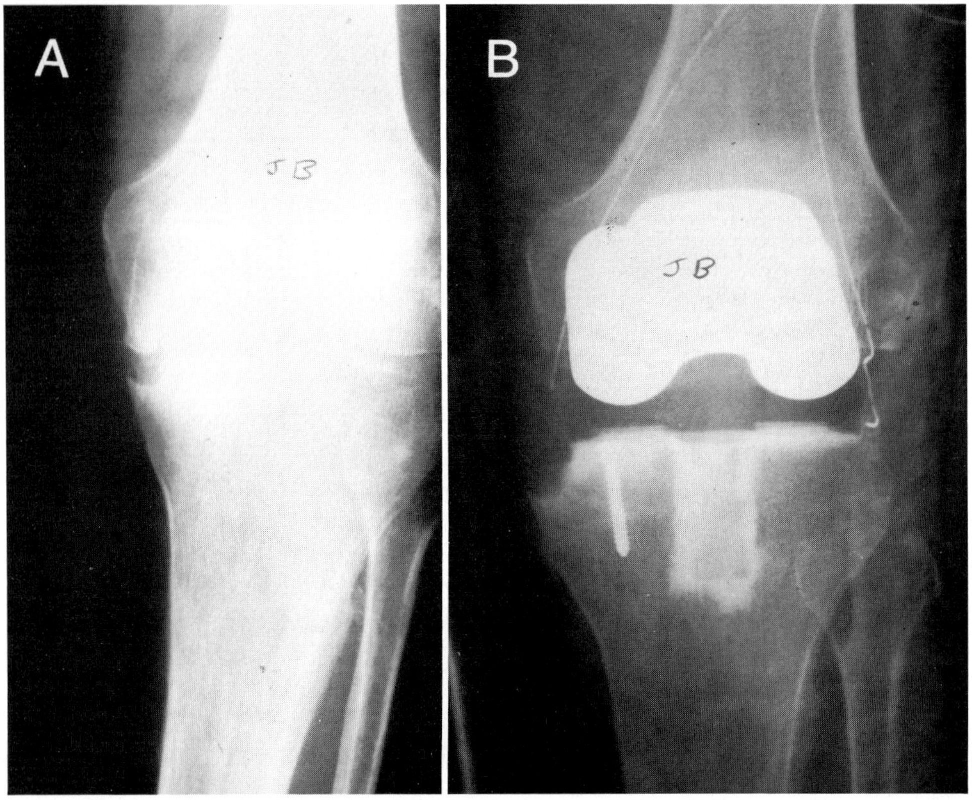

FIG 13–13.
A,B, intermediate bone loss on medial tibial plateau treated with screw and methylmethacrylate composite.

seat on bone of less than good quality[4, 23] and this may lead to problems of subsidence and mechanical loosening. Sizing of the implant may also be affected because of the reduced cross-sectional area on the upper portion of the tibia now available for implant seating. For all of these reasons the concept of augmentation of tibial deficiency is preferred over resection to the floor of the bony deficit.

For defects in the 8- to 13-mm range encompassing less than one half of the tibial plateau surface, several choices are available. Resection of the less involved portion of the tibia will usually be on the order of 8 mm and therefore the bone resected will approach the bed of the deficit. The floor of the involved tibial plateau will tend to be sclerotic even in the rheumatoid patient, and therefore fenestration of the surface should be performed to allow penetration of methylmethacrylate into the subchondral bone of the tibia. If several millimeters of bone deficit remain, this can easily be filled with methylmethacrylate alone. Unsupported large columns of methylmethacrylate in this range have not been liable to fracture and loss of implant support. Larger columns of methylmethacrylate may fracture and should not be used to fill bony defects. They are especially liable to failure when alignment is suboptimal and there is increased loading in an asymmetric manner across the tibial surface.

Where defects are present on the order of 3 to 5 mm after resection of the upper tibia, the methylmethacrylate may be reinforced with cortical screws. These screws are placed just below the metal tray of the tibial implant and the cement incorporates these screws to fill the bone defect. If there is a tendency for the implant to tilt into the defect when the trial tibial component is inserted, the screws may be placed so that their heads abut the tibial tray and prevent subsidence into the bony defect. It must be remembered that synergistic metals must be used if this technique is to be employed.

In larger tibial surface deficits, i.e., greater than 13 to 15 mm and encompassing greater than one third of the tibial surface, bone grafting or augmented tibial implants should be used. A prosthetic implant may be customized with a wedge to fill the void on the affected tibial side (Fig 13–14). Problems may arise with regard to the fabrication and fitting of custom implants. The implant may not fit at the time of surgery and there is little recourse to the surgeon should this occur. Additionally, custom implants are expensive and take a minimum of 6 to 8 weeks to make. More recently, modular implants of

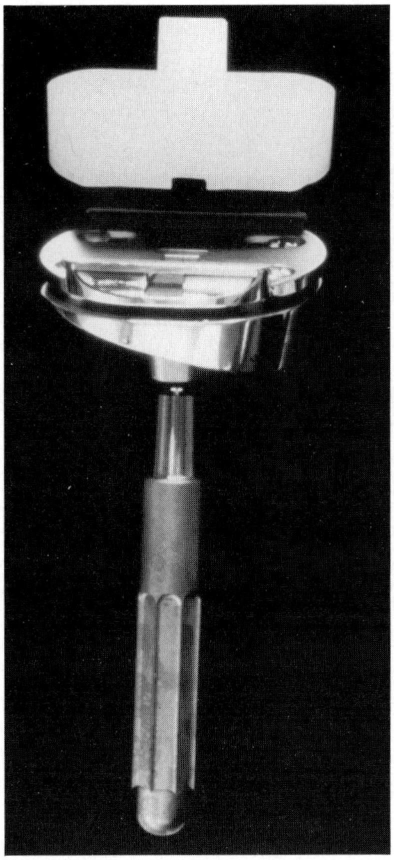

FIG 13–14.
Modular tibial component with wedge augmentation for asymmetric tibial bone loss.

various sizes that provide augmentation to the undersurface of the tibia have allowed the surgeon to construct the configuration that is required. The opportunity to restore bone stock by grafting the deficient tibia is lost if a modular wedge is used. Bone grafting also allows flexibility in fashioning the bone graft to the defect encountered.

Technique of Bone Grafting for Tibial Deficiency

Bone grafting of the proximal tibia for tibial deficiency seen in severe angular deformity in rheumatoid arthritis may be performed without difficulty utilizing bone removed as part of the knee arthroplasty procedure.[66] I prefer to use a technique[2] which employs bone removed from the distal femoral condyles to fill tibial defects (Fig 13–15,A–F). It is important to first prepare the recipient bed which may be quite sclerotic. Using an oscillating saw a planar oblique cut is made extending to the floor of the defect. It is important that this oblique cut be deep enough to expose cancellous bone. Generally, the medial femoral condylar bone is greater in size than the lateral condylar bone and is therefore used to fill the tibial defect. The cancellous surface of the condyle is rotated until the defect is covered. The graft is then cancellous surface to cancellous surface of the recipient bed and is held in place by two Kirschner wires. Using the tibial surface on the more normal side of the tibia which has been osteotomized at right angles to the axis of the tibia as a guide, the overhanging bone graft is removed in line with the upper tibial osteotomy. Once this has been performed two cancellous screws are used to fix the graft to the bed. When the upper tibial surface is now observed it will be seen that the subchondral rim of the femoral graft acts as a peripheral rim for the tibia and essentially the upper surface of the tibia has been reconstituted. The tibial peg hole should be made prior to the grafting and in this way the screws can be monitored to prevent their entering the area of the peg hole. Bone cement is used to caulk the interface of the graft and the adjacent tibia during the cementing of the femoral component. This step is important in preventing cement from entering the bone graft–recipient bed interface and interfering with consolidation of the graft to the underlying bed.

This technique has been used by me in 32 patients over the past 12 years. There has to date been no resorption of the graft, failure of the graft to consolidate, or loss of implant position with mechanical failure (Fig 13–16,A and B). These patients have needed no change in postoperative rehabilitation.

Similar bone grafting procedures have been performed for bone loss on the femoral condylar surface. Bone may be shaped to fill these voids and larger corticocancellous grafts can be fixed with screws. Local bone removed at the time of the arthroplasty may be used to fill cystic deficiencies both on the femoral and on the tibial side. These cystic areas are particularly common in the rheumatoid patients in whom there is significant osteopenia. Corticocancellous bone from the iliac crest may be used if large deficiencies are present and bone harvested during the arthroplasty is inadequate. Allograft bone can also be used if autograft bone is insufficient.

The Patellofemoral Joint

Because valgus deformity is more common in the rheumatoid patient there is a greater need for lateral retinacular release of the patella to improve tracking

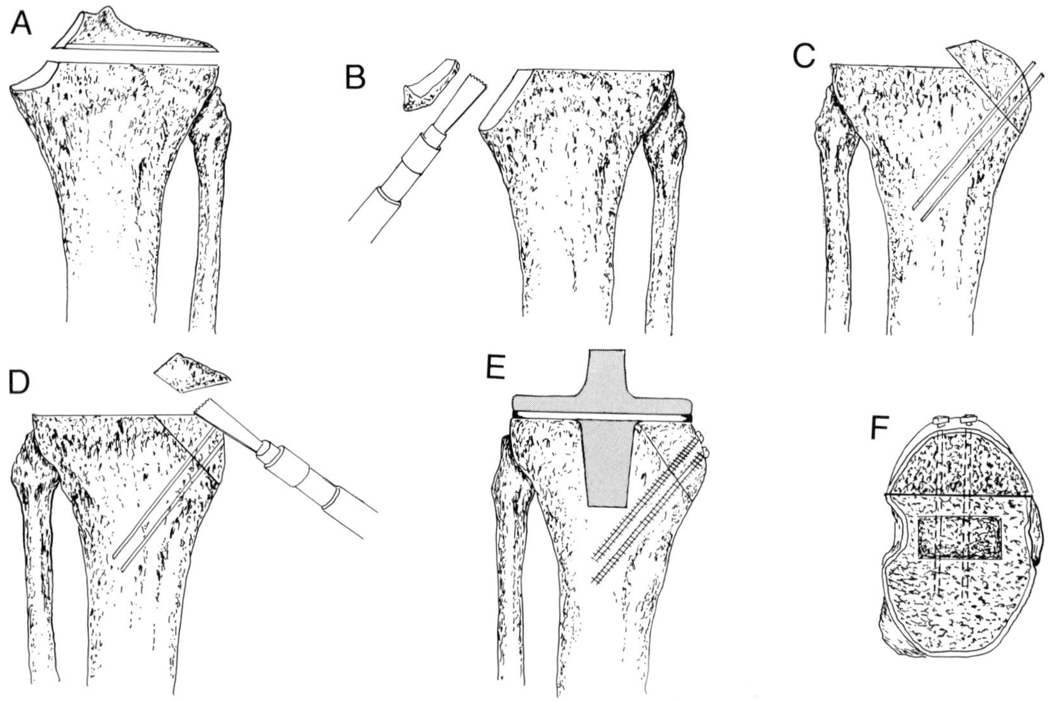

FIG 13–15.
Bone grafting technique for the proximal tibia. **A,** proximal tibial resection. **B,** planar resection of sclerotic tibial defect. **C,** femoral condylar bone apposed to cancellous tibial bed. **D,** resection of overhanging femoral condylar bone. **E,** graft fixed with cancellous screws and prosthesis implanted. **F,** proximal tibial reconstitution with subchondral femoral bone graft reproducing the tibial rim.

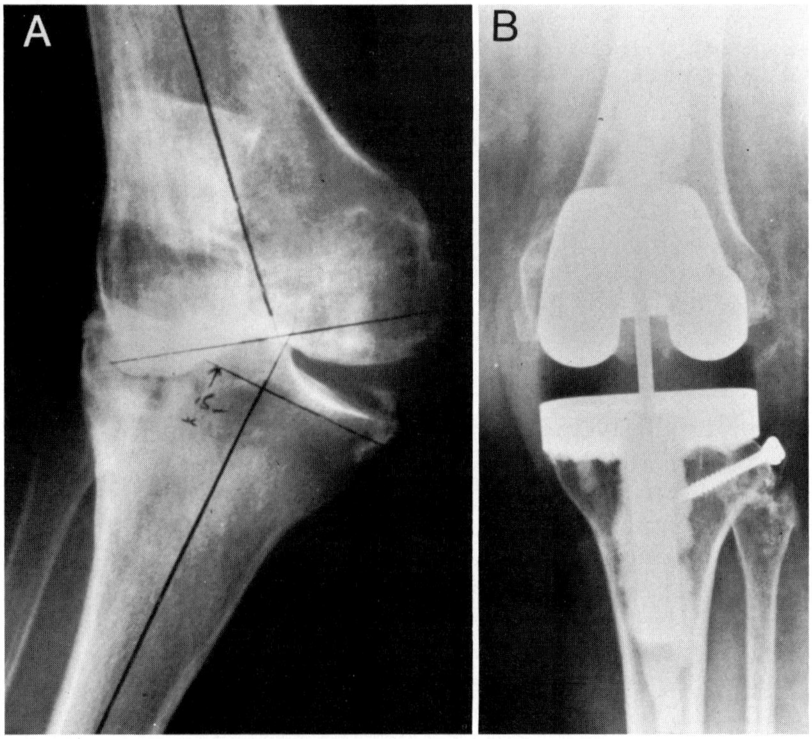

FIG 13–16.
A,B, valgus deformity with lateral tibial bone loss treated with the total condylar III prosthesis and proximal tibial bone grafting.

at the time of total knee arthroplasty. This should be performed if there is any tendency for the patella to sublux laterally after the trial components have been inserted and the knee is flexed. The lateral release is best done from the inside of the knee joint by releasing all tight structures lateral to the patella. The subcutaneous fat will usually be visible once the lateral release has been extended through the retinaculum and this indicates that the release has been adequately performed. Dissection of the subcutaneous tissue from the patella and then releasing the lateral retinaculum external to the joint should not be performed, particularly in the rheumatoid patient. This dissection further devascularizes the skin flaps and may jeopardize wound healing. The superior lateral geniculate artery should be avoided when the lateral release is effected, although in my experience transection of this vessel has not led to problems of patellar blood supply.

The patellofemoral joint should always be replaced in total knee replacement in the patient with rheumatoid arthritis. The joint is universally affected as part of the disease process and trying to preserve it will lead to pain and functional disability. Mechanical failure related to the patella prosthesis has been rare when a polyethylene prosthesis was used.

POSTOPERATIVE REHABILITATION

Rapid return of range of motion and overall recovery of function is assisted with the use of the CPM.[36] Although the CPM may be placed on the knee in the recovery room immediately after surgery, in the rheumatoid patient I usually place it on 24 hours after surgery. Wound healing can be a major problem in the patient with rheumatoid arthritis and therefore the wound is not stressed immediately.[29] A bulky knee dressing is applied in the operating room with medial and lateral plaster splints and the knee is placed in full extension. Additionally, there is generally a hemarthrosis despite intraarticular drainage postoperatively and a flexion contracture may persist if a CPM is applied too soon. The patient will tend to keep the knee in the flexed position to accommodate this swelling and this may be difficult to correct.

The patient is allowed to stand at the bedside and ambulate on postoperative day 2. Ambulation has progressed from use of a walker to a single cane at the time of discharge. If bilateral knee replacements have been performed, the patient will generally be advanced to use of two canes at the time of discharge. Range of motion is continued with the CPM increasing about 10 degrees per day depending upon the patient's tolerance. The patient is expected to achieve 90 degrees of knee flexion prior to discharge. Stair climbing is also taught for independence at home. Depending on the nature of the remaining joints, various modifications of the assistive devices may be necessary. The physical and occupational therapists play an integral role in the rehabilitative recovery. Home physical therapy is arranged for most patients with rheumatoid arthritis undergoing knee replacement to maintain range of motion, strengthen the knee, and improve gait. Bilateral patients are advanced to one cane at 2 to 3 weeks and are generally ambulatory without external support at 6 to 8 weeks after surgery.

PROSTHETIC SELECTION

Cemented Prostheses and Porous Implants

After the success demonstrated in hip replacement, efforts were directed toward studying the applicability of noncemented designs to the knee joint. Long-term studies have shown that the use of cemented knee implants are attended by fewer mechanical failures than hip arthroplasty.* If knee replacement is performed accurately, excellent long-term results can be expected from a cemented implant. Radiolucent areas are common, particularly below the tibia, but tend to be nonprogressive. Loosening and implant positional shifts are uncommon.

Porous implants require precise technique and implant-bone coaptation must be absolute. In a cemented total knee arthroplasty small voids in coaptation, although not common with current instrumentation, can be filled by methylmethacrylate and fixation is not impaired. This is not the case with a porous implant. For bone ingrowth to occur there must be intimate contact. This requires instrumentation that offers a high degree of accuracy and a high degree of surgical skill.

A number of fixation methods utilizing porous systems have been developed. These rely on a press fit of the femoral component and the patella. On the tibial side various types of pegs and screw fixation have been used. Histologic evaluation has raised the question as to how good bone ingrowth is. In a histologic and radiographic analysis of 85 porous-

*References 13, 17, 19, 25, 29, 43, 45, 47, 52–54, 64.

coated knee implants, Cook et al.[9] found little bone ingrowth. In 52% of components there was no evidence of bone ingrowth, in 29% it was minimal, in 12% it was moderate, and in only 7% was it considerable. Ingrowth was universally poor on all components, femoral, patellar, and tibial alike. The little bone ingrowth that did occur was present around the fixation pegs or screws. No one design was superior over another in this respect, nor did type of porous surface make a difference. Clinical studies have also demonstrated inferior results with noncemented designs with a higher reoperation rate and reduced range of motion.

Because of the excellent long-term results with cemented implants and the poor[50] quality of bone in rheumatoid arthritis, porous implants should be utilized infrequently and only in a closely controlled prospective manner by investigators with extensive experience with noncemented technology and knee replacement surgery.

COMPLICATIONS OF TOTAL KNEE ARTHROPLASTY IN RHEUMATOID ARTHRITIS

Because rheumatoid arthritis is a systemic disease affecting multiple organ systems, complications are common. Local complications related to delayed wound healing or infection can jeopardize the success of the arthroplasty and must be treated aggressively.

Local Complications

Many patients with rheumatoid arthritis are treated with corticosteroid and immunosuppressive medications and these may interfere with wound healing after total knee arthroplasty. There is often a marked deficiency in subcutaneous fat which provides blood flow to the skin, and undue traction during knee replacement may damage this blood supply and the skin margins. Additionally, when angular deformity is severe, soft tissue releases will be extensive and knee manipulation may cause trauma to wound edges and impair healing. Long-term studies indicate an incidence of wound problems in the range of 4% to 10%.[3, 5, 6, 48]

Local complications may be defined as any problem related to the healing of the knee incision or its immediate environment. These complications may then be classified as (1) delayed wound healing, (2) wound slough, (3) hematoma, (4) seroma, (5) superficial wound infection. Both superficial and deep infections occur more frequently in rheumatoid arthritis and this may in part be related to defective functioning of phagocytosis by leukocytes.[20, 67] Deep wound infection is discussed separately.

Delayed Wound Healing

Delayed wound healing refers to marginal skin necrosis which may affect a variable length of the incision but generally encompasses a distance of several centimeters. Most commonly the central portion of the incision is affected where soft tissue coverage tends to be less abundant. Also, subcutaneous fat is deficient in this area, particularly if a straight incision over the patella has been used. The wound edges will appear necrotic for a width of several millimeters and drainage as a rule does not occur. An eschar will develop and the tissue loss is superficial. Generally, this eschar may be left intact and it will slough when new epithelium is present beneath it. If purulence develops around this area of necrotic tissue the eschar must be debrided and skin grafting may be necessary. Continued physical therapy and use of the CPM is allowed in these patients unless deterioration of the wound develops and knee flexion generates excessive wound stresses. Sterile dressings should be placed over the wound until the local area is dry.

Wound Slough

Wound slough connotes a full-thickness loss of skin and subcutaneous tissue and is a serious local complication (Fig 13–17). The extent of these sloughs may range from 6 to 10 cm and they may encompass the entire prepatellar area. The most serious potential danger when a wound slough of this order has occurred is contamination of the subfascial structures with extension to the knee joint itself. This will result in deep infection with loss of the arthroplasty and need for prolonged parenteral antibiotics and reimplantation.

It is imperative that when a wound slough has occurred plastic surgery consultation be obtained immediately. Early aggressive debridement and gastrocnemius muscle pedicle flaps to cover the resultant defect are often necessary and are best done immediately. Hallock[22] has recently reported on the use of local fasciocutaneous flaps which are rotated to cover defects anteriorly without having to resort to a full muscle pedicle flap. The skin is mobilized with its subcutaneous tissue and fascia and accompanying blood supply. In six patients reported to date the technique has been successful.

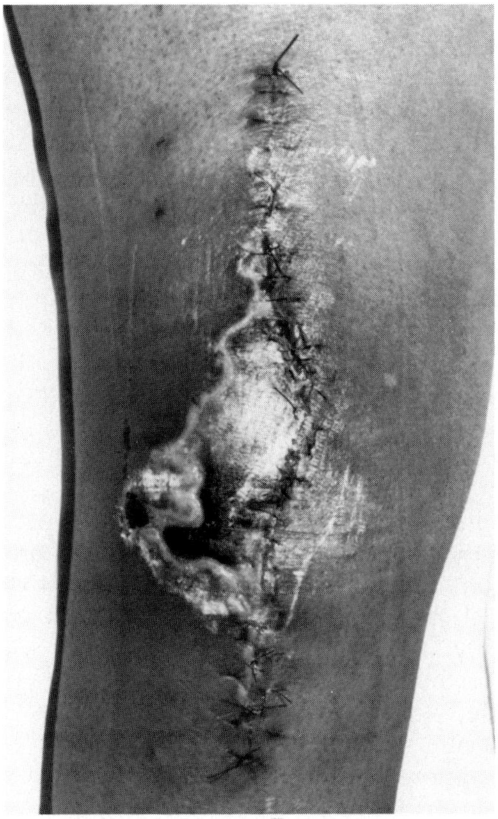

FIG 13–17.
Wound slough after total knee replacement. Patient was on corticosteroid therapy.

Range-of-motion exercises and other knee joint rehabilitation are postponed until the integrity of wound coverage has been safely reconstituted. It cannot be overemphasized that the early recognition and treatment of a wound slough can salvage a knee arthroplasty from deep infection and the possible total loss of the knee replacement.

Wound Hematoma

Knee joint hematoma occurs after every knee arthroplasty and is generally decompressed with suction drainage systems postoperatively. However, if the drainage system malfunctions or bleeding is considerable, a persistent bloody effusion may occur. This will lead to pain and difficulty with range of motion and may impede physical therapy and knee rehabilitation. The knee should be packed in ice and range of motion restrained until acute swelling has subsided. If the patient is not in significant pain, the CPM may be maintained at a range not to exceed 30 to 45 degrees depending upon the degree of swelling and the pain. Formal range of motion by physical therapy should be postponed for several days until pain and the acute swelling have subsided.

Postoperative hematoma may also result in patients placed on anticoagulation therapy in whom the prothrombin level becomes excessive. If swelling is severe the knee is immobilized and range of motion restrained. If the hematoma remains tense and nonresolving and limits physical therapy, the patient may be brought back to the operating room for surgical evacuation and wound closure.

One of the most serious complications related to hematoma formation is the development of bloody drainage from the wound. This generally occurs as range-of-motion exercises are begun and may be copious. It may also be persistent and nonresolving. Additionally, seroma formation may occur days after surgery and also lead to persistent and heavy drainage. Drainage from the wound postoperatively, which may begin as a benign problem, can lead to wound infection with ultimate development of a deep periprosthetic infection.[51]

Treatment of a draining hematoma or seroma must be aggressive. Frequent sterile dressing changes should be performed and drainage should not be allowed to saturate the outer surface of the dressing. Care must be taken to maintain a sterile environment at all times when treating these draining wounds. The knee should be immobilized and physical therapy and range-of-motion exercises put off until drainage ceases. If drainage persists the patient should be returned to the operating room for a formal debridement of the hematoma or seroma. Hemostasis should be obtained and closure of the wound effected. Once the draining wound has been converted into a dry wound with a secure closure, postoperative physical therapy can commence as in the primary knee arthroplasty.

Superficial Wound Infection

Superficial wound infection is defined as a bacterially induced infection not extending below the deep fascia or retinaculum of the knee joint. These occur in the immediate postoperative period and are seen in conjunction with wound healing disorders or wound drainage. Since they may extend into the knee joint if untreated, it is mandatory that treatment be appropriate and without delay. Antibiotics should not be administered until cultures have been obtained. Cultures must be from fresh drainage in an attempt to most accurately determine the infecting organism. Broad-spectrum antibiotics are given until final cultures have been reported and administered intravenously for 7 to 10 days or until all evidence of infection has passed. Dressings should be changed sterilely several times daily as necessary. Physical therapy and range-of-motion exercises are put off. If drainage continues despite local wound care and antibiotics, the patient should be returned to the operating room for formal debridement of the wound. If infection continues with persistent purulent drainage, deep periprosthetic infection should be suspected.

Deep Infection

One of the most catastrophic complications that can occur after total knee arthroplasty is deep infection extending to the knee joint itself (Fig 13–18). Although the incidence of this complication is uncommon in most series of knee arthroplasty, in the range of 1%, the rheumatoid patient is more susceptible. In a review of long-term results of knee replacement in our polyarthritic rheumatoid patients, the infection rate was 7%.[51] Of the nine deep infections in our series, five occurred after 5 years from initial knee replacement. Laskin,[32] in his long-term review of total knee arthroplasty in rheumatoid patients, reports similar findings. The infection rate in Laskin's patients was 6.3% with all five of the infections arising after 3 years from the initial procedure.

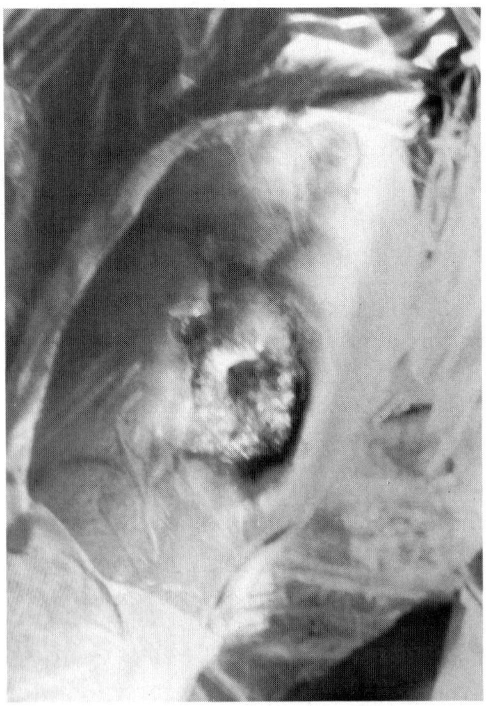

FIG 13–18.
Draining sinus and infected knee replacement through a previously skin-grafted wound.

Diagnosis

The diagnosis of deep infection after total knee replacement must be suspected in any painful knee after arthroplasty in which the cause of pain is unclear. The presenting features may be subtle with mild to moderate swelling within the knee joint and intermittent pain. Temperature elevation may be migratory but if present should reinforce the diagnosis of infection. In more advanced and severe infections purulent drainage may occur through a sinus either in the knee incision itself or below the knee joint in the area of the patellar tendon.

When infection is suspected, routine radiographs are useful and may demonstrate bone resorption under the implant in the area of the bone-cement interface (Fig 13–19,A–C). This resorption represents invasion of this interface by infected granulation tissue and is characteristic of prosthetic knee joint infection. The sedimentation rate is generally high but the white blood cell count may, remarkably, be normal unless there is an acute element to the infection. Bone scans will demonstrate increased activity about the knee and as a rule are nonspecific. Indium 111–labeled scans may be helpful in differentiating whether increased activity is due to mechanical failure with loosening or to infection.

The definitive diagnosis of infection within the knee joint is obtained by aspiration and recovery of organisms from the periprosthetic environment. It must be remembered that these aspirations and cultures will be of little use if the patient has been taking antibiotics and therefore the surgeon must resist the tendency to place the patient on antibiotics immediately. The patient with rheumatoid arthritis may, because of the immunosuppressive medication, demonstrate little systemic or local signs of deep infection or bacteremia. Only when the infection has become severe and life-threatening with sepsis may the diagnosis become obvious.

Because the rheumatoid patient is susceptible to infection, metastatic spread of infection from another visceral origin may occur and involve the knee joint. All urinary tract infections, dental abscesses, and soft tissue infections must be treated aggressively with antibiotics to prevent spread to the knee joint. Additionally, because of the vasculitis that may accompany rheumatoid arthritis, and the poor quality of the epithelium and subcutaneous tissue, skin breakdown may occur with ulceration on the lower legs. These may progress to secondary infection with later seeding to the knee joint. Ulcerations must therefore be treated with frequent dressing

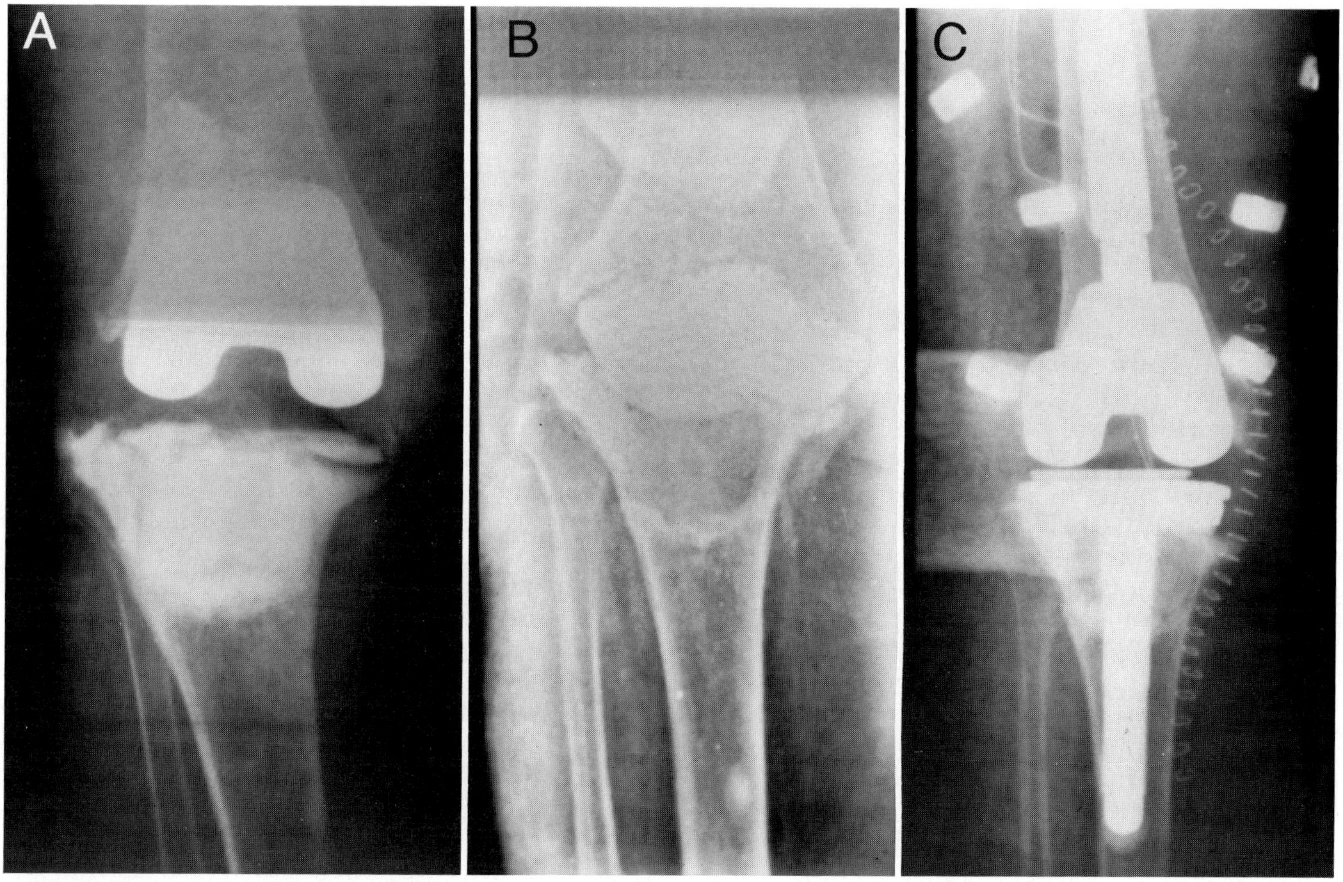

FIG 13–19.
A, loose infected total knee replacement with medial tibial bone loss. **B,** after implant removal, marked tibial medullary bone loss. **C,** postoperative radiograph demonstrating allograft femoral head bone graft into the tibial defect and tibial component wedge augmentation.

changes and prevention of infection in these lesions must be paramount in their management.

If initial aspiration of the knee joint is negative and yet the explanation for knee pain and swelling is not defined, further aspiration should be performed. If suspicion remains that infection is present and repeated aspirations are negative, arthroscopic synovial biopsy can be performed and tissue cultures obtained.

Treatment

Once the diagnosis of deep infection has been made, treatment consists of removal of the implant, appropriate parenteral antibiotic treatment, and reimplantation of the prosthetic knee joint. The protocol[26] at The Hospital for Special Surgery recommends a 6-week course of parenteral antibiotics with significant bactericidal levels being established as treatment progresses. Careful monitoring of antibiotic levels is performed to ensure that proper and adequate antibiotic levels are being maintained. A Broviac-type catheter is implanted at the time of implant removal and this greatly facilitates the mobilizing of the rheumatoid patient from bed. Additionally, peripheral vein access may be extremely poor in these patients and the central venous line obviates the need for repeated futile attempts at venipuncture.

The reimplantation is performed at the completion of the 6-week course of antibiotics. Generally the patient is maintained in the hospital during this period. If insurance coverage is adequate to allow home antibiotic treatment, the patient may be treated at home with visiting nurse services. At the time of the reimplantation the quality of the tissues is evaluated and if there is any question of possible continued infection a debridement is performed and the knee closed awaiting negative cultures and then reimplantation. This course of treatment is rarely necessary. Frozen section of the local tissues can also be obtained at the time of the reimplantation and if there is no evidence of acute inflammatory cells or organisms, reimplantation may be performed.

Utilizing this protocol of implant removal, a 6-week course of parenteral antibiotics, and then reimplantation, the success rate with absence of recurrent infection has been 98% in over 150 infected total knee replacements performed at The Hospital for Special Surgery. The nature of the infecting organism has not altered the end result as long as appropriate bactericidal levels of antibiotics are maintained during the antibiotic period. After reimplantation, antibiotics are administered for 48 hours, as is done routinely for a primary total knee replacement.

There are instances when reimplantation is not recommended and knee arthrodesis is the procedure of choice. In rheumatoid patients in whom there is a major loss of skin and soft tissue coverage over the implant, reimplantation may not be possible. Significant damage to the extensor apparatus of the knee joint with dissolution of the patellar tendon will make knee function difficult after knee arthroplasty. In patients in whom bone loss is extensive and irretrievable by grafting or implant methods, arthrodesis is the procedure of choice. Arthrodesis should also be considered in patients in whom the infecting organism(s) cannot be controlled with antibiotics or intolerance to the necessary antibiotic regimen prevents proper antimicrobial coverage. H.E. Figgie et al.,[14] in a review of the results of arthrodesis at our institution, reported successful fusion in 20 of 27 patients. Success was correlated with absence of sepsis, correct alignment, and the use of a stable fixation construct. In this group of patients resection arthroplasty led to unsatisfactory results because of lack of stability, persistent pain, and loss of independent ambulation.

Deep Vein Thrombosis

Deep vein thrombosis after total knee replacement remains a serious and frequent problem. The incidence of deep vein thrombosis after total knee replacement in patients who received no prophylaxis has been reported to be as high as 84% by Stulberg et al.[62] and others.[16, 21, 35, 38, 39] The causative agents are multiple but the most significant is probably trauma to the deep vein system during the manipulation required for total knee replacement. The rheumatoid patient appears to be equally at high risk although most patients are receiving anti-inflammatory medications which may provide some degree of protection. In a recent review[38] of 92 knee replacements in 65 patients, venograms were performed immediately after surgery or on the first postoperative day and again at 5 to 7 days after surgery. There was a 30% incidence of positive venograms in the immediate postoperative period (first postoperative day) which increased to 58% on the later venograms. This is further evidence that deep venous thrombosis is initiated in the operating room, and treatment should be directed toward reducing the incidence of intraoperative clot formation.

Current regimens are directed at the postoperative period and there are reported series which demonstrate reduction in the rate of deep vein thrombosis with the use of sequential-compression boots,[21] antithrombin III and low-dose heparin,[16] aspirin, or warfarin,[62] or the CPM.[35] Although the deep vein thrombosis rate is high, most clots occur in the calf and rarely progress to the femoral vein. Our current regimen for prophylaxis after knee replacement is to place patients on aspirin postoperatively unless they are considered to be at high risk to develop deep vein thrombosis. Those who are considered at risk include patients undergoing bilateral procedures at one operative setting; patients with a history of deep vein thrombosis or pulmonary embolism; obese patients; patients who are slow to ambulate or who cannot be mobilized from bed; and patients with severe local venous disease (stasis, edema, or ulceration). The patient who falls into one of the above categories is treated with warfarin which is begun on the day before surgery and is continued for 6 to 8 weeks. The prothrombin time is maintained in the range of 14 to 16 seconds. All patients undergo venography on the fourth or fifth postoperative day and if clot formation is present they are begun on warfarin which is continued for 6 to 8 weeks.

RESULTS WITH TOTAL KNEE ARTHROPLASTY IN RHEUMATOID ARTHRITIS

Patients with rheumatoid arthritis have an inferior biological substrate when total knee arthroplasty is performed when compared with the patient with osteoarthritic knee involvement. Soft tissue coverage is often of poorer quality, ligamentous stability may be inadequate, the deformity is often fixed and severe, and bone quality is suboptimal. These factors also make rehabilitation more complex. On the other hand, owing to the nature of the disease and the

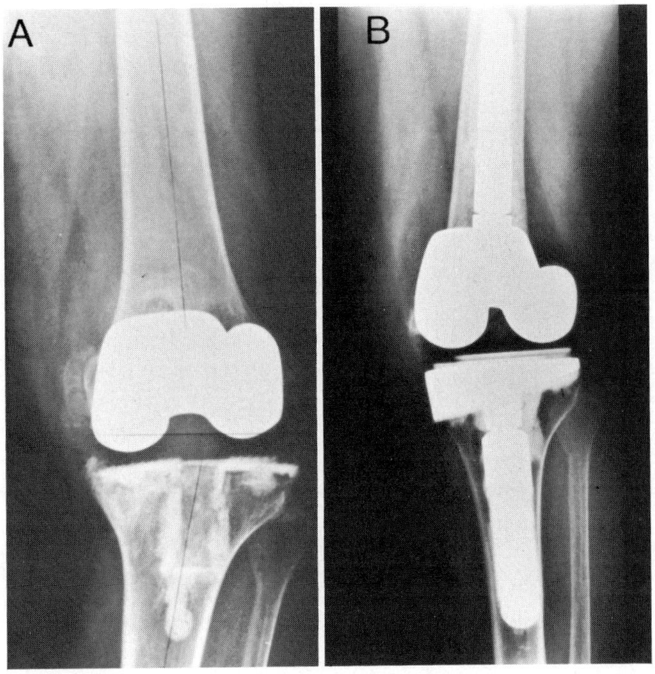

FIG 13–20.
A, tibial component subsidence and loosening 7 years after knee replacement. **B,** wedge-augmented tibial prosthesis utilized to replace tibial bone loss.

lesser functional and mechanical demands placed on the arthroplasty, good long-term results may be expected.[49]

In our long-term follow-up[51] of 80 patients undergoing 129 total knee arthroplasties, mechanical failure necessitating revision was uncommon. Eighty (90%) of these patients were American Rheumatism Association (ARA) class III or IV and 43 patients (54%) either were or had been receiving corticosteroids. This group was followed an average of 6 years with a range of 2 to 10 years. There were no failures for loosening although seven patients demonstrated a shift in implant position, four on the tibial side (Fig 13–20,A and B) and three on the femoral side (Fig 13–21,A and B). Only one patient complained of mild pain and no patient needed revision because of limited ambulation. There were 20 wound complications (13.8%), 12 of which were culture-negative drainage and 8 delayed wound healing. Of note is that 4 of these 20 wound problems went on to a later deep periprosthetic wound infection. Overall, there were 7.8% deep infections requiring implant removal. In this group of 9 patients the onset of infection occurred 5 years postoperatively or later in 5 patients. The overall results when evaluating patients after treatment of their complications (reimplantation in the case of deep infection) yielded 85% good to excellent results, 11% fair, and 4% poor. Twenty-four percent of patients were not ambulatory prior to their total knee arthroplasty; all but 1 were ambulatory after knee replacement.

Hvid et al.[25] reported on 119 total condylar replacements in rheumatoid patients followed 4 to 6 years and noted good to excellent results in 87% of patients. There were two late infections, one at 3 and another at 5 years postoperatively. There were

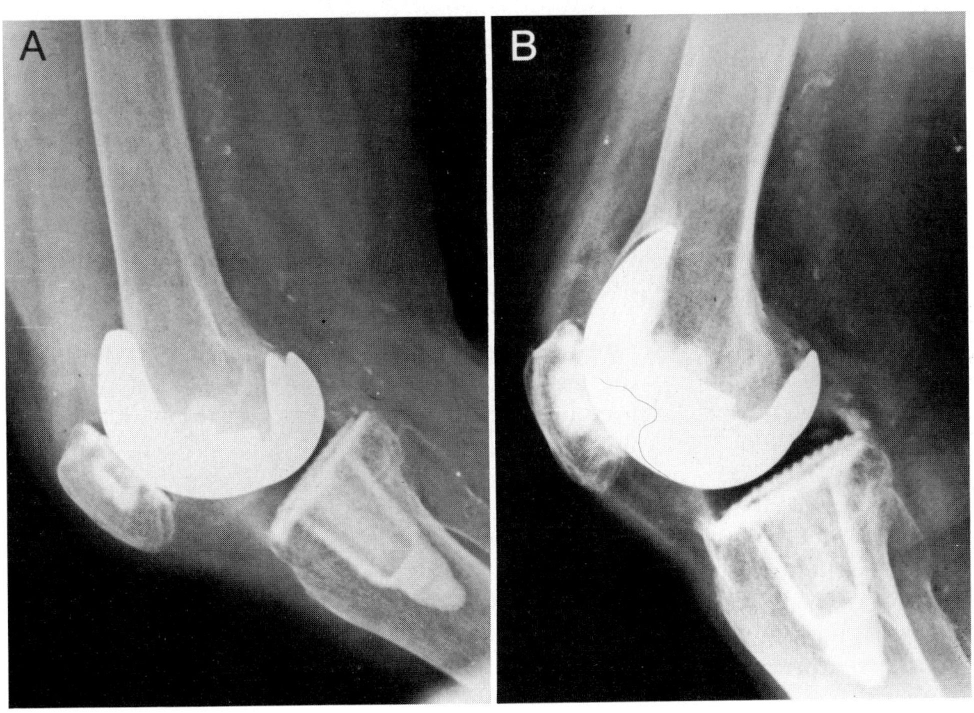

FIG 13–21.
A, a 72-year-old woman 3 years after total knee replacement. **B,** the prosthesis still appears well fixed but the femoral component has shifted into an extended position secondary to failure of osteopenic bone.

no revisions for loosening but two patients demonstrated loose implants. In a comparison study of 247 total knee arthroplasties followed at least 2 years, Nielsen et al.[43] reported similar results with their rheumatoid and osteoarthritic knee replacements. Knutson et al.,[31] in a monumental review of 4,505 knee replacements in osteoarthritis and 3,495 replacements in rheumatoid arthritis in Sweden, found 87% implant survival in the osteoarthritic group and 90% implant survival in the rheumatoid group at 6-year follow-up evaluation. This was in patients in whom two or three compartment replacements were used. Failure rates were much higher in the hinge and severely constrained implants. There was a significantly increased incidence of deep prosthetic infection in the rheumatoid patients—3% compared to 2% in the osteoarthritic group.

Tauber,[63] in a review of 71 total condylar prostheses with an average follow-up of 3.5 years, found "good" or "excellent" results in 85% of osteoarthritic knees (45/53 patients) and in 50% (9/18 patients) of rheumatoid knees although the patient population is too small to draw strong conclusions. An earlier review of geometric knee replacement by Hunter et al.[24] also showed poorer results but these may have been related to the implant itself. The authors found a 9% infection rate with 38% of patients developing late deep infections having had delayed wound healing after knee replacement.

Sledge and Walker[59] followed 563 duopatellar replacements for 5 years in a rheumatoid population and found that 17 underwent revision. Seven revisions were necessary due to implant loosening and ten because of patellofemoral pain. The authors described only three infections in this series. Eighty-five percent of results were good to excellent.

Laskin,[32] in a 10-year follow-up of 80 total knee replacements in rheumatoid arthritis, described 19 revisions, 12 necessitated by loosening of the tibial component. All of these failed tibial components had been placed in varus alignment initially, and collapsed on bone of poor quality.

In younger patients with rheumatoid arthritis results have tended to be somewhat better. Stuart and Rand[61] reviewed 44 total knee arthroplasties in 28 patients aged 19 to 39 years and found 24 excellent, 14 good, 6 fair, and zero poor results at average follow-up of 5 years postoperatively. There were no revisions in this group. Sarokhan et al.[52] documented good to excellent results in 20 of 21 younger rheumatoid patients followed for 5 years. Carmichael and Chaplin[8] reported on 21 total knee replacements in 11 younger patients with rheumatoid arthritis at 5-year follow-up. They found no infections, no loosening, and no revisions.

REVISION KNEE REPLACEMENT

Primary knee replacement may fail in the rheumatoid patient because of (1) infection, (2) loosening of components, (3) instability, (4) patellofemoral dysfunction, or (5) bony collapse beneath a well-fixed implant. When failure has occurred it is paramount that the reason for failure be carefully defined and, preoperatively, a plan of management developed. Infection must be eliminated as a possible source of implant failure and this is best done by aspiration of the knee and evaluation as described earlier in this chapter.

The problems which confront the surgeon in revision knee replacement surgery are similar to those in the primary knee operation, but more complex, and the task of implant removal further complicates the procedure. Exposure must be ample and not jeopardize soft tissue investment of the knee and overlying skin. Soft tissue imbalance must be corrected. Bone deficits can be addressed either with bone graft or modular prostheses. Patellofemoral tracking must be reestablished in a stable manner. The implant must be removed without increased damage to the underlying bony substrate which is tenuous in the rheumatoid patient.

Implant Removal

When the knee joint has been fully exposed and flexed without undue tension on skin and soft tissues, attention is turned to implant removal. It is important that all soft tissue be removed from the periphery of the prosthesis-bone interface to allow chisels to be inserted into the implant-cement–bone interface. In patients in whom the implant is well fixed to the underlying cement, these chisels are used to loosen the cement around the periphery of the implant. Care must be exercised to avoid levering on the underlying osteoporotic bone. Damage to the supporting femoral and tibial surfaces can occur easily if force is exerted during implant removal. Once the interface has been clearly defined, a distraction device with a slaphammer (Fig 13–22,A and B) attachment may be attached to the prosthesis and the implant may be removed with several firm distracting forces. If considerable force is needed, and the implant remains well fixed, it is necessary

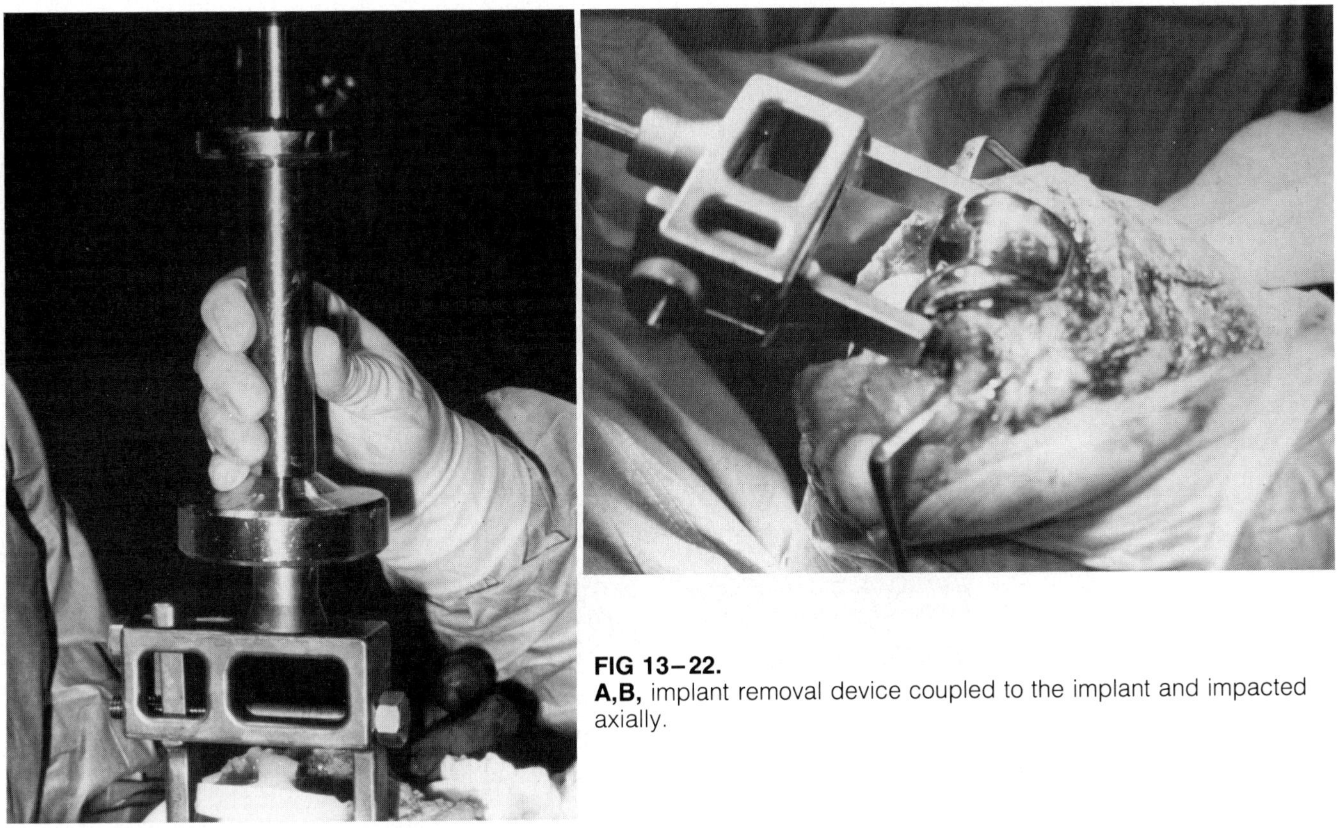

FIG 13–22.
A,B, implant removal device coupled to the implant and impacted axially.

to further loosen the implant-cement–bone interface. Once the implants have been removed methylmethacrylate should be removed from the femur and tibia. The patellar component, if well-fixed and not damaged and compatible with the revision component, may be left in place. Hand-operated cement-removing instruments are preferred; a mosaic should be created on the cement surface and fragments of methylmethacrylate removed. Power drill devices such as the Midas can be used to remove cement from tibial peg holes.

Bone Deficits

Bone deficits are common in revision knee procedures and tend to be of several types. The most common deficits encountered are those which are cystic and multiple. They are most often found on the surface of the tibia and femur after implant removal. These are best managed by impacting cancellous bone that is removed as part of the revision procedure into their craterlike surfaces. The second type of bone deficit involves the tibial plateau and is seen when the implant has collapsed into the tibial surface with malalignment and loss of supporting bone beneath the implant. The tibial component will lift off the contralateral surface and compress tibial bone on the side of the collapse (see Fig 13–20). These defects can be managed by using an allograft or iliac crest bone to fill the defect. A modular implant with a wedge augmentation, which is available in differing angle configurations, can also be used to fill the deficient tibial surface. The metal augmentation of the tibial implant will fill the defect and allow proper alignment of the tibial component.

The third type of tibial deficiency encountered in revision knee replacement is the severe funnel defect of the upper tibia (Fig 13–23). Marked bone loss is present in the entire upper tibia and its medullary canal. Bone support to the tibial component is poor at the upper surface of the tibia because of the large area of bone loss. In these settings a stemmed implant must be used to transfer the load more distally into the tibial shaft. Bone grafting is also necessary around the deficient upper tibia.

Femoral defects are treated in a similar fashion, using autogenous bone when possible. Augmentation of the distal and posterior femoral component can be used in clinical situations where there is severe distal femoral bone loss. A stemmed implant is again recommended when there is severe damage to the face of the distal femur.

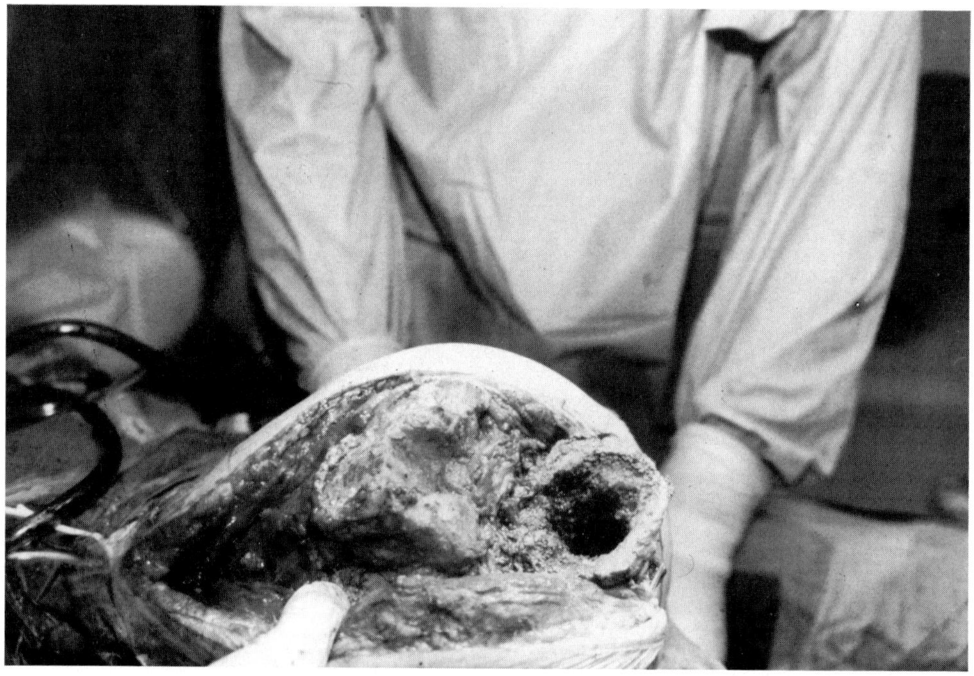

FIG 13–23.
Severe bone loss of a funnel defect on the upper tibial surface.

IMPLANT SELECTION AND TECHNIQUE OF IMPLANTATION

Some of the principles of selection of a more constrained implant have been alluded to previously in this chapter. The criteria for selection of a constrained implant are the following in knee revision surgery: (1) marked medial-lateral instability with an inability to balance the soft tissues and create a stable environment for a less constrained implant; (2) instability in the anteroposterior plane which cannot be corrected by augmenting the implants to alter stability in flexion and extension; (3) severe bone loss on the distal femoral or upper tibial surface with associated instability.

The total condylar III (see Fig 13–12) implant was among the first constrained condylar design implants to be used to provide stability in complex revision knee replacement surgery. The design includes a deepened femoral intercondylar box into which a square elongated polyethylene column inserts. It is a stemmed component on the femoral side and the peg is longer on the tibial side than in the standard condylar designs. Newer modular knee replacement designs allow custom fabrication of an implant to deal with the individual clinical problems encountered at the time of revision. These modular designs allow the following adaptation: (1) femoral and tibial stems of varying lengths and diameters; (2) femoral configurations with mated polyethylene components which may provide significant constraint (similar to the total condylar III), or a posterior stabilized version; (3) augmentation inserts which may be used to augment the distal and posterior femoral component; (4) augmentation of the undersurface of the tibial component with wedges for plateau deficits.

The concept of modularity in both constraint and customization of the implant has been a major advance in the surgical management of the failed total knee arthroplasty. It must be emphasized that the implant is only as good as the underlying biological substrate and what has been done to prepare it for the prosthesis. Without adequate and atraumatic exposure, soft tissue balancing, bone deficit management, proper alignment, and an adequately aligned and functioning extensor mechanism, the chance of recurrent failure is increased.

Technique of Modular Constrained Condylar Revision Surgery

Once the failed implant has been removed, bone cuts can be made on the tibia and femur to ensure proper coaptation of the implant to the remaining underlying bone. Correct knee joint alignment must be established. The proximal tibia is addressed first. Tibial cutting jigs are used against the anterior tibia and the alignment guide which is at right angles to the cutting jig should be directed to the medial ankle area toward the intermetatarsal space between the first and second metatarsals. A minimal amount of bone is removed and in general the upper tibia is simply leveled and debrided of poor-quality bone and fibrous tissue. Additional bone removed from the upper tibia will increase the flexion and extension gaps and increase the need for a thicker tibial implant. If a plateau deficit requires a wedge tibial component augmentation, a cutting block should be used which accounts for the wedge and the tibia should be resected to allow a secure fit between the augmented tibial implant and the underlying deficient bone.

After preparation of the upper tibia, a T-square device (a spacer block with an alignment rod through its end can be used) should be placed on the tibial surface and alignment perpendicular to the tibia confirmed. If the surface is poor and an intramedullary rod is to be used, sequential reaming with Küntsher-type reamers is performed. The ultimate diameter is determined by the largest reamer that is broaching cortical tibia and is usually in the range of 14 to 16 mm.

Femoral preparation is made using the appropriate jig system. In the constrained condylar knee system, femoral cutting instruments must provide a femoral surface that will allow secure and close apposition of implant to underlying bone. Jigs utilize an intramedullary femoral rod for alignment and ensure a valgus cut on the distal femur of 5 to 7 degrees. The distance from the most anterior edge of the collateral ligaments and the femoral condylar articular surface is in the range of 17 to 20 mm and this relationship must be achieved when the femoral implant trial is placed on the femur. If there are areas of bone deficiency on the distal femur and this relationship is not reconstituted, then augmentation of the condyle should be performed with bone graft or metal wedges attached to the distal portion of the femoral component. Intramedullary stems should be added to the femoral prosthesis if the femoral surface is inadequate for femoral component fixation. The constrained condylar knee system allows for intramedullary reaming through centering drill guides which fit onto the distal femoral surface. This maintains the increasing diameter of the intramedullary reamers in the central axis of the femur and significantly reduces the possibility of femoral perforation. Reaming should continue until broaching of the femoral cortical bone is appreciated, generally in the range of 15 to 17 mm. Additional intercondylar bone has to be removed if the constrained polyethylene tibial component is to be used. There may be a need to augment the posterior femoral condylar surface if there is significant bone loss posteriorly on the femur. This will allow better apposition of the femoral component against the posterior femur if there is bone deficiency in this area. The femoral component should be placed as posterior as possible to reduce the flexion gap on the femoral side. This reduces the need for an extremely thick tibial component to fill the flexion gap yet not allow full extension. The joint line will be more accurately repositioned if the flexion and extension gaps are filled by augmentation on both the femoral and tibial side and not solely by utilizing a thicker tibial component. If tibial augmentation alone is used, impingement may occur between the patellar and the tibial polyethylene components because the patella will descend into an inferior position.

The femoral and tibial components are then assembled and a reduction is performed. The knee should be stable in flexion and extension and allow a range of flexion greater than 90 degrees. The type of constraint to be incorporated into the knee replacement should be based on knee joint stability. If there is instability still present despite all attempts at soft tissue balancing and augmentation, a constrained polyethylene component should be used and this will require the use of a constrained femoral component. If stability is satisfactory, the posterior stabilized polyethylene component can be used with the standard posterior stabilized femoral component. Alignment can be checked at this point using an extramedullary alignment rod which should bisect the ankle joint and knee joint and be approximately 2 to 3 cm medial to the anterosuperior iliac spine. Patellar tracking must be stable at this point and, if there is a tendency toward subluxation, lateral patellar release is performed.

Bone is lavaged with a pulsatile spray and dried thoroughly. Methylmethacrylate is mixed and used only on the upper tibial surface and the distal femoral surface just beneath the implant. Care is taken that the cement does not penetrate deeply into the intramedullary canals. The stemmed implants are inserted (usually the femoral component is positioned first) and the intramedullary rods on the implants should be of a length and diameter to gain adequate purchase into femoral and tibial bone. The knee is extended to allow further pressurization of the methylmethacrylate. The tourniquet is deflated prior to closure and hemostasis obtained. Suction drainage is used postoperatively for 24 hours.

The modular nature of revision knee replacement systems has allowed customization of the components at the time of the surgical procedure. Stems of varying lengths and diameters can be added, femoral posterior and distal augmentation in different thicknesses and tibial wedges can be used, and tibial configurations with varying constraints can be selected, depending on the pathologic conditions present in the knee.

CONCLUSIONS

The knee joint is involved in the vast majority of patients presenting with rheumatoid arthritis. The treatment depends on the severity of knee joint involvement and the response to less invasive methods of treatment. When these are not successful and the disease is progressive yet not severely destructive to the joint surface, synovectomy may be a surgical treatment option. Joint replacement is the procedure of choice once the knee joint has become significantly impaired. Because of the special problems of soft tissue, ligament imbalance, angular deformity, and poor-quality bone, the surgical plan, technique of arthroplasty, perioperative care, and rehabilitation must be comprehensive and precise if catastrophic complications are to be avoided.

REFERENCES

1. Aglietti P, Windsor RE, Buzzi R, et al: Arthroplasty for the stiff or ankylosed knee. *J Arthroplasty* 1989; 4:1–5.
2. Altchek D, Sculco TP, Rawlins B: Autogenous bone grafting for severe angular deformity in total knee arthoplasty. *J Arthroplasty* 1989; 4:151–155.
3. Attenborough CG: The Attenborough total knee replacement. *J Bone Joint Surg [Br]* 1978; 60:320–326.
4. Bargren, JH, Day WH, Freeman, MA, et al: Mechanical tests on the tibial components of non-hinged prostheses. *J Bone Joint Surg [Br]* 1978; 60:256–261.
5. Bengtson S, Blomgren G, Knutson K, et al: Hematogenous infection after knee arthroplasty. *Acta Orthop Scand* 1987; 58:529–534.
6. Bengtson S, Carlsson A, Relander M: Treatment of the exposed knee prosthesis. *Acta Orthop Scand* 1987; 58:662–665.
7. Bradley GW, Freeman MA, Albrektsson BEJ: Total prosthetic replacement of ankylosed knees. *J Arthroplasty* 1987; 2:179–183.
8. Carmichael E, Chaplin DM: Total knee arthoplasty in juvenile rheumatoid arthritis. *Clin Orthop* 1986; 210:192–200.
9. Cook SD, Barrach RC, Thomas DA, et al: Quantitative histologic analysis of tissue growth in porous knee components. *J Arthroplasty* 1989; 4(suppl):33–43.
10. Doets H, Bierman BT, Soesbergen R: Synovectomy of the rheumatoid knee does not prevent deterioration. *Acta Orthop Scand* 1989; 60:523–525.
11. Donaldson WF III, Sculco TP, Insall JN: The total condylar III knee prosthesis, long term follow-up. *Clin Orthop* 1988; 226:22–27.
12. Dorr LD, Ranawat CS, Sculco TP: Bone grafting for tibial defects in total knee arthroplasty. *Clin Orthop* 1986; 205:153–165.
13. Ecker M, Lotke PA, Windsor RE, et al: Long term results after total condylar knee arthroplasty. *Clin Orthop* 1987; 216:151–158.
14. Figgie HE III, Brody G, Inglis AE. Knee arthrodesis following total knee arthroplasty in rheumatoid arthritis. *Clin Orthop* 1987; 224:237–243.
15. Fleming A, Crown JH, Corbett M, et al: Early rheumatoid disease, 1. Onset. *Ann Rheum Dis* 1976; 35:357–365.
16. Francis C, Pellegrini VD, Stulberg BN, et al: Prevention of venous thrombosis after total knee arthroplasty. *J Bone Joint Surg [Am]* 1990; 72:976–982.
17. Garner RW, Nowat A, Hazleman BL: Wound healing after operations on patients with rheumatoid arthritis. *J Bone Joint Surg [Br]* 1973; 55:134–143.
18. Geen S, Clayton ML, Leidholt JD, et al: Synovectomy and debridement of the knee in rheumatoid arthritis. *J Bone Joint Surg [Am]* 1967; 51:626–642.
19. Goldberg VM, Figgie MP, Figgie HE, et al: Use of the total condylar knee prosthesis for treatment of osteoarthritis and rheumatoid arthritis: Long term results. *J Bone Joint Surg [Am]* 1988; 70:802–811.
20. Goldenberg D: Infectious arthritis complicating rheumatoid arthritis and other chronic rheumatic disorders. *Arthritis Rheum* 1989; 32:496–502.
21. Haas SB, Insall JN, Scuderi G, et al: Pneumatic sequential compression boots compared with aspirin prophylaxis of deep venous thrombosis after total knee arthroplasty. *J Bone Joint Surg [Am]* 1990; 72:27–31.
22. Hallock GG: Salvage of total knee arthroplasty with local fasciocutaneous flaps. *J Bone Joint Surg* 1990; 72:1236–1239.
23. Hoffman AA, Daniels AV, Wyatt RY: Clinical and laboratory comparison of the tibial cut for total knee arthroplasty. *Orthop Trans* 1987; 11:79.
24. Hunter JA, Zoma AA, Scullion FE, et al: The geometric knee replacement in polyarthritis. *J Bone Joint Surg [Br]* 1982; 64:95–98.
25. Hvid I, Kjaesgaard-Andersen P, Wethelund JO, et al: Knee arthroplasty in rheumatoid arthritis. *J Arthroplasty* 1987; 2:233–239.
26. Insall JN, Thompson FM, Brause BD: Two stage reimplantation for the salvage of infected total knee arthroplasty. *J Bone Joint Surg [Am]* 1983; 65:1087–1098.

27. Ishikawa H, Ohno O, Hirohata K: Long term results of synovectomy in rheumatoid arthritis. *J Bone Joint Surg [Am]* 1986; 68:198–205.
28. Johnson DP: Midline or parapatellar incision for knee arthroplasty. *J Bone Joint Surg [Br]* 1988; 70:656–658.
29. Johnson DP: The effect of constant passive motion on wound healing and joint mobility after knee arthroplasty. *J Bone Joint Surg [Am]* 1990; 72:421–426.
30. Kennedy AC, Smith DA, Anton HC, et al: Generalized and local bone loss in patients with rheumatoid arthritis. *Scand J Rheumatol* 1975; 4:209–215.
31. Knutson D, Lindstrand A, Lidgren L: Survival of knee arthroplasties. *J Bone Joint Surg [Br]* 1986; 68:795–803.
32. Laskin RS: Total condylar knee replacement in patients who have rheumatoid arthritis. *J Bone Joint Surg [Am]* 1990; 72:529–535.
33. Laurin CA, Desmarchais L, Daziano L, et al: Long term results of synovectomy of the knee in rheumatoid arthritis. *J Bone Joint Surg* 1974; 56:521–531.
34. Lotke PA, Wong R, Ecker ML: The management of large tibial defects in primary total knee replacement. Presented to the American Academy of Orthopaedic Surgeons, Las Vegas, Feb, 1985.
35. Lynch AF, Bourne RB, Rorabeck CH, et al: Deep venous thrombosis and constant passive motion after total knee arthroplasty. *J Bone Joint Surg [Am]* 1988; 70:11–14.
36. Maloney WJ, Schurman DJ, Hanger D, et al: The influence of constant passive motion on outcome in total knee arthroplasty. *Clin Orthop* 1990; 256:162–168.
37. Matsui N, Taneda Y, Ohta H, et al: Arthroscopic versus open synovectomy in the rheumatoid knee. *Int Orthop* 1989; 13:17–20.
38. Maynard M, Sculco TP, Ghelman B: Progression and regression of deep vein thrombosis after total knee arthroplasty. Presented to the Knee Society, Anaheim, Calif. March 1991.
39. McKenna R, Bachmann F, Kaushal S, et al: Thromboembolic disease in patients undergoing total knee replacement. *J Bone Joint Surg [Am]* 1976; 58:928–932.
40. Myllyla T, Peltonen L, Pirranen J, et al: Consequences of synovectomy of the knee joint: Clinical, histopathological and enzymatic changes in two components of complement. *Ann Rheum Dis* 1983; 42:28–35.
41. Nicholls DW, Dorr LD: Revision surgery for stiff total knee arthroplasty. *J Arthroplasty* 1990; 5(suppl):73–77.
42. Nielsen PT, Jorgensen LN, Albrecht-Beste E, et al: Lower thrombosis risk with epidural blockage in knee arthroplasty. *Acta Orthop Scand* 1990; 61:29–31.
43. Nielsen S, Hvid I, Sneppen TC: Total condylar knee arthroplasty: A report of two year follow-up on 247 cases. *Arch Orthop Trauma Surg* 1985; 104:227–233.
44. Ritter MA: Screw and cement fixation of large defects in total knee arthroplasty. *J Arthroplasty* 1986; 1:125–129.
45. Rooser B, Torsten B, Knutson K, et al: Revision knee arthroplasty in rheumatoid arthritis. *Clin Orthop Rel Res* 1987; 219:169–173.
46. Ranawat CS, Desai K: Role of early synovectomy of the knee joint in rheumatoid arthritis. *Arthritis Rheum* 1975; 18: 117–121.
47. Ranawat CS, Hansraj KK: Effect of posterior cruciate ligament sacrifice on durability of the cement-bone interface, a nine year survivorship study of 100 total condylar knee arthroplasties. *Orthop Clin North Am* 1989; 20:63–70.
48. Rand JA, Chao EYS, Stauffer RM: Kinematic rotating hinge total knee arthroplasty. *J Bone Joint Surg [Am]* 1987; 69:489–497.
49. Rand JA, Ilstrup DM: Survivorship analysis in total knee arthroplasty. *J Bone Joint Surg [Am]* 1991; 73:397–409.
50. Robinson DR, Tashjiuan AH, Levine C: A possible mechanism for bone destruction in rheumatoid arthritis. *J Clin Invest* 1975; 56:118–1186.
51. Rosa R, Sculco TP, Inglis AE, et al: Total knee arthroplasty in rheumatoid arthritis: A long term follow-up. Presented to the Knee Society, Feb, 1983, Anaheim, California.
52. Sarokhan AJ, Scott RD, Thomas WH, et al: Total knee arthroplasty in rheumatoid arthritis. *J Bone Joint Surg [Am]* 1983; 65:1071–1080.
53. Scott RD, Volatile TB: 12 year experience with posterior cruciate retaining total knee arthroplasty. *Clin Orthop* 1986; 205:100–107.
54. Scuderi G, Insall JN: The posterior stabilized knee prosthesis. *Orthop Clin North Am* 1989; 20:71–77.
55. Sculco TP: Condylar III prosthesis in ligament instability. *Orthop Clin North Am* 1989; 20:221–227.
56. Sculco TP: Soft tissue balancing in total knee arthroplasty, in Goldberg V (ed): *Controversies of Total Knee Arthroplasty.* New York, Raven Press, 1991, pp 167–174.
57. Sculco TP, Faris P: Total knee replacement in the stiff knee. *Techn Orthop* 1988; 3:5–10.
58. Sharrock NE, Haas SB, Hargett MJ, et al: Effects of epidural anesthesia on the incidence of deep vein thrombosis after total knee arthroplasty. *J Bone Joint Surg [Am]* 1991; 73:502–506.
59. Sledge CB, Walker PS: Total knee arthroplasty in rheumatoid arthritis. *Clin Orthop* 1984; 182:127–136.
60. Sledge CB, Zuckerman JD, Shortkroff S, et al: Synovectomy of the rheumatoid knee using intraarticular injection of dysprosium-165-ferric hydroxide macroaggregates. *J Bone Joint Surg [Am]* 1987; 69:970–975.
61. Stuart MJ, Rand JA: Total knee arthroplasty in young adults who have rheumatoid arthritis. *J Bone Joint Surg [Am]* 1988; 70:84–87.
62. Stulberg BN, Insall JN, Williams GW, et al: Deep vein thrombosis following total knee replacement, an analysis of 638 arthroplasties. *J Bone Joint Surg [Am]* 1984; 66:194–201.

63. Tauber C, Bar-On EB, Ganel A, et al: The total condylar prosthesis, a review of 71 operations. *Arch Orthop Trauma Surg* 1986; 104:252–256.
64. Thomas BJ, Cracchiolo A, Lee YF, et al: Total knee arthroplasty in rheumatoid arthritis, a comparison of the polycentric and total condylar prosthesis. *Clin Orthop Rel Res* 1991; 265:129–136.
65. Tillman K: Recent advances in the surgical treatment of rheumatoid arthritis. *Clin Orthop* 1990; 258:62–71.
66. Windsor RE, Insall JN, Sculco TP: Bone grafting of tibial defects in primary and revision total knee arthroplasty. *Clin Orthop* 1986; 205:153–165.
67. Wilton JM, Gibson T, Church CM: Defective phagocytosis by synovial fluid and blood polymorphonuclear leukocytes in rheumatoid arthritis. *Rheum Rehabil* 1978; 17:25–35.

CHAPTER 14

Bilateral Hip and Knee Replacement

Thomas P. Sculco, M.D.

INTRODUCTION

The polyarticular nature of rheumatoid arthritis contrasts it sharply from osteoarthritis. The manifestation of multiple joint involvement may be in noncontiguous joints of both the lower and upper extremities. In the most severe form of the disease, however, both major weightbearing joints in both lower extremities may be affected. These patients may require bilateral hip and knee replacement surgery and are discussed separately because of the subset of clinical concerns related to these patients. Should such extensive surgery be performed at all? How and in what priority should these joints be replaced? Do the surgical results, risks, and expense justify these procedures? These are but a few of the questions raised when surgery is contemplated in these disabled patients.

As important as the technical success of their reconstructive surgery is the requirement that these patients be willing to cooperate and work assiduously at rehabilitation after surgery. Patients needing bilateral hip and knee replacements but whose desire to recover ambulatory function is lacking may become surgical successes but functional failures. The surgeon confronted with these complex arthritic patients tends to recommend surgical treatment without exploring more deeply the patient's wishes and motivation. A frank discussion between surgeon and patient regarding the difficult rehabilitative course is necessary prior to proceeding along a surgical course.

These patients, because of the severe functional disability related to impairment of both hip and knee joints, rapidly become household ambulators or lose ambulatory capacity completely. As sitting becomes more commonplace and walking deteriorates, pathologic changes occur which contribute to the complexity of surgical correction. Flexion deformities of hips and knees increase if ambulation is minimal and sitting time is significant (Fig 14–1). These contractures, which are initially reversible, become intractable. Prosthetic replacement of these arthritic joints requires correction of these deformities by soft tissue release and in the most severe cases alteration in bone cuts to compensate for the flexion deformity (e.g., resection of additional femur in knee replacement with marked flexion deformity).

Osteopenia is also more apparent in these patients because many are receiving steroids and because of the severity of the disease process itself (Fig 14–2). Bone mass is further reduced because of the failure to ambulate and the disuse phenomenon. Osteopenia complicates surgical treatment by providing a poor substrate for insertion of the implant. Additionally, there is an increased risk of intraoperative fracture during the procedure itself when the limb is manipulated to promote exposure. Not only is the quality of bone poor but the surrounding investment of soft tissues is of suboptimal quality and this complicates implant coverage and restoration of muscle, tendon, and ligament function.

Muscle loss is greater the longer the patient is nonambulatory and this will definitely delay recovery and walking ability. When severe deformities are corrected there is often a need to reconstruct muscle-tendon relationships. The ability to recover from

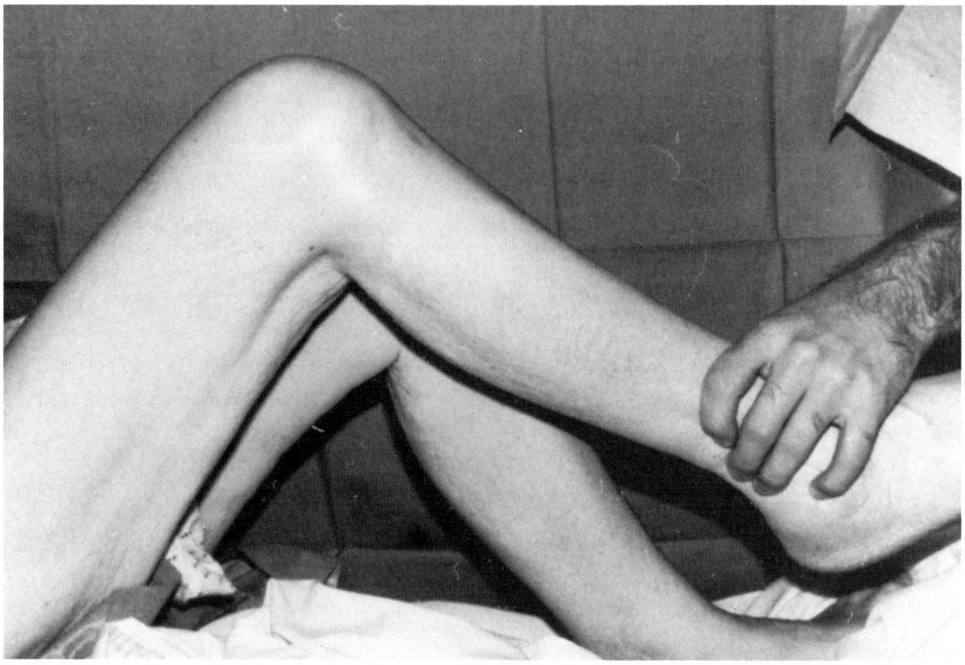

FIG 14–1.
Severe bilateral hip and knee flexion contractures in a patient undergoing bilateral hip and knee replacement.

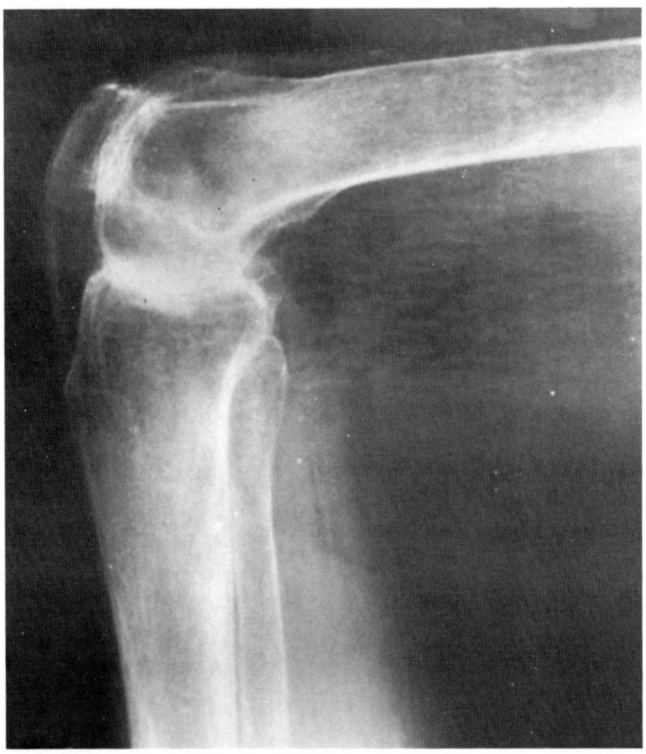

FIG 14–2.
Marked periarticular osteopenia in a nonambulatory patient undergoing replacement of four lower extremity joints.

these intricate procedures may be prolonged and full return of function may not be possible.

The surgeon must also consider the possibility of increased ankle and foot pain once ambulatory function has returned. These more distal joints, having been spared the loads of weightbearing during the period the patient is not walking, may be markedly arthritic and interfere with the ability to walk. Marks[5] in a review of 21 patients undergoing bilateral hip and knee replacement, found that the ability to walk had improved in all patients but many noted an increase in ankle and foot pain that limited walking.

SURGICAL APPROACH

The question frequently raised when contemplating the correction of both hip and knee joints is in what order and priority should the various joints be addressed. It is strongly recommended that both hip joints be replaced at one operative setting followed approximately 10 to 14 days later by replacement of both knee joints at another single operative setting. This interim period allows wound healing to progress and confirms stable, uncompromised wounds prior to proceeding with knee replacements. By submitting the patient to two operative procedures, only two anesthetica inductions are required and also only the trauma of two surgical events. Rehabilitation can then proceed with all affected joints having been surgically corrected. Piecemeal treatment by delayed staging of unilateral procedures will greatly prolong recovery. In addition, the still affected joints will hinder rehabilitation of the replaced joints and ultimate function will be jeopardized.

When hip joints are replaced before knee joints in patients in whom both areas are symmetrically affected, rehabilitation tends to be less cumbersome for the patient. Recovery is more rapid after hip replacement surgery and ambulatory function returns quickly. Manipulation of the knee is necessary during hip replacement surgery, particularly if the posterior approach is used, and this may produce undue stress on a fresh knee replacement. Hemarthrosis within the knee after manipulation during hip replacement will adversely affect the result of the knee replacement. The surgeon must avoid excessive flexing of the hip when performing knee replacement surgery in a patient in whom both hips have been replaced. The hip can easily and inadvertently be flexed beyond 60 to 70 degrees when obtaining full flexion of the knee for exposure at knee replacement. This may put the hip into an unstable zone and the risk of dislocation is significant.

In patients in whom there is a significant asymmetry of symptoms between hip and knee joints, there are a number of factors that should be considered before deciding which to proceed with first, hip replacement or knee replacement. As a rule the most painful joints are treated first. Should complications intervene between surgeries it is best to have the most painful joints reconstructed and comfortable. A second consideration in surgical planning is replacement of those joints with severe deformity as a priority. In a patient who has severe flexion deformities of both knees, ambulation will not be possible if the hips are corrected first. The converse is generally not the case in that severe hip flexion contractures, although they will impede ambulation, will be compensated for by increased lumbar lordosis and walking may proceed. If hip flexion contractures are not corrected first and knee flexion contractures are present, the knee deformities will tend to recur after knee replacement until the hip contractures are released. This return of knee flexion contracture is particularly apt to occur if ambulation is not restored and a sitting posture again becomes predominant.

CLINICAL RESULTS

In two clinical reviews of bilateral hip and knee replacement surgery at The Hospital for Special Surgery in New York, the first in 1985[7] and an updated study in 1991,[1] the clinical results were encouraging. In both study groups 90% of the patient population was female. The average age at the time of the first joint replacement was in the early fourth decade. The duration of disease prior to surgical treatment was 13 years, evidence of the chronic deteriorating nature of the disease in these patients. Half of the patients in the earlier study were receiving corticosteroids at the time of their initial procedure. Follow-up averaged 6.3 years in the earlier study and 9.4 years in the later study with some of the earlier patients being lost to follow-up evaluation.

Overall results indicated an improvement in function in the earlier study in 73% of patients. In the later review, 82% of patients were rated as good or excellent in function and 90% had good to excellent pain relief. In the study by Sculco et al.[7] the American Rheumatism Association (ARA) classification was considered inadequate for evaluation of function after surgical treatment and therefore a new grading system was developed. Patients were staged accordingly:

Level A: patients able to walk independently outside the home
Level B: patients limited to walking in the home
Level C: patients limited to walking a few steps only
Level D: patients who were wheelchairbound
Level E: patients who were bedbound

Figures 14–3, 14–4, and 14–5 demonstrate the marked improvement in patient function and ambulatory capacity. Patients were asked to place themselves in a functional category preoperatively, immediately postoperatively, and at the time of final follow-up evaluation. Figures 14–6 and 14–7 demonstrate the level of functional improvement in these patients. If, for example, a patient improved from taking a few steps in the home (level C) to an independent ambulator in the community (level A), that patient is represented as +2 level improvement.

Seventy-three percent of patients demonstrated sustained functional improvement, 21% showed no

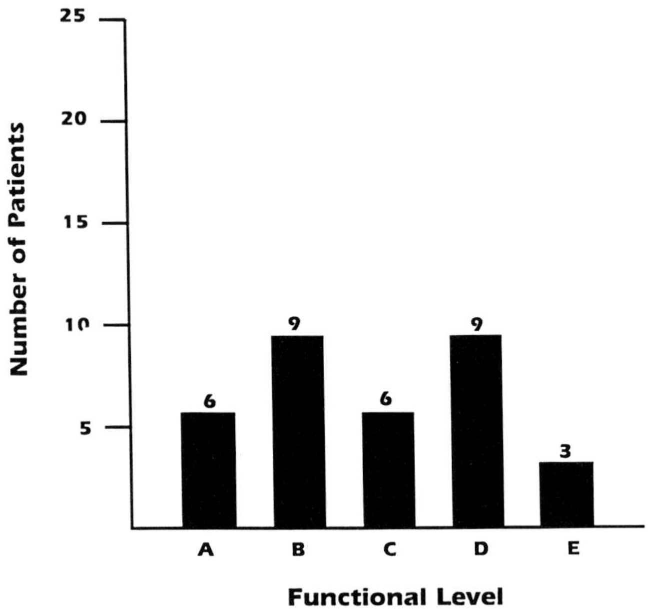

FIG 14–3.
Preoperative functional level.

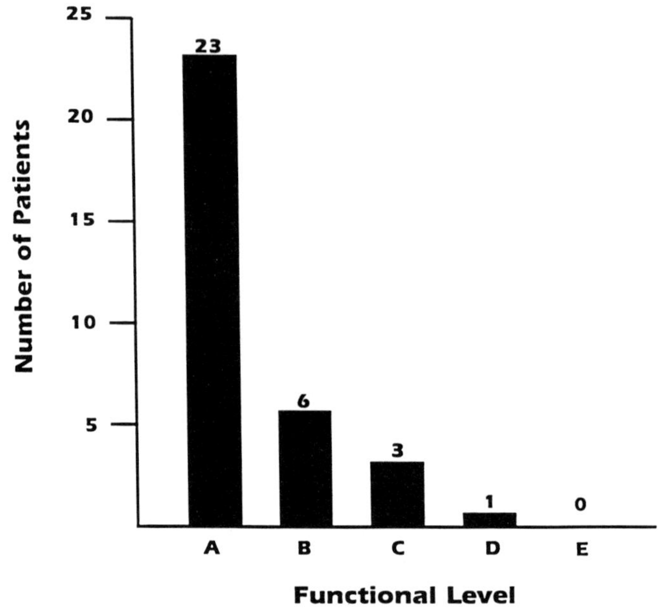

FIG 14–5.
Long-term functional level.

change, and 6% actually became worse. In the group that was worse or showed no change, the average age was just slightly higher than the average age for the entire group, 48 years vs. 45 years. Most of the unchanged group began in level A or B preoperatively and were satisfied with their pain relief, although functional level did not improve dramatically. The one patient that decreased three functional levels was a patient with three deep periprosthetic *Escherichia coli* infections.

When asked which surgery was more beneficial, 48% elected the hips, 21% the knees, and 31% thought that both were equally helpful. McDonald,[6] in his review of bilateral hip and knee replacement in rheumatoid patients, obtained similar appreciation of the hip replacement procedure although the knee replacements were performed without problem, as in our series. Eighty-nine percent of the patients would undergo the surgery again, 9% would not, and 2% undecided.

Of the 76 arthroplasties in the earlier study three were revised: one T-28 prosthesis for a broken femoral stem, and two surface replacements (Fig 14–8) because of loosening. Three of the knee arthroplas-

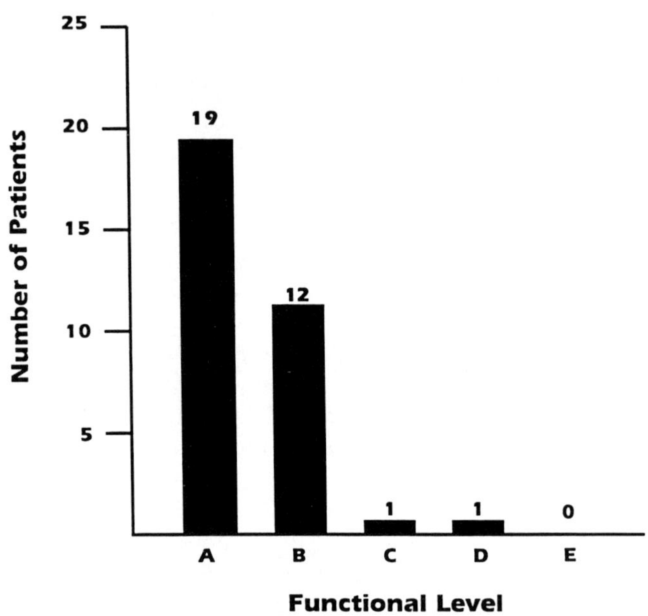

FIG 14–4.
Immediate postoperative functional level.

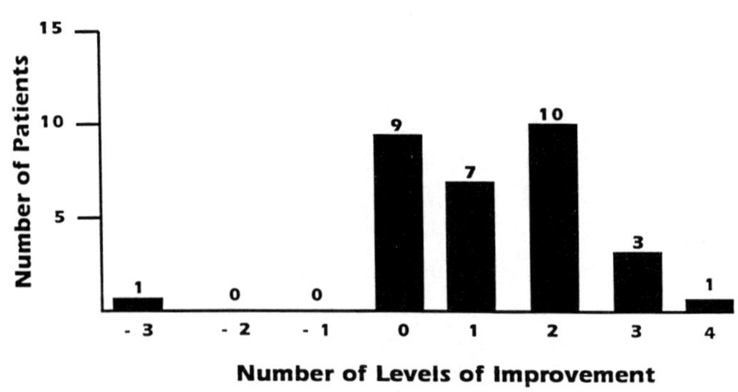

FIG 14–6.
Comparison of preoperative and postoperative functional level.

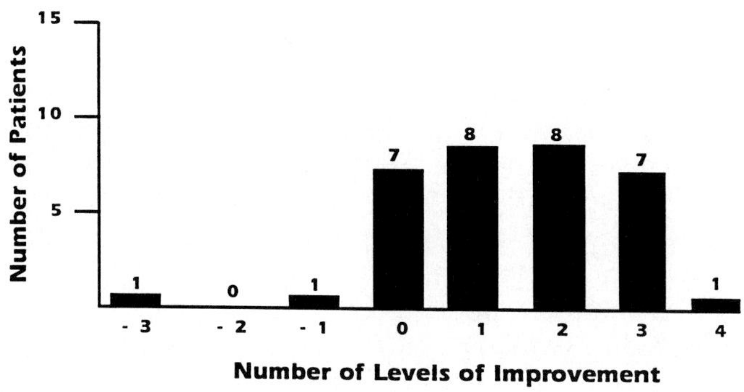

FIG 14–7.
Preoperative and long-term functional level.

ties were revised. Both were earlier designs—one geomedic and two duocondylar for loosening and patellofemoral pain.

In the study of Dossick et al.[1] of 280 hip and knee replacements, there were 14 failed hip replacements and 9 failed knee replacements. The cause of failure for the hip replacements was loosening of components. In the knees failure was due to a variety of causes including patellofemoral instability, loosening, and knee joint instability. Of note in this study is that three hip and three knee revision arthroplasties went on to further failure. Additionally, six as yet unrevised components demonstrate evidence of loosening.

In the earlier series there were a total of four deep infections, two after hip replacement and two after knee replacement. Both deep hip infections were in the same patient and were caused by *E. coli* organisms. Of the two knees infected, the causative organism was also *E. coli* and in the same patient who had both hip infections. In this patient there was major loss of soft tissue with exposure of the implant and the knee subsequently underwent arthrodesis (Fig 14–9). The other deep knee infecting organism was beta streptococcus. In the later review, eight deep infections were equally divided between hips and knees.

The results from both series support functional improvement and pain relief in the vast majority of patients. Patient satisfaction with the procedures is high and complication rates were generally low. Deep infection was in the range of 3% to 5%, high in comparison with most series of joint replacements but consistent with rheumatoid patient groups. Of note in both series was that although the patient population tends to be younger than most joint replacement series, return to work was poor in these patients. This signifies the severe polyarticular nature of the disease and the many limitations put upon patients by the disease.

Johnson,[4] reporting in 1975 on results from the Mayo Clinic, reviewed 11 patients with bilateral hip and knee replacements. He noted improvement in pain relief and increased function in the majority of patients although the study was performed using earlier implant designs. Jergensen et al.[3] followed 16 patients an average of 23 months, noting improvement in most except that older patients, those with

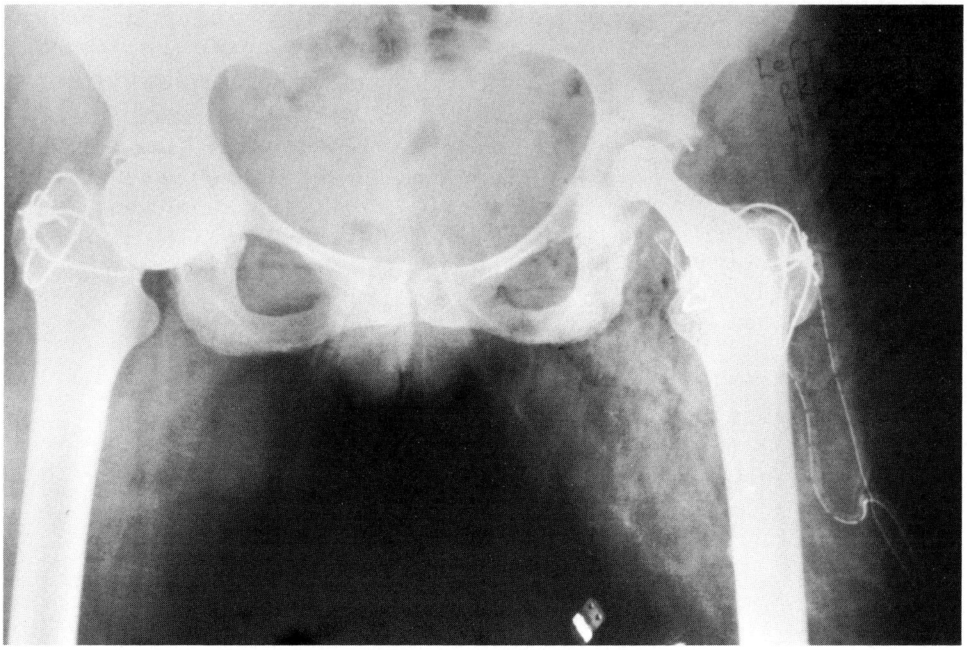

FIG 14–8.
Failed surface replacement with resorption of the femoral neck under the prosthesis.

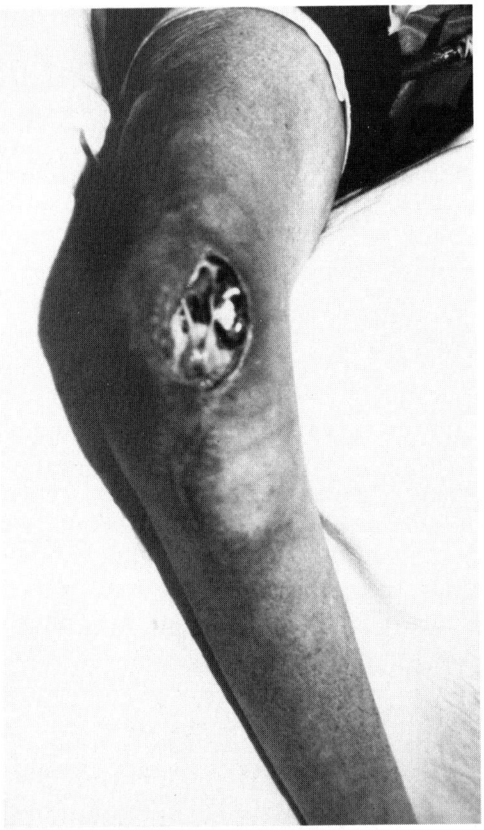

FIG 14–9.
Infected total knee replacement caused by *E. coli* and loss of all soft tissue coverage over the knee implant.

prolonged rheumatoid arthritis and more active disease, did less well. Additionally, the authors noted that 190 degrees of combined flexion of the hip and knee was necessary for ease in climbing stairs and rising from the seated position.

McDonald[6] noted in his review of 26 patients that the pattern of the disease played a significant role in resultant hip and knee flexion with the ankylosing type of disease leading to less hip and knee flexion independent of the implant used. He noted that a combined hip and knee flexion of greater than 180 degrees was only achieved in 32 of the 52 limbs operated upon. His overall results were similar to those for other surgeons with 97% of hip replacements achieving good to excellent pain relief, and 85% of knee replacements good to excellent in terms of pain relief. Four knees required revision for loosening of a component and one patient had tuberculosis of the knee joint. There were no other deep infections in his series.

Hoekstra et al.[2] developed a complex 200-point rating system to evaluate preoperative and postoperative function. Only 13 patients were available for review. They noted that all patients demonstrated a marked pain relief, and function good as demonstrated by an improved score. Walking ability did not always improve in their series, primarily owing to the severe nature of the patients' polyarticular disease. All patients were pleased with their operations, however, and were enthusiastic as to the benefit of the procedures.

Yoshino et al.[8] reported on 18 patients and noted that walking ability was improved in 16 patients. Activities of daily living were easier and the authors noted that 7 of the 14 married patients were able to perform sexual intercourse as prior to their disease. Pain relief was excellent and patient satisfaction, as in all previous studies, was high.

CONCLUSIONS

Clinical data from multiple centers in this country and abroad have demonstrated the overwhelming relief in pain and improvement in function in patients undergoing bilateral hip and knee replacement surgery. The patients affirmed that the risks and results justified these extensive procedures. The economic impact of these procedures is significant and the consumption of medical resources is high in the treatment of these patients. The surgery is complex, the medical care expensive, and the intensive physical and occupational therapy needed is labor-intensive and time-consuming. The functional improvement has in some cases reduced the need for full-time home care assistance and this does provide some saving of expenditure for the health care system. The major benefit remains the relief of pain which allows patients to live their lives more comfortably. The incremental improvement in function and in activities of daily living provides a more meaningful and independent life. The risk-benefit ratio is heavily tilted toward the benefit side in these patients.

REFERENCES

1. Dossick PH, Falatyn S, Alexiades MP, et al: Four joint replacement in rheumatoid arthritis. Submitted for publication, 1991.
2. Hoekstra HJ, Veth RP, Nielsen HF, et al: Bilateral total hip and knee replacement in rheumatoid arthritis patients. *Arch Orthop Trauma Surg* 1989; 108:291–295.
3. Jergensen HE, Poss R, Sledge CB: Bilateral total hip

and knee replacement in adults with rheumatoid arthritis. *Clin Orthop* 1978; 137:120–128.
4. Johnson KA: Arthroplasty of both hips and both knees in rheumatoid arthritis. *J Bone Joint Surg [Br]* 1975; 57:901–904.
5. Marks JS: Benefits of multiple joint replacement in rheumatoid arthritis. *Scand J Rehabil Med* 1984; 16:43–46.
6. McDonald I: Bilateral replacement of the hip and knee in rheumatoid arthritis. *J Bone Joint Surg [Br]* 1982; 64:465–468.
7. Sculco TP, Adams W, Fried S, et al: Four joint replacement in rheumatoid arthritis. Presented at the American Academy of Orthopaedic Surgeons Meeting, Las Vegas, February, 1985.
8. Yoshino S, Fujimori J, Morishige T, et al: Bilateral joint replacement of hip and knee joints in patients with rheumatoid arthritis. *Arch Orthop Trauma Surg* 1984; 103:1–4.

CHAPTER 15

The Hindfoot

Mark P. Figgie, M.D.

Mark Sobel, M.D.

Mark J. Geppert, M.D.

INTRODUCTION

Rheumatoid arthritis may affect all joints, bones, vessels, nerves, and other connective tissue components of the foot and ankle. Rheumatoid involvement of the hindfoot can become the single most important deterrent to ambulation,[1] and failure to assess hindfoot involvement may severely compromise the results of surgical intervention of the hip, knee, or forefoot.[94] Vaino[104] has stated that the hindfoot may be involved in up to 70% of patients with rheumatoid arthritis.

The normal biomechanics of the ankle, subtalar, and midfoot joints are intimately related and critical to smooth bipedal gait. The frequency of operative intervention on the hip, knee, and forefoot in the rheumatoid patient warrants a greater understanding of the normal function of the ipsilateral joints. One must understand the normal function of the hindfoot in order to appreciate the pathologic effects of rheumatoid arthritis and its consequences on distal (forefoot) and proximal (hip and knee) structures. This awareness promotes timely, comprehensive, and appropriate care for the entire lower extremity in the rheumatoid patient.

BIOMECHANICS

The osseous structures of the foot and ankle are linked by ligaments, crossed by muscles and tendons, and divided for descriptive purposes into ankle, hindfoot, midfoot, and forefoot regions.

The ankle joint consists of the tibial plafond, its posterolateral border (posterior malleolus), the medial malleolus, distal fibula (lateral malleolus), and the talus. Stability of the ankle joint is determined by the saddle shape of the distal tibia and the medial deltoid and lateral ligament complexes. Anteriorly, the talus is widened, which provides greatest ankle stability in dorsiflexion. In addition, as the foot moves from plantar flexion to dorsiflexion, an external rotation of the distal tibiofibular joint occurs.

The axis of the ankle joint, determined by the work of Inman,[45] is oblique, courses posterolaterally in the transverse plane and inferolaterally in the coronal plane. Palpation of the tips of the malleoli gives an approximation of the ankle axis.[57] Analysis of motion of the ankle is complicated by the translational movement or gliding of the domed talus on the tibial plafond. The axis of the ankle joint is therefore not fixed, is dependent on the position of the foot,[43] and is obliquely oriented to all three anatomic planes. The obliquity of the axis allows rotation of the foot or leg with movement of the ankle, as described by Mann: from heel strike to foot flat, the ankle plantar flexes with apparent intoeing of the foot. At midstance, the foot is fixed; dorsiflexion of the ankle is accompanied by internal rotation of the leg.[57] The amount of observed rotation of the leg and foot at the ankle during normal gait cannot, however, be explained by the obliquity of the ankle axis alone. Motion at the subtalar joint and rotation about the transverse tarsal (Chopart's) joint permits increased rotation. Mann effectively utilizes the concept of a mitered hinge to demonstrate this complex relationship.[57]

The talus is suspended without muscular attachment and therefore passively transmits force and motion between the calcaneus and tibia through its ligamentous attachments and articular contacts. The subtalar joint is comprised of three facets (posterior, middle, and anterior) which are located on the calcaneus and articulate with the undersurface of the talus.

Stability of the subtalar joint is dependent upon the muscles and tendons that traverse the joint; the ligamentous attachments connecting the tibia, talus, and calcaneus; and articular congruity between the facets of the subtalar joint. The axis of the subtalar joint, like the axis of the ankle joint, is obliquely orientated with respect to the three planes of orientation. It averages 23 degrees medial to the transverse plane and 41 degrees superior to the horizontal plane,[46] passing from the dorsomedial aspect of the talus and exiting the plantar lateral surface of the calcaneus. Together, the ankle–subtalar joint complex has been likened to a universal joint.

Motion of the subtalar complex intimately affects the transverse tarsal (Chopart's) joint which is comprised of the talonavicular and calcaneocuboid joints.[29] With heel strike, the calcaneus everts, which aligns the transverse tarsal joint in parallel, resulting in a flexible forefoot. The hindfoot thereby allows a plantigrade accommodation to uneven terrain. When footflat is reached, the swing of the contralateral limb imparts an external rotation of the stance leg. The external rotation of the tibia is transmitted across the ankle joint and is translated into subtalar inversion. Inversion of the subtalar joint causes a nonparallel alignment of the transverse tarsal joint which contributes to the rigidity needed for toe-off.[63]

The axes of the two components of the transverse tarsal joint (talonavicular and calcaneocuboid) are therefore dependent on the position of the subtalar joint. When in heel varus, their axes are nonparallel, resulting in a rigid foot lever which is a necessary component of normal gait. Permanent heel varus (subtalar arthrodesis malaligned in varus) results in a rigid transverse tarsal joint requiring increased compensatory motion stressing adjacent joints.

The navicular, cuboid, and three cuneiforms and their articulations form the midfoot.[22] The osseous geometry of the midfoot, strong interligamentous connections, support from the inflexible plantar fascia, and action of the foot intrinsic and extrinsic musculature all combine to form the longitudinal and transverse arches of the foot. The arches distribute the forces of ambulation and their position is dependent upon the motion of adjacent joints. According to Mann,[59] the longitudinal arch is elevated by the following sequence of events: external rotation of the tibia, inversion of the calcaneus, and adduction of the forefoot. The arch depresses with the opposite sequence: external rotation of the tibia, eversion of the calcaneus, and adduction of the forefoot.[59] Dorsiflexion of the metatarsophalangeal joints causes tension on the plantar fascia which inserts on the calcaneus. This elevates the longitudinal arch through the windless mechanism described by Hicks.[42, 43] Another major factor in the stability of the arch is the geometric configuration of the talonavicular joint. In both the sagittal and transverse planes, the concentric convex articular end of the talus locks into the concave surface of the navicular during weightbearing.[60]

Normal foot and ankle function is clearly dependent upon an intricate interplay of the osseous structures, position, ligament stability, and coordinated movement of component parts via muscle contractions and tendon movements. The complex interrelationship of normal structural anatomy and physiology indicate that pathologic changes in one component can have far-reaching sequelae.

PATHOPHYSIOLOGY

Rheumatoid arthritis is a systemic inflammatory condition of uncertain etiology which, at the cellular level, involves an activation of the inflammatory cascade leading to the enzymatic destruction of tissues. Proliferative synovitis can lead to attenuation of ligaments and joint capsules, thus altering normal biomechanical function and kinematics of the foot and ankle. All structures of the foot, including skin, nerves, vessels, bones, ligaments, and tendons can be affected by rheumatoid arthritis. Additionally, though the disease progresses by similar periarticular and peritendinous pathophysiologic mechanisms as in the hand, progression in the ankle and hindfoot is aggravated by the repetitive weightbearing forces of ambulation. The predominant deformity of the rheumatoid hindfoot, as described by Vahvanen,[102, 103] is pes planovalgus (Fig 15–1). Other deformities in his study of 202 preoperative rheumatoid patients include forefoot varus (19.4%), pes calcaneovarus (9.2%), and pes cavus or calcaneocavus (6.9%). Combined deformities were noted in 22.9%.

Tillman[99, 100] states that the tarsal joints, particularly the important "medial chain" of supporting ligaments and capsules, are attenuated by rheumatoid inflammation. This inflammatory slackening of the ligaments, coupled with tenosynovitis of the posterior tibial tendon, weakness of the intrinsic musculature, and the dynamic and persistent downward weightbearing forces of the body[99, 100] results in a pes planovalgus deformity. Both Tillman and Vahvanen agree that the first and most frequently involved joint in the hindfoot is the talonavicular joint.[99, 100, 103] Loss of the arch can also occur at the cuneonavicular joint as described by Vaino.[104]

The hypermobility of all joints evidenced in early rheumatoid arthritis results in progressive deformity of the hindfoot and midfoot due to excessive joint motion and loss of normal biomechanics. Increased motion at the talonavicular joint due to ligamentous laxity allows increased forefoot pronation

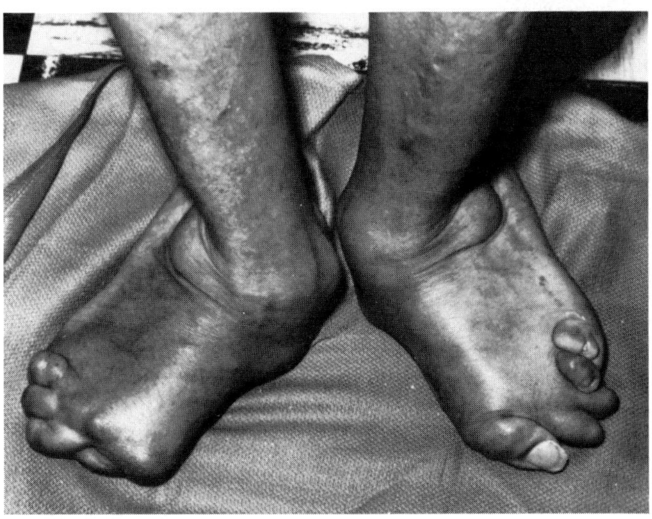

FIG 15–1.
A severe pes planovalgus deformity.

with weightbearing. Increased forefoot pronation results from increased lateral rotation of the calcaneus about its long axis (eversion)[66] which is seen in rheumatoid arthritis. Stockley and colleagues[94] have documented, in pedographic studies, increased medial forefoot pressures in subjects with hindfoot valgus.

Abnormal mechanics due to ligamentous laxity can result in articular and osseous changes. The articular cartilage and bone is directly susceptible to enzymatic degradation due to the inflammatory reactions of rheumatic arthritis. Tillman[99] states that the tibial plafond is more susceptible to degradation than the talus, and a lateral softening would result in progressive valgus deformity.

Virtually every combination of deformity is seen in rheumatoid arthritis.[87] As synovitis subsides and soft tissue contractures increase, stiffness and secondary degenerative arthritis occur. Clayton[14] describes two types of rheumatoid arthritis: the stiff and loose form. Involvement of various combinations of joints, with either an increased (ligamentous laxity) or decreased (fibrosed) character, would yield a highly variable clinical presentation understandable in the context of an alteration in normal biomechanics.

Tenosynovitis can occur in rheumatoid arthritis leading to dysfunction or eventual tendon rupture. The predominantly affected tendons are the posterior tibial and peroneal tendons,[10] though the anterior tibial tendon and extensor and flexor tendons can also be affected. The most obvious evidence of tenosynovitis involves unilateral rupture or attenuation of the posterior tibial tendon as reported by Downey et al.[26] Because the posterior tibial tendon inserts on the navicular, medial cuneiform, and first metatarsal base, and is a primary dynamic stabilizer of the longitudinal arch, its disruption provides a dramatic example of pathomechanics. The ligamentous laxity of the talonavicular joint coupled with the loss of posterior tibial tendon function leads to a lateral slide of the navicular, a medial and plantar drift of the talar neck, abduction and pronation of the forefoot, loss of the longitudinal arch, increased motion at the transverse tarsal joint, and increased hindfoot valgus. Increasing valgus hindfoot deformity may result in weightbearing on the medial malleolus. With progressive flattening of the feet, tension on the inelastic plantar fascia creates a painful hindfoot.

Tarsal tunnel syndrome, or entrapment of the posterior tibial nerve at the tarsal tunnel, has been reported as an initial presentation of rheumatoid arthritis.[56] The posterior tibial nerve can be stretched with a progressive planovalgus foot deformity accounting for the tarsal tunnel syndrome. Anatomic crowding at the tarsal tunnel can occur due to proliferative tenosynovitis of the posterior tibial tendon. It is unlikely that anatomic crowding plays a significant role because the lateral border of the tarsal tunnel, the laciniate ligament (flexor retinaculum), is attenuated in rheumatoid arthritis. Primary affliction of the nerve, or a secondary interference with its blood supply owing to vasculitis, could also explain the finding of tarsal tunnel syndrome in rheumatoid arthritis.

Understanding the intricacy of normal foot and ankle mechanics, pathomechanics, and the variable effects of rheumatoid arthritis on all tissues of the foot and ankle helps one understand the significance of physical findings, formulate a diagnosis, and plan a therapeutic intervention.

PHYSICAL EXAMINATION

The foot and ankle are systemically examined after inspecting the hip, knee, and gait patterns. With the patient standing, the mechanical axis of the leg is determined. While the patient is bearing weight, the maintenance of the longitudinal arch is inspected in addition to any forefoot abnormalities. Hindfoot position is determined with the patient standing and the tibiocalcaneal angle is measured with a goniometer. The patient is then asked to rise on the toes with one leg elevated. Heel inversion is inspected to assess competence of the posterior tibial tendon and eversion is performed to evaluate the peroneal tendons.

The patient is then asked to walk and gait is assessed. Forefoot pain generally causes a voluntary external rotation of the forefoot to decrease pressure on the metatarsal heads. Clinically, the gait is usually an antalgic, steppage gait with the specific gait abnormalities of rheumatoid arthritis as demonstrated in formal gait laboratory studies.[66]

The patient is then seated with the legs dangling free. The posterior calf and Achilles tendon are palpated for swelling, tenderness, or other signs of Achilles tendinitis or the presence of rheumatoid nodules. The retrocalcaneal region is then palpated to rule out retrocalcaneal bursitis. Passive and active

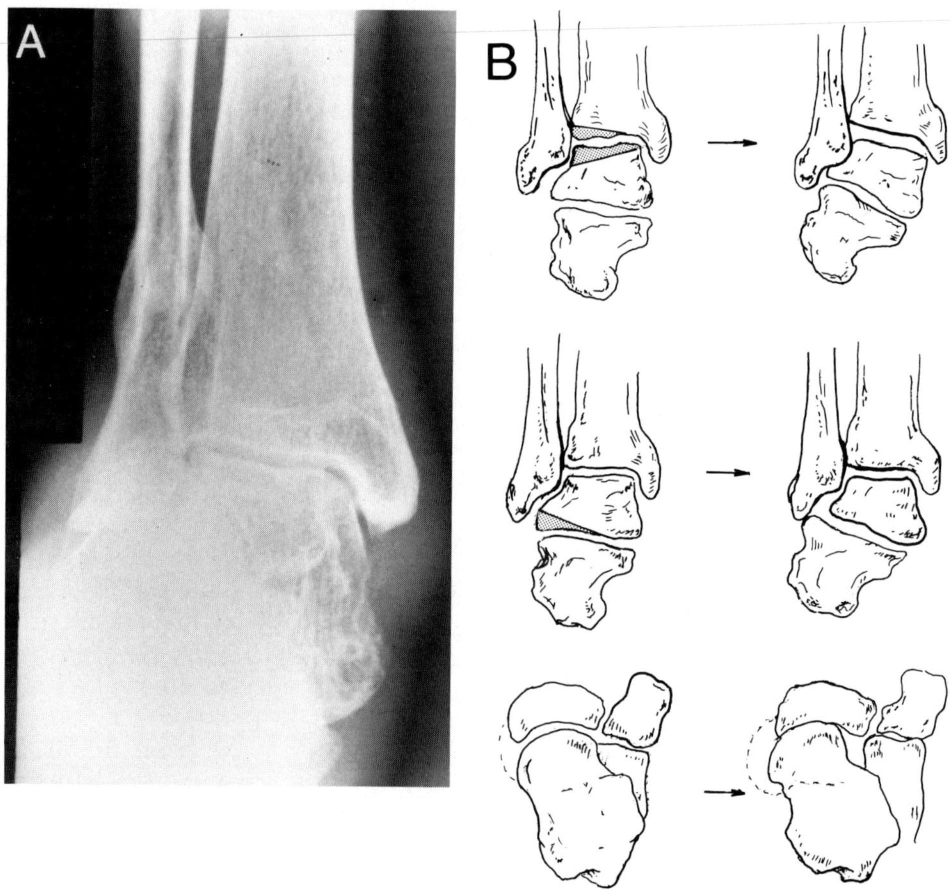

FIG 15–2.
A, fibular stress fractures due to significant hindfoot valgus deformity. **B,** the valgus deformity can be secondary to bone loss at the ankle or subtalar joint.

ankle motion is then determined. The ankle is inspected for evidence of joint effusion and tenosynovitis of the peroneal, tibialis anterior, or posterior tibial tendons. The medial and lateral ligaments of the ankle and the regional tendons are palpated for tenderness. Pain on palpation several centimeters proximal to the distal end of the fibula may indicate a stress[111] fracture due to excessive hindfoot valgus or lateral migration of the talus (Fig 15–2). These two mechanisms may cause distal fibular tenderness indicating calcaneofibular impingement.[51, 52] A history of a sudden painful onset of symptoms suggests a possible stress fracture, whereas sudden deformity suggests tendon rupture.

A history of painful ambulation, particularly on uneven terrain, suggests subtalar joint involvement. Patients often mistakenly attribute their pain to the ankle joint. Subtalar involvement is indicated by palpable tenderness at the sinus tarsi, restricted hindfoot inversion, and painful peroneal spasm when the tibia is stabilized and the heel rapidly inverted.[95, 96]

After examining the ankle and subtalar joint for range of motion, the dorsalis pedis and posterior tibial pulses should be palpated. The sole of the foot is inspected for rheumatoid nodules (Fig 15–3), ulcerations, and callus formation. Physical examination for signs of rheumatoid vasculitis (splinter hemorrhages, etc.) is performed.

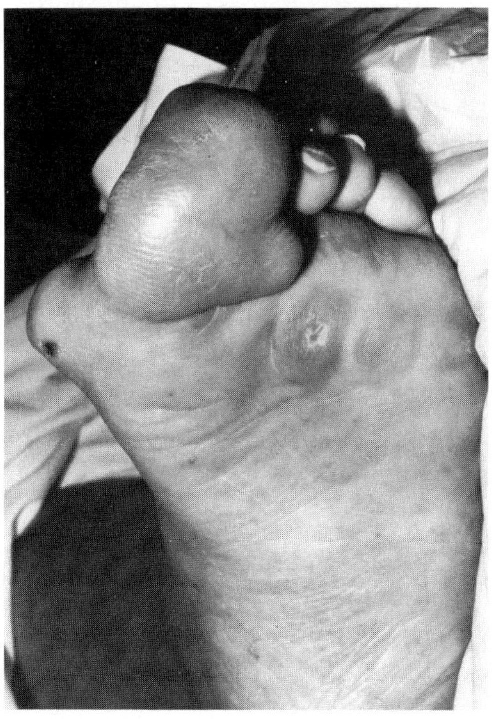

FIG 15–3.
Rheumatoid nodules of the forefoot.

A neurologic examination includes a careful sensory examination. Deficits in the medial or lateral plantar distribution can indicate a tarsal tunnel syndrome or an entrapment of the medial or lateral plantar nerves. Neurologic symptoms of a bilateral nature may indicate a more central deficit as the increased incidence of cervical myelopathy is well documented in the rheumatoid patient. Reflexes, proprioception, and vibratory sense should be evaluated.

An abnormal motor examination of the strength of the tibialis anterior, tibialis posterior, Achilles, or peroneal tendons often indicates a painful tenosynovitis as electromyographic examination of patients with rheumatoid feet indicates only minor electromyographic abnormalities.[68]

Normally, there is little movement of the midfoot structure owing to their interlocking geometric configuration and strong ligamentous structures. While grasping the heel with one hand, a pronation-supination maneuver to the midfoot region that elicits pain may signal synovitis of the transverse tarsal or midfoot joints.

RADIOGRAPHIC FINDINGS

Many patients with rheumatoid arthritis complain of diffuse pain in the foot and ankle and exact localization of the primary site of pathologic change can be difficult. Appropriate radiographic examination helps provide diagnostic information.

All films, except for oblique views, must be weightbearing to assess alterations in foot mechanics due to ligamentous laxity and to assess the status of joint spaces. Recommendations include: weightbearing anteroposterior (AP) ankle and foot; oblique foot; lateral weightbearing foot including the ankles; and a weightbearing tibiocalcaneal view.[53]

The earliest radiographic sign of rheumatoid arthritis is periarticular soft tissue swelling that corresponds to the proliferative synovitis stage of rheumatoid arthritis. Resnick states that the fusiform periarticular swelling involves a hyperemia that results in regional or periarticular osteoporosis—the second radiographic sign of rheumatoid arthritis.[78, 79] These changes are more evident in the forefoot and hand. Thould and Simon[97] found that in an examination of 105 patients with definite rheumatoid arthritis, 91% revealed radiographic changes in the foot and hand, while 16% had normal hand radiographs with definite findings in the foot. While some asymptomatic feet revealed rheumatoid erosions, there was, in general, good correlation between the severity of radiographic changes and the clinical severity of the disease. The authors stated that radiographic examination of the feet was more useful than examination of the hand.[98]

Persistent synovial inflammation affects cartilage nutrition and activates the inflammatory cascade resulting in enzymatic degradation of cartilage. This is reflected in a loss of joint space indicating more advanced rheumatoid arthritis. Pannus formation and enzymatic destruction results in marginal erosions, again more evident in the forefoot. With advanced disease, subchondral cysts occur.

Bursae and tendons are also affected in rheumatoid arthritis. For example, the persistent inflammation of the retrocalcaneal bursae can result in erosions of the calcaneus. Tendon attenuation or rupture can result in recognizable alterations in the normal alignment of bones. The altered mechanics from rheumatoid arthritis can result in secondary osteoarthritis.[33]

Cracchiolo,[19] Elboar et al.,[28] and Wigren[110] warn that the frequent complaint of ankle pain is often due to involvement of the subtalar or talonavicular joint. Vidigal and colleagues[105, 106] noted that only half of their patients who complained of ankle pain had radiographic evidence of ankle involvement. The reverse pattern was found in the tarsal joints where the incidence of definite radiographic evidence of rheumatoid arthritis doubled the incidence of midfoot symptoms.[105, 106] Anteroposterior and lateral weightbearing ankle films will assess the status of the ankle joint. Synovitis of the ankle joint is radiographically evidenced by soft tissue masses and a displacement of the normal pericapsular fat. Later changes include subchondral erosions or cysts at the tibia, talus, or articular surfaces of the malleoli.

Articular destruction is evidenced as a loss of joint space. A unilateral destruction of a joint can lead to a progressive valgus deformity as the talus impacts into the lateral portion of the tibial plafond. Rarely, complete bony ankylosis at the ankle joint is evident. If the patient retains ankle motion, a spherical deformity of the talus can result. Buck et al.[7] have described a standing tibiocalcaneal view to help assess varus-valgus hindfoot alignment. Samuelson and colleagues[85] also utilize a double exposure technique of the hindfoot to determine whether clinical deformity emanates from the ankle or subtalar joint.

The subtalar joint[27] is frequently involved in rheumatoid arthritis. When there is clinical suspicion of subtalar involvement, the radiographic views described by Isherwood, the lateral oblique, medial oblique axial, and lateral oblique axial views of the foot, allow visualization of the subtalar joint. Broden's views, a series of four radiographs varying at 10-degree increments from 10 to 40 degrees visualize the posterior facet well. The series has the advantage of movement of the x-ray tube with a stationary patient (important in intraoperative assessment or with severely painful feet). The supine patient rotates the dorsiflexed foot medially to 45 degrees. The central beam is directed at the lateral malleolus and angled 10 to 40 degrees cephalad. The posterior tangential view, or Harris axial view of the calca-

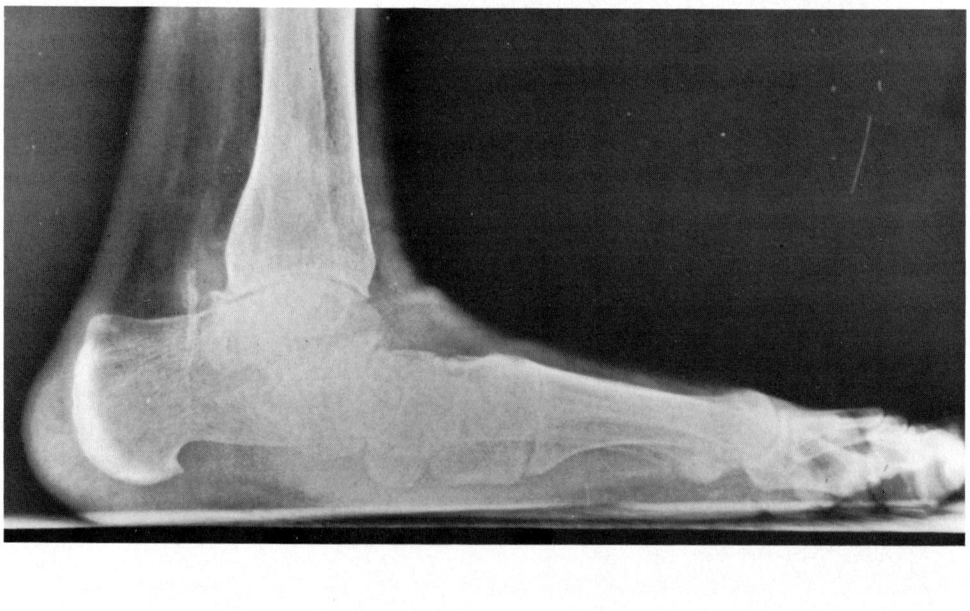

FIG 15–4.
Pes planovalgus deformity with loss of arch.

neus, visualizes the posterior and middle facets. The anterior facet of the subtalar joint is best seen on an oblique radiograph of the foot. For definitive visualization of the subtalar joint, coronally orientated computed tomography (CT) is required.[89] The talonavicular and calcaneocuboid joints are well visualized on the AP, lateral, and oblique views of the foot.

Radiographic visualization of the joints of the foot and ankle allows evaluation of cartilaginous or osseous changes resulting from the inflammation of rheumatoid arthritis. Measurement of standard radiographic lines can indicate malalignment and deformity. The lateral radiograph of the foot reveals useful angles that help localize the site of deformity. The calcaneal pitch measures the angle of inclination of the base of the calcaneus with respect to the plantar surface of the foot. A calcaneal pitch of less than 20 degrees is considered indicative of a flattened longitudinal arch. Gould described a variation of the lateral talus–first metatarsal angle greater than 4 degrees in either direction as an indication of pes cavus or pes planus.[35]

The most common foot deformity in rheumatoid arthritis is pes planovalgus. On the lateral foot view, the break in the longitudinal arch can be noted at the talonavicular joint (Fig 15–4). The lateral foot radiograph also reveals talonavicular beaking when subtalar motion is restricted.

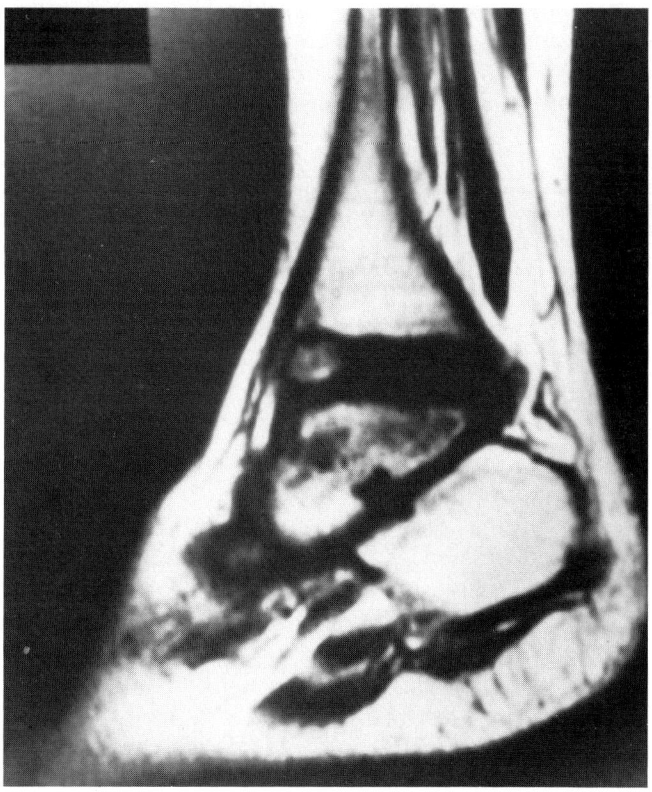

FIG 15–5.
MRI of the ankle and hindfoot revealing subchondral cysts in the talus.

The AP view of the foot helps assess the talonavicular and calcaneocuboid joints in addition to revealing the relationship of the forefoot to the hindfoot. Progressive medial displacement of the talar head with lateral movement of the navicular indicates forefoot abduction. The talocalcaneal angle assesses hindfoot alignment. The normal angle varies between 20 and 35 degrees: an angle greater than 35 degrees indicates hindfoot valgus and an angle less than 20 degrees indicates hindfoot varus.

Routine radiographs can also indicate rheumatoid involvement of bursae and tendons. Retrocalcaneal bursitis initially obliterates the radiolucent retrocalcaneal fat triangle between the posterior calcaneus and the Achilles tendon.[33] Chronic bursitis results in an erosion of the superior portion of the calcaneus. If the Achilles tendon is involved clinically, radiographic findings include soft tissue swelling and sometimes spurs or erosions at the insertion site. Similarly, the attachment of the plantar fascia on the medial tubercle of the calcaneus can be associated with spurring, though less prominently than seen in psoriatic or Reiter's disease.

Unexplained hindfoot pain may be due to calcaneus stress fractures. Increased vertical sclerosis in the calcaneus on a lateral view is evidence of a calcaneal stress fracture. On a weightbearing AP view of the ankle, lateral migration of the talus or valgus malalignment may create a stress fracture of the fibula. Bone scans are helpful if a stress fracture is suspected but not demonstrated on plain films.

The role of newer radiographic techniques such as magnetic resonance imaging (MRI) is not yet defined. Certainly, tenosynovitis, intratendinous abnormalities, rupture, or other soft tissue abnormalities are well demonstrated but at a significant cost (Fig 15–5). This information can usually be ascertained by a careful clinical examination, radiographs, and a knowledge of the rheumatoid process. For example, a ruptured posterior tibial tendon is an obvious physical finding. Significant tenosynovitis is evident on palpation. Failure to improve on medical and conservative (brace and injection) therapy warrants surgical exploration and the appropriate operative procedure.

The combination of appropriate routine radiographs should confirm a clinical diagnosis. Bone scans should be obtained when a stress fracture is suspected but cannot be demonstrated. Bone scans will also confirm inflammation of joints that appear radiographically normal. CT scans or MRI can provide helpful information to confirm a suspected diagnosis or rule out involvement of adjacent joints. Their role in the routine diagnosis and management of rheumatoid arthritis of the foot and ankle is still evolving.

CONSERVATIVE TREATMENT

Treatment of the patient with rheumatoid arthritis requires coordinated optimal medical management with nonsteroidal drugs and, if necessary, second-line agents under the supervision of a rheumatologist. Rest during periods of inflammation and mobilization and exercise during periods of quiescence, in addition to medical management, form the mainstay of conservative management.

Pathologic consequences of rheumatoid arthritis of the foot and ankle predominantly manifest themselves as abnormalities in the forefoot including plantar ulcerations and callosities, hallux valgus, hammering, clawing, or dislocation of the lesser toes. Hindfoot malalignment (excessive valgus) has been demonstrated to increase forefoot pressures[94] and therefore control of hindfoot alignment is a critical component of the conservative care of the rheumatoid foot and ankle.

Initial measures of nonoperative care of the rheumatoid foot include appropriate shoewear.[17] The shoe must be extrawide and extradeep to accommodate the forefoot deformities and appropriate inserts. A medial longitudinal arch support with an insert distributes the weight and decreases focal pressure. In more advanced foot disease, distal migration of the fat pad and plantar skin atrophy can lead to skin ulceration. Plastizote inserts give the most contoured support. The medial arch support contributes to maintenance of the longitudinal arch and decreases forefoot pressure. It must, however, be accompanied by a firm shoe counter; otherwise, the hindfoot slides into valgus.

The supple hindfoot can be controlled with a University of California Bioengineering Laboratory (UCBL) insert, which corrects for hindfoot valgus. Unfortunately, the skin in many rheumatoid patients will not support such a rigid orthosis. An ankle orthosis with a lateral support and medial T-strap or a double upright brace are other options to control hindfoot valgus.

Acute inflammatory periods of rheumatoid arthritis can result in significant pain. Resting the joint and even short-term casting may result in a resolution of mechanical pain or inflammatory synovitis. Persistent pain despite immobilization suggests a vasculitic or neurologic component and must be investigated.

Selective injections of local steroids into the joints is helpful in obtaining a diminution of the synovial inflammation. The inclusion of a local anesthetic helps to confirm that the painful joint is correctly identified and therefore is a useful diagnostic test. Cracchiolo[18] and Goldberg[34] have recommended no more than three injections per joint per year as a general guideline.

Acute episodes of proliferative synovitis of the posterior tibial tendon often warrant operation or the careful use of peritendinous steroids. With or without steroid injections, a short leg walking cast with some hindfoot inversion and arch support may resolve the painful episode. Casting periods should be followed with mobilization of joints, strength exercises, and support with appropriate arches, shoes, braces, or orthoses as indicated. Casting is also an instructive preoperative tool and is confirmatory that the patient's pain is mechanical in nature.

The earlier discussion of normal mechanics and pathology of rheumatoid arthritis emphasized the interrelationship of the ankle, hindfoot, midfoot, and forefoot regions. An awareness of the natural history of rheumatoid arthritis and of its effect on neighboring structures emphasizes the importance of appropriate and timely intervention.

SURGICAL TREATMENT OF THE RHEUMATOID HINDFOOT

INTRODUCTION

Surgical treatment of the rheumatoid hindfoot must be influenced by other pathologic abnormalities present in the ipsilateral hip and knee. Coughlin and Mann and colleagues,[15, 58, 62, 64] Figgie et al.,[31] and Manoli[65] have emphasized the importance of realigning the knee prior to hindfoot and ankle surgery (Fig 15–6,A and B). Mann and collegues[58, 62, 64] and Johnson[48, 49] have emphasized that the position of ankle arthrodesis be chosen based upon the ipsilateral knee alignment, and the contralateral normal rotation of the foot with respect to the knee. Both Tillman[99, 100] and Keenan et al.[50] have reported the common association of a valgus knee with a plano-

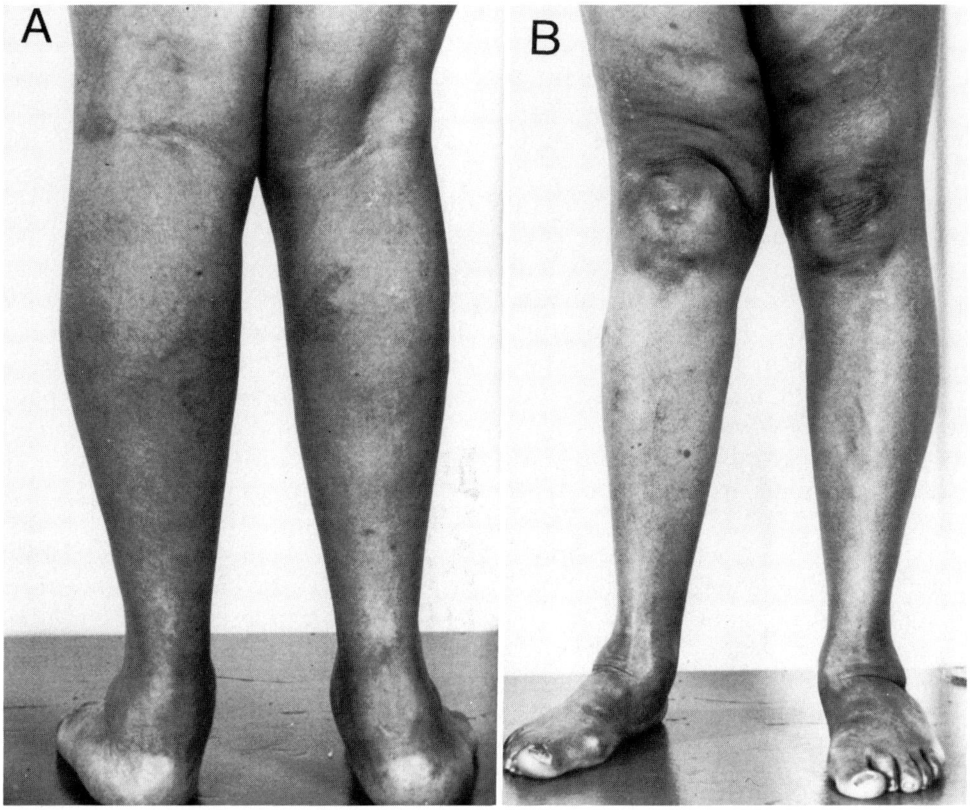

FIG 15–6.
A, B, significant valgus deformity of the knee may complicate hindfoot reconstruction and should be addressed prior to surgery.

valgus hindfoot in the rheumatoid patient. It has also been emphasized that ankle and hindfoot reconstruction precede forefoot reconstruction as the result of the forefoot reconstruction may be negatively influenced by abnormal valgus of the hindfoot or ankle. Stockley et al.[94] have demonstrated increased pedobarograph pressures on the forefoot if the hindfoot is in valgus position.

Accordingly, prior to embarking on complex hindfoot and ankle reconstructions in the rheumatoid patient, careful attention must be paid to the remainder of the patient's limb. Results of hindfoot and ankle arthrodesis may be negatively influenced owing to abnormal knee alignment and may become malaligned if there is significant knee deformity when the hindfoot or ankle is fused.

As emphasized in Chapter 16, the vascular status of the foot must be carefully evaluated prior to surgical treatment, as many of these patients will have an underlying rheumatoid vasculitis. This can be determined by inspecting the foot carefully (especially near the medial malleolus in the planovalgus foot) for areas of skin breakdown or previous ulceration. Since the rheumatoid patient is at an increased risk for infection and wound problems, it is best to address any local areas of infection and skin breakdown prior to hindfoot and ankle reconstruction. Epidural anesthesia is preferred, and has the advantage of allowing postoperative patient-controlled analgesia through an epidural catheter for the first 48 hours after surgery.

It is not uncommon for the rheumatoid patient to become severely disabled by involvement of the hindfoot or ankle. The talonavicular joint is most commonly involved at an early stage. Adam and Ranawat[1] and Elboar et al.[28] reported that in the disease process, hindfoot involvement can be just as disabling to the patient's functional status as involvement of other more proximal, larger joints.

In patients that have persistent disabling pain despite an adequate trial of conservative therapy, surgical treatment may become necessary to correct the deformity and restore function. The indications for stabilizing procedures of the hindfoot, as outlined by Patterson et al.,[77] include relief of pain and correction of deformity so that the foot can be properly fitted into a shoe or brace to achieve equal weightbearing and correction of instability. Although there have been advances in total joint arthroplasty for the ankle[48] as well as the hindfoot,[83] arthrodesis continues to be the major surgical procedure to address these painful joints.[62, 70, 91] The limited indications and technique for ankle joint arthroplasty are discussed later in this chapter.

ANKLE JOINT

Synovectomy

Synovectomy of the ankle joint is indicated when medical management fails to eliminate the synovitis or if ankle symptoms persist despite an initial good response to medical management. It is important to emphasize that this procedure be performed early in order to maximize success rates. The combination of ankle synovectomy with tenosynovectomy of the posterior tibial and peroneal tendons has been used successfully by both Tillman[99, 100] and Mohing et al.[72] The ideal candidate, as described by Mohing et al.,[72] is one with early swelling around the posterior tibial and peroneal tendons and ankle joint pain with weightbearing and motion.

In 1982, Mohing et al.[72] reported on 123 open ankle synovectomies in 99 patients. The procedure was performed through two longitudinal incisions: one medial and one lateral. A radical synovectomy was performed which included debridement of any osteophytes present on the tibia or talus. Additionally, if there was swelling along the course of the peroneal or posterior tibial tendons, the diseased tenosynovium was debrided from behind the medial and lateral malleolus as well. Patients were started on range-of-motion exercises on the first postoperative day.

At an average follow-up of 4 years, the authors reported a significant decrease in pain and swelling and improved range of motion and gait pattern in more than 80% of the joints. Unfortunately, the authors found that ankle joint synovectomy did not improve the walking distance or dependency on walking aids. They pointed out that this was most likely due to multiple joint involvement of the lower extremity. Furthermore, there was a 20% rate of recurrence of pain and swelling of the ankle joint following synovectomy. The authors concluded that the best results were obtained in patients with involvement of the ankle joint alone or with minimal involvement of the subtalar and talonavicular joints. The prognosis was poor when subchondral bone cysts were present on the weightbearing surface of the tibia and talus (Fig 15–5). No benefit can be expected if the patient has evidence of severe deformity.[72]

Ankle Arthrodesis

Since ankle arthrodesis was first described by Albert[2] in 1879, more than 30 different techniques have been described with fusion rates that range from 65% to 100%. Scranton[88] suggests that the reason for so many techniques is that the ankle joint is not always easily fused, owing to varying degrees of normal multiplane motion of the ankle. Carrier and Harris[11] noted that the large number of techniques suggests that no one technique is universally applicable to all patients. Scranton[88] notes that the basic types of ankle arthrodesis techniques include tibiotalar coaptation, sliding or bridging graft involving the tibia and fibula, iliac crest graft, internal compression plate, internal screws, external compression pins, and arthroscopic abrasion and external compression pins. The use of supplemental autogenous bone graft has been supported by the literature[48] although Mann et al.[64] report excellent fusion rates in the absence of the bone graft. The concept of compression across the fusing joint has been emphasized[1, 12, 16, 20, 21] and the trend has been toward internal fixation to achieve this end.[19, 16, 21, 62, 64] The Calandruccio external fixation device has been used with good success by Johnson[48, 81]; reports by Cracchiolo,[16] Moekel et al.,[71] and Holt et al.,[44] however have pointed out that there are inherent problems with external fixation. These include: (1) increased patient dissatisfaction with the concept and appearance of the external fixator, (2) increased sepsis, (3) the need for increased pin and wound care, (4) more consideration to the timing of protected vs. unprotected ambulation, (5) instability of the construct under sheer stresses, (6) inability of the construct to maintain exact position of the foot in the sagittal plane, (7) lower rate of successful union, (8) compromise of the subtalar and midfoot joint motion secondary to longer periods of nonweightbearing and time to union, and (9) patient dissatisfaction with the appearance of the feet and poor gait mechanics when fusions do not consolidate.

In considering the technique of fusion, one must consider that patients with severe rheumatoid arthritis have osteopenia and decreased bone density, unlike patients with posttraumatic or degenerative arthritis. It is imperative, therefore, to adapt the fusion technique to each individual patient. The factors to consider when deciding on the technique of ankle arthrodesis include the amount of deformity, bony deficiency or insufficiency, and the patient's ambulatory needs.

Achieving the optimal position of ankle arthrodesis is of paramount importance and the work of Mazur et al.[67] and Buck et al.[7] has shown that when optimal position is achieved, a virtually normal walking gait in an appropriate shoe can be achieved.

The optimal position for ankle arthrodesis has been defined as: neutral flexion, 0 to 5 degrees of valgus of hindfoot angulation, 5 to 10 degrees of external rotation of the foot (matched to contralateral foot rotation), and slight posterior translation of the talus on the tibia, if possible (i.e., positioning the foot along the weightbearing line of the tibia in relation to the dome of the talus, or slightly posterior to that line).

Very few reports on ankle arthrodesis focus solely on the rheumatoid population. Accordingly, it is difficult to compare techniques of ankle arthrodesis for rheumatoid arthritis. There are, however, several excellent reports on techniques that have been used with consistent results.

Indications and Contraindications

The primary indication for ankle arthrodesis in the rheumatoid patient is pain secondary to inflammatory destruction.[1, 62] Rheumatoid involvement of the ankle may also cause malalignment of the ankle joint and this should be corrected at the time of surgery.

Contraindications for ankle arthrodesis include acute or chronic infection, inadequate vascular supply, or severe vasculitis.[62] A relative contraindication is a neuropathic joint.

Biomechanics

It is important to recognize the concept described by Mann and Coughlin,[62] that when arthrodesis of a joint or series of joints is performed, the motion that normally occurs within that joint is effectively eliminated, requiring adjacent joints to compensate. It is important, therefore, to attempt to maintain the mobility of the adjacent joints, whenever possible, as these aid in the ability of the limb to absorb shock; produce stability for heel strike, toe rise, and toe-off; and allow for dorsiflexion and plantarflexion (ankle) and inversion and eversion (hindfoot) during ground contact of gait. Mann and Coughlin have advocated that only the symptomatic painful joints be fused.[62]

Thordarson et al.[97] and Cracchiolo and colleagues[13, 16] have studied the biomechanics of the fibular strut graft in the laboratory on cadaveric feet. In the study of Thordarson et al.[97], 18 fresh-frozen cadaveric ankles were arthrodesed using a fibular strut graft. The fibula was osteotomized 6 to 7 cm above the tip of the malleolus. The tibiotalar joints were then fixed with two 6.5-mm cancellous bone screws. A fibular strut graft was then fixed with two 6.5-mm cancellous bone screws in some of the specimens. The bending movement was applied manually to the tibia by the instrumented load handle. Results showed that for all specimens, with and without bone graft, the greatest amount of motion at the site of arthrodesis was seen with tibial torque, and the least motion was seen with medial-lateral bending. Removal of the fibular strut graft allowed for increased tibiotalar motion.

Thordarson et al. concluded that two-screw fixation of ankle arthrodeses is more effective in resisting plantar flexion and dorsiflexion bending moments than internal-external rotation.[97] The addition of the fibular strut graft added stability to the specimens of good bone quality, but contributed more significantly to the construct when bone quality was poor. Cracchiolo et al. further emphasized the difficulty of achieving good cancellous bone screw fixation in patients with poor bone quality and in these cases recommended either the Calandruccio external fixation device or the addition of a fibular strut graft.[13, 20] They also emphasized the use of the external compression device in cases requiring extensive bone grafting for large defects. However, Mann and colleagues[58, 62, 64] reported that the use of a fibular graft can contribute to a widened heel, which may cause problems with shoewear.

Thordarson et al.[97] compared internal and external fixation of the tibiotalar joint in 15 fresh-frozen ankles. The first group of ankles underwent ankle arthrodesis using two cancellous bone screws, and were then loaded with 8 nm of manually applied tibial torque, and plantar flexion-dorsiflexion and medial-lateral bending moments. Next, the screws were removed and the Calandruccio external compression device was applied to the threaded pins through the tibia and talus. The above series of tests was then repeated. Thordarson et al.[97] found that the biomechanical strength of both internal and external fixation was dependent upon bone quality. The two cancellous bone screws were most effective in preventing tibiotalar motions produced by plantar flexion-dorsiflexion and medial-lateral bending moments. The two screws were least effective against torque. The Calandruccio clamp was most effective in resisting rotations produced by medial-lateral bending moment and tibial torque. Based upon these findings, Thordarson et al.[97] concluded that cancellous bone screws provided more biomechanically sound fixation in patients with good bone quality. They further recommended that an external fixator be used when bone quality is poor or low-insertion torque indicates the poor thread purchase of cancellous bone screws.

Surgical Approaches

The surgical approaches described include the anterior, anterolateral, and the posterior approach. Each has its advantages. The anterior approach provides an excellent wide exposure although extreme care must be taken to avoid injury to the neurovascular bundle. The anterolateral approach is especially useful if additional procedures on the hindfoot are necessary. Moving this incision closer to the fibula enables fibular exposure if a strut graft technique is employed (Fig 15–7,A and B). Advantages of the posterior approach include excellent exposure of the posterior facet of the subtalar joint (the presence of the flexor hallucis longus and flexor digitorum communis cover the bone graft nicely) and easy access to the posterior iliac crest for autogenous bone graft. Care should be taken to avoid the sural nerve with this approach.

The transfibular approach is preferred by Mann[58, 64] because it offers excellent exposure of the ankle joint and allows for direct visualization while inserting bone screw fixation. Mann emphasizes that the ideal position of the arthrodesis is (1) neutral dorsiflexion–plantar flexion; (2) approximately 5 degrees of valgus alignment; and (3) rotation in the transverse plane matched to the normal contralateral ankle. This plane is usually somewhat external and can be approximated by flexing the knee and ankle to 90 degrees and visualizing the anatomic relationship between the center of the patella and the bases of the toes.

First, the contralateral extremity is inspected for its alignment in the varus-valgus and transverse

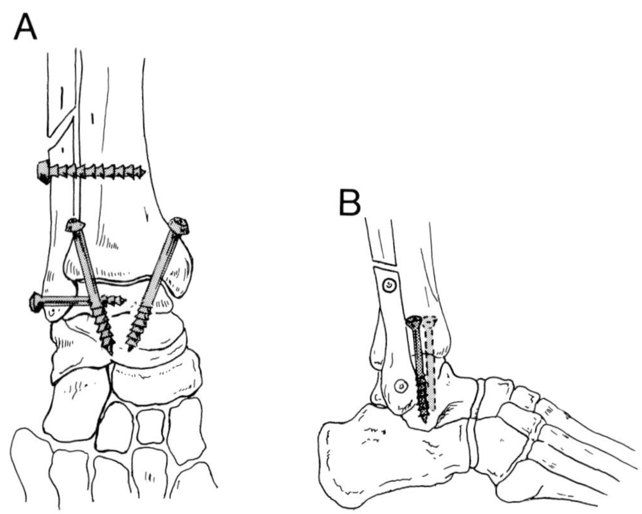

FIG 15–7.
A, fibular strut graft techniques in the AP view. **B,** lateral view.

plane. Next, a tourniquet is placed around the proximal thigh and a sandbag is placed under the involved ankle to enhance lateral ankle exposure. Next, the skin incision is made from approximately 10 cm proximal to the distal tip of the fibula down along the fibula and then gently curved along the lateral aspect of the foot toward the base of the fourth metatarsal. Care is taken to take the incision directly down to bone so that one full-thickness flap of tissue is created. Next, the fibula is fully exposed by subperiosteal dissection, which is taken anteriorly and medially across the tibia. This exposes the medial aspect of the ankle joint as well as the lateral aspect of the talus and talar neck. The distal fibula is then removed by making an oblique osteotomy with a power saw at a point 1.5 cm above the ankle joint. Next, the posterior aspect of the ankle joint is exposed to prepare for the distal tibial cut, which is made under direct vision. Now, using a power saw, the distal tibial cut is made as perpendicular to the long axis of the bone as possible. This cut is taken medially to the point where the curve of the medial malleolus begins. Mann[64] emphasizes that just enough bone be removed to create a broad flat surface of cancellous bone. Next, the foot is positioned in neutral dorsiflexion-plantar flexion, and 5 degrees of valgus. The dorsal talar cut is then made parallel to the tibial cut. After the bone is removed, the medial aspect of the ankle joint is further exposed by placing a lamina spreader into the joint. A curette is used to decorticate the medial aspect of the joint. Next, the tibia and talus are juxtaposed to check alignment in the dorsiflexion-plantar flexion and varus-valgus planes.

Mann emphasizes that if the joint surfaces do not come together easily, the medial malleolus is likely impinging and accordingly recommends that the distal 1 cm of the medial malleolus be excised. This is done through a 3-cm incision which is made over the anterolateral aspect of the malleolus. The distal 1 cm of medial malleolus is then exposed subperiosteally and excised. Mann emphasizes that care be taken not to harm the posterior tibialis tendon which lies directly under the medial malleolus. Next, attention is again focused on the tibiotalar arthrodesis site and both bony surfaces are feathered with a 4-mm osteotome to enhance contact of a broad surface of cancellous bone. Next, the arthrodesis site is aligned in proper position as described above. In addition, rotation is corrected to agree with the uninvolved side. A towel clamp or Bishop clamp is then used to temporarily hold the osteotomy site. Next, the arthrodesis is internally fixed with two 6.5-mm AO long-threaded screws. The first screw is placed in the hard cortical bone of the plantar aspect of the base of the neck of the talus, and is directed medially and almost parallel to the floor and across the tibia. The 3.5-mm drill is left in place and a second hole is made just above the lateral process of the talus and is directed slightly posteriorly and medially across the tibia. This drill bit is also left in place. The drill bits are next exchanged for screws of appropriate length. A third screw may be added if the arthrodesis site is not rigidly fixed. This third screw can be placed from the lateral aspect of the tibia downward into the talus, but Mann emphasizes that care be taken to prevent drill or screw penetration into the posterior facet of the subtalar joint. Mann does not routinely use bone graft for this arthrodesis, as there is usually excellent coaptation of cancellous bony surfaces with little, if any, room for bone graft. Next, the wound is closed over a Hemovac drain.

Postoperatively, a compression dressing with plaster splints is used for the first 10 days. The patient is then placed into a short leg nonweightbearing cast for approximately 6 weeks and radiographs are taken. If there is evidence of early union, the patient is allowed to bear weight. Union is usually achieved by 12 weeks and the patient is then permitted to walk without support.

Inglis[76] prefers the anterolateral approach to the ankle joint which was initially described by Hallock[40] and later by Morris et al.[73] The incision is made over the anterior aspect of the distal tibia in the interval between the extensor hallucis longus and the tibialis anterior tendons (Fig 15–8,A). The incision runs from approximately 8 cm proximal to 5 cm distal to the ankle joint. The superficial peroneal nerve is identified and retracted laterally. After the extensor retinaculum is sharply divided, the interval between the extensor hallucis longus and the tibialis anterior is developed.

The neurovascular bundle is identified and carefully retracted medially. Next, the lateral malleolar vessels at the level of the tibiotalar joint are ligated to enhance exposure. Next, the inferior retinaculum, joint capsule, and periosteum are sharply divided in line with the skin incision. Inglis emphasizes preservation of the periosteum during careful subperiosteal dissection to allow for better closure after arthrodesis. Next, an anterior synovectomy is performed to enhance exposure, and then the tibia and talus are denuded of all cartilage and fibrous tissue using curettes and a power burr. A lamina spreader may be placed within the joint to enhance exposure.

Inglis emphasizes that it is important to maintain or recreate the normal concentricity of the tibial plafond and talar dome during the debridement. A small dental burr is very helpful in the preparation of compatible surfaces. He further notes that the creation of two planar surfaces using an oscillating saw may compromise bony apposition when the foot is placed in the appropriate position for internal fixation. Next, the anterior tibial graft is harvested with an oscillating saw. The graft measures approximately 1.5 cm wide by 5.0 cm long. A small quantity of cancellous bone may be removed from the superior portion of the graft site to augment the arthrodesis. Next, the corticocancellous strut graft is removed and the tibiotalar joint is positioned for arthrodesis. There should be good bony contact between the talar dome and the denuded tibial surface. The ideal position for fusion is neutral dorsiflexion–plantar flexion, and 5 degrees of valgus alignment. After the talus is aligned with the tibia in proper position, a quadrilateral space of approximately 1.2 cm deep is marked out with methylene blue in the talar–neck-body junction.

The defect in the anterior tibia serves as a template for the talar hole. The bone is then removed from the talus using an osteotome and saved for bone graft (Fig 15–8,B and C). The talar dome and tibial plafond are then compressed using two 6.5-mm cancellous bone screws which are placed from the medial and lateral aspect of the tibia down into the talus (Fig 15–8,D). Next, the anterior tibial graft is placed in the anterior tibial slot and advanced downward into the quadrilateral defect in the talus (Fig 15–8,E). The strut graft is then compressed with one or two 3.5-mm bicortical screws placed in an anteroposterior direction. The bone graft from the talus is then packed around the tibiotalar junction and the top two corners of the tibial slot are rounded off with a rongeur to reduce the stress riser effect of a sharp corner. Inglis notes that prior to routinely performing this step, there were instances of stress fractures at the top of the slot.

The wound is then closed in layers beginning with the periosteum and then the retinaculum. The wound is not routinely drained. A compressive dressing with incorporation of plaster splints is applied and changed after approximately 1 week. A short leg nonweightbearing cast is then applied for the following 6 weeks, at which time the wound is inspected and a short leg walking cast is applied. Weightbearing as tolerated is permitted for the next 6 weeks, at which time the short leg cast is removed and the patient is permitted to continue weightbear-

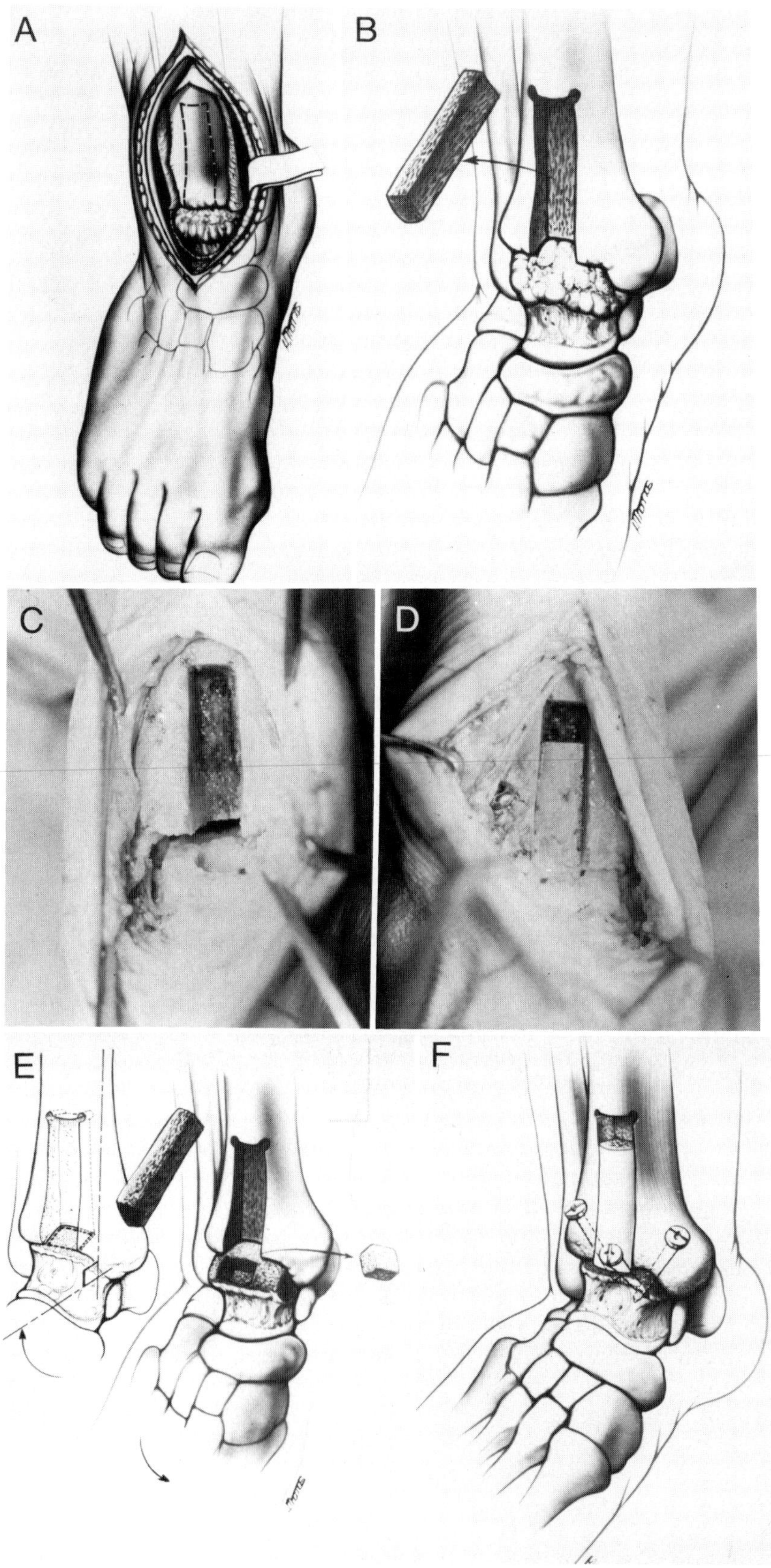

FIG 15–8.
A, anterior sliding tibial graft. An anterior approach to the ankle is used. **B,** the ankle is debrided and the correct position is obtained. An anterior slot is cut in the tibia and the bone is removed and saved. **C,** the bone removed. **D,** after the ankle is fixed with two crossing screws, a trough is cut in the talus. **E,** the bone graft is impacted into the talus. **F,** the graft is fixed in place with a cortical screw.

ing as tolerated in a molded plastic air splint. A sliding anterior graft performed in a patient with inflammatory arthritis is shown in Figure 15–9,A–C.

Results

Adam and Ranawat,[1] in 1976, reviewed the experience at The Hospital for Special Surgery in New York City with 21 ankle arthrodeses for rheumatoid arthritis (15 unilateral, 3 bilateral). All patients were graded according to the American Rheumatism Association classification as stage III or IV and functional class 3 or 4. A variety of methods were used to achieve fusion. There were 11 sliding tibial grafts, 4 compression arthrodeses, 3 fibular strut grafts, 4 transcalcaneal Steinmann's pin fixation procedures, 2 bone dowel grafts, and 1 staple fixation. The authors emphasized that the different techniques shared a common need for meticulous dissection, re-

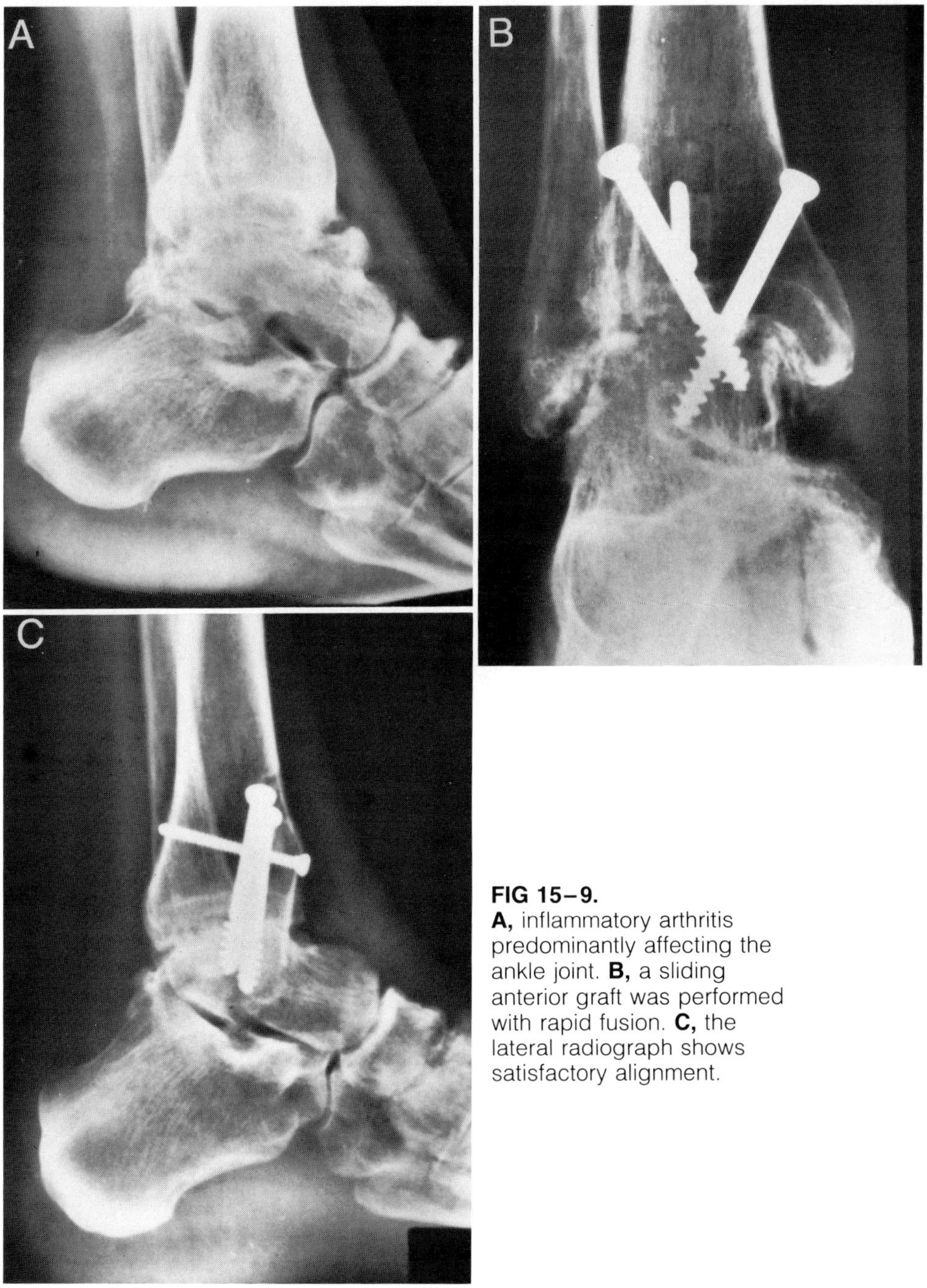

FIG 15–9.
A, inflammatory arthritis predominantly affecting the ankle joint. **B,** a sliding anterior graft was performed with rapid fusion. **C,** the lateral radiograph shows satisfactory alignment.

moval of all articular cartilage, and adequate approximation of bony surfaces. The authors prefer the anterior approach today as they believe this offers the best visualization of the joint. In all 11 cases with anterior sliding tibial grafts with or without screw fixation, a stable pain-free ankle was achieved. However, they had two poor and two fair results which were attributed to lack of graft fixation in one, and improper seating of the graft at surgery in another. This technique is still the authors' procedure of choice at The Hospital for Special Surgery, and cancellous bone screws are used to achieve compression fixation in all cases.

In four of the cases, Charnley compression arthrodesis of the ankle was carried out and a solid arthrodesis was achieved in all cases. The authors believed that this technique was advantageous when a significant preoperative deformity existed which required correction. They did, however, have one patient in whom skin ulceration occurred at the site of the incision which was attributed to vascular insufficiency. A second patient developed subsequent marked subtalar subluxation which negatively impacted on the ankle arthrodesis. The authors believed that this patient would have best been treated initially with a pantalar arthrodesis. Moeckel et al.,[71] in a more recent follow-up at the same institution, have noted a statistically significant increase in wound problems and infection rate with external vs. internal fixation.

A bone dowel technique was used in two cases with good results, and a fibular strut graft as described by Adam and Ranawat was used in 3 cases with good results.[1] The authors pointed out that the advantage of the latter technique was wide exposure of the ankle joint with a large surface for firm fixation.

In four other cases of ankle arthrodesis in which a rotational deformity was present, Adam and Ranawat used a transcalcaneal Steinmann's pin for supplemental fixation.[1] This technique is advantageous in cases with minimal deformity and severely poor bone which precludes adequate compression. Three of these patients went on to fusion with excellent results. However, one patient developed a painful pseudarthrosis which was thought to be due to the poor bone quality and inadequate fixation. This technique was also recently reported by Carrier and Harris[11] in five patients with severe rheumatoid involvement of the ankle. The authors reported a 100% fusion rate with all patients being fully satisfied at an average follow-up of 6 years. Despite the fact that the authors had three patients in whom pin migration occurred, causing plantar ulceration of the skin in one patient, they recommended this technique in the rheumatoid ankle with severely decreased bone density. They argued that in this subpopulation of rheumatoid patients, success of the Charnley compression device would be hampered by the inability to obtain good pin fixation.[12]

The transfibular approach of Adam and Ranawat[1] and Mann et al.[64] has been used in the rheumatoid ankle by Iwata et al.[47] who reviewed their experience with 9 patients. The authors noted the advantages of a wide exposure of the ankle joint without any damage to the nearby vessels and nerves, the ability to perform an easy synovectomy, and easy correction of alignment. The authors achieved fusion with satisfactory results and complete relief of pain in all patients at an average follow-up of 4 to 5 years. The authors emphasized their concern about the use of an external fixation device to achieve compression in patients who have an inherently lowered resistance to infection as a result of steroid therapy and vascular disease.

Cimino et al.[13] reviewed 25 ankle fusions in 22 rheumatoid patients. External fixation was performed in 14 ankles and internal fixation was done in 11 ankles. The two groups were comparable with respect to age, sex, preoperative medications, and severity of disease. Average follow-up for both groups was 33 months with a minimum of 24 months. The average time to fusion was 24 weeks in the external fixation group compared to 17 weeks in the internal fixation group. The fusion rate was 79% in the external fixation group and 77% in the internal fixation group. There were six complications in the external fixation group (three infections) and four complications in the internal fixation group (two infections). Of the seven failures, four were taking 7 mg/day of prednisone preoperatively. In this limited study, the authors concluded that the method of fusion did not affect the fusion rate, complication rate, or functional outcome of ankle arthrodesis in the rheumatoid population.

Gschwend and Steiger[39] reported on 28 ankle arthrodeses in which the compression technique of Charnley[12] was used. They were very satisfied with this method and with their results. They did note, however, that in their patients with severe osteoporosis, migration of the clamps occurred which propagated late union or even nonunion. They also reiterated the increased risk of pin tract infection and the need for careful observation during the early postoperative period. For these reasons, the authors adopted the internal fixation technique of Wagner and Pock[107] using cancellous bone screws and a fibular strut graft. They reported on the use of this technique in 35 patients. However, only five of these patients had rheumatoid arthritis. Although more technically demanding than the Charnley compression technique,[12] the authors believed that the internal fixation technique using cancellous bone screws and fibular strut graft provided for shorter time to fusion, better patient satisfaction, reduced hospital stay, and a lower complication rate.

Benson and Johnson[5] advocated the compression technique of Charnley as it assured them a high rate of success. They cautioned, however, that when a triple arthrodesis is performed in conjunction with an ankle arthrodesis, i.e., a pantalar arthrodesis, the time to union and percentage of nonunions increased.

Smith and Wood[90] reviewed 14 patients with rheumatoid arthritis who underwent ankle arthrodesis utilizing the Charnley compression technique. There were two deaths and one patient was lost to follow-up, leaving 11 patients available for review. The average age at the time of surgery was 50.6 years and follow-up averaged 58 months. Results were assessed using the Fries score and the ankle evaluation grading system of Mazur et al.[67] All patients eventually obtained fusion of the ankle joint, although there was one delayed union necessitating prolonged use of the Charnley fixator for 1 year. Two other patients required reoperation at 9 and 27 months for delayed unions. Four patients developed pin tract sepsis and *S. aureus* was isolated in all four. Delayed wound healing occurred in one patient who was taking corticosteroids. The authors noted that decreased subtalar and midtarsal motion was seen in all of their patients but that this loss of mobility was compensated for by proximal joints. The authors concluded that although Charnley compression arthrodesis may be associated with pin tract infections and delayed union, a pain-free, stable ankle joint may be achieved with this method and offers a more reliable long-term option than total ankle arthroplasty.

Mann et al.[64] reviewed 15 ankle fusions that were performed through a transfibular approach between the sural nerve and the lateral branch of the superficial peroneal nerve. The patients' ages ranged from 21 to 68 years. Internal fixation was used and included two or more 6.5-mm AO screws. Bone graft was not utilized. Postoperatively, patients were managed nonweightbearing in a short leg cast for 6 weeks and then weightbearing in a short leg cast for 6 weeks. At follow-up (range 6–48 months), 100% of the fusions healed with an average period of 3½ months of immobilization. There were no wound or nerve complications. The authors concluded that this approach is a simple one which allows excellent visualization of the ankle joint through a safe internervous interval, provides good bone apposition, rigid fixation, and does not necessitate bone graft.

Dennis et al.[24] reported on 16 patients who underwent ankle arthrodesis using internal fixation with compression. This technique was originally described by Wagner and Pock[107] and was modified by Gschwend and Steiger.[39] There were eight women and eight men with an average age of 50.8 years (range 23–72 years). The preoperative diagnosis was posttraumatic osteoarthritis in 13 patients and rheumatoid arthritis in 3 patients. A lateral transfibular approach was utilized with an anterior capsulotomy. The fibula was reflected posteriorly, leaving the peroneal tendon sheath intact. The articular surfaces were prepared using currettes and a power burr, unless significant malalignment existed and then appropriate wedges were resected to correct the deformity. Fixation of the ankle in the neutral position (0 degrees equinus) was done using two 6.5-mm cancellous bone screws. One screw (32-mm thread) was directed from the sinus tarsi, across the talus, into the posteromedial cortex of the distal tibial metaphysis, and another screw (16-mm thread) was inserted from the lateral cortex of the distal tibial metaphysis (1.5 in. above the joint line) to the medial aspect of the body of the talus. If fixation was not rigid (i.e., in rheumatoid or osteopenic bone), the authors supplemented the screws with staples which were placed anterolaterally and posterolaterally to avoid a hinging effect. Additional bone graft was obtained from the articular one half of the fibula and the outer one half was secured to the lateral aspect of the tibia and talus with 4-cm cancellous screws. Dennis et al.[24] noted that the distal fibula can be discarded if narrowing of the ankle is required. In the rheumatoid group, concomitant surgery included a triple arthrodesis in one patient, and a subtalar arthrodesis in another. The third patient in this group had a previous triple arthrodesis several years before the ankle arthrodesis.

Follow-up was obtained in 15 of 16 patients and the Mazur ankle score[67] was used to assess the results. Union was achieved in 15 of 16 patients (94%) in an average of 9.2 weeks (range 7–22 weeks). The average ankle score was 77 points (range 53–88 points). There were 8 patients (53.3%) with an excellent score, 4 patients (26.7%) with a good score, 2 patients (13.3%) with a fair score, and 1 patient

(6.7%) with a nonunion rated poor. In the patients without concomitant hindfoot arthrodeses, the subtalar motion was less than the contralateral subtalar joint in all cases, with 5 patients having loss of subtalar motion greater than 50% and 6 patients having less than a 50% loss compared to the contralateral extremity. Midtarsal motion averaged 18 degrees (range 13–25 degrees) and there were three complications. In 1 patient, a nonunion was attributed to screw threads bridging the arthrodesis site. In another, a distally directed screw entered the subtalar joint, eventually causing subtalar joint pain and necessitating later removal. The third complication occurred in a patient with rheumatoid arthritis who had skin ulceration over the head of a screw in the heel placed for a pantalar arthrodesis. Two reoperations were performed: one for removal of the screw that had entered the subtalar joint and the second was a subtalar arthrodesis in a patient who developed persistent subtalar pain after ankle arthrodesis.

Good or excellent results were achieved in 80% of their patients. The advantages of this technique include: (1) rigid fixation allows early mobilization of adjacent hindfoot and midfoot joints; and (2) the lateral approach avoids neurovascular structures other than the sural nerve and allows distal fibula removal if necessary to narrow the contour of the ankle.

Moeckel et al.[71] reviewed 65 patients who underwent ankle arthrodesis and compared internal fixation (36 cases) with external fixation (29 cases). Average follow-up was 6 years. The external fixation group had significantly more complications, including infection and nonunion, than the internal fixation group. The authors concluded that external fixation for ankle arthrodesis was poorly tolerated because of the limited soft tissue envelope and subcutaneous nature of the bone in this area. They found that internal fixation (screws) provided excellent stabilization with minimal complications and lower postoperative morbidity.

Patterson et al.[76] reported their results with the anterior sliding graft technique for tibiotalar arthrodesis in nine patients with rheumatoid arthritis. They achieved a 95% fusion rate and concluded that this technique is easily performed with readily available resources, is associated with a high rate of rapid union, and avoids the routine use of iliac crest bone graft.

Cracchiolo's[16] recent paper gives an in-depth review of the current trends in ankle arthrodesis. The position of the arthrodesis should place the foot neutral to the leg when viewed laterally. The heel should be between neutral and 7 degrees of valgus and the foot should be in 5 to 10 degrees of external rotation. One can use the contralateral limb as a guide. Cracchiolo cautions against a varus hindfoot as this position will lock the transtarsal joints and accordingly decrease the plantar flexion motion that is normally provided by these joints. Careful attention should be focused on the knee for deformity and malalignment which, if present, should be addressed prior to ankle arthrodesis. Cracchiolo recommends the use of external fixation for arthrodesis requiring extensive bone grafting for large defects, for patients with poor-quality bone which makes cancellous bone screw internal fixation difficult, or if a tibiocalcaneal arthrodesis is performed. The disadvantages of this technique include the need for a cooperative patient, additional nursing care to keep the pins clean, and the added risk of infection. Cracchiolo prefers the Calandruccio clamp for this technique which was described by Russotti et al.[81] Internal fixation is recommended for most cases in which good bone stock is present. Screw selection for the tibiotalar joint includes two 6.5-mm cancellous bone screws which are passed from the tibia into the talus (Fig 15–10). Depending on the size of the talus, either a 16-mm or a 32-mm screw thread is chosen. The screw threads should not cross the arthrodesis site. Intraoperative radiographic assessment is necessary to rule out penetration of the posterior facet of the subtalar joint.

The preferred method of Hansen[16] includes placement of the same-size screw through the posterior malleolus and into the lateral neck of the talus, with the advantage of excellent-quality bone of the posterior tibia and lateral neck of the talus. The pre-

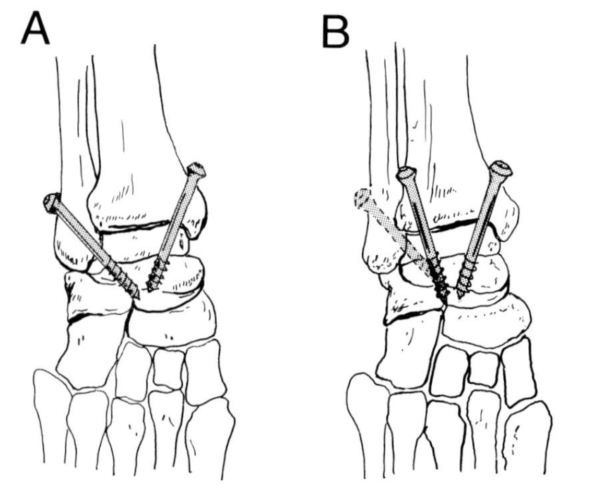

FIG 15–10.
Internal compression fixation may be achieved utilizing 6.5-mm cancellous bone screws across the tibiotalar and fibular joints **(A)** or across the tibiotalar joint above **(B).**

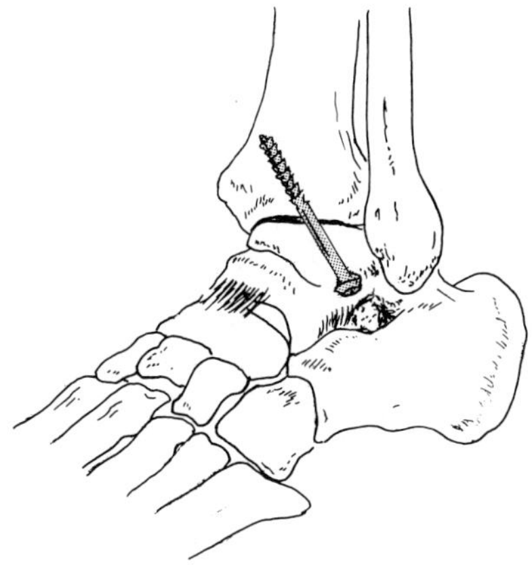

FIG 15–11.
The preferred method of Mann utilizes two 6.5-mm cancellous bone screws directed from the sinus tarsi across the tibiotalar joint. (This procedure usually utilizes two screws, and the fibula is excised.)

ferred method of Mann et al.[64] includes placing both screws from the lateral side through the talus beginning at the sinus tarsi and directing both into the superomedial tibia (Fig 15–11). The advantage of this technique includes avoidance of possible subtalar penetration, and accordingly eliminates the need for an intraoperative radiograph to inspect the subtalar joint.

Complications
Complications include nonunion or delayed union, malalignment, wound problems, and infections.[61, 62] Wound problems may often be treated with antibiotics and immobilization, but sometimes soft tissue procedures to achieve coverage of exposed tendons may be necessary. Pin tract infection occurs with external compression devices. Fortunately, the occurrence of deep infection is infrequent.

Reported nonunion rates range from 0% to 20%. The rates may be higher in patients with avascular necrosis of the talus. Mann and Coughlin[62] suggest that supplemental iliac crest bone grafting may be used in these cases. Often, nonunions should be investigated for infection. If the nonunion is symptomatic, it can be treated by repeat arthrodesis with bone grafting and internal fixation. Malalignment following ankle arthrodesis may be difficult to treat. Mann and Coughlin note that excessive valgus places increased stress on the medial aspect of the knee.[62] A residual varus deformity leads to increased subtalar joint stress with increased pressure under the fifth metatarsal head. Placing the ankle in plantar flexion creates an abnormal vaulting gait pattern with a back knee thrust. This can be managed using a heel lift. If the ankle arthrodesis is in too much dorsiflexion, increased heel pad stress will result. This can be managed with a rocker-bottom sole.[62]

Total Ankle Arthroplasty

Introduction
Total ankle arthroplasty may have application in patients with multiple joint involvement from rheumatoid arthritis. In these patients, maintenance of tibiotalar motion is often beneficial, especially when they have involvement of the ipsilateral forefoot, hindfoot, and knee. However, the long-term durability of ankle replacements has not been established, and the complication rates are high, including problems with wound healing, infection, loosening, impingement, malleolar fractures, and subsidence. Despite these potential problems, total ankle replacement may be a viable alternative for well-selected patients who require tibiotalar motion.

Indications
The ideal patient for a total ankle replacement is one with rheumatoid arthritis who is older and has low demands. The patient should have near–anatomic alignment of the hindfoot in order to allow for even stress distribution. In addition, the patient will often have ipsilateral involvement of the knee or midfoot, or both, such that an ankle arthrodesis would create an abnormal gait pattern, thus increasing stress on other joints (Fig 15–12,A). Patients with isolated involvement of the tibiotalar joint may be better candidates for arthrodesis.[3]

Contraindications
Contraindications include patients with local or remote sepsis, a neuropathic joint, marked neuromuscular disorders, or severe peripheral vascular disease. Relative contraindications for total ankle replacement include a high activity level in a younger or obese patient. These factors may put a higher stress on the implant causing higher rates of loosening. In addition, patients with avascular necrosis of the talus may not be good candidates for implant arthroplasty. They have higher risks for subsidence of their talar components. Patients with marked malalignment of the hindfoot are also relatively poor candidates for ankle replacement, as the malalignment will cause increased edge loading on the ankle replacement and may lead to loosening. In these patients, correction of a hindfoot malalignment to an anatomic position may allow for later ankle replacement. Another relative contraindication is

conversion of a failed arthrodesis to an ankle replacement.

Preoperative Assessment

Careful preoperative assessment is essential for a successful ankle arthroplasty. The patient's neurovascular status, muscle balance, and skin condition should be evaluated. Preoperative vascular evaluation may consist of noninvasive studies including Doppler ultrasonography, thermography, and fluorescein testing. Arteriography may be indicated if the arterial supply of the foot is compromised.

Patients should also be examined for neuropathy, especially patients with rheumatoid arthritis with cervical spine disease. Hyperreflexia, spasticity, and loss of proprioception may be indicative of myelopathy. Loss of proprioceptive feedback allows abnormal transmission of load, leading to early failure of the implant.

The alignment of the foot and leg should be carefully evaluated. The goal of surgery is to provide a painless, well-aligned ankle with approximately 30 degrees of motion. The mechanical alignment of a leg should be restored such that the centers of rotation of the hip, knee, and ankle are in alignment. If imbalance occurs, higher stresses will be placed across the ankle. Those patients with marked knee deformity should have their knee realigned prior to ankle surgery. In addition, patients with hindfoot malalignment and forefoot problems should have these addressed before an ankle arthroplasty is considered.

Technical Considerations

Prior to arthroplasty, AP, and lateral weightbearing radiographs should be obtained. Foot films should also be performed. These are assessed for the preoperative varus or valgus deformity of the hindfoot

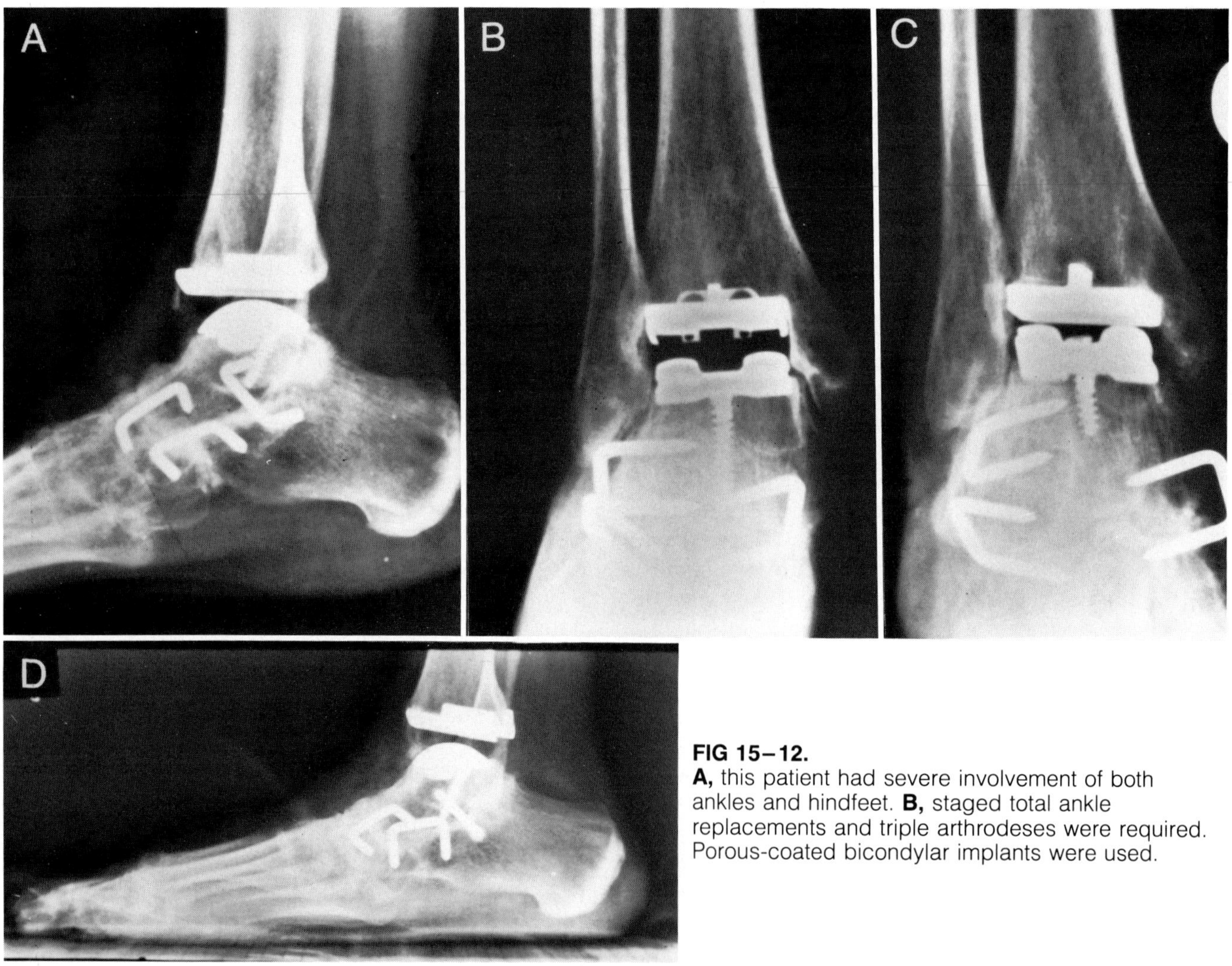

FIG 15–12.
A, this patient had severe involvement of both ankles and hindfeet. **B,** staged total ankle replacements and triple arthrodeses were required. Porous-coated bicondylar implants were used.

and tibiotalar joint and to determine the center of rotation of the tibiotalar joint. Patients with marked valgus or varus deformity of the tibiotalar joint may not be good candidates for arthroplasty. The goal of surgery should be to restore the center of rotation of the ankle no matter which type of implant is used. The center of rotation can be determined from the radius of curvature of the talar dome in the lateral view. Posterior positioning of the implant will result in decreased dorsiflexion, while anterior positioning may result in limitations of plantar flexion. Patients with multiple planes of deformity at the tibiotalar joint are not good candidates for arthroplasty and should be considered for arthrodesis.

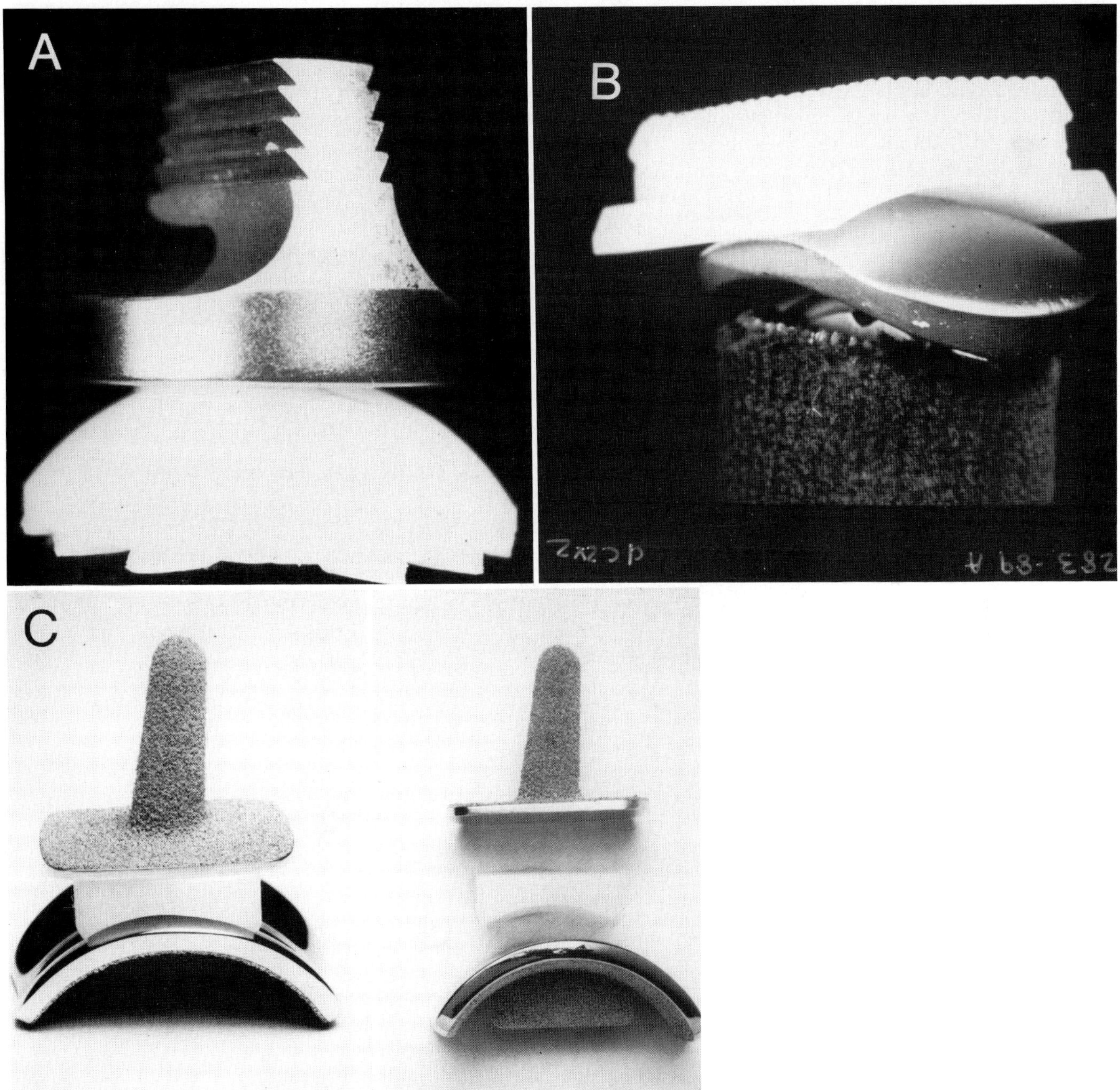

FIG 15–13.
Nonconstrained total ankle prostheses: **A,** Smith. **B,** Newton. **C,** LCS. (From Morrey BF: *Joint Replacement Arthroplasty*. New York, Churchill Livingstone Inc, 1991, p 1163. Used by permission of the Mayo Foundation.)

Implant Design

Implant design can be subdivided into two general groups: nonconstrained and semiconstrained prostheses. Each of these groups can be further subdivided into congruent vs. incongruent designs based upon the conformity of the metal and polyethylene. Incongruent designs may have different radii of curvature between the concave and convex surfaces or may have trochlear surfaces or convex surfaces which result in high loads on the polyethylene.[75] Most current designs are congruent with the nonconstrained-type implants having either a spherical or spheroidal-type articulation which allows for multiaxis motion without inherent stability. The implants include the Waugh, Smith, Newton, and LCS prostheses[8, 25, 30, 69, 74, 109] (Fig 15–13). Theoretically, stress distribution is better in the nonconstrained devices compared with semiconstrained implants, but they are inherently less stable and may result in problems such as impingement against the malleoli and instability.[9] There are multiple semiconstrained-type devices available which vary in their relative amounts of constraint. These include the Mayo, Conoidal, Conaxial, Oregon, TPR, St. George-Buchholz, ICLH, Scholz, and The Hospital for Special Surgery ankles[36, 37, 41, 55, 84, 86, 93, 101] (Figs 15–14 and 15–15). The semiconstrained devices are less apt to subluxate and may provide more protection against malleolar impingement and subsequent fracture. However, the increase in stability may also result in increased loosening rates as greater rotational torque is transferred to the bone-cement interfaces. In order

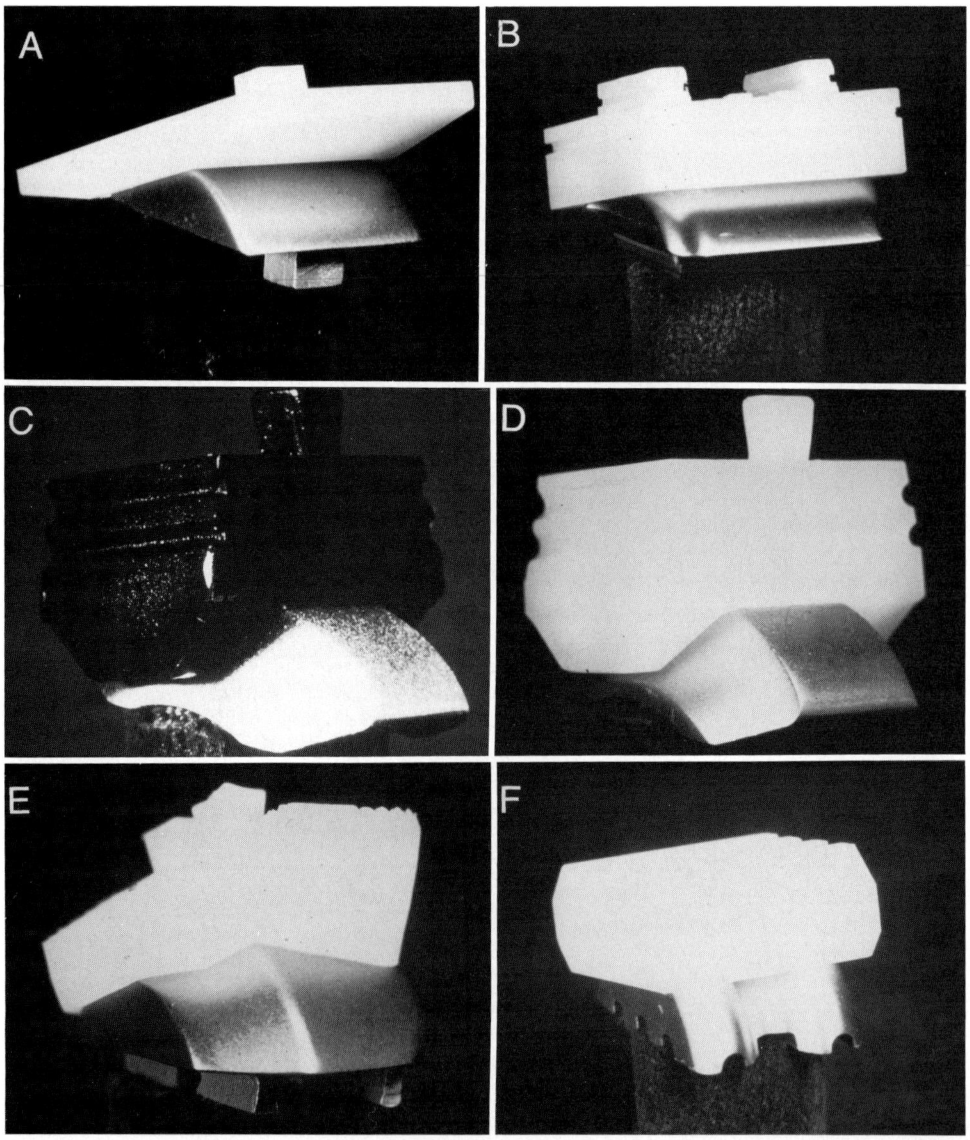

FIG 15–14.
Semiconstrained total ankle prostheses: **A,** ICLH. **B,** Mayo. **C,** Oregon I. **D,** Oregon II. **E,** Conoidal. **F,** Conaxial. (From Morrey BF: *Joint Replacement Arthroplasty*. New York, Churchill Livingstone Inc, 1991, p 1164. Used by permission of the Mayo Foundation.)

to circumvent this, some of the implants have less constrained designs. The current Hospital for Special Surgery design is bicondylar which allows for rotation, eversion, and inversion as well as flexion and extension (Fig 15–15,A and B). In order to address the problem of malleolar impingement, several designs have attempted to resurface the malleoli including the Oregon ankle.[36, 37] In an attempt to decrease loosening rates, several implants have been designed for implantation with porous ingrowth surfaces, including the Scholz, LCS, and The Hospital for Special Surgery implant.[8, 86]

Surgical Technique

Most authors describe an anterior approach for implantation of a total ankle replacement. However, a posterior approach, as described by Unger et al.[101] may be used. With either approach, excellent exposure of the ankle can be obtained with exposure of the malleoli. The advantage of the anterior approach is its ease and the relative low risk to neurovascular structures. The rate of wound problems may, however, be higher. The posterior approach has excellent visualization, especially of both malleoli and of the posterior aspect of the talus. The posterior tibial artery and tibial nerve must be identified and carefully retracted, however.

Anterior Approach.—The patient is placed upon an operating table and a pneumatic tourniquet is applied. An anterior incision is made along the crest of the tibia in line with the second metatarsal. It should be equidistant from the medial and lateral malleoli. The skin is then sharply divided down to the deep fascia. The extensor retinaculum is opened longitudinally. The extensor hallucis longus and tibialis anterior are retracted medially. The extensor digitorum communis and neurovascular bundle are retracted laterally. Sharp dissection is made to identify the capsule of the ankle joint. A careful dissection is made to identify the medial and lateral malleoli. The lateral collateral and deltoid ligaments must be carefully protected. Retractors can be placed to improve exposure. Then, the anterior margin of the tibia must be carefully identified, often by performing a cheilectomy. At this point, the surgical techniques will be different, depending upon the type of implant used, but most require resection of the talus and distal to the tibia. The malleoli must be carefully protected to prevent fracture. In addition, with the posterior cuts, the flexor hallucis longus is at risk. The cuts should be checked by radiograph for assurance that they are parallel and that the alignment is not in valgus or varus. Then, appropriate-sized spacing blocks can be used to determine the size of the prosthesis. If a polyethylene spacer is used that is too thick, inadequate motion will result. If the polyethylene is too thin, instability may occur. In

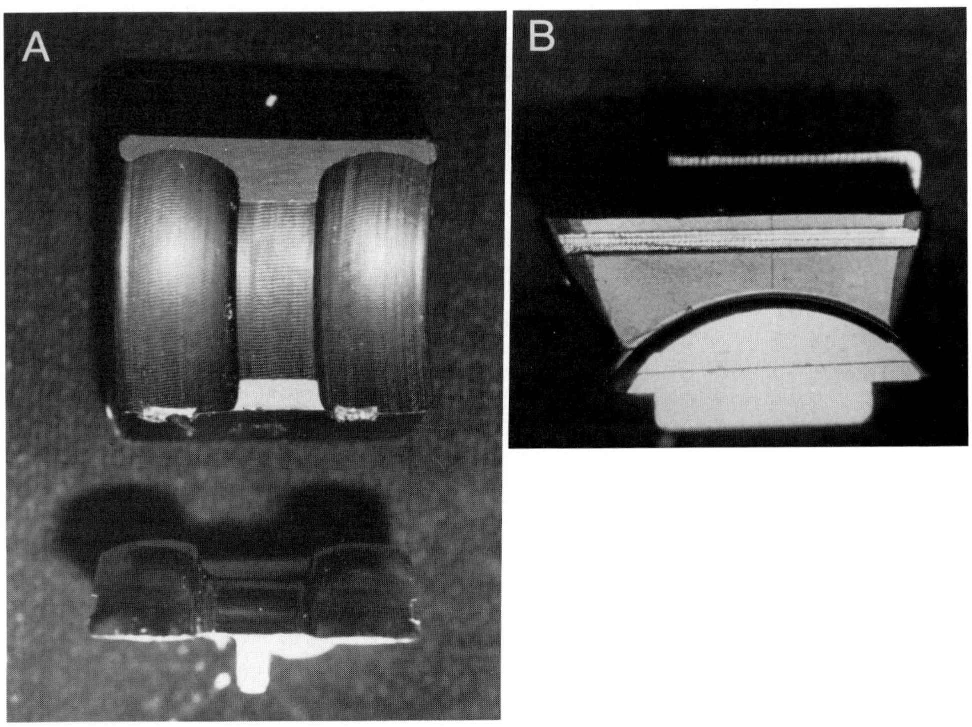

FIG 15–15.
A, B, The Hospital for Special Surgery bicondylar implant.

addition, positioning of the implant should be checked to ensure that the center of rotation is restored. This is especially true with the talar component, which, if placed too far anteriorly, will block plantar flexion, and if placed too far posteriorly, will limit dorsiflexion. Once the positioning has been checked, the implants should be placed. If cement fixation is required, both components should be cemented simultaneously. Excess cement must be carefully removed. A drain can then be placed deep in the wound and the superficial fascia is closed with interrupted absorbable sutures. Skin and subcutaneous tissues are closed in the standard fashion and the ankle is placed in the well-padded soft dressing with a posterior U-splint.

Posterior Approach.—The posterior approach may result in fewer soft tissue and wound complications and offers wider exposure and visualization of the malleoli. In addition, the center of rotation of the arthroplasty can be better assessed because the anatomy of the posterior cortex in the tibia and the os calcis remains constant. It is also easier to identify hindfoot alignment.

The patient is placed prone and draped in sterile fashion. All pressure points must be well padded. A pneumatic tourniquet is used. The skin incision is made using a medial zigzag incision, starting 10 cm proximal to the medial malleolus, paralleling the medial border of the Achilles tendon (Fig 15–16,A), and carried down to the medial border of the Achilles tendon insertion. The crural fascia is identified and opened longitudinally (Fig 15–16,B). The plantaris tendon is identified and may be released from its insertion on the medial aspect of the calcaneus. The flexor group is identified and retracted and the deep posterior fascia is identified on the posterior aspect of the tibia (Fig 15–16,C). The posterior periosteum can be split. The flexor hallucis longus is subperiosteally reflected around the medial malleolus. This preserves the medial flexor group and the neurovascular bundle. Blunt Bennett retractors can be used medially around the malleolus. The Achilles tendon is reflected laterally. Subperiosteal dissection is performed laterally around the lateral malleolus. A Bennett retractor can be placed. The posterior capsule is then easily identified and both malleoli are well visualized. The capsule can be resected and the appropriate cuts can be made. Often, the talar cut can be made first as the posterior cartilage surface is easily identified. In addition, the malleoli can be well protected, as they are well visualized using this approach. The implant can be placed as with the anterior approach, again using either biologic or cement fixation (Fig 15–16,D). Upon closing, a drain is placed deep in the wound and the crural fascia is closed. Skin and subcutaneous tissues are again closed and an ankle is placed in a well-padded dressing with a posterior or U-splint.

Postoperative Care

The patient should be treated with 3 to 4 days of elevation of the ankle. Suction drainage should be continued until drainage ceases, usually after 24 to 48 hours. At 3 to 4 days postoperatively, a short leg walking cast can be applied. With a cemented implant, the patient may begin weightbearing as tolerated. Often, the cast is worn for a 2- to 3-week period and then discontinued. In the case of biologic fixation, from 6 to 12 weeks of cast immobilization has been recommended.[8, 86] Once the cast is discontinued, an ankle stirrup may be worn for an additional 2 to 4 weeks. Active, resistive flexion and extension exercises may begin at that time, although walking alone is usually adequate therapy.

Results

Nonconstrained Implants.—In 1977, Evanski and Waugh[30] evaluated 28 patients with nonconstrained implants, predominantly using the Waugh prosthesis. The average follow-up was 9 months and only five procedures were performed for rheumatoid arthritis. The results of the patients with rheumatoid arthritis were not isolated and the average ankle score postoperatively was 74 points. Complications included 3 patients with delayed wound healing, 2 patients with malalignment of the prosthesis, 1 patient with oversizing of the prosthesis, and 1 patient with arterial thrombosis that required amputation.

In 1977, Wiedel[109] reported on 11 Smith prostheses, 7 of which were for rheumatoid arthritis. The average follow-up was 17 months. There were no deep infections, but 3 patients with rheumatoid arthritis had increasing valgus deformity that required further bracing and also resulted in lateral impingement. In 1979, Demottaz et al.[23] reported on a series of 21 ankle replacements of which 14 were semiconstrained prostheses and 7 multiple axis prostheses (Waugh or Smith). In this study, 16 replacements were performed for rheumatoid arthritis with six good, seven fair, and three poor results. The average follow-up was 15 months and there were four wound problems in the patients with rheumatoid arthritis. In this series, there was no correlation with

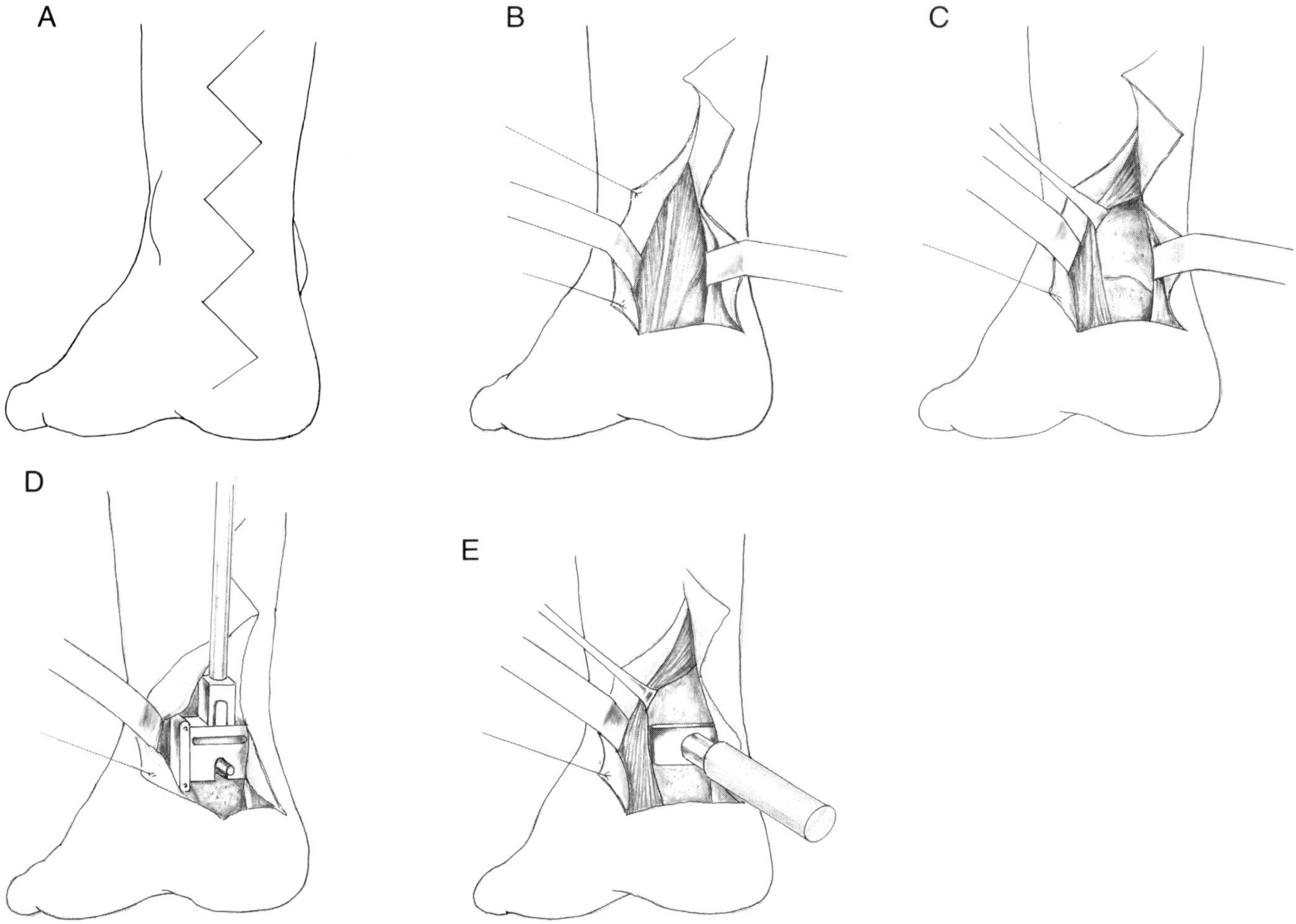

FIG 15–16.
Posterior approach for total ankle replacement. **A,** a zigzag incision is made. **B,** the posterior medial structures are exposed. **C,** the flexor group is retracted medially while the Achilles tendon is reflected laterally. **D,** jigs are used in making the cuts. **E,** a spacer block aids in choosing the proper implant thickness.

the type of prosthesis used and the incidence of mechanical complications. However, the types of mechanical complications did relate to the implant type. This was based on the fact that 2 of the 14 semiconstrained prostheses became loose and 1 of the 7 multiple-axis prostheses became unstable.

In 1980, Dini and Bassett[25] reviewed 21 replacements using Smith prostheses. Five were performed for rheumatoid arthritis. Of these, two had a good result, two had a fair result, and one required removal. Despite the fact that the Smith prosthesis is nonconstrained, there were 3 failures out of the 21 implants due to loosening.

In 1982, Newton[74] reported on 50 Newton prostheses at an average follow-up of 42 months. Ten of these were performed for rheumatoid arthritis and three had good results and seven had poor results including three patients who had loose prostheses, one of which was revised and another converted to an arthrodesis. The third patient had a wound dehiscence and developed a deep infection requiring an arthrodesis and later amputation. In addition, three other patients had stress fractures which were treated conservatively.

In 1988, Buechel et al.[8] reported on 23 noncemented LCS implants, 6 of which were performed for rheumatoid arthritis. Of the patients with rheumatoid arthritis, three had good to excellent results, two had fair results, and one was a failure. The average follow-up for patients with rheumatoid arthritis was 38 months. Two of the six patients with rheumatoid arthritis had wound problems including one with a deep wound infection that was successfully treated with repeat surgery and antibiotic suppression. The results of nonconstrained total ankle arthroplasty are summarized in Table 15–1.

TABLE 15–1.
Results of Total Ankle Arthroplasty (Nonconstrained)*

Author	Year	Implant Type	No. of Patients: Total	RA	Follow-up (mo)	RA Results (G/F/P)
Evanski & Waugh	1977	Waugh-Smith	28	5	9	NA
Wiedel	1977	Smith	11	7	NA	NA
Demottaz et al.	1979	Multiple	21	16	14.7	6/7/3
Dini & Bassett	1980	Smith	21	5	30	2/2/1
Newton	1982	Newton	50	10	42.5	3/0/7
Buechel et al.	1988	LCS	23	6	38.3	3/2/1

*RA = rheumatoid arthritis; G = good; F = fair; P = poor; NA = not available.

Semiconstrained Implants.—In 1977, Groth[36] reported on 16 Oregon ankle prostheses, three for rheumatoid arthritis, with a follow-up ranging between 9 and 21 months. One patient had a delayed wound infection. Groth[37] reported on a larger series in 1983 consisting of 44 replacements, ten of which were for rheumatoid arthritis. There were nine good and one fair results with no failures in this group.

In 1981, Stauffer and Segal[93] reported on a series of 102 Mayo prostheses, 43 of which were performed for rheumatoid arthritis. Of the patients with rheumatoid arthritis, 38 had good to excellent results, 1 had a fair result, and there were 4 failures. Three of these failures were due to deep infection. Each required implant removal and arthrodesis. In addition, the overall complication rate for the patients with rheumatoid arthritis was 23%. Other complications included medial or lateral impingement, loosening, delayed wound healing, and intraoperative fracture. In 1984, Lachiewicz et al.[55] reported on 15 ankle replacements for rheumatoid arthritis, 14 of which were Mayo prostheses. All 15 had a satisfactory result. However, 11 (73%) of the ankles showed radiolucent lines at the bone-cement interface. A longer follow-up on the same patients was reported in 1988 by Unger et al.[101] The series included 23 patients, all with rheumatoid arthritis. The average follow-up was 67 months and the patients had shown a deterioration: 15 had good results, 4 had fair results, and 4 had poor results. In addition, the authors identified talar component subsidence in 14 of 15 patients with sequential radiographs and tibial component radiolucency in 14 ankles.

Herberts et al.,[41] in 1982, and Bolton-Maggs, et al.[6] in 1985, reported on the ICLH prosthesis. In the earlier study, 21 ICLH prostheses were reviewed, 7 of which were performed for rheumatoid arthritis. The average follow-up of 36 months revealed 2 good, 2 fair, and 3 failed results. Two of the failures were revisions to arthrodesis. In addition, there was one wound complication among the 7 cases.[41] In the series of Bolton-Maggs et al., 54 ICLH prostheses were implanted, 27 of which were for rheumatoid arthritis. There were 6 good, 13 fair, and 8 poor results, including 5 which were converted to arthrodesis. In the overall series, there was a 40% wound healing complication rate.[6] The results of semiconstrained total ankle arthroplasty are summarized in Table 15–2.

Complications

Early complications include intraoperative problems, including fractures of the malleoli, and early postoperative problems, including delayed wound healing or drainage. Later complications may include dislocation and subluxation, especially of nonconstrained implants, which may be accompanied by stress fractures of the malleoli (Fig 15–17,A and B). Avascular necrosis of the talus with subsidence of the talar component may contribute to impingement of the malleoli. This can also occur with instability of the ankle joint. Loosening may be related to implant constraint. Late infection may result from hematogenous spread of bacteria.

Delayed wound healing, skin edge necrosis, and drainage may be prevalent in patients with rheumatoid arthritis who are taking high-dose steroids. Bolton-Maggs et al.[6] reported a 40% wound complication rate in their series. Wound complications should be treated aggressively, including debridement and immobilization with possible correcting procedures to cover exposed tendons or implants. The use of the posterior approach to the ankle may help to lessen these complications.

Despite the high wound complication rate, the deep infection rate in the larger series approaches 5% to 6%. In the series of Stauffer and Segal,[93] there were three deep infections in 43 patients with rheu-

TABLE 15–2.
Results of Total Ankle Arthroplasty (Semiconstrained)*

Authors	Year	Implant Type	No. of Patients Total	RA	Follow-up (mo)	RA Results (G/F/P)
Groth	1977	Oregon	16	3	9–21	NA
Stauffer & Segal	1981	Mayo	102	43	23	38/1/4
Herberts et al.	1982	ICLH	21	7	36	2/2/3
Groth	1983	Oregon	44	10	24–84	9/1/0
Lachiewicz et al.	1984	Mayo (n = 14) Buchholz (n = 1)	15	15	39	15/0/0
Bolton-Maggs et al.	1985	ICLH	54	27	42.5	6/3/8
Unger et al.	1988	Mayo (n = 22) Buchholz (n = 1)	23	23	67	15/4/4

*RA = rheumatoid arthritis; G = good; F = fair; P = poor; NA = not available.

matoid arthritis. However, in the series of Unger et al.,[101] there were no deep infections at 5½-year follow-up of 23 patients. In this series, half of the implants were performed using a posterior approach. Although Buechel et al.[8] reported the ability to suppress deep infection, most patients will require removal of the implant with arthrodesis. Arthrodesis may be difficult to obtain and a bone graft may be required in order to maintain leg length.[38, 92]

Implant dislocation is a very rare complication, especially with semiconstrained implants. With nonconstrained implants, subluxation may occur, resulting in medial or lateral malleolar fracture. If subluxation or dislocation occurs early, it may be treated with immobilization and a cast for a 6-week period. If dislocation occurs late, it will most likely mean that the implant will require revision or removal with arthrodesis.

Loosening with talar subsidence may also occur. Symptomatic loosening may require revision surgery, either to a new implant or more frequently to an arthrodesis. All cases of loosening should be evaluated for possible infection by aspiration and bone scan. With talar component subsidence, malleolar impingement may result. This can also occur with a nonconstrained implant. Malleolar impingement may be treated by excising the tip of the malleoli, but if the problem is due to ligamentous instability, excision of the tip of the malleoli alone will not solve the problem. Malleolar impingement may occasionally be treated conservatively using steroid injections and bracing. Other infrequently reported

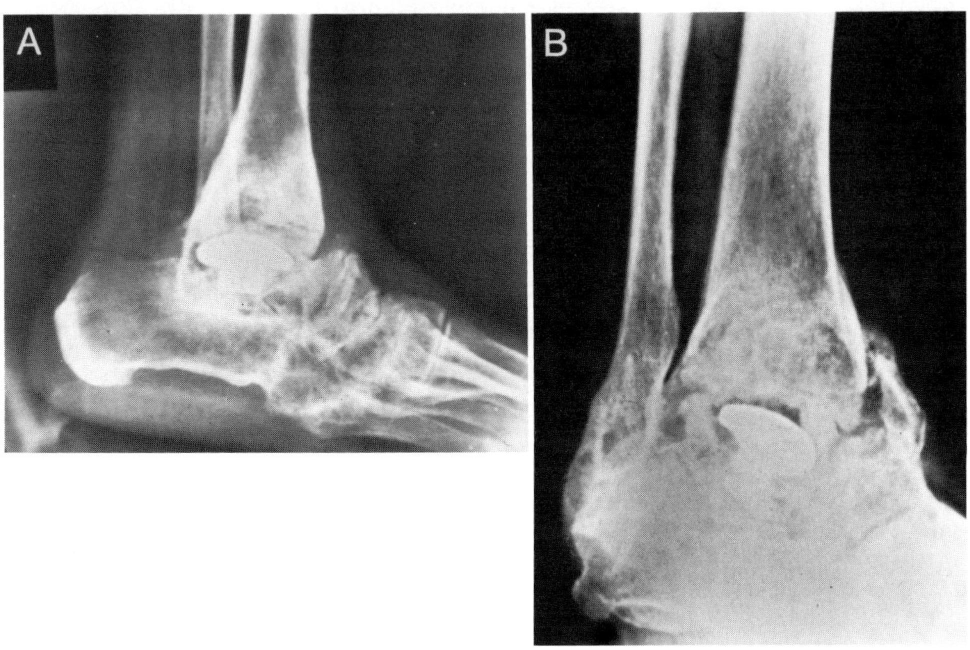

FIG 15–17.
A, a patient with a nonconstrained Smith prosthesis had failure secondary to implant loosening, instability, and resultant medial malleolus fracture **(B).**

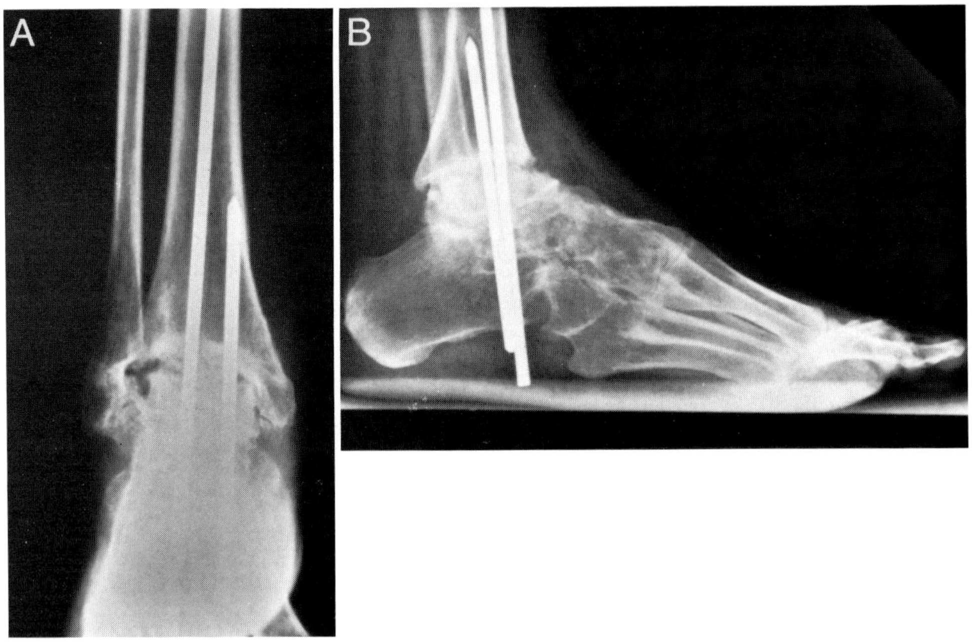

FIG 15–18.
A, B, this patient had a failed total ankle replacement which was treated by implant removal and interposition iliac crest bone grafting to maintain length.

complications include thrombosis of the posterior tibial artery requiring amputation, reflex sympathetic dystrophy, damage to the superficial peroneal nerve, and retained intraarticular methymethacrylate.

Revision Procedures

Failed total ankle arthroplasty is usually best treated by arthrodesis.[38, 92] However, in selected cases, if adequate bone stock is available, a revision implant may be considered. The difficulties of arthrodesis are usually centered around the fact that there is marked bone loss and arthrodesis would result in marked shortening. In addition, the presence of the medial and lateral malleoli will often prevent adequate compression. Thus, interposition bone grafting is often used in a Chuinard and Peterson–type arthrodesis as modified by Stauffer[92] (Fig 15–18,A and B). Surprisingly, despite the use of a large-segment bone graft for a compression arthrodesis, the fusion is usually successful. If the revision is for a septic joint, then osteotomy of the malleoli and fusion without bone graft has been recommended.[38] Another option would be performing a resection, treating with antibiotics, and later arthrodesis with bone graft. While this would require two operations, it would also help maintain leg length. The third option is to perform an astragalectomy by excising the remainder of the talus. This may often allow for a functional resection arthroplasty.

Summary

Total ankle arthroplasty may be a successful procedure in carefully selected patients. Arthroplasty should be limited to sedentary patients with multiple joint involvement. Surgical technique is demanding, requiring careful selection of an implant, thorough preoperative planning, and a patient who will comply with the postoperative regimen. While the chief advantage of the operation is maintenance of motion in the tibiotalar joint, the durability of implant arthroplasty is still in question.

Current implant design is currently directed at minimizing bone stresses and improving stability while decreasing constraint. Biologic fixation with porous ingrowth surfaces may provide advantages over cement fixation and may lessen talar subsidence and resulting impingement. Clinical trials are currently under investigation of a bicondylar or variable-center-of-rotation implant, employing a metal backing, variable joint height, and biologic fixation. In addition, the use of a posterior approach to the ankle may decrease wound healing problems and lower the infection risk.

HINDFOOT

The advancements in reconstruction of the hip and knee in rheumatoid patients have yielded gratifying

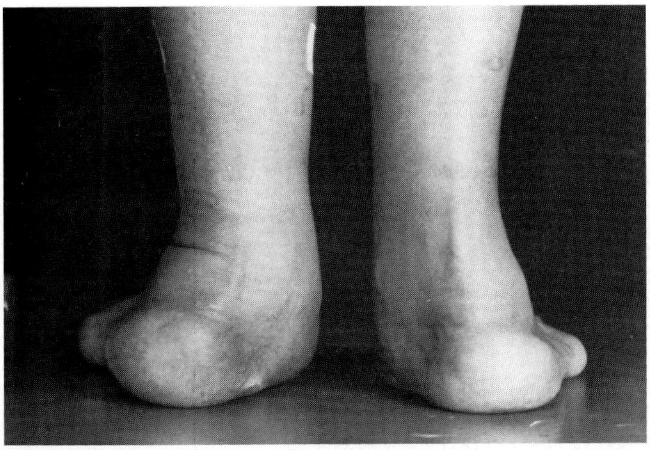

FIG 15–19.
Severe hindfoot valgus deformity.

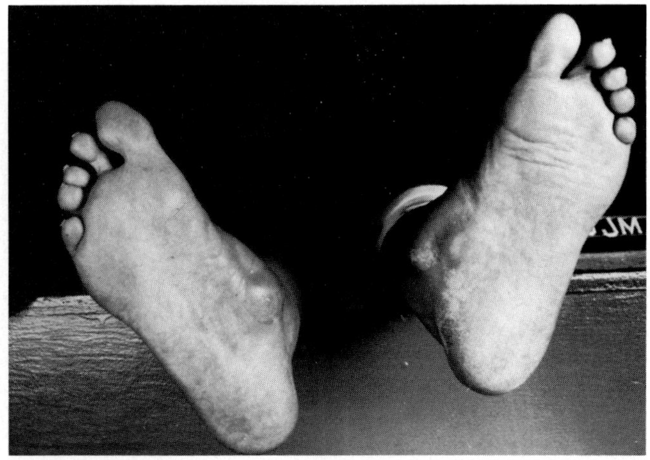

FIG 15–20.
Dislocation of the talonavicular joint results in loss of arch, valgus deformity, forefoot abduction, and pressure over the talar head.

results. Accordingly, the increased activity permitted by these reconstructions has placed increased demands for a more functional and pain-free foot in order to encourage optimal rehabilitation of the lower extremities. For these reasons, arthrodesis of the hindfoot may become necessary to stabilize the foot before a severe hindfoot valgus deformity develops (Fig 15–19). Radiographic studies of rheumatoid patients have emphasized that the talonavicular joint is frequently the first to be involved and often the major source of pain and deformity (Fig 15–20). For this reason, Elboar et al.[28] recommend early isolated talonavicular arthrodesis in these patients (Fig 15–21). Both Elboar et al.[28] and Fogel et al.[32] have reported satisfactory results with isolated talonavicular arthrodesis. This concept of isolated hindfoot fusions is further supported by Mann and Coughlin[62] who state that this procedure is indicated in the rheumatoid patient with only a moderate degree of deformity of the foot. They note that the surgeon must carefully evaluate the foot to determine whether an isolated talonavicular fusion can achieve an acceptable realignment of the foot.[21] If this is not the case, then the calcaneocuboid or subtalar joint, or both, may also need to be incorporated.

Indications and Contraindications

The indications for hindfoot arthrodesis, as outlined by Patterson et al.[77] and Adam and Ranawat[1] are primarily pain relief and correction of the deformity to provide a plantigrade foot. This allows the foot to be properly fitted to a shoe or brace. Also, the patient may achieve a more normal weightbearing capacity, which improves ambulation. Isolated talonavicular joint disease may be treated with an isolated talonavicular arthrodesis (Fig 15–22,A and B). Isolated subtalar arthrodesis can be considered when the valgus deformity of the hindfoot can be passively corrected and there is a relatively uninvolved transverse tarsal joint.

Chronic infection or the presence of wound breakdown are contraindications to midfoot and hindfoot surgery. The skin breakdown associated with severe hindfoot deformity should be adequately treated prior to hindfoot surgery. An inadequate vascular supply or severe vasculitis is also a contraindication to hindfoot surgery.[62]

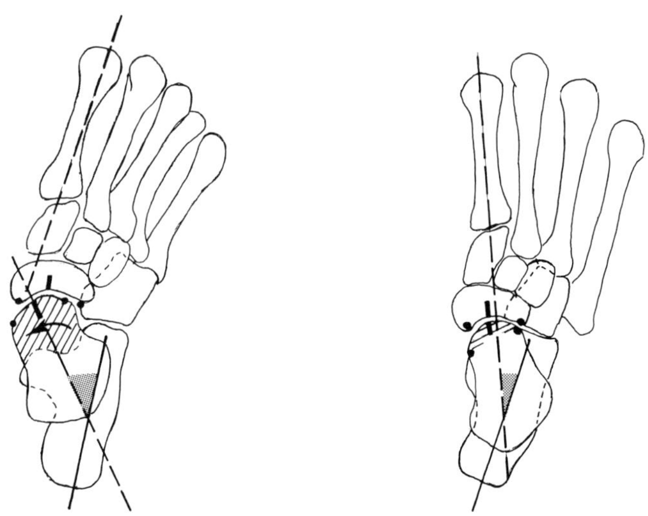

FIG 15–21.
When early changes occur at the talonavicular joint, the foot may be reduced and corrected by an isolated talonavicular fusion.

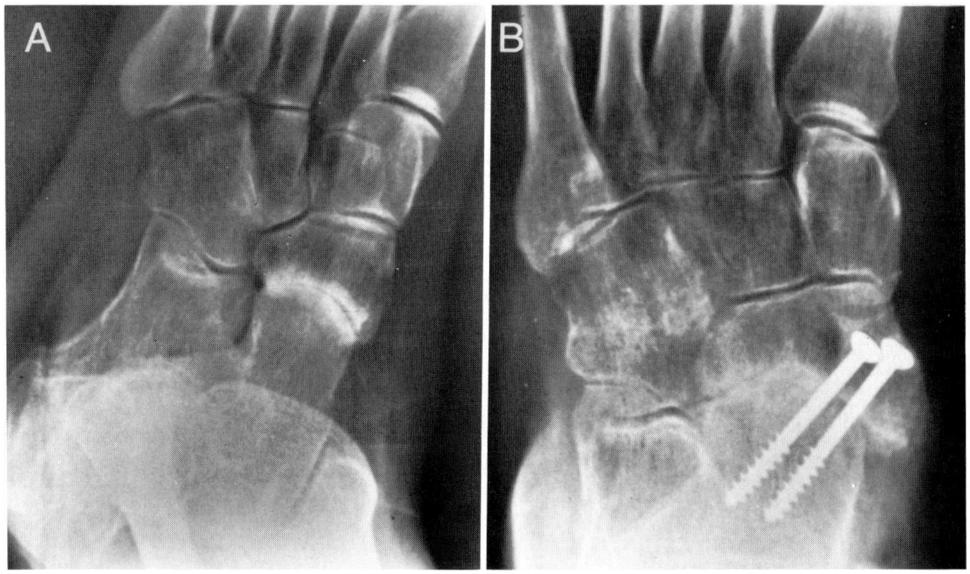

FIG 15–22.
A, B, a patient with early disease and minimal deformity. An isolated talonavicular fusion was performed.

Isolated Talonavicular Arthrodesis

Elboar et al.[28] reported on 35 isolated talonavicular arthrodeses on 31 patients with an average follow-up of 5 years. Twenty six of the 31 patients had rheumatoid arthritis and the remainder had osteoarthritis. At follow-up, complete relief of hindfoot pain was achieved in 75% of patients, mild relief in 11%, and additional surgery of some type was required in 14%. Subsequent operations included an ankle fusion in 1 patient for progressive ankle deterioration and repeat bone grafting for a nonunion in 1 patient in whom no form of internal fixation was used. The nonunion persisted despite an additional bone graft but went on to spontaneous subtalar fusion with relief of symptoms. Removal of subcutaneous staples was necessary in 2 patients and in 1 patient the navicular first cuneiform joint was fused by mistake. A subsequent operation was required to fuse the talonavicular joint. However, the patient continued to have mild pain. In the 5 patients with only mild improvement in symptoms, the pain was less than it was preoperatively, and 2 of these patients had progressive ankle deterioration.

Overall, 28 (89%) patients showed a definite improvement in ambulation with successful arthrodesis of the talonavicular joint. Elboar et al.[28] specifically studied the effect of isolated talonavicular arthrodesis on the adjacent hindfoot joints. They found progression of disease in five ankles, two of which had arthritic changes preoperatively, and three of which had normal-appearing ankles preoperatively. Additionally, there was postoperative progression of deformity in 11 other tarsal joints (37%), including 5 subtalar, 3 calcaneocuboid, and 3 naviculocuneiform. Eleven calcaneocuboid and 3 subtalar joints were narrowed preoperatively, but no progression was seen following isolated talonavicular arthrodesis. The authors concluded that there appeared to be no causal relationship between isolated fusion of the talonavicular joint and the initiation or progression of degenerative changes in adjacent hindfoot joints.[28]

Surgical Technique

The talonavicular joint is approached through a longitudinal medial incision which starts approximately 1 cm distal to the tip of the medial malleolus and is carried distally along the midline of the foot to the region of the naviculocuneiform joint (Fig 15–23). The incision is carried down through the subcutaneous tissue. If one chooses to carry the incision slightly more dorsal, care should be taken to avoid the saphenous nerve which courses with the saphenous vein. It is important to carefully palpate and identify the talonavicular joint as the naviculocuneiform joint can be mistakenly exposed. After the talonavicular joint is exposed, the capsular tissue along the dorsal, medial, and plantar aspects is stripped, taking care not to damage the posterior tibial tendon. Mann and Coughlin[62] recommend avoiding excessive stripping over the dorsal aspect of the talonavicular joint for an arthrodesis in situ. However, in the presence of more advanced deformity with dorsal spurs, more extensive exposure is warranted. To perform an arthrodesis in situ, the foot is positioned and held in the plantigrade position and a rectangular slot of bone is removed from the talonavicular joint using a small oscillating saw. It is important to be sure that the saw blade is sufficiently long to cross the entire talonavicular joint. If this blade length is unavailable, the authors recommend the alternative technique of decortication of the talonavicular joint instead of using an osteotome to complete the cut. In this way, one avoids the chance of fracture of the fragile talar head.

Next, after the slot is cut, the bone is removed. The slot should extend from 7 to 8 mm on each side of the talonavicular joint and should remove from one half to two thirds of the bone in the dorsiplantar direction. After the bone is removed, the defect is filled with a bone graft from either the iliac crest or medial malleolus. Another alternative is to simply reverse the bone block that is removed, and reinsert it into the defect. Before filling the slot, the remaining articular cartilage of the talonavicular joint should be removed with a small curette. Next, the talonavicular joint and graft are internally fixed with a staple across the arthrodesis.

Alternatively, one can simply decorticate the articular surfaces, feather the talonavicular subchondral bone, and internally fix the arthrodesis site with one or preferably two cancellous bone screws. After the wound is closed, the foot is placed into a short leg compression dressing with plaster splints. At 10 days, the initial dressing is removed and the foot is placed into a short leg nonweightbearing cast for 6 weeks or until there is radiographic evidence of union, and is then placed into a short leg walking cast for another 6 weeks. In the authors' experience, arthrodesis is usually achieved in 12 to 16 weeks.

In Johnson's[49] recent paper on hindfoot arthrodesis, he notes dissatisfaction with textbook diagrams as a guideline for bony cuts as these are difficult to fit together to achieve an anatomically correct position. To address this problem, he has developed the "moldable bone graft" concept which, in a previous report by Russotti et al.,[81] attained a union rate of 98% for isolated subtalar arthrodeses. In performing an isolated subtalar arthrodesis, the classic sinus tarsi approach is used and after the extensor digitorum brevis origin is reflected from the calcaneus distally, the sinus tarsi is cleared of soft tissue. The anteroinferior process of the posterior facet of the talus is identified and excised (Fig 15–24,A). The articular cartilage and subchondral bone are denuded from the talocalcaneal joint surfaces (Fig 15–24,B). Alignment of the hindfoot in approximately 5 degrees of valgus is then achieved and a 0.4-cm smooth Steinmann's pin or a 6.5-mm cancellous bone screw of appropriate length is directed through the neck of the talus into the calcaneus (Fig 15–24,C).

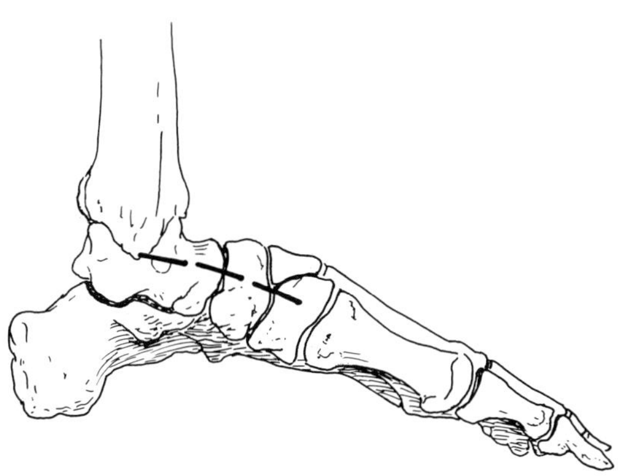

FIG 15–23.
Medial incision for talonavicular arthrodesis.

The moldable bone graft is applicable to both the varus and valgus hindfoot deformity and precludes the need for medially based wedge resections of the subtalar joint. In this fashion, each aspect of the hindfoot deformity is corrected through a separate joint rather than at a single arthrodesis site. Internal fixation is achieved with stout Steinmann's pins which are subsequently removed and therefore cannot cause later problems for the patient.

If a triple arthrodesis is required, the moldable bone graft technique can be used. In this instance, enough of the calcaneocuboid surface should be removed that any forefoot adduction deformity can be straightened by shortening the lateral column of the foot. The talonavicular joint is prepared by removing the talar dome at the level of the dorsal joint line and the navicular is osteotomized beyond the depth of its concave joint apex in order to obtain good bone apposition. Morsellized bone graft slurry is placed at the three joints. Next, a second Steinman pin or screw is placed through the cuboid into the calcaneus (realigning forefoot abduction and adduction), and a third is placed across the talonavicular joint (realigning forefoot rotation so that the line of metatarsal weightbearing is transverse to the tibia). When the foot is correctly positioned, additional bone graft is packed into each resection area with finger pressure and Steinman pins are cut off just beneath the skin.

Triple Arthrodesis

In the majority of patients with rheumatoid arthritis of the hindfoot, isolated talonavicular joint arthrode-

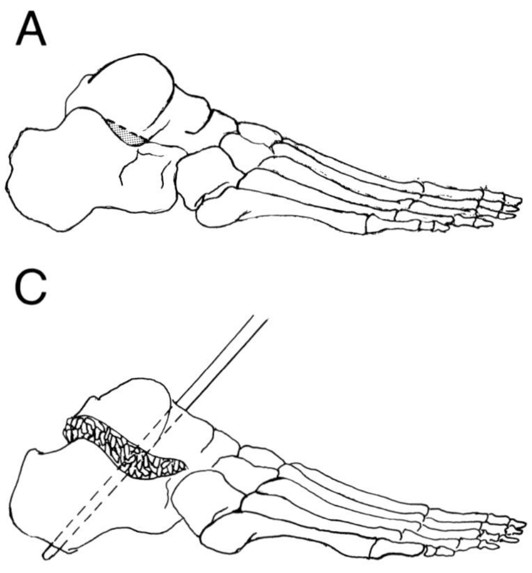

FIG 15–24.
A, isolated subtalar arthrodesis. Excision of the anterior process of the posterior talar facet allows visualization of the subtalar joint. **B,** the subtalar joint is denuded. **C,** a Steinman pin or screw can be used to fix the alignment once the morselized bone graft is placed.

sis will not suffice, as the subtalar joint will be involved. A triple arthrodesis is indicated in these instances. In addition, a triple arthrodesis is required when a significant deformity exists. Russotti et al.[81] emphasize that pain is the primary indication for hindfoot arthrodesis, and the surgeon must consider the patient's personality, occupation, and recreational desires. The authors also state that if the technique of arthrodesis causes malalignment of the other hindfoot joints in the triad, then subsequent painful joints and eventual additional fusions are likely.

Russotti et al. emphasize that 5 degrees of valgus alignment of the hindfoot is only appropriate if the forefoot is mobile. With a rigid forefoot, the hindfoot is placed in a position that places the metatarsal heads parallel to the floor in the plantigrade position. Excessive bone graft should not be placed laterally as it may subsequently cause symptoms by impinging on the distal fibula. The Steinman pin or

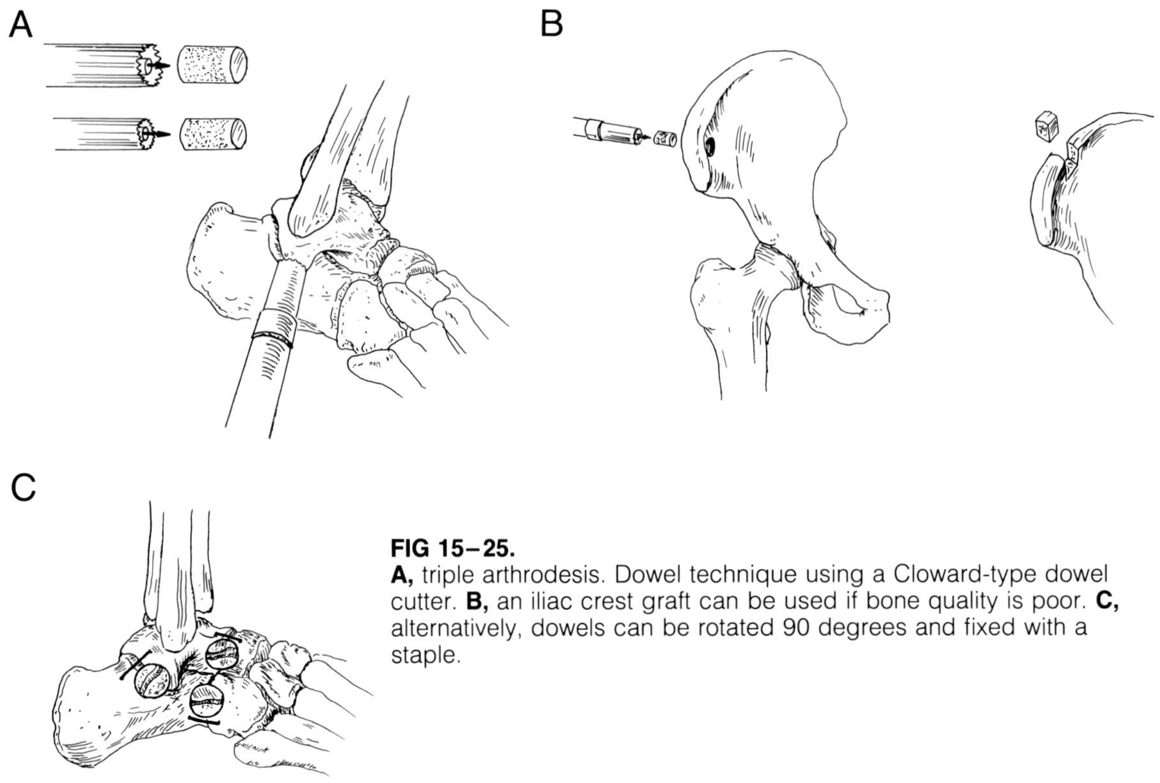

FIG 15–25.
A, triple arthrodesis. Dowel technique using a Cloward-type dowel cutter. **B,** an iliac crest graft can be used if bone quality is poor. **C,** alternatively, dowels can be rotated 90 degrees and fixed with a staple.

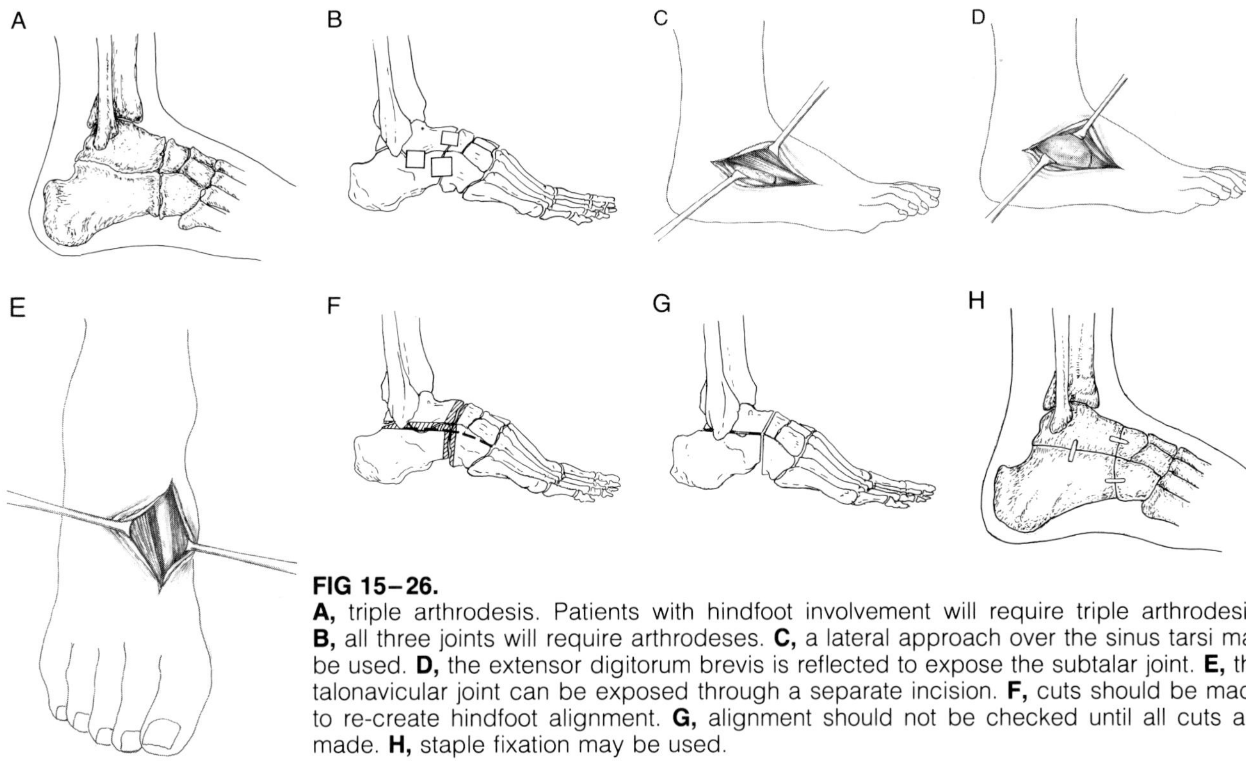

FIG 15–26.
A, triple arthrodesis. Patients with hindfoot involvement will require triple arthrodesis. **B,** all three joints will require arthrodeses. **C,** a lateral approach over the sinus tarsi may be used. **D,** the extensor digitorum brevis is reflected to expose the subtalar joint. **E,** the talonavicular joint can be exposed through a separate incision. **F,** cuts should be made to re-create hindfoot alignment. **G,** alignment should not be checked until all cuts are made. **H,** staple fixation may be used.

cancellous bone screw is removed under local anesthesia at approximately 6 weeks.

Adam and Ranawat[1] reviewed 16 cases of triple arthrodesis to correct hindfoot deformity and relieve pain. The technique of Ryerson,[82] modified by the addition of staple fixation, was used in 9 cases. In 7 cases, a dowel technique similar to that described by Cracchiolo et al.[21] was used (Fig 15–25,A–C). With the dowel technique, the exposure of the subtalar and calcaneocuboid joints was similar to that described by Ryerson.[82] The Morera dowel cutter is used to harvest full-thickness bone plugs while the foot is held in a corrected position. A full-thickness 2-cm dowel is cut from the subtalar joint and a 1.5-cm dowel is cut from the calcaneocuboid joint. The talonavicular joint is approached through a separate incision as described above for the isolated talonavicular arthrodesis (see Fig 15–23). A 1.5-cm dowel is then cut from the talonavicular joint as well. At this point, while the foot is held in the same position, the bone plugs are rotated 90 degrees and impacted in their rotated position. Staple fixation is used for all three joints. Postoperatively, all patients are placed in a patellar tendon-bearing cast. Protected weightbearing is started at 6 weeks and continued until there is radiographic evidence of union. Weightbearing to tolerance is then begun and patients are fitted with a molded orthopaedic shoe.

Figgie et al.[31] reported on the long-term follow-up results of 49 triple arthrodeses performed for rheumatoid arthritis. The operative technique utilized medial and lateral incisions as described by Mann and Coughlin[62] (Fig 15–26,A–H). For an arthrodesis in situ, the bony surfaces were prepared by removing cartilage with curettes and burrs. For patients with moderate to severe deformity, the incision was often changed from an oblique incision over the sinus tarsi to a more vertical incision. Patterson et al.[76] intiated this modification to prevent tension on the wound after correction of more advanced valgus hindfoot deformities. Correction of deformity was accomplished with closing wedge osteomies when necessary[77] (Fig 15–27).

Internal fixation was achieved with hand-driven staples and the use of local supplemental autogenous bone grafting was routine (Fig 15–28,A and B). In no cases was exogenous or iliac crest bone grafting required. The postoperative regimen was similar to that described by Adam and Ranawat[1] above. At an average 5-year follow-up, 94% of patients had significant pain relief with 83% experiencing no pain at all. Ambulation was improved in 80% of patients. While more than half of the patients were limited to household ambulation preoperatively, 90% of the patients were community ambulators or better at the time of latest follow-up. The average time to a radio-

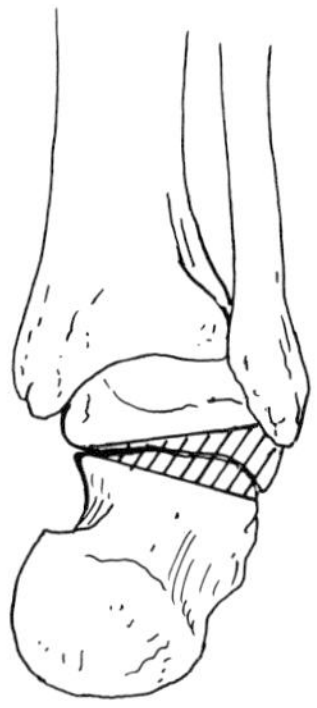

FIG 15–27.
Closing wedge osteotomies may be required to correct alignment after triple arthrodesis.

graphic union was 3½ months (range 2–8 months).

Complications included four wound infections, all of which responded to antibiotics and local care. Two wound separations healed adequately with local care. There were two patients with pseudarthrosis of the talonavicular joint, one of whom was symptomatic and required two operations with bone grafting to achieve fusion (Fig 15–29). Additional surgery was needed in three patients who developed progressive ankle pain after their triple arthrodesis (Fig 15–30,A–C). These patients were converted successfully to pantalar arthrodeses. There was no evidence of progression of forefoot or knee symptoms. There was no significant progression of ankle symptoms in patients who were corrected to hindfoot valgus between 0 and 10 degrees. The authors found triple arthrodesis in the rheumatoid arthritis population to yield a high union rate with significant improvement in ambulation.[31]

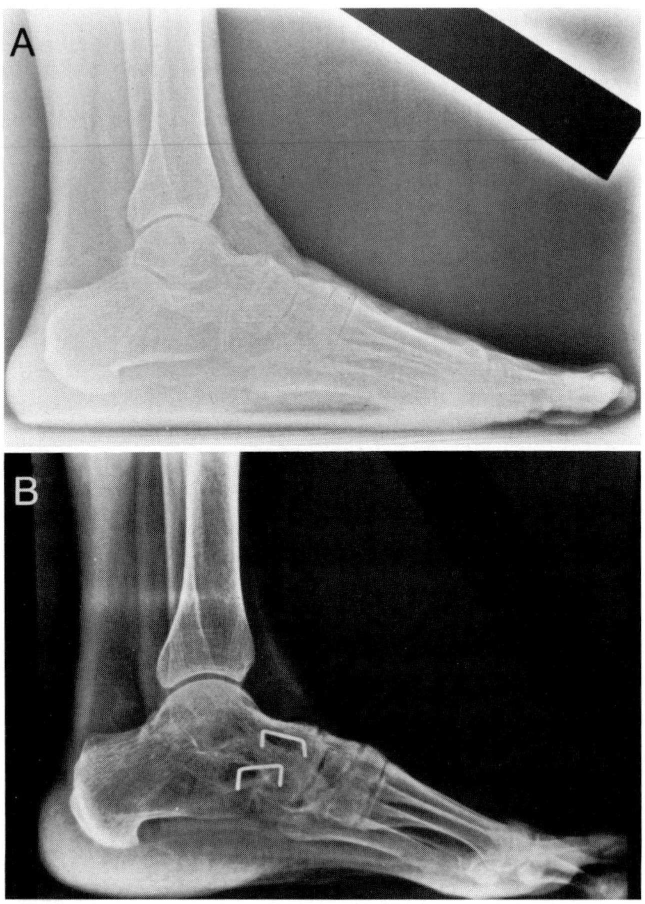

FIG 15–28.
A, minimal perioperative deformity. **B,** triple arthrodesis in anatomic alignment preserved the ankle joint.

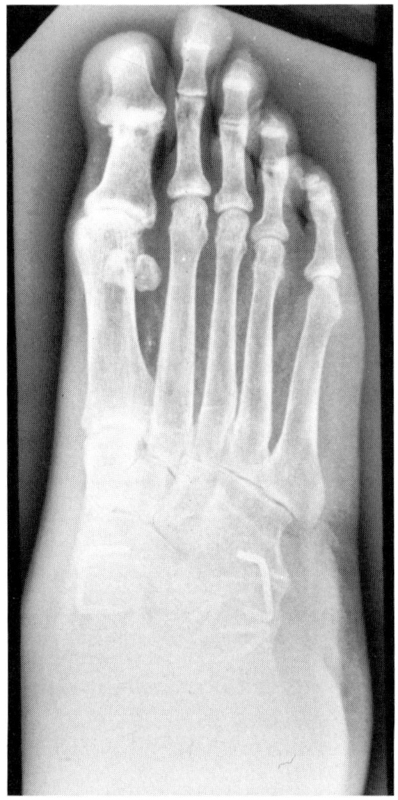

FIG 15–29.
A patient with incomplete correction of his valgus deformity developed pseudarthrosis of the talonavicular joint.

Ruff and Turner[80] reported on 15 patients who underwent 21 selective hindfoot arthrodeses for rheumatoid arthritis. Ten patients underwent isolated talonavicular arthrodesis, 8 underwent a triple arthrodesis, 2 had a calcaneocuboid arthrodesis, and 1 had a naviculocuneiform arthrodesis combined with another fusion. Follow-up averaged 3½ years (range 9 months to 7¾ years). At follow-up, 7 of the 10 talonavicular arthrodeses were rated good and 3 were fair. Of the 3 fair results, 2 had radiographic evidence of a lucent line at the site of fusion, but

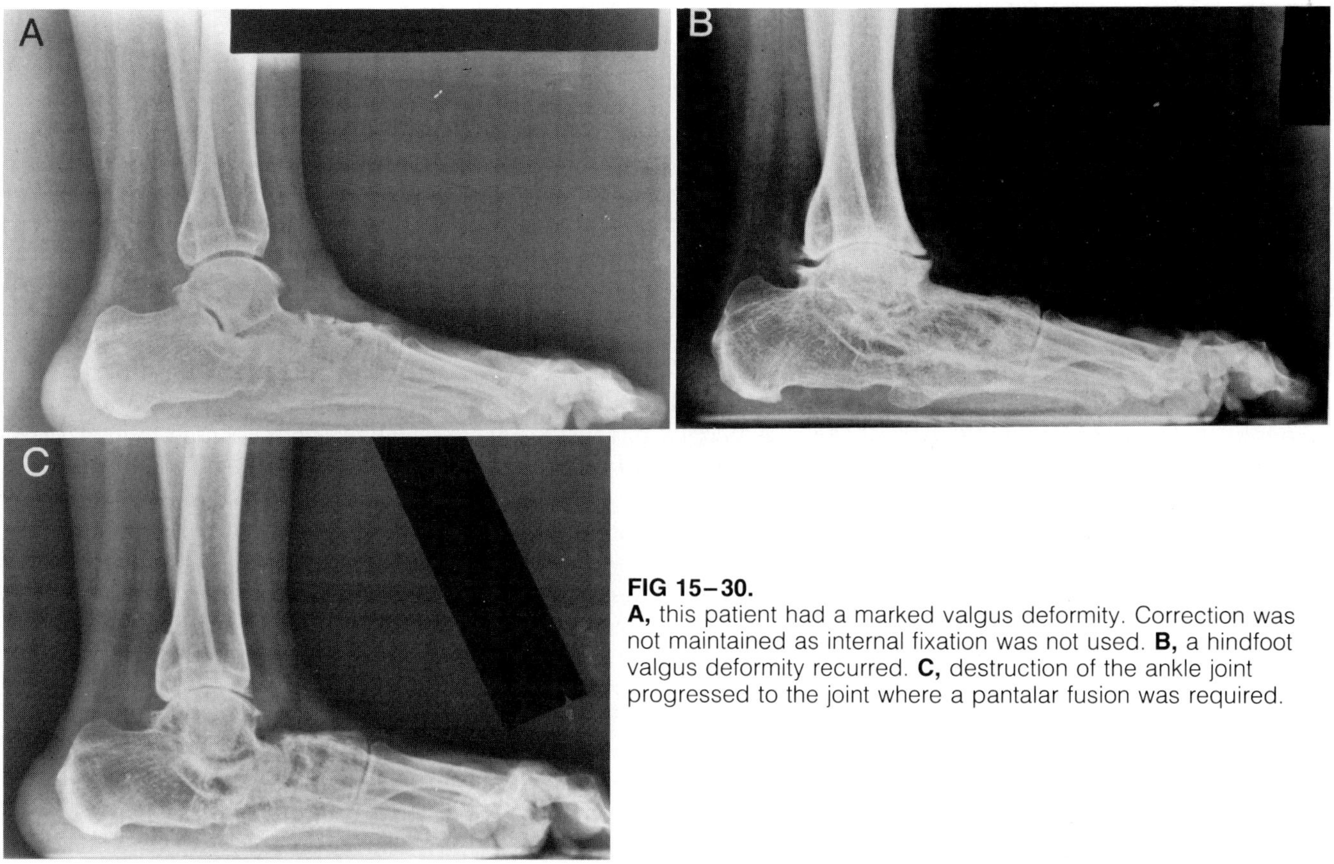

FIG 15–30.
A, this patient had a marked valgus deformity. Correction was not maintained as internal fixation was not used. **B,** a hindfoot valgus deformity recurred. **C,** destruction of the ankle joint progressed to the joint where a pantalar fusion was required.

had no clinical evidence of motion. Of the 8 triple arthrodeses, 7 were rated good and 1 was fair. The patient with the fair result had radiolucent lines at the talonavicular and calcaneocuboid joints with solid fusion of the subtalar joint. This patient was painfree, however. The 2 patients with calcaneocuboid and talocuneiform arthrodeses were also rated as good. There were no reoperations and there was one superficial wound infection which resolved with oral antibiotics and local wound care through a windowed cast. Ruff and Turner concluded that limiting the extent of hindfoot fusion provided for a more anatomically correct position of the foot with preservation of adjacent hindfoot joints. This enhanced the overall shock-absorbing capacity of the foot. They also noted no progression of deterioration of adjacent joints due to abnormal mechanical stress imposed by fusion.[80]

Gschwend and Steiger[39] reported on hindfoot arthrodesis in the rheumatoid foot. They utilized the technique of Wagner and Puck[107] in which internal compression fixation is achieved with large cancellous bone screws. They noted that "subtalar and pantalar arthrodesis was a most rewarding procedure." It should be noted that in their study, only 5 of the 35 feet were afflicted by rheumatoid arthritis.

Wigren[110] reported on 25 triple arthrodeses in 21 patients with rheumatoid arthritis. He divided his patients into two groups: group 1 were those patients with minimal deformity and a normal mechanical axis and with narrowing of the joint space (9 feet), and group 2 were those patients with a marked varus or valgus deformity with a loose unstable foot (16 feet). The author performed a triple arthrodesis in situ for the group 1 patients and a triplane osteotomy and triple arthrodesis for patients in group 2. Internal fixation was achieved using staples, and a plaster cast was applied for 10 to 12 weeks. This was followed by wearing a supportive shoe.

At an average follow-up of 4½ years, pain relief was achieved in all patients. All feet with a varus or valgus malalignment preoperatively were fully corrected to an acceptable mechanical axis postoperatively. Wigren concluded that a triple arthrodesis can reduce the need for ankle joint arthroplasty as only one third of the patients initially felt to need an ankle joint replacement before triple arthrodesis subsequently underwent ankle surgery. Accordingly, they stated that a triple arthrodesis should be considered as the first step in the preoperative planning for a total ankle arthroplasty.

Cracchiolo et al.[21] reviewed 26 patients (30 feet) after hindfoot arthrodesis using a dowel graft technique. Twenty-seven triple arthrodeses and 3 isolated subtalar arthrodeses were performed on 20 women and 6 men. Average age at the time of surgery was 53.5 years (range 27–73 years). The preoperative diagnosis was inflammatory arthritis in 24 feet (i.e., rheumatoid arthritis in 20 feet, juvenile rheumatoid arthritis in 3 feet, Reiter's syndrome in 1 foot), posttraumatic arthritis in 2 feet, polio in 1 foot, posterior tibialis tendon rupture in 2 feet, and developmental flatfoot in 1 foot. Of the 30 feet, 24 had staple fixation with dowel grafts and 6 had dowel grafts without internal fixation.

The dowel graft technique was similar to that previously described by Cracchiolo in 1984.[19] The dowel fusion technique consisted of either rotating a dowel graft 90 degrees across the joint being fused, placing a dowel of bone from the iliac crest into a joint (usually the subtalar joint), or using the dowel graft technique supplemented with hand-driven staples. (see Fig 15–25). Postoperatively, a nonweightbearing short leg cast was used for 6 weeks and then a weightbearing short leg cast for 6 weeks. Average total cast immobilization was 11.8 weeks (range 8–17 weeks). At an average follow-up of 44.1 months (range 24–80 months), 24 patients (92%) were completely satisfied with their result. One patient had pain in the sinus tarsi area. One patient with rheumatoid arthritis was graded unsatisfactory. He had an uncorrected valgus deformity which required additional surgery.

Cracchiolo and colleagues described the use of dowel grafts, cancellous screws, and power-driven titanium staples to stabilize the talonavicular, calcaneocuboid joints, and subtalar joints.[16, 19, 20, 21] They state that any of the three techniques is effective in achieving a solid hindfoot arthrodesis as long as several basic principles are adhered to: (1) surgeon familiarity with the technique and instrumentation; (2) correction of the hindfoot deformity, and if necessary; supplemental bone graft in the subtalar joint to restore height; and (3) good stability at the arthrodesis sites with internal fixation as described above.[16, 19, 20, 21]

For subtalar joint bone grafting, Cracchiolo and colleagues describe three techniques. The first is a dowel method in which a Cloward drill is used to harvest a 12-mm dowel which removes only 80% of the posterior facet of the subtalar joint from lateral to medial. A dowel cutter of the same or slightly larger size is then used to harvest a dowel from the iliac crest. The dowel graft is then packed into the defect created by the drill. The second grafting procedure includes a bicortical or tricortical iliac crest graft which is impacted into a slot fashioned in the subtalar joints, similar to the Grice procedure. This graft is usually stabilized with power-driven staples, or a 0.062-in. Kirschner wire. The third type is the "moldable" bone graft described by Johnson.[49]

Weltmer and Cracchiolo[108] reviewed 35 patients (40 operations) in which a powered metaphyseal stapler was used for reconstructive procedures in the adult foot. The staples are made of titanium and have slightly divergent prongs, which, when fired into the bone, tend to spring together, providing some compression. There are several key technical points to remember: (1) If possible, flat bony surfaces provide increased stability; (2) the position of the staple should be perpendicular to the bone surface to be stapled, in order to obtain maximum rigidity and compression; (3) the stapler is designed for use in metaphyseal bone but the authors have found that it can also be used in bones with a large cancellous content, such as the bones of the midfoot and hindfoot; (4) at least two staples are required to control rotation and they should be parallel to each other; (5) the staples work as a tension band and accordingly should be placed in a tension mode; (6) three to four hits are usually required for completely seating a large staple; (7) the legs of the staple should not penetrate the opposite sides of the bones in which they are being used; (8) the ideal size for the hindfoot is the 16 × 20 mm or 16 × 25 mm. The staple should have a sufficiently wide bridge to provide compression across the fusion site as well as increase stability.

Weltmer and Cracchiolo[108] noted several complications. Four staples in three patients backed out and required removal. Two patients had broken staples on routine follow-up radiographs. The authors recommend that multiple staples be used across any arthrodesis or osteotomy site in case of staple fracture. Staple fixation may not be optimal for hindfoot arthrodesis using dowel or other inlay graft techniques. Additionally, young active patients with dense bone may not accept a power-driven staple and, accordingly, an alternative form of fixation (i.e., a screw) should be considered[108] (Fig 15–31,A and B).

Bennett et al.[4] reviewed 22 triple arthrodeses of the hindfoot in adults. The preoperative diagnoses included six patients with posttraumatic arthritis, eight with posterior tibialis tendon rupture, three

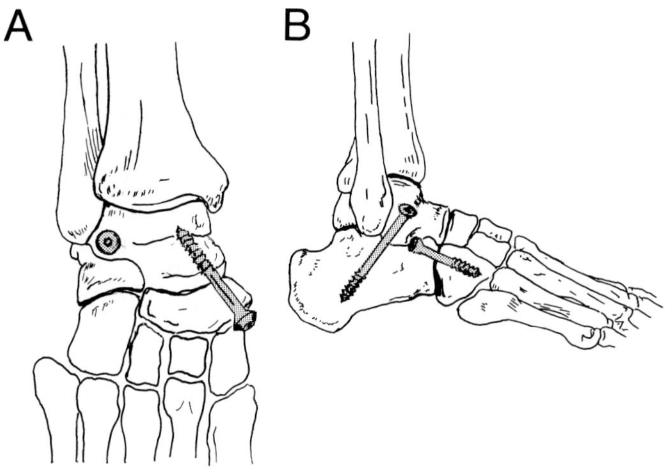

FIG 15–31.
A, B, screw fixation may be done in lieu of staples.

with rheumatoid arthritis, four with polio and clubfoot sequelae, and one with painful pes planus. Average age at the time of surgery was 51 years (range 18–75 years). Surgical technique included medial and lateral incisions, appropriate bony and soft tissue correction, and internal fixation of the fusion sites with staples. At minimum follow-up of 3 years, 20 patients had radiographic union of all three joints. There were two talonavicular nonunions (both asymptomatic). There were no infections or wound problems. Eleven patients had ankle pain and three had midfoot pain postoperatively. Eleven patients had radiographic evidence of ankle joint arthritis and 11 patients had midfoot arthritic changes that had progressed postoperatively. Fifteen of the 22 patients (68%) had some pain in the foot and ankle with activity. Twenty-one of the 22 patients (95%) were satisfied with the procedure and felt that they were improved overall. The authors concluded that triple arthrodesis is a useful procedure for treating painful conditions of the hindfoot in adults which yields high patient satisfaction and a low complication rate if proper surgical technique is used. They stated that longer follow-up is needed to ascertain whether hindfoot arthrodesis predisposes patients to the development of symptomatic tibiotalar or midfoot arthritis.

Pantalar Arthrodesis

The decision to perform a pantalar arthrodesis may be complex. Often, it is difficult to determine if the tibiotalar or hindfoot joints are causing the greatest disability. Sometimes, this decision can be aided by selective injections of bupivacaine (Marcaine) into either the ankle joint or sinus tarsi.

The options for patients with ankle and hindfoot arthritis include staged ankle and triple arthrodeses, one-stage pantalar arthrodesis, and either staged or simultaneous ankle arthroplasty and triple arthrodesis. In patients with marked hindfoot deformity, correction of alignment by performing a triple arthrodesis may decrease the ankle stress enough to avoid the need for ankle fusion.[31, 110] However, if a subsequent ankle fusion is required, this would mean additional cast immobilization. An ankle arthroplasty may be performed with a triple arthrodesis in either a staged or simultaneous procedure, in order to maintain ankle motion (see Fig 15–12). This may allow for a more normal gait pattern than a pantalar arthrodesis does. With a pantalar arthrodesis, the stride length will shorten and greater stress may be placed upon the forefoot (Fig 15–32). However, the pantalar arthrodesis will provide a more durable result.

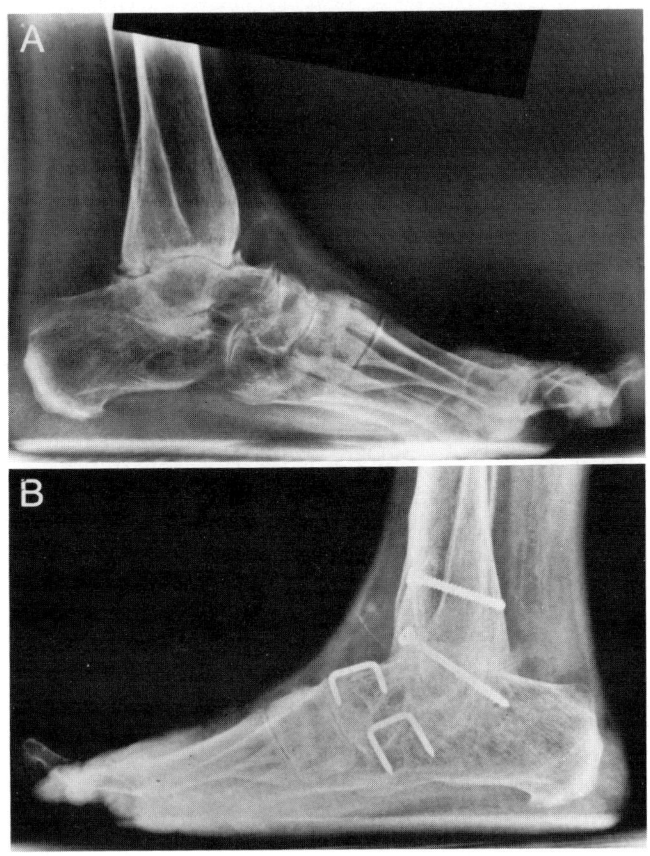

FIG 15–32.
A, a patient with ankle and hindfoot involvement. **B,** a pantalar arthrodesis was performed. Owing to increased forefoot pressure, a subsequent Hoffmann procedure was required.

Techniques of pantalar arthrodesis vary, depending upon the type of fixation. We prefer an anterior ankle approach that curves laterally over the subtalar and calcaneocuboid joint. This can be combined with a medial incision to expose the talonavicular joint. We perform the ankle arthrodesis using the anterior sliding graft technique with screw fixation, and use staple fixation for the triple arthrodesis. Alternatively, exposure can be obtained by osteotomizing the fibula and utilizing it as a strut graft.

There is relatively little in the literature with regard to the results of pantalar arthrodesis. Adam and Ranawat[1] reported on six pantalar arthrodeses and all achieved a solid fusion. However, all were severely limited by multiple joint involvement and were household ambulators. A pantalar arthrodesis does provide pain relief but limits motion such that increased stress is placed on the ipsilateral joints. Further gait analysis is required to study the extent of these limitations.

Complications

Malunion.—Salvage of the malaligned hindfoot or midfoot arthrodesis is a difficult problem, and accordingly, one should be careful to prevent this problem from the start. Varus position of the heel after triple arthrodesis may lead to an abnormal and painful gait pattern. One may also experience difficulty in shoewear and ambulation if the forefoot is placed in an abduction-adduction deformity or varus-valgus deformity. It should be emphasized that the surgeon should carefully address the position of the forefoot, midfoot, hindfoot, and ankle at the time of fixation and at the conclusion of surgery in order to avoid malunion. Excessive resection at the talonavicular joint may lead to varus positioning. In addition, one must ensure that the forefoot is plantigrade after hindfoot correction in order to avoid high stress loading of the medial or lateral foot.[62]

Wound Problems.—The incidence of wound problems is often increased in patients with rheumatoid arthritis due to steroid therapy. Patients with significant hindfoot deformities are at risk for wound problems when correction is obtained. In order to prevent this problem, a vertical skin incision should be used in patients with marked valgus deformities. This reduces the tension on the wound.[62]

Nonunion.—The most frequent site of nonunion after triple arthrodesis is the talonavicular joint. If this occurs, it may lead to a valgus deformity or loss of the arch. If nonunion is symptomatic, it should be treated by iliac crest bone grafting and internal fixation.[62]

In summary, the presence of painful hindfeet in patients with rheumatoid arthritis often indicates advanced hindfoot disease. Hindfoot arthrodesis is effective in relieving pain and restoring the foot to ambulatory capacity. The complication rate is low and nonunions occur infrequently. The hindfoot should be realigned to restore the mechanical axis of the leg. This may reduce the progression of ankle and forefoot disease.

REFERENCES

1. Adam W, Ranawat C: Arthrodesis of the hindfoot in rheumatoid arthritis. *Orthop Clin North Am* 1976; 7:827–840.
2. Albert E: Zur Resektion des Kniegelenkes. *Med Press* 1879; 20:705.
3. Alexakis P, Smith RC, Wellish M: Indications for ankle fusion versus total ankle replacement versus pantalar fusion. *Orthop Trans* 1977; 1:87.
4. Bennett GL, Graham CE, Mauldin DM. Triple arthrodesis in adults. Presented at the American Orthopaedic Foot and Ankle Society Sixth Annual Summer Meeting, Banff, Canada, June 1990.
5. Benson GM, Johnson EW Jr: Management of the foot in rheumatoid arthritis. *Orthop Clin North Am* 1971; 2:733.
6. Bolton-Maggs BG, Sudlow RA, Freeman MAR: Total ankle arthroplasty: A long-term review of the London Hospital Experience. *J Bone Joint Surg [Br]* 1985; 67:785.
7. Buck P, Morrey BF, Chao EYS: The optimum portion of arthrodesis of the ankle: A gait study of the knee and ankle. *J Bone Joint Surg [Am]* 1987; 69:1052.
8. Buechel FF, Pappas MV, Cloris LJ: New Jersey law contact stress total ankle replacement, biomechanical rationale and review of 23 cementless cases. *Foot Ankle* 1988; 8:279.
9. Burge P, Evans M: Effect of surface replacement arthroplasty on stability of the ankle. *Foot Ankle* 1986; 7:10.
10. Calabro JJ: A critical evaluation of the diagnostic features of the feet in rheumatoid arthritis. *Arthritis Rheum* 1962; 5:19–29.
11. Carrier DA, Harris CM: *Ankle arthrodesis with vertical Steinmann's pins in rheumatoid arthritis.* 1991; 268:10–14.
12. Charnley J: Compression arthrodesis of the ankle and shoulder. *J Bone Joint Surg [Br]* 1951; 33:180–191.
13. Cimino WR, Lian G, Cracchiolo A: Comparison of internal fixation and external fixation for ankle fusions in rheumatoid arthritic patients. Presented at the American Orthopaedic Foot and Ankle Society

Sixth Annual Summer Meeting, Banff, Canada, June 1990.
14. Clayton ML: Surgical treatment of the rheumatoid foot, in Giannestras NJ (ed): *Foot Disorders: Medical and Surgical Management*, ed 2. Philadelphia, Lea & Febiger, 1973.
15. Coughlin MJ: The rheumatoid foot, in Chapman MW: *Operative Orthopedics*, vol. 3. New York, JB Lippincott Co, 1988, pp 1845–1855.
16. Cracchiolo A: Surgical arthrodesis technique for foot and ankle pathology. *Instr Course Lect* 1990; 39:49–63.
17. Cracchiolo A III: The use of shoes to treat foot disorders. *Orthop Rev* 1979; 8:73–83.
18. Cracchiolo A III: Management of the arthritic forefoot. *Foot Ankle* 1982; 3:17–23.
19. Cracchiolo A III: Surgery for rheumatoid disease. *Instr Course Lect* 1984; 33:386–411.
20. Cracchiolo A III, Kitaoka HB, Pearson S: Treatment of the painful, arthritic hindfoot (abstract). *Orthop Trans* 1988; 12:765.
21. Cracchiolo A, Pearson S, Kitaoka H, et al: Hindfoot arthrodesis in adults utilizing a dowel graft technique. *Clin Orthop* 1990; 257:193–203.
22. Daniels AU, Samuelson KM, Rusin KA: Talonavicular joint surface anatomy and prototype resurfacing protheses. *Foot Ankle* 1981; 2:5.
23. Demottaz JD, Mazur JM, Thomas WH, et al: Clinical study of total ankle replacement with gait analysis: A preliminary report. *J Bone Joint Surg [Am]* 1979; 61:976.
24. Dennis DA, Clayton M, Wong DA, et al: Internal fixation compression arthrodesis of the ankle. *Clin Orthop* 1990; 253:212–220.
25. Dini AA, Bassett FH: Evaluation of the early result of Smith total ankle replacement. *Clin Orthop* 1980; 146:228.
26. Downey DJ, Simkin PA, Mack LA, et al: Tibialis posterior tendon rupture: A cause of rheumatoid flat foot. *Arthritis Rheum* 1988; 31:441–446.
27. DuVries HL: *Surgery of the Foot,* ed 2. St Louis, Mosby–Year Book, Inc, 1965.
28. Elboar JE, Thomas WH, Weinfeld MS, et al: Talonavicular arthrodesis for rheumatoid arthritis of the hindfoot. *Orthop Clin North Am* 1976; 7:821–826.
29. Elftman H: The transverse tarsal joint and its control. *Clin Orthop* 1960; 16:41.
30. Evanski PM, Waugh TR: Management of arthritis of the ankle. *Clin Orthop* 1977; 122:110.
31. Figgie MP, Ranawat CS, O'Malley MJ, et al: *Triple Arthrodesis in Rheumatoid Arthritis.* Presented at the American Orthopaedic Foot and Ankle Society 56th Annual Meeting, Las Vegas, February 1989.
32. Fogel GR, Katoh Y, Rand JA, et al: Talonavicular arthrodesis for isolated arthrosis: 9.5-year results and gait analysis. *Foot Ankle* 1982; 3:105.
33. Gold RH, Basset LW: Radiologic evaluation of the arthritic foot. *Foot Ankle* 1982; 2:332–341.
34. Goldberg VM: Early management of the rheumatoid joint. *Instr Course Lect* 1984; 33:404–411.
35. Gould N: Graphing the adult foot and ankle. *Foot Ankle* 1982; 2:203–219.
36. Groth HE: The Oregon ankle: A total ankle designed to replace all three articular surfaces. *Orthop Trans* 1977; 1:86.
37. Groth HE: Total ankle replacement with the Oregon ankle: Evaluation of 44 patients followed two to seven years. *Orthop Trans* 1983; 7:488.
38. Groth HE, Fitch HF: Salvage procedures for complications of total ankle arthroplasty. *Clin Orthop* 1987; 224:244.
39. Gschwend N, Steiger U: Stable fixation in hindfoot arthrodesis: A valuable procedure in the complex rheumatoid arthritis foot. *Rheumatology* 1987; 11:114–125.
40. Hallock H: Arthrodesis of the ankle joint for old painful fractures. *J Bone Joint Surg [Am]* 1945; 27:49–58.
41. Herberts P, Goldie IF, Kornsi L, et al: Endoprosthetic arthroplasty of the ankle joint. *Acta Orthop Scand* 1982; 53:687.
42. Hicks JH: The mechanics of the foot. I. The Joints. *J Anat* 1953; 87:345.
43. Hicks JH: The mechanics of the foot. II. The plantar aponecrosis and tahe arch. *J Anat* 1954; 88:25.
44. Holt ES, Hansen ST, Mayo KA, et al: Ankle arthrodesis using internal screw fixation. *Clin Orthop* 1991; 268:21–28.
45. Inman VT: *The Joints of the Ankle.* Baltimore, Williams & Wilkins Co, 1976, p 35.
46. Isman RE, Inman VT: Arthropometric studies of the human foot and ankle. *Bull Prosthet Res* 1969; 10:97.
47. Iwata H, Yasuhara N, Kwashima K, et al: Arthrodesis of the ankle joint with rheumatoid arthritis: Experience with the transfibular approach. *Clin Orthop* 1980; 153:189–193.
48. Johnson K: *Surgery of the Foot and Ankle.* New York, Raven Press, 1989.
49. Johnson KA: Hindfoot arthrodesis. *Instr Course Lect* 1990; 39:65–69.
50. Keenan MAE, Peabody TD, Gronley JK, et al: Valgus deformities of the foot and characteristics of gait in patients who have rheumatoid arthritis. *J Bone Joint Surg [Am]* 1991; 73:237–247.
51. King JB, Burke D, Freeman MAR: The incidence of pain in the rheumatoid hindfoot and the significance of calcaneo-fibular impingement. *Int Orthop* 1978; 2:255–257.
52. King JB, Levack B: Hindfoot disorders. in Helal B, Wilson D (eds): *The Foot,* vol. 1. Edinburgh, Churchill Livingstone, 1988, pp 542–549.
53. Kitaoka HB: The rheumatoid hindfoot. *Orthop Clin North Am* 1989; 201:593–604.
54. Kitaoka HB: Salvage of non-union following ankle arthrodesis for failed total ankle arthroplasty. *Clin Orthop* 1991; 268:37–43.

55. Lachiewicz PF, Inglis AE, Ranawat CS: Total ankle replacement in rheumatology arthritis. *J Bone Joint Surg [Am]* 1984; 66:340.
56. Lloyd K, Agarwal A: Tarsal tunnel syndrome, a presenting feature of rheumatoid arthritis. *Br Med J [Clin Res]* 1970; 3:32.
57. Mann RA: Biomechanics of the foot and ankle, in Mann RA (ed): *Surgery of the Foot,* ed 5. St Louis, Mosby–Year Book, Inc, 1985, pp 1–30.
58. Reference deleted by author.
59. Mann RA: Overview of foot and ankle biomechanics, in Jahss MH (ed): *Disorders of the Foot and Ankle: Medical and Surgical Management,* ed. 2. Philadelphia, WB Saunders Co, 1991, pp 37–67.
60. Mann RA: Biomechanics of the foot and ankle, in Sammarco GH (ed): *Foot and Ankle Manual.* Philadelphia, Lea & Febiger, 1991, pp 32–41.
61. Mann RA, Coughlin MJ: The rheumatoid foot: Review of the literature and method of treatment. *Orthop Rev* 1979; 8:105–112.
62. Mann RA, Coughlin MJ: *The Video Textbook of Foot and Ankle Surgery.* St Louis, Medical Video Productions, 1991.
63. Mann RA, Inman VT: Phasic activity of intrinsic muscles of the foot. *J Bone Joint Surg [Am]* 1964; 46:469.
64. Mann RA, Van Mannen JW, Wapner K, et al: Ankle fusion. *Clin Orthop* 1991; 268:49–55.
65. Manoli A III: Personal communication, 1991.
66. Marshall RN, Myers DB, Palmer DG: Disturbance of gait due to rheumatoid disease. *J Rheumatol* 1980; 7:617–623.
67. Mazur JM, Schwartz E, Simon SR: Ankle arthrodesis: Long-term follow-up with gait analysis. *J Bone Joint Surg [Am]* 1979; 61:964–975.
68. McGuigan L, Burke D, Fleming A: Tarsal tunnel syndrome and peripheral neuropathy in rheumatoid disease. *Ann Rheum Dis* 1983; 42:128–131.
69. McGuire MR, Kyle RF, Gustilo RB, et al: Comparative analysis of ankle arthroplasty versus arthrodesis. *Clin Orthop* 1988; 226:174.
70. Mizel M, Sobel M: Arthrodesis and disorders of the talus and calcaneous: Part II. *Curr Opin Orthop* 1991; 2:558–567.
71. Moeckel BH, Patterson BM, Inglis AE, et al: Ankle arthrodesis: A comparison of internal and external fixation. Presented at the American Academy of Orthopaedic Surgeons 57th Annual Meeting of the New Orleans, February 1990.
72. Mohing W, Kolher G, Coldeway J: Synovectomy of the ankle joint. *Int Orthop* 1982; 6:117–121.
73. Morris HD, Hand WL, Dunn AW: The modified Blair fusion for fractures of the talus. *J Bone Joint Surg [Am]* 1971; 53:1289–1297.
74. Newton StE III: Total ankle arthroplasty: Clinical study of fifty cases. *J Bone Joint Surg [Am]* 1982; 64:104.
75. Pappas M, Buechel FF, DePalma AF: Cylindrical total ankle replacement: Surgical and biomechanical rationale. *Clin Orthop* 1976; 118:82.
76. Patterson BM, Inglis AE, Moeckel B: Anterior sliding graft technique for tibiotalar arthrodesis. *J Bone Joint Surg* (accepted for publication).
77. Patterson RL, Parrish FF, Hathaway EN: Stabilizing operations on the foot: A study of indications, techniques used, and end results. *J Bone Joint Surg [Am]* 1950; 32:1–26.
78. Resnick D: Roentgen features of the rheumatoid mid- and hindfoot. *J Can Assoc Radiol* 1976; 27:99.
79. Resnick D, Niwayama G: Rheumatoid arthritis, in Resnick D (ed): *Diagnosis of Bone and Joint Disorders,* ed 2, vol 2. Philadelphia, WB Saunders Co 1988.
80. Ruff ME, Turner RH: Selective hindfoot arthrodesis in rheumatoid arthritis. *Orthopedics* 1984; 7:49.
81. Russotti GM, Cass JR, Johnson KA: Isolated talocalcaneal arthrodesis: A technique using moldable bone graft. *J Bone Joint Surg [Am]* 1988; 70:1472–1478.
82. Ryerson EW. Arthrodesing operations of the feet. *J Bone Joint Surg [Am]* 1923; 5:453–464.
83. Samuelson KM, Freeman MA, Tuke MA: Implant arthroplasty in the adult hindfoot. *Clin Orthop* 1983; 177:67.
84. Samuelson KM, Freeman MAR, Tuke MA: Development and evolution of the ICLH ankle replacement. *Foot Ankle* 1982; 2:32.
85. Samuelson KM, Harrison R, Freeman MAR: A roentogenographic technique to evaluate and document hindfoot position. *Foot Ankle* 1981; 1:286–289.
86. Scholtz KC: Total ankle arthroplasty using biological fixation components compared to ankle arthrodesis. *Orthopedics* 1987; 10:125.
87. Schwartzman JR: The surgical management of foot deformities in rheumatoid arthritis. *Clin Orthop* 1964; 36:86–95.
88. Scranton PE Jr: An overview of ankle arthrodesis. *Clin Orthop* 1991; 268:96–101.
89. Seltzer SE, Weissman BN, Braunstein FM, et al.: Computed tomography of the hindfoot and rheumatoid arthritis. *Arthritis Rheum* 1985; 28:1234–1242.
90. Smith EJ, Wood PRL: Ankle arthrodesis in the rheumatoid patient. *Foot Ankle* 1990; 10:252–256.
91. Sobel M, Mizel M: Arthrodesis and disorders of the talus and calcaneus: Part I. *Curr Opin Orthop* 1991; 2:547–557.
92. Stauffer RN: Salvage of painful total ankle arthroplasty. *Clin Orthop* 1982; 170:184.
93. Stauffer RN, Segal NM: Total ankle arthroplasty: Four years' experience. *Clin Orthop* 1981; 160:217.
94. Stockley I, Betts RP, Rowley DI, et al: The importance of valgus hindfoot in forefoot surgery in rheumatoid arthritis. *J Bone Joint Surg [Br]* 1990; 72:705–708.
95. Thomas WH: Surgery of the foot in rheumatoid arthritis. *Orthop Clin North Am* 1975; 6:831–835.
96. Thomas WH: Rheumatoid arthritis of the ankle and foot. *Instr Course Lect* 1979; 28:325–336.

97. Thordarson DB, Markolf KL, Cracchiolo A: Arthrodesis of the ankle with cancellous bone screws and fibular strut graft. *J Bone Joint Surg [Am]* 1990; 72:1359–1363.
98. Thould AK, Simon G: Assessment of radiological changes in the hands and feet in rheumatoid arthritis: Their correlation with prognosis. *Ann Rheum Dis* 1966; 25:220–228.
99. Tillman K: *The Rheumatoid Foot: Diagnosis, Pathomechanics, and Treatment*. Littleton, Mass, PSG Publishing Co, 1979.
100. Tillman K: Recent advances in the surgical treatment of rheumatoid arthritis. *Clin Orthop* 1990; 258:62–72.
101. Unger AS, Inglis AE, Mow ES, et al: Total ankle arthroplasty in rheumatoid arthritis: A long-term follow-up study. *Foot Ankle* 1988; 8:173.
102. Vahvanen V: Arthrodesis of the TC or pantalar joints in rheumatoid arthritis. *Acta Orthop Scand* 1969; 40:642.
103. Vahvanen VAJ: Rheumatoid arthritis in the pantalar joints: A follow-up study of triple arthrodesis on 292 adult feet. *Acta Orthop Scand Suppl* 1967; 107:9.
104. Vainio K: Rheumatoid foot: Clinical study with pathological and roentgenographical comments. *Ann Chir Gynaecol Suppl* 1956; 45:1.
105. Vidigal E, Jacoby RK, Dixon A St J, et al: The foot in chronic rheumatoid arthritis. *Ann Rheum Dis* 1975; 34:292–297.
106. Vidigal EC: Forefoot in chronic rheumatoid arthritis. *Orthop Rev* 1978; 7:43–46.
107. Wagner H, Pock HG: Die Verschraubungs-Arthrodese der Sprunggelenke. *Unfallheilkunde* 1982; 85:280.
108. Weltmer JB Jr, Cracchiolo A III: The use of the powered metaphyseal stapler for reconstructive procedures in the adult foot. *Foot Ankle* 1990; 11:12–15.
109. Wiedel JD: Total ankle arthroplasty with Smith prosthesis. *Orthop Trans* 1977; 1:154.
110. Wigren A: Operative treatment with special regard to the hindfoot. *Arthritis Rheum* 1987; 11:100–103.
111. Young A, Kinsella P, Boland P: Stress fractures of the lower limb in patients with rheumatoid arthritis. *J Bone Joint Surg [Br]* 1981; 63:239–243.

CHAPTER 16

The Forefoot

Thomas P. Sculco, M.D.

Mark J. Geppert, M.D.

Mark Sobel, M.D.

INTRODUCTION

The orthopaedic surgeon usually sees the pathologic rheumatoid foot long after the diagnosis of chronic rheumatoid arthritis has been established. Johnson[40] states that virtually 100% of patients with a 10-year history of rheumatoid arthritis have clinically apparent involvement of the feet. Sixteen percent of rheumatoid patients, however, have foot problems presenting as the initial manifestation of their disease.[78] The prevalence of initial foot and hand involvement is approximately equal (15.7% vs. 14.7%),[73] yet the lay population, rheumatologists, and orthopaedic surgeons seem more familiar with the well-known deformities of the more visible rheumatoid hand. Attention to and familiarity with rheumatoid foot and ankle problems will parallel the improved quality of care and expectations of chronic rheumatoid arthritic patients.

The recent advances in total knee and hip arthroplasty have placed increased importance on the preservation or improvement of weightbearing tolerance in the rheumatoid foot and ankle to allow functional ambulation. Pain relief is still the primary indication for surgical intervention in the rheumatoid foot and ankle. Yet the orthopaedic surgeon must be aware of more than just appropriate operative technique. An understanding of the pathogenesis and clinical presentation allows intelligent intervention with the goals of preserving function, delaying disease progression, and correcting the deformity at the appropriate time and in the correct manner. Pathogenesis and clinical presentation, in addition to physical examination, radiographic findings, diagnosis, nonoperative management, operative indications, and surgical techniques of the rheumatoid forefoot are reviewed in this chapter.

PATHOPHYSIOLOGY

Rheumatoid arthritis is an autoimmune systemic disease resulting from a production of globulin antibodies against tissue antigens. These IgM antibodies, known as rheumatoid factor, have a particular affinity for synovium, explaining the involvement of diarthrodial joints, bursa, and para- or peritendinous synovial tissue in rheumatoid arthritis. The high incidence of forefoot abnormalities in rheumatoid arthritis may, in part, be due to the large number of bones, joints, ligaments, and tendons which occupy a small anatomic area yet are subjected to enormous physiologic loads.[4]

The pathologic effects of rheumatoid arthritis can be understood as a consequence of hypertrophy and inflammation. The anatomic effects of stored rheumatoid factor result from synovial hypertrophy, joint swelling and distention, and secondary ligamentous laxity. The intraarticular release of rheumatoid factor from synovial tissue incites an inflammatory cellular response involving macrophages, complement, leukocytes, and lysozymes. Once released, lysozymes secondarily digest and destroy articular cartilage.

Rheumatoid arthritis therefore affects the foot in two ways. First, synovial hypertrophy and hyperplasia lead to stretching of normal capsular restraints causing ligamentous laxity, secondary muscle imbalances, and resultant joint subluxation and dislocation. The second mechanism is the activation of the inflammatory cascade causing an enzymatic destruction of cartilage, periarticular tissues, and normal supportive structures.

If the metatarsophalangeal (MTP) joint is considered, synovial proliferation distends the MTP joint capsule and stretches the collateral ligaments. This attenuation of the supporting structures, coupled with the dorsiflexion ground reaction force of ambulation, eventually leads to dorsal subluxation of the digits. Displacement of the digital flexors into the intermetatarsal space causes the tendons to pass dorsal to the MTP joint axis. The flexors now act as functional extensors at the MTP joint.[4, 55, 78] An additional MTP joint extensor force is produced by the unopposed action of the extrinsic extensors at the MTP joint, which, coupled with forefoot dorsiflexion forces during ambulation, results in gradual and progressive dorsal phalangeal dislocation. Intrinsic weakness results which prevents extension of the interphalangeal joint leading to claw, hammer, and mallet toe deformities. With time, these flexible deformities become fixed and result in fibrous ankylosis and severe soft tissue contractures (Fig 16–1,A–C).

The plantar fat pad is attached to the plantar aspect of the proximal phalange. Dislocation of the proximal phalanx causes distal migration of the fat pad and a plantar-directed force on the metatarsal head.[1, 47] The plantar-flexed metatarsal head has inadequate plantar soft tissue coverage secondary to atrophy of the local tissues and distal migration of the fat pad. Inflammatory cells and their byproducts also erode the normal osseous anatomy, and the metatarsal head may become quite abnormal and distorted. With ambulation, the decreased surface area of the remaining metatarsal head increases focal pressure on the plantar soft tissues. These factors all contribute to metatarsalgia and callus formation under the transverse metatarsal arch. In the most severe cases, skin breakdown under the prominent metatarsal heads can occur with subsequent drainage and infection (Fig 16–2).

Dorsal dislocation of the lesser toes removes a lateral stabilizing force on the great toe.[55] Additionally, capsular laxity secondary to synovial proliferation leads to instability of the great toe. Shoewear, and attritional attenuation or rupture of the abductor hallucis tendon also contribute to the hallux valgus deformity in rheumatoid arthritis.

Hallux valgus deformity results also from MTP joint distention and loss of both dynamic and static stabilizers (Fig 16–3). As the hallux shifts laterally, the extensor hallucis longus tendon also shifts laterally and acts more as an adductor than an extensor. The metatarsal drifts into a varus position facilitated by laxity and damage at the tarsometatarsal joint of the great toe. The medial aspect of the metatarsal head then becomes more prominent and a redundant inflammatory bursa develops over this exostosis (Fig 16–4).

Deformity of the forefoot is complex and results from direct destruction of the metatarsophalangeal joint by an inflammatory cellular interaction and additionally by the mechanical forces produced by

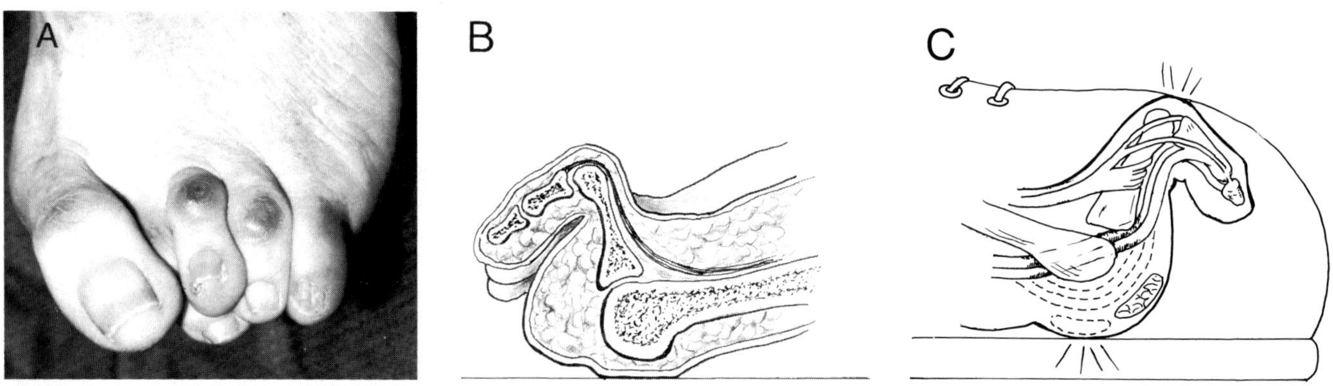

FIG 16–1.
A, rheumatoid forefoot with marked hallux valgus deformity and fixed dislocation of metatarsophalangeal joints. **B, C,** schematic demonstrating dislocation of metatarsophalangeal joint with distal retraction of metatarsal fat pad, dorsal and plantar areas of painful callosity, and increased contact weightbearing.

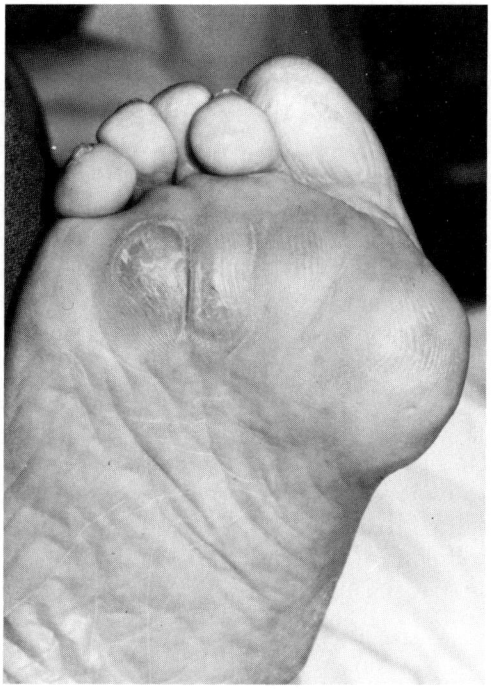

FIG 16–2.
Marked plantar callosity with distal fat pad retraction and metatarsal head prominence.

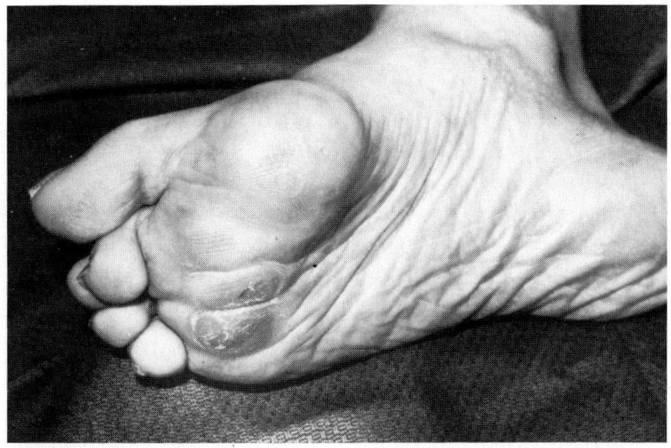

FIG 16–4.
Large bursa over prominent metatarsal head and metatarsal exostosis. Bursae are filled with fluid and rheumatoid synovial tissue.

weightbearing, shoewear, and soft tissue and tendon malposition.

The pathologic processes involved in joint destruction, instability, and dislocation are familiar articular manifestations of rheumatoid arthritis. Less commonly appreciated but potentially devastating is the nonarticular and nonosseous involvement in the rheumatoid foot, i.e., rheumatoid involvement of vascular and nerve structures. Rheumatoid vasculitis is due to immune complex deposition in various-sized vessels with activation of the complement cascade and resultant inflammation. According to Spiegel and Spiegel,[74] vasculitis is the primary extraarticular manifestation of rheumatoid arthritis. Clinical vasculitis in patients with rheumatoid arthritis manifests two forms: (1) a bland obliterative endarteritis involving digital vessels, and (2) an inflammatory focal and segmental vasculitis. The former manifests itself as self-limited nail bed or periungual hemorrhages generally not requiring treatment. The latter may involve major vessels with infarctions, gangrene, and even death.[33] Vasculitic disease may also produce major delay with wound healing, and in severe cases frank wound sloughs may occur.

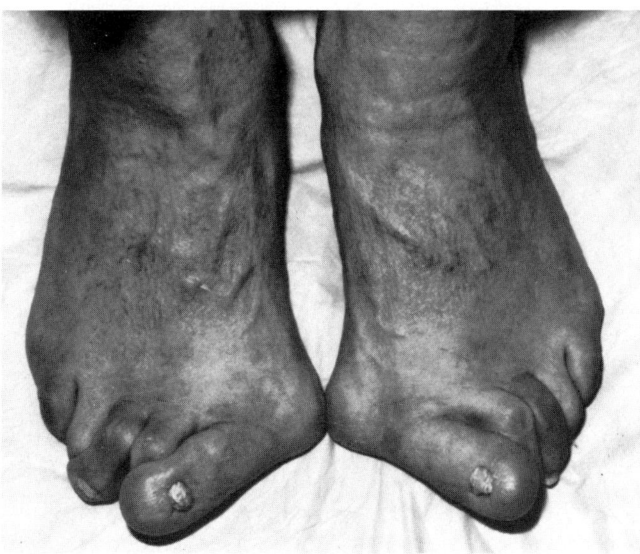

FIG 16–3.
Severe hallux valgus with pronation of hallux and lateral deviation of lesser toes with claw deformities.

Peripheral nerves also may be secondarily involved by rheumatoid arthritis. Vasculitis of the nerves' blood supply will impair blood flow and lead to secondary neurologic involvement. Rheumatoid neuropathy may present in the foot as a peripheral sensory neuropathy, sensorimotor neuropathy, or an entrapment neuropathy and is discussed in the next section.

CLINICAL PRESENTATION AND PHYSICAL EXAMINATION

Clayton[12] has described two types of joint involvement in rheumatoid arthritis. The first, seen in young patients, is a progressive stiffening with eventual fibrosis or bony ankylosis known as the stiff (dry) type. The second, loose (wet) type, involves laxity of soft tissues and resultant deformity due to mechanical stress. The loose type is accompanied by greater synovial hypertrophy and recognizable deformity of the greater and lesser toes. It is more easily diagnosed clinically whereas the stiff type is confirmed by radiographic analysis. Those patients with the ankylosing form of rheumatoid arthritis will also often demonstrate contractures of supporting soft tissues (ligaments, tendons) as well as the skin itself.

The physical examination of the rheumatoid forefoot is a continuation of the examination of the entire lower extremity. Malalignments or arthritic involvement of the more proximal joints affect the foot and ankle. The foot and ankle can compensate for a more proximal deformity so that an isolated evaluation of foot and ankle function without considering the entire leg may lead to an error in therapeutic intervention. A valgus deformity at the knee may aggravate the tendency toward heel valgus and pronation of the forefoot with pes planus.

Physical examination requires the removal of shoes and stockings with only shorts or a gown worn to allow full access to the lower extremity. After examination of the hip and knee, the patient is placed in a standing position. Weightbearing accentuates foot and ankle deformities in addition to providing a check on total limb alignment (Fig 16–5). Hindfoot alignment is evaluated by observing the patient's stance from behind. Normally, the heel is neutrally aligned with the longitudinal axis of the leg. If there is a varus or valgus deviation of the hindfoot it should be recorded. The patient is then asked to stand and walk on his or her toes to assess heel inversion. Patients with rheumatoid arthritis frequently have posterior tibial insufficiency or rupture which prevents this inversion of the heel or interferes with their ability to walk on their toes.

Maintenance of the longitudinal arch also is inspected while standing. The patient is then asked to ambulate and gait is assessed. Severe forefoot abnormalities prevent efficient toe-off[10] and the patient ambulates with an antalgic, flatfooted, steppage gait[20] (Fig 16–6). Visual gait analysis is important as it also indicates the patient's functional capacity. Severely involved rheumatoid patients may not have the ability to stand. The early evaluation of stance and ambulation provides a quick assessment of the functional capacity of the patient, directs attention to specific regions for detailed examination, and forms a conceptual framework for further evaluation and therapeutic intervention.

Hindfoot

The patient is seated with the legs dangling free. Symptomatic subtalar joint involvement is the most frequently affected part of the hindfoot in rheumatoid arthritis.[22, 66] The forefoot is held in neutral position and the heel is cupped with the opposite hand. A gentle eversion and inversion movement assesses subtalar motion. Pain or reduction in range

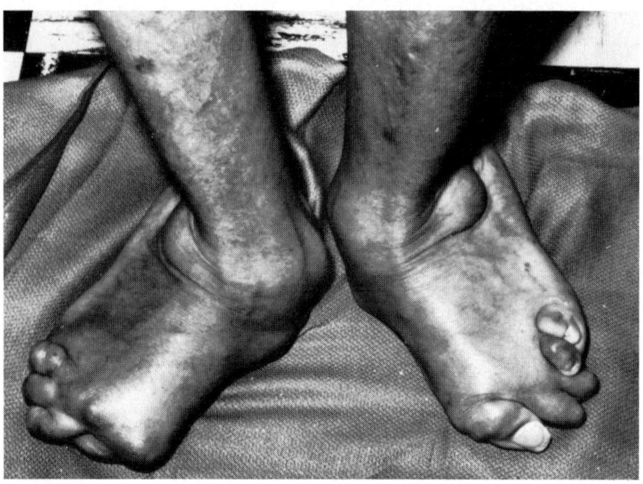

FIG 16–5.
A 46-year-old woman with advanced polyarticular rheumatoid arthritis, combined severe planovalgus, and forefoot deformity.

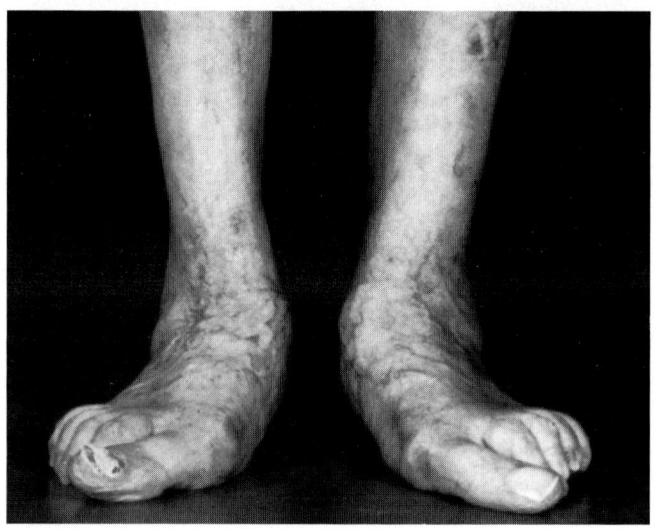

FIG 16–6.
Combined forefoot and hindfoot deformity produces a severe flatfoot weightbearing pattern.

of motion indicates subtalar involvement. The subtalar joint normally inverts slightly greater than it everts with a total range of motion varying between 24 and 44 degrees.[38] Evaluation of contralateral hindfoot motion, if less symptomatic, may provide useful information regarding the patient's customary range of motion. Hindfoot valgus is a common deformity of the rheumatoid patient and may be due to posterior tibial tendon insufficiency.[44] The subtalar rigidity or arthritic involvement causes painful ambulation as the accommodation to uneven surfaces is lost. This increases stress on adjacent joints.

Ankle range of motion and pain with motion is assessed to check for arthritic involvement of the ankle joint. This is also performed by cupping the heel and evaluating hindfoot dorsiflexion and plantar flexion. The sinus tarsi and ankle ligaments are next palpated for tenderness, swelling, or other signs of synovitis.

Hindfoot evaluation includes examination of the Achilles, tibialis anterior, and peroneal tendons, and the posterior tibial tendon for continuity, tenderness, and strength. A lack of motor power may be secondary to an inflammatory involvement of the tendon with pain on tendon use or to frank rupture of the tendon itself. Articular pain or neurologic involvement (both peripheral and myelopathic) may also produce hindfoot weakness.

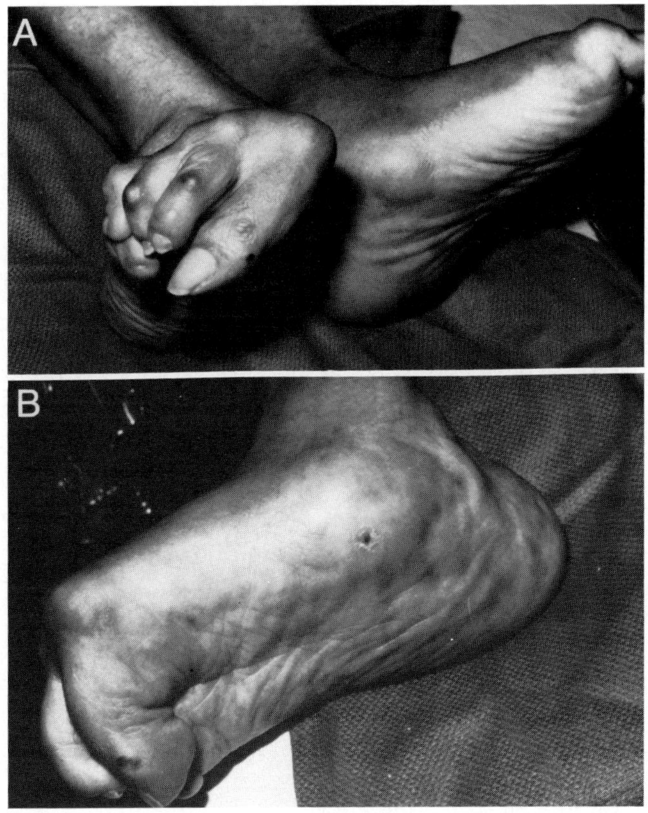

FIG 16–7.
A, B, severe hallux valgus deformity in rheumatoid arthritis with overriding dislocated second toe.

Forefoot

Great Toe

The pathologic attenuation of the soft tissue support of the MTP joint is a prime factor leading to clinical deformity of the great toe as the rheumatoid disease progresses.

The predominant deformity of the great toe is hallux valgus. A number of factors associated with the rheumatoid forefoot may contribute to the occurrence of hallux valgus: (1) the presence of a splay foot with metatarsus primus varus[80]; (2) loss of lateral stabilization secondary to lesser toe subluxation[55]; (3) shoewear with a tight, crowded toe box; (4) pronation of the first metatarsal and hallux secondary to hindfoot valgus; (5) bowstringing of the extensor hallucis longus tendon which adducts rather than extends the hallux; and (6) synovitis and articular destruction of the MTP joint with loss of ligamentous support. The great toe usually rides under the dorsally subluxed second toe; however, an overriding great toe is occasionally seen (Fig 16–7,A and B). Mechanical and other factors described above favor development of a hallux valgus deformity, but other abnormalities such as hallux varus are infrequently seen. In contrast to the lesser toes, complete dislocation of the phalanges of the great toe is rare, probably because of the sesamoid attachment to the proximal phalanx.[48]

The two sesamoids are embedded in the two tendons of the flexor hallucis brevis which inserts into the plantar base of the proximal phalanx. Severe hallux valgus will also produce an external rotation of the hallux with subluxation of the sesamoids. The subluxed sesamoids are not subjected to compression between the metatarsal and the ground, and the metatarsal head is subjected to loading without the sesamoid interface. Sesamoiditis is therefore rare in patients with rheumatoid arthritis.

The soft tissue bunion that accompanies hallux valgus and metatarsus primus varus differs from that seen in the nonrheumatoid patient. In a study of 196 great toes in hospitalized patients with rheumatoid arthritis, Jacoby et al.[39] found 99 cases of hallux valgus, but only four with enlarged bursae and bony exostoses. In these patients, the bunion deformity was confined to the skin only, and was smaller than those of nonrheumatoid patients. The authors attributed the difference in size and the underlying pathologic changes to decreased ambulation and the avoidance of tight conventional shoes by patients with rheumatoid arthritis.

Physical examination frequently demonstrates limitation of dorsiflexion in the first MTP joint. Hallux rigidus, defined as dorsiflexion of 20 degrees or less of the MTP joint,[48] was the second most common deformity of the great toe reported by Kirkup et al.[48] In rare instances, spontaneous fusion of the MTP joint of the great toe can occur. Whether fused or restricted, abnormal kinematics and loading of the MTP joint can lead to abnormal stresses on the interphalangeal joint of the great toe.

Jacoby et al.[39] defined two deformities of the phalanges and interphalangeal joint of the great toe. The first involves a pathologic medial rotation of the hallux greater than 20 degrees measured as the angle of the nail plate with respect to the horizontal plane. The phalanges usually pronate with symptoms arising under the medial aspect of the interphalangeal joint due to contact forces with the floor or shoe. They termed this rotation with callus beneath the interphalangeal joint *hallux tortus*.[39] When the interphalangeal joint is hyperextended with no rotation, plantar callosities may be evidenced beneath the interphalangeal joint. More important, nail dystrophic change with paroncyhia, fungal infection, or ingrown toenails can result from dorsal shoe pressure. They termed this symptom complex *chisel toe*.[39]

Lesser Toes

The earliest signs of rheumatoid arthritis include soft tissue swelling of the forefoot[83] with initial involvement of the lateral MTP joints. Eventually, all the digits and MTP joints are involved. Tenderness to palpation or painful motion of the phalanx indicates synovitis of the MTP or interphalangeal joints. Pain on metatarsal head compression may be the only positive sign in the earliest involvement with rheumatoid arthritis.[77] Chronic synovitis coupled with ligamentous laxity and intrinsic muscle weakness is thought to contribute to splaying of the forefoot.[81]

Dorsal stress on the second proximal phalanx may elicit tenderness or instability signaling significant synovitis of this joint. Usually, however, the physical examination of the rheumatoid foot reveals severe forefoot involvement with gross abnormality due to the capsular laxity with joint dislocation. Physical appearance of the forefoot reveals lateral shift of the digits with subluxation or dislocation at the MTP joints. A clawtoe deformity is often present with marked hyperextension at the MTP joint and flexion at the proximal and distal interphalangeal (DIP) joints (Fig 16–8). Isolated mallet toe (DIP flexion deformity) or hammer toe, a proximal interphalangeal (PIP) flexion deformity, occurs less frequently (Fig 16–9). Extrinsic shoe pressure on the dorsum of the elevated interphalangeal joint (PIP in particular) can cause painful calluses or ulceration (Fig 16–10).

Neurovascular

The neurologic examination of the rheumatoid forefoot may be abnormal with multiple causative factors. Spinal cord compression may produce a myelopathy that results in diffuse yet often subtle neurologic findings. Proprioception and vibratory examination is often abnormal and Babinski's sign may be present as well as clonus. Peripheral neuropathy with severe motor weakness or footdrop may indicate motor neuropathy secondary to necrotizing arteritis of the vasa vasorum of the nerves.[74] Sensory nerve vasculitis presents as paresthesias in a stocking distribution. The dorsalis pedis and posterior tibial pulse examination provides a gross evaluation of

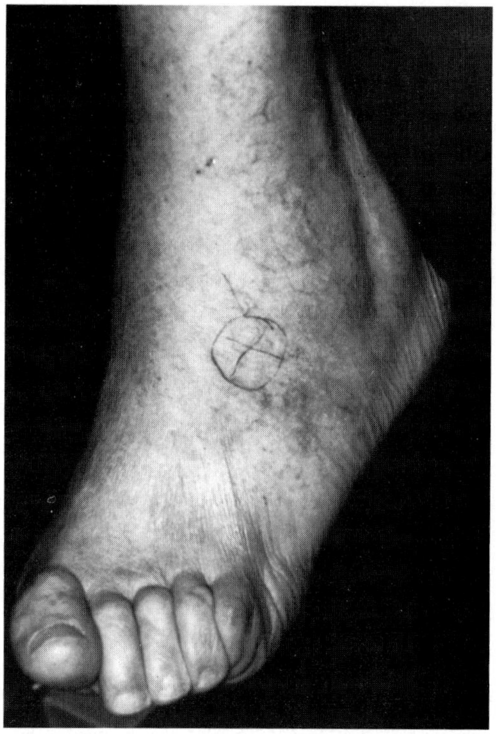

FIG 16–8.
Clawtoe deformity with dorsal subluxation at metatarsophalangeal joint and flexion deformity at proximal and distal interphalangeal joint.

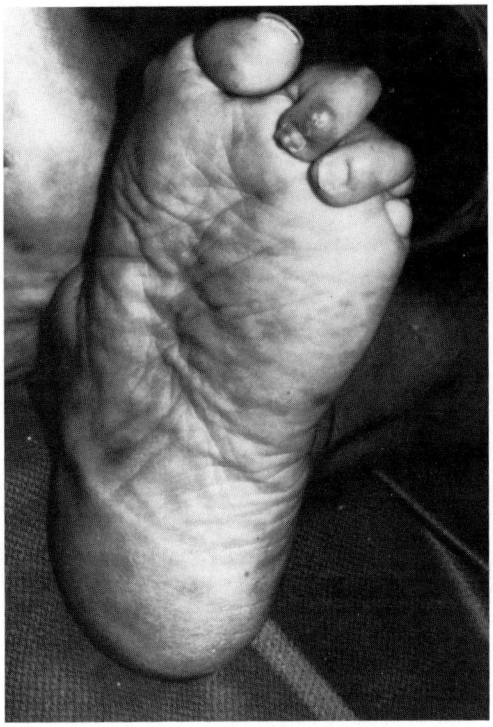

FIG 16–9.
Fixed flexion deformity at proximal and distal interphalangeal joints.

vascular sufficiency though these tests cannot evaluate the adequacy of the blood supply at the level of the nerve. Local compression of peripheral nerves may produce abnormal sensory findings. Crowding within confined anatomic spaces due to exuberant tenosynovitis can also cause an entrapment neuropathy with sensory or motor symptoms.[65]

The tarsal tunnel region can be compressed or tapped to elicit a Tinel's sign which may indicate a tarsal tunnel syndrome. Partial tarsal tunnel syndrome involves a distal medial or lateral plantar nerve entrapment. It is indicated by sensory sparing of the heel with symptoms radiating along the anatomic regions of innervation. More proximal nerve involvement (sciatic, peroneal, etc.) may be due to lumbar spine involvement, secondary to a Baker's cyst, or signal a mononeuritis multiplex. Frequently, rheumatoid feet have subluxations or dislocations of the phalanges which cause traction on the neurovascular bundle. This traction of the common digital nerve against the plantarly displaced intermetatarsal ligament causes a Morton's neuroma. Interdigital compression of the web space will elicit pain and strongly suggests this diagnosis.

Gross peripheral pulses may be palpable, but small vessel involvement secondary to vasculitis may still be present. Clinical signs of obliterative endarteritis include nail splinter hemorrhages, and digital gangrene. Major vessels can be involved in focal and segmental vasculitis resulting in skin ulceration, infarction, and purpura. These physical findings reveal severe involvement with rheumatoid vasculitis. Accordingly, vasculitis may severely impair wound healing and the clinical results of forefoot reconstruction.

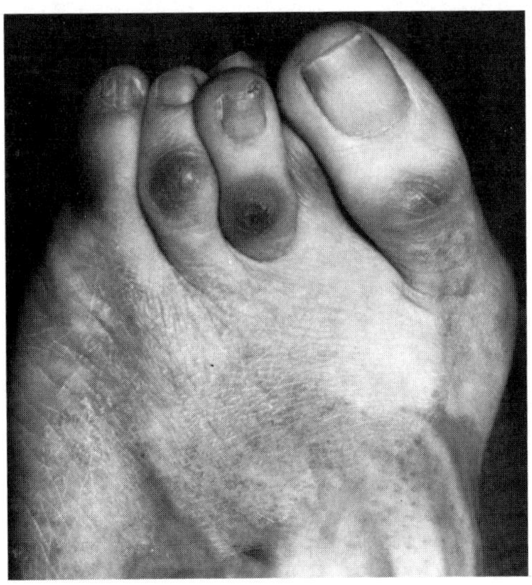

FIG 16–10.
Ulceration and marked callus formation over lesser toe interphalangeal deformities.

SKIN AND SOFT TISSUES

The skin overlying the forefoot in rheumatoid arthritis is often thin and fragile, secondary to both inactivity and medication (corticosteroid) use. In those patients with the ankylosing form of the disease, the skin may be extremely attenuated over contracted MTP and PIP joints.

Other disorders of the soft tissues include synovial cysts and rheumatoid nodules. The latter are actually due to vasculitis of the subdermal connective tissue. Chronic inflammatory cells surround the centrally necrotic arteriole and account for the palpable mass. They may be painful, particularly if located in high-load areas during weightbearing. Nodules usually occur on the extensor surface of joints, bone, or tendon. As in the hand, nodular infiltration occurs in tendons of the foot.

The sole of the foot should be carefully examined and the distribution of calluses, plantar kerato-

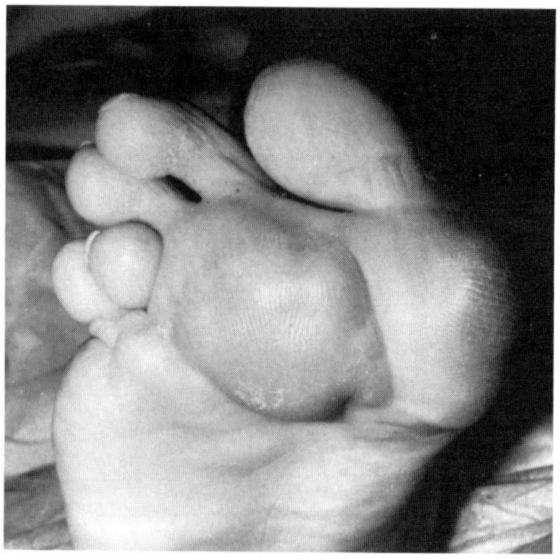

FIG 16–11.
Marked plantar nodular disease over prominent metatarsal heads.

sis, and even ulceration beneath the pronounced metatarsal heads noted. Nodules and synovial cysts can ulcerate and become infected (Figs 16–11 and 16–12). Erosion may occur, particularly over metatarsal head prominences. Metatarsal head resections will improve this problem by removing abnormal nodules and prominent metatarsal heads. These areas of callus or nodular breakdown are attributed to the distal migration of the plantar fat pad, plantar angulation of the metatarsal head, atrophy of the plantar skin secondary to corticosteroids and rheumatoid vasculitis, and increased weightbearing on the metatarsal head due to phalangeal dislocation.

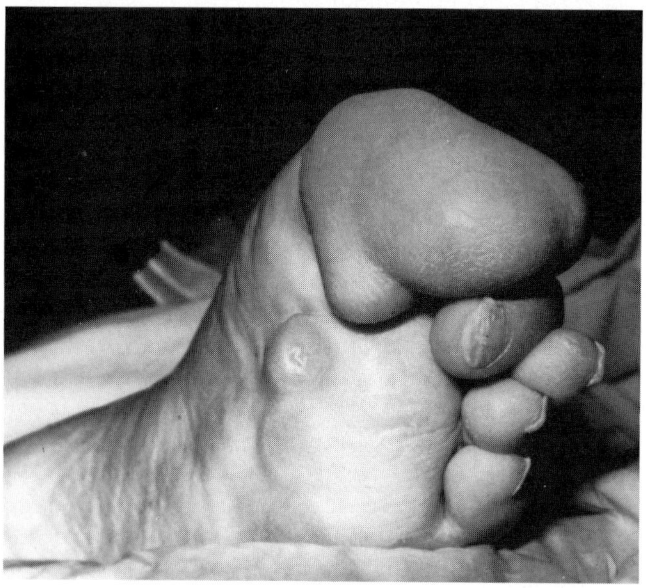

FIG 16–12.
Ulceration through callosity over prominent metatarsal head.

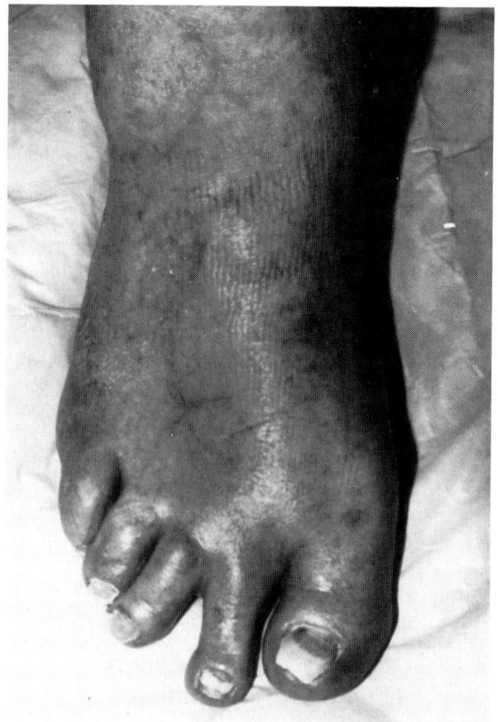

FIG 16–13.
Interdigitial splaying in rheumatoid forefoot. Note atrophic soft tissue quality.

Progressive asymptomatic spreading of the toes can also be secondary to a rheumatoid nodule[21] which may be palpable and the initial manifestation of rheumatoid arthritis (Fig 16–13).

Tendon dysfunction in the rheumatoid forefoot and hindfoot occurs in many different ways. Any tendons of the foot may demonstrate tenosynovitis but the predominant tendons are the posterior tibial and peroneal tendons.[7] Rarely, triggering of a toe digit is secondary to rheumatoid tenosynovitis.[68] Tendon rupture and tenosynovitis of the tendons of the foot and ankle are far less frequent than tenosynovitis or rupture in the rheumatoid hand.[7] Careful attention on physical examination should be given to the continuity of tendinous structures by examining strength in inversion-eversion, and dorsi- and plantar flexion. Increased pes planus deformity with a valgus hindfoot is the hallmark of posterior tibial tendon rupture or dysfunction.

RADIOGRAPHIC EVALUATION

Radiographs of the forefoot with the exception of the oblique view should always be weightbearing to best evaluate the alignment and extent of forefoot

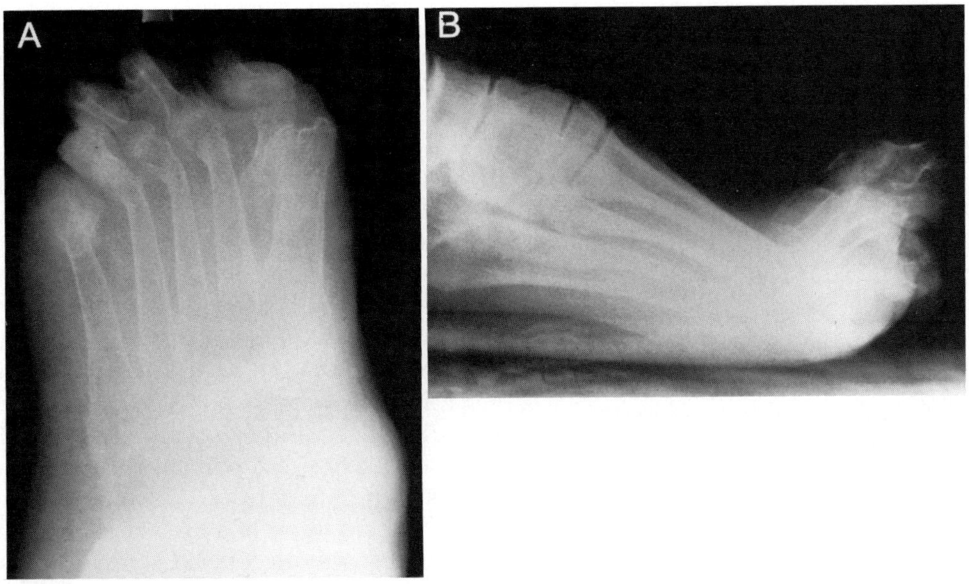

FIG 16–14.
A, B, radiographs demonstrating severe hallux valgus, dislocation of metatarsophalangeal joints, and joint destruction.

disease. Dorsoplantar, lateral, and oblique radiographs of the foot should be routine in the examination of the forefoot. The earliest radiographic forefoot sign in the rheumatoid patient is soft tissue swelling[83] and periarticular osteoporosis secondary to the hyperemia of synovial hypertrophy.[35] Initially, the swelling involves the fifth MTP joint but it extends rapidly and symmetrically to the other four digits. The inflamed synovium is initially confined to the intracapsular but nonarticular recesses within the joint. This exposed bone is unprotected from destruction by inflammatory pannus which leads to marginal erosions[30] (Fig 16–14). Both medial and lateral aspects of the fifth metatarsal head demonstrate early osseous changes. These changes, according to Resnick and Niwayama,[69] are limited to the medial side of the metatarsal heads of digits 1 through 4. The distal medial aspect of the proximal phalanx of the first toe is also involved early in the disease process. As the disease progresses, the plantar aspect of the metatarsal head is eroded.[30]

Later radiographic features of rheumatoid involvement include joint space narrowing secondary to cartilage destruction. Generalized osteoporosis reflecting a systemic inhibition of osteogenesis is also a finding that indicates significant rheumatoid activity.[24] Even in the stiff type of forefoot disease described by Clayton,[12] osteophytes, subchondral sclerosis, and intraarticular bone ankylosis are unusual and indicative of secondary osteoarthritis in the rheumatoid forefoot.

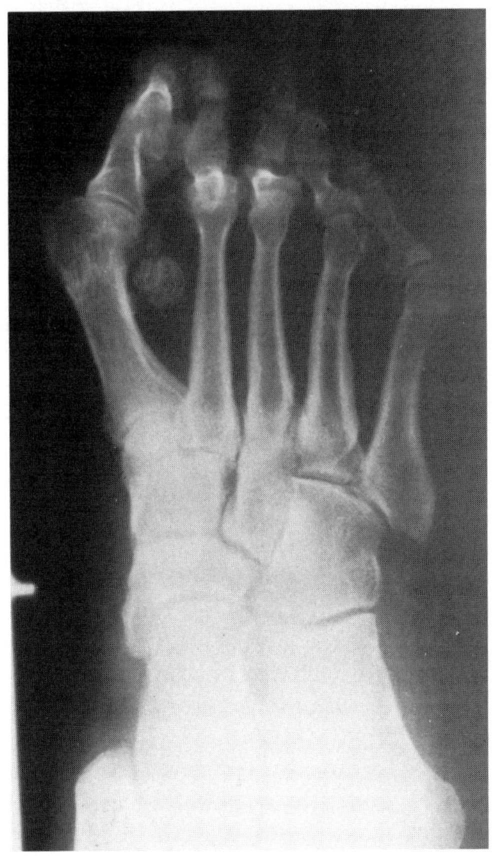

FIG 16–15.
Radiograph demonstrating complete dislocation of metatarsophalangeal joints with end-on view of phalanges.

Positional abnormalities secondary to ligamentous laxity and MTP joint destruction include fibular deviation and subluxation of all five MTP joints. With complete dislocation of the phalanges, an anteroposterior radiograph of the foot reveals a "gun barrel" sign of the proximal phalanx.[12] The end-on view of the proximal phalanx in anteroposterior radiographs is a very late sign in severe rheumatoid arthritis (Fig 16–15).

TREATMENT

Treatment of the rheumatoid patient with forefoot involvement must address both relief of pain and either correction or accommodation of the deformity. Forefoot involvement is but one component of the systemic disease of rheumatoid arthritis. Primary attention must be directed at optimal control of the disease process which is supervised by the rheumatologist. Orthopaedic care encompasses both conservative (nonsurgical) and surgical treatment.

CONSERVATIVE TREATMENT

The goals of conservative measures are to provide pain relief, delay the progression of the disease, which may be inevitable, or accommodate the structural abnormalities in a nonoperative manner. A thorough understanding of the principles of conservative care can delay or prevent operative intervention and also enhance postoperative recovery and results in the event of surgery. Nonoperative measures are most beneficial during stage I and stage II rheumatoid involvement.[31]

Pain in the forefoot in rheumatoid arthritis is due to both inflamed synovitis and structural abnormality. During acute exacerbations, rest is the primary therapeutic measure. Orthotic shoe devices can be utilized to decrease positional deformity and provide a relative immobilization of the painful area of the forefoot.

Gould[34] outlined the mechanisms by which these devices help the rheumatoid foot: (1) to decrease plantar shear forces; (2) to diffuse weightbearing by providing more contact area; (3) to eliminate pressure effects from contact areas; (4) to shift weightbearing areas; (5) to support unstable joints; and (6) to restrict motion.

Shear forces on the tender plantar surface are dissipated with a cushioned insole (e.g., Spenco) (Fig 16–16). This padded insole also supplements the atrophied skin of the rheumatoid forefoot. The increased focal weightbearing on the metatarsals with more severe rheumatoid involvement can be diffused through deformable Plastazote material which increases weightbearing over a larger surface area. In addition, focal deformities such as a rheumatoid nodule or an area of skin compromise necessitate the addition of cutouts or reliefs to the Plastazote (Fig 16–17) to decrease the forces on these prominent painful areas and accommodate the abnormalities. Simple longitudinal (nonrigid) arch supports provide support and decrease motion of the collapsing arch.

The addition of a metatarsal bar, metatarsal pad, or other orthotic device shifts the load proximally, away from painful or compromised metatarsal areas. Nodules or underlying bony deformities should be protected from increased focal weightbearing so that ulceration and infection can be prevented.

Low-heeled shoes with soft leather uppers of ad-

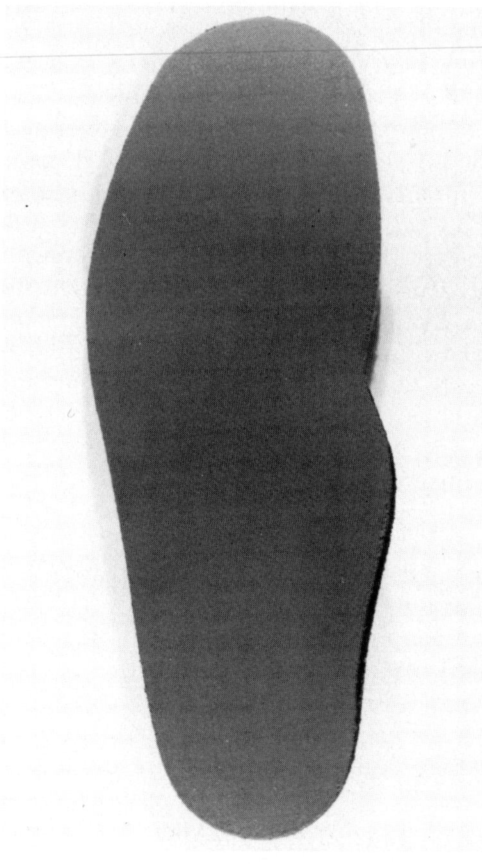

FIG 16–16.
Padded insole with metatarsal and scaphoid support.

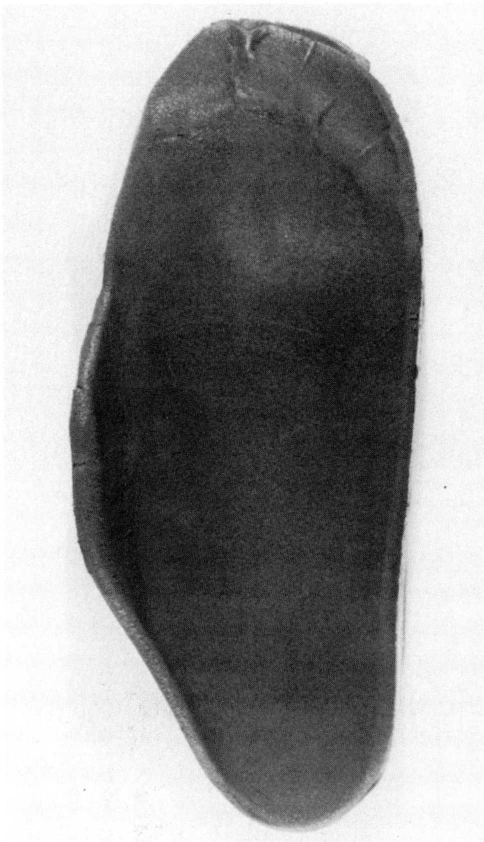

FIG 16–17.
Plastazote custom-molded insole.

equate forefoot width decrease forefoot pressure and are the initial shoes advised for mild rheumatoid involvement. As the claw toe and hammer toe deformities of the lesser toes progress, dorsal shoe pressure causes painful callosities over the interphalangeal joints and increases plantar-directed forces on the metatarsal head. Extradepth shoes, soft leather uppers, open-toed shoes, or sandals decrease this pressure (Fig 16–18,A–C).

Hindfoot deformities such as heel valgus or posterior tibial insufficiency can exacerbate forefoot pronation. Control of position of the hindfoot with a UCBL insert can delay forefoot abnormalities; however, skin tolerance and comfort limit the use of these devices to patients with early rheumatoid involvement. When fixed deformities of the hindfoot or forefoot occur, accommodative devices such as lateral or medial heel wedges can be used which will share the weightbearing load and decrease focal pressure areas. The last concept of conservative care is to restrict joint motion by the use of braces.

Specific recommendations for conservative management depend on the type and severity of the rheumatoid abnormality. Once the diagnosis of rheumatoid arthritis is made, all patients are instructed in foot care and inspection. If the patient is unable to reach his or her feet, family members are recruited to assist in proper nail cutting and foot inspection. Softening lotions applied at home between office visits can decrease the crusted character of hyperkeratotic lesions.

Splaying of the forefoot may require a shoe with a last modified to accommodate the widened forefoot. Early forefoot symptoms require shoe inserts and modifications that require an extradepth shoe. Cushioning to decrease frictional shear forces can be accomplished with a simple neoprene liner. Early hammer toes are treated with a metatarsal pad and medial longitudinal arch support in an extradepth shoe. A full-length shank will decrease toe-off forces and metatarsalgia, and the tendency to dorsally dislocate the phalanges. Difficulty in heel slippage out of the widened shoe is corrected with a pillow collar.[15] External shoe modifications include a metatarsal bar or rocker-bottom sole for severe metatarsalgia. Severe deformity requires custom-made space shoes which are cast from a plaster mold of the foot.

Measures other than shoe or orthotic modifications include a regimen of rest during exacerbation, stretching to improve or maintain range of motion and strengthen the foot, and exercise. Gripping exercises with the foot, standing on toes, heel-rocks, and inversion-eversion exercises are important to maintain strength in the foot and ankle. Exercise sandals are also useful early in the rheumatoid patient. Short-term casting may help during acute rheumatoid flares. Weight control, modified crutches, or canes can reduce weightbearing on affected joints. Rheumatoid involvement of the upper extremities may preclude effective use of ambulatory supports. Platform or Canadian crutches may help if conventional canes cannot be grasped.

Acutely inflamed joints may benefit from the intraarticular injection of steroids.[3] Cracchiolo[17] advocates the more frequent use of aspiration and injection therapy in the conservative management of rheumatoid arthritis. In the forefoot, painful MTP joints and bursae may be aspirated and then injected with small amounts of corticosteroids. Cracchiolo advocates no more than one injection per month during 3 consecutive months over a 9- to 12-month period as a safe guideline.[17] The risk of tendon rupture precludes injection therapy near the insertion of tendons. The judicious use of aspiration and steroid injection may delay the need for surgical treatment.

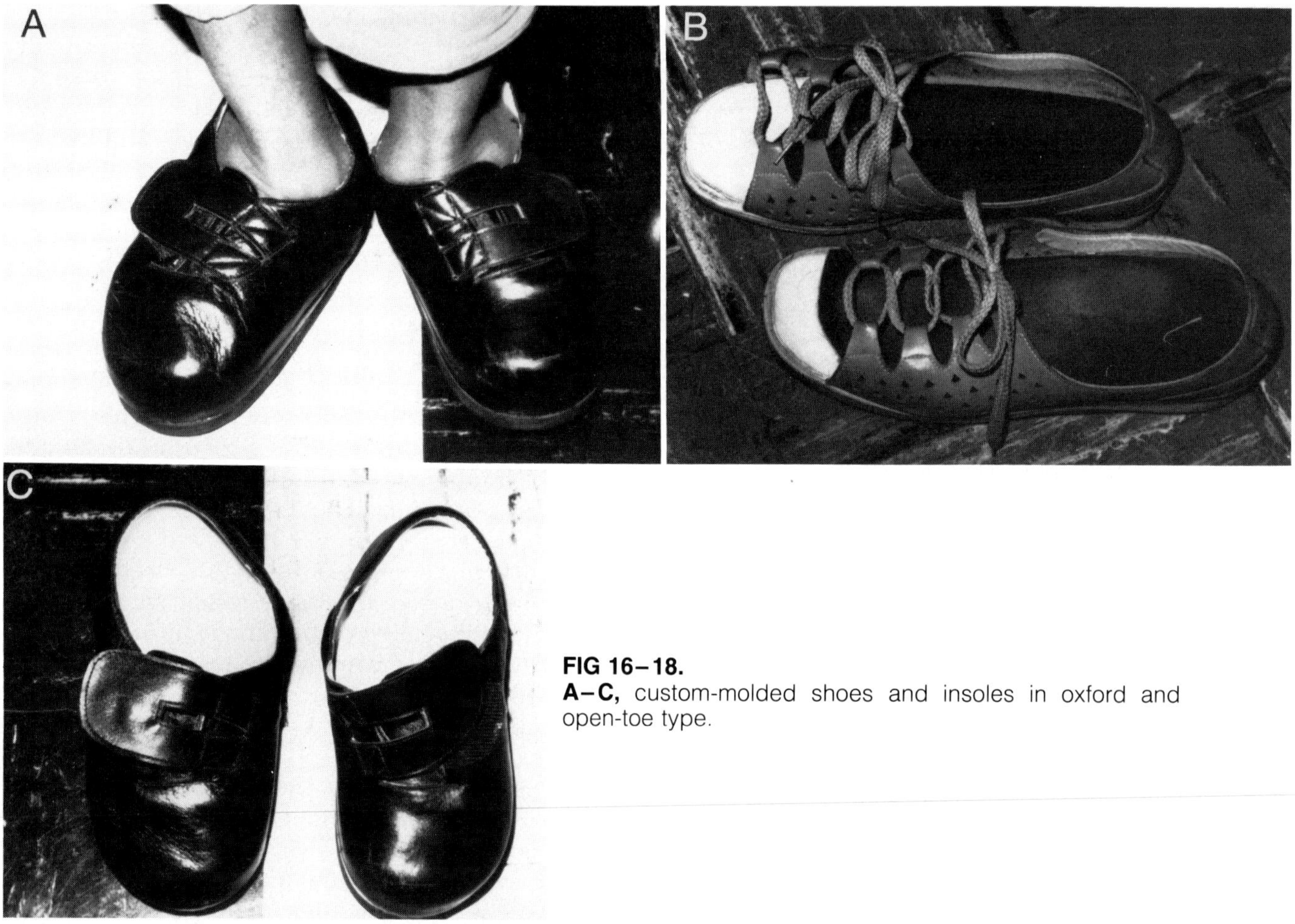

FIG 16–18.
A–C, custom-molded shoes and insoles in oxford and open-toe type.

SURGICAL TREATMENT

The approach to the rheumatoid forefoot must be influenced by other pathologic abnormalities present in the knee, midfoot, and hindfoot. Coughlin,[13] Figgie et al.,[27] and Manoli[58] have emphasized the importance of realigning the knee prior to hindfoot or forefoot surgery. Stockley et al.[75] have demonstrated increased pedobarograph pressures on the forefoot if the hindfoot is in valgus position. Results with forefoot arthroplasty may be negatively influenced as a result of this abnormal hindfoot position. Therefore, prior to embarking on complex forefoot reconstructions in the rheumatoid forefoot, careful attention must be paid to the remainder of the foot and ankle.

As in other areas of the musculoskeletal system, in patients with rheumatoid arthritis factors both local and systemic may deleteriously influence the result of forefoot surgery. This is particularly true of the vascular status of the forefoot which must be carefully evaluated prior to surgical treatment. It is of importance to monitor the posterior tibial and dorsalis pulses but care must also be taken to consider the small vessel flow, as many of these patients will have an underlying vasculitis. This can be determined by looking carefully at the foot for areas of skin breakdown or previous ulceration and questioning the patient whether healing has been a problem with injuries to the foot and ankle. A history of Raynaud's-type symptoms or acrocyanosis may herald a significant wound healing problem postoperatively.

Nodular disease is common when there is forefoot involvement and these areas may drain and become secondarily infected. Since the rheumatoid patient is at higher risk for infection,[74] wound healing may be compromised and deep infection may occur from these locally contaminated areas. The metatarsal heads may be so prominent after atrophy and distal displacement of the metatarsal fat pad that erosions occur through skin with secondary infection extending not only to the subcutaneous tissues but on occasion to the metatarsal head itself. Ideally, these local areas of infection and skin breakdown are addressed prior to surgical treatment and forefoot reconstruction. In some cases these areas may be eradicated only as part of the forefoot arthroplasty and, although suboptimal, if healing is to be achieved the only choice may be to remove the underlying bony prominences and reposition the fat pad for better soft tissue coverage for the metatarsal shafts.

Rheumatoid arthritis tends to be symmetric in nature, and forefoot deformity is usually bilateral with similar pathologic findings on both feet. It is highly recommended that both feet be reconstructed during the same operative setting. Ankle block or epidural anesthesia is preferred. The advantage of ankle block anesthesia is that it is less systemic; however, the rheumatoid patient will generally require some form of sedation because lying in one position for a prolonged surgical procedure may be uncomfortable. Epidural anesthesia has the additional benefit of allowing postoperative patient-controlled analgesia through an epidural catheter for the first 48 hours postoperatively.

In patients with disabling pain or fixed deformity of the forefoot that is refractory to conservative measures, surgical treatment may become necessary to correct the deformity and restore function. The surgical options for the rheumatoid forefoot can be divided into treatment of the hallux valgus and options for the lesser toes.

Surgical treatment for the destructive hallux valgus deformity of the MTP joint must be directed at dealing with all aspects of the pathologic process damaging the joint. This embodies a realignment of the metatarsal varus alignment, correction of the soft tissue imbalance across the MTP joint, lengthening and repositioning of the extensor hallucis longus tendon, and correction of the arthritic process at the MTP joint. At the conclusion of the procedure, attention must be given to obtaining excellent skin coverage. This complex series of procedures for the great toe is generally performed in combination with a forefoot arthroplasty of the lesser toes and this is discussed in the next section. Single correction of the great toe without concomitant correction of the lesser toes will lead to an unsatisfactory result and persistent foot pain in the rheumatoid patient. It should further be emphasized that attempts at less comprehensive surgical treatment will lead to the need for multiple procedures and prolonged rehabilitation in the rheumatoid patient. Because of the multiple joint involvement in these patients, a thorough approach is recommended.

Surgical options for hallux valgus include resection arthroplasty, Silastic arthroplasty, and arthrodesis.

Great Toe—Surgical Treatment

Resection Arthroplasty

Resection arthroplasty is reserved for patients who are low-demand or housebound. Patients with poor circulation also fit into this category. Amuso et al.,[1] Clayton,[8–12] Larmon,[50] and Peterson[66] have advocated the Keller arthroplasty. The problems with resection arthroplasty have been recurrence of deformity, cock-up deformity, loss of push-off power, and metatarsalgia.

McGarvey and Johnson[61] reported on the results of the Keller arthroplasty[45, 46] and resection of metatarsal heads 2 through 5 in 49 feet with an average follow-up of 4.9 years. There was recurrent hallux valgus in 53%, forefoot instability in 27%, and continuing metatarsalgia in 20%.

A possible explanation for these discouraging results was offered by Henry and Waugh[36] who used footprints to compare the results of resection arthroplasty with arthrodesis. They found that after resection arthroplasty only 40% of patients loaded the great toe compared with 80% in the arthrodesis group. They concluded that the inability to bear weight on the great toe was related to the presence of metatarsalgia in the resection group and excessive weightbearing on the lesser metatarsal heads. These complications were seen more commonly after resection arthroplasty than after arthrodesis.

Keller Procedure[45, 46] (Technique of Mann[54]).—A dorsomedial incision is made in the skin over the first MTP joint. The incision is taken down to the joint capsule with care to protect the underlying dorsomedial nerve. Next, the MTP joint capsule and periosteum are released from the medial side of the base of the proximal phalanx creating a proximally based rectangular flap with a base on the metatarsal shaft. An osteotomy of the proximal phalanx is performed at the level of the metaphyseal proximal flare using an oscillating saw (Fig 16–19,A). Approximately 30% to 40% of the proximal phalanx is removed. The amount of proximal phalanx resected is

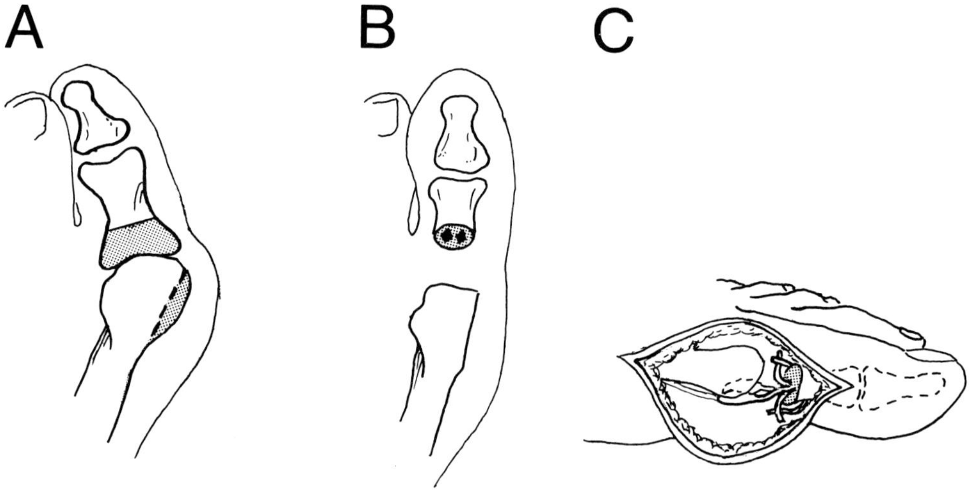

FIG 16–19.
A, *shaded areas* indicate levels of bone resection in Keller arthroplasty. **B,** drill holes made into the medial and plantar aspect of the remaining proximal phalanx. **C,** medial capsule and flexor hallucis brevis attached to the proximal phalanx.

critical as overresection can lead to a cock-up deformity due to intrinsic-extrinsic tendon imbalance. If, however, insufficient motion (dorsiflexion) is obtained after the proximal phalanx cut, further bone may be removed from the dorsal aspect of the metatarsal head to decompress the joint further. The medial eminence is resected in line with the metatarsal shaft. A rongeur or small rasp is used to smooth down the remaining osteophytes on the metatarsal head.

Next, a pair of drill holes are made in the medial and plantar aspects of the diaphysis of the proximal phalanx for repair of the medial capsular structures (i.e., the medial capsule with plantar plate and attached sesamoids) (Fig 16–19,B). The tendons of the flexor hallucis brevis are also attached to the remaining proximal phalanx to provide some intrinsic plantar flexion strength and add stability to the hallux (Fig 16–19,C). A 5/64-in. Steinmann's pin is driven distally through the proximal phalanx, interphalangeal joint, and distal phalanx, out through the tip of the hallux, and then in a retrograde fashion through the metatarsal head. In this way, the great toe is stabilized with a gap of approximately 5 mm at the osteotomy site. Next, the distal tip of the pin is bent to prevent proximal migration and the capsular structures are repaired. The foot is dressed with a soft compression dressing and the patient is permitted to ambulate in a bunion shoe. The pin is removed at 3 to 4 weeks and motion is begun. Dressings are discontinued after 6 weeks.

Techniques of Clayton and Johnson.—Clayton[8–12] popularized the use of the Keller procedure (excision of bunion and the proximal portion of the proximal phalanx) for the treatment of hallux valgus in the rheumatoid foot. He used a dorsal transverse incision at the base of the toes because, as a general rule, the lesser MTP joints were addressed at the same operation. Other authors have preferred multiple dorsal incisions to achieve the same purpose. No internal fixation was used by Clayton because early ambulation was desired; however, he noted that the use of Kirschner wire fixation was the surgeon's choice.

Johnson[40] recommends a straight dorsal longitudinal incision and the decision to perform a Keller or Mayo-type resection arthroplasty is based upon the size of the preoperative intermetatarsal angle. He prefers a Keller procedure in which resection of the base of the proximal phalanx is done for deformities with an intermetatarsal 1–2 angle of less than 20 degrees. If, however, the intermetatarsal 1–2 angle is greater than 20 degrees, and metatarsus primus varus is present, he prefers the Mayo procedure in which the first metatarsal head is resected. He emphasizes that care must be taken to insure that the plane of resection is angled plantarward and medially to avoid prominent sharp bony edges postoperatively (Fig 16–20,A–C).

When performing the Keller procedure, it is critical that neither too much nor too little bone be resected. If too little bone is removed from the proximal phalanx, a painful, stiff pseudarthrosis may result. On the other hand, excessive removal of bone from the proximal phalanx may result in overshortening and instability of the toe with decreased push-off power in the take-off phase of gait or possibly a cock-up toe deformity. Furthermore, excessive shortening of the great toe may also decrease the load taken by the first metatarsal head with resultant transfer of pressure onto the second toe. Because of these potential difficulties, Johnson prefers arthrodesis to resection arthroplasty of the great toe.

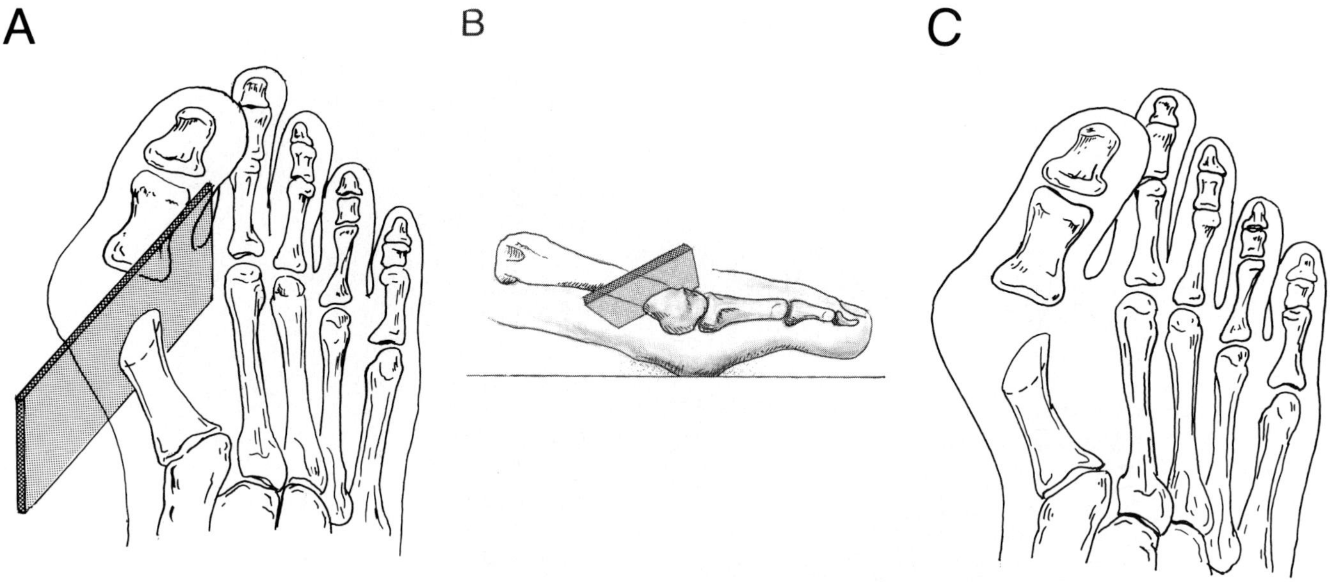

FIG 16–20.
A–C, Mayo procedure utilizing Johnson technique with plantar and medial osteotomy of the first metatarsal.

Implant Arthroplasty

To address the shortcomings of the Keller resection arthroplasty, Swanson et al.[76] introduced silicone implant arthroplasty which they hoped would improve the predictability of results in this procedure. Silastic arthroplasty has been used particularly as an alternative to resection arthroplasty for hallux valgus in the low-demand rheumatoid patient.

Swanson and colleagues[19, 76] popularized silicone implant arthroplasty of the great toe. More recently, Cracchiolo and co-workers[16, 18, 52, 67] and Wenger and Whalley[84] reported good early success with these implants. Early designs of Silastic implants replaced only the base of the proximal phalanx and there was a small incidence of implant fracture after many years of use.[17] These implant failures were thought to be due to (1) the quality of silicone elastomer, which was not as durable as present-day high-peformance elastomers, and (2) the shape of the arthritic metatarsal head, which may have been irregular, leading, in some cases, to implant wear.

Subsequently, the silicone implant evolved to a flexible double-stem design made from high-performance silicone elastomers. The good early success with these new implants has been tempered, however, by reports of fracture, foreign body giant cell synovitis with resultant bony resorption, recurrence of deformity, and loss of push-off power.[32]

Gordon and Bullough[32] reported a foreign body giant cell synovitis together with foci of foreign body giant cells and chronic inflammation in the intramedullary bone in six patients with failed silicone rubber prostheses. Shereff and Jahss[72] reported seven complications of Silastic implant arthroplasty in the hallux secondary to acute inflammatory reactions in five feet with subsequent delayed wound healing, skin necrosis, and superficial infection. Three feet developed implant fracture or erosion, or both, through the articulating surface of the prosthesis. All of these patients exhibited late radiographic findings of resorption of bone around the implant. These complications necessitated removal of the implants in five feet (Fig 16–21,A–C).

In 1990, Lian and Cracchiolo[52] presented their long-term results with double-stem silicone implant arthroplasty of the hallux metatarsophalangeal joint. At an average follow-up of 68 months, 47 feet were reviewed. Pain, walking, and function were improved with 86% of patients being "fully satisfied," 11% "satisfied with some reservations," and 3% "slightly worse" after surgery. Complications included implant fractures in six cases. There was no evidence of silicone synovitis necessitating removal of implant or loss of correction. The authors concluded that at long-term follow-up, the double-stem silicone implant appeared to be a satisfactory option for the treatment of an arthritic hallux MTP joint.

Cracchiolo,[17] and Moeckel et al.[63] have described their large surgical experience with the use of these implants.

Technique of Cracchiolo[17] and Sculco[63].—The surgical technique should emphasize careful soft tissue

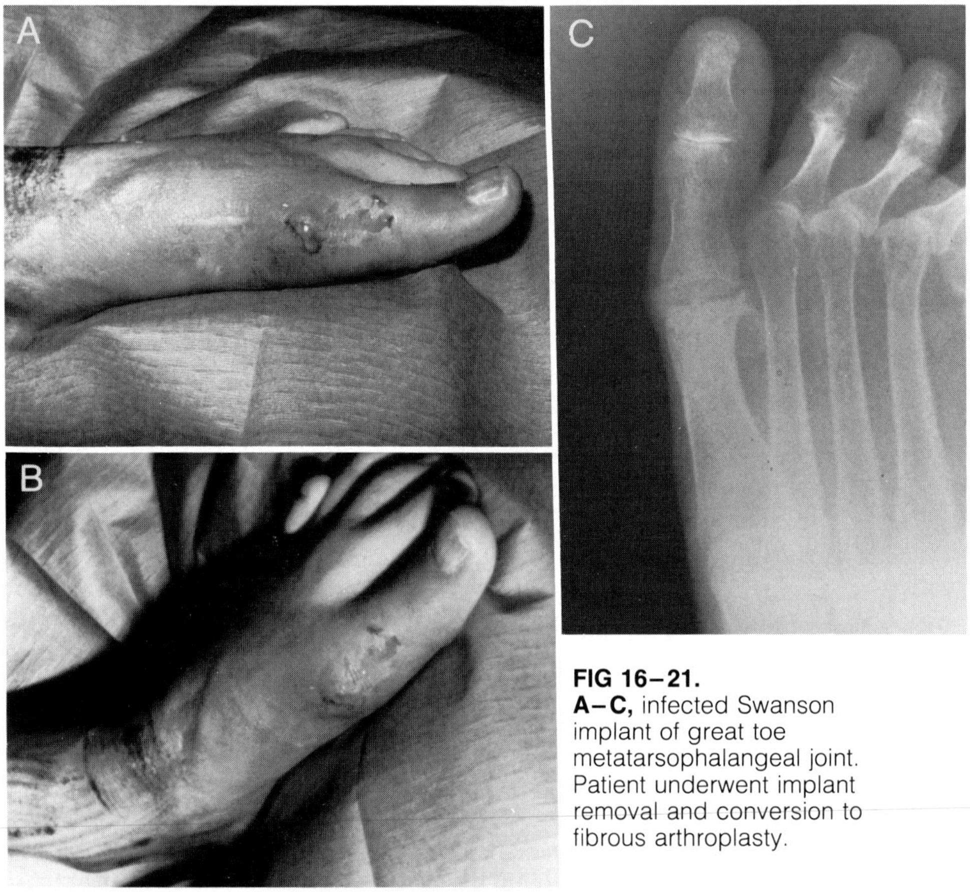

FIG 16–21.
A–C, infected Swanson implant of great toe metatarsophalangeal joint. Patient underwent implant removal and conversion to fibrous arthroplasty.

handling. All patients receive prophylactic antibiotics intravenously (IV) approximately 45 minutes before the limb is exsanguinated and the tourniquet is inflated.

A dorsal longitudinal incision is made over the hallux metatarsal. Exposure of the first MTP joint is achieved either through a goblet capsulotomy based proximally or through a longitudinal incision in the medial joint capsule (Fig 16–22,A–C). The metatarsal head is freed from its capsular and collateral ligament attachments. Care is taken not to strip any of the soft tissue attachments to the base of the proximal phalanx. Soft tissue releases are performed to balance the MTP joint of the hallux. The structures released include the adductor hallucis, the lateral capsule, and adhesions from both the metatarsal head and the sesamoids (Fig 16–22,D). The exostosis is excised (Fig 16–22,E). In the presence of a severely deformed metatarsal head, the bony cut is made in the metatarsal head before soft tissue releases are performed. Next, the appropriate-size double-stem implant is chosen (usually a no. 0, 1, 2, or 3 implant) and the bony cuts are made with an oscillating saw. Only enough bone is removed to allow accommodation of the hinged portion of the implant (Fig 16–22,F–H). The base of the proximal phalanx is simply shaved flat from its normal concavity. It is important to maintain the integrity of the medial and lateral heads of the flexor hallucis brevis tendon. If they are inadvertently released, they should be reattached to the base of the proximal phalanx through drill holes in the cortex to prevent a postoperative hammer toe or cock-up deformity.

Next, the intramedullary canals of the proximal phalanx and metatarsal are prepared gently with appropriate broaches or special power pilot burrs. A trial reduction is performed to confirm that adequate correction has been accomplished. Additional releases may now be necessary, including the extensor hallucis brevis and lengthening of the extensor hallucis longus.

Before final placement of the implant, 1-mm holes are drilled in the dorsal medial cortex and a no. 0 polyglactin 910 (Vicryl) suture on a curved cutting needle is passed through these holes and used to reattach the capsule after placement of the implant. The capsulorrhaphy is performed by advancing the plantar side of the capsular flap dorsally (re-

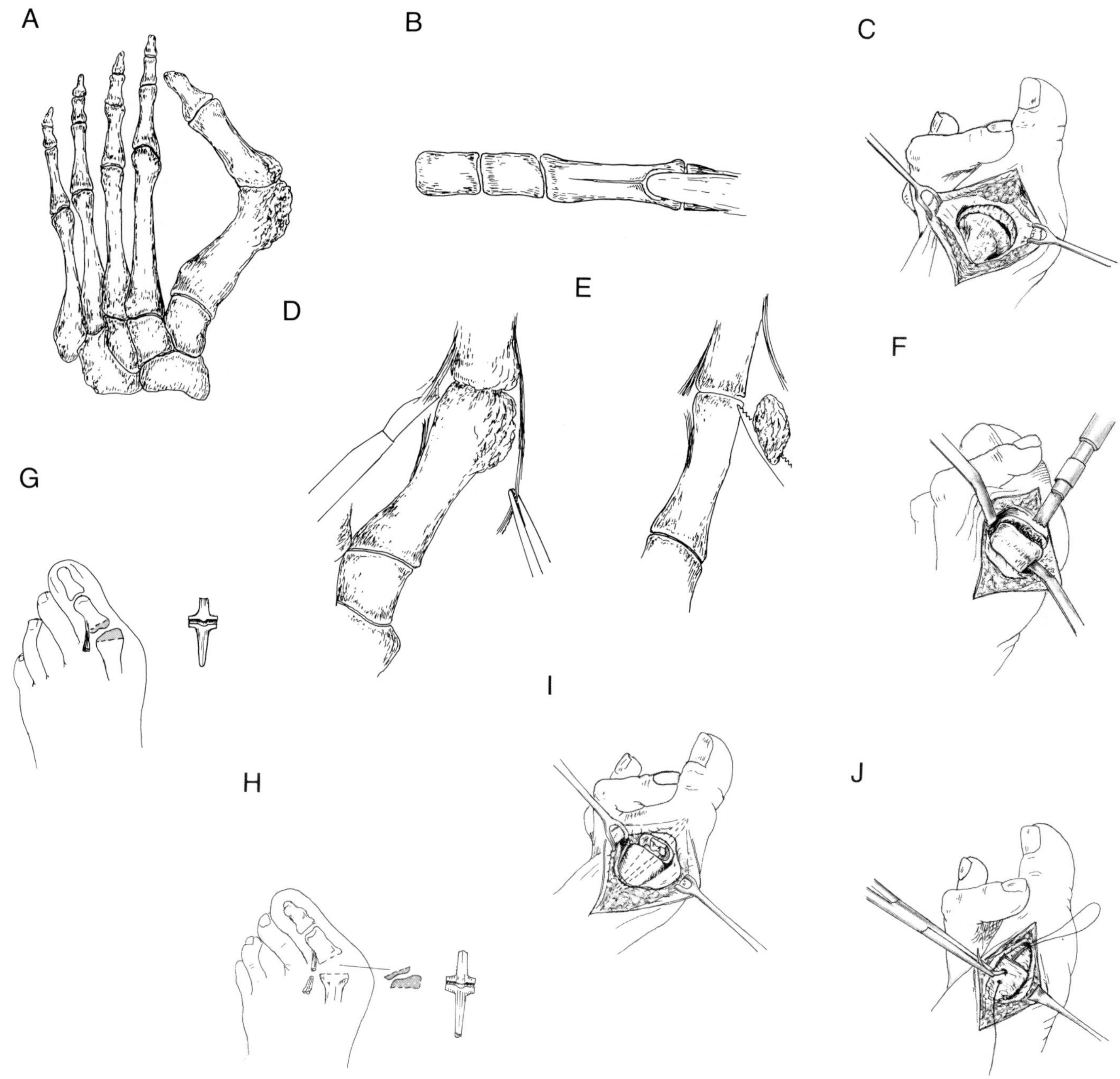

FIG 16–22.
A, hallux valgus deformity in rheumatoid arthritis with joint destruction and metatarsus primus varus. **B,** lateral view of metatarsophalangeal joint demonstrating goblet-shaped capsulotomy. **C,** metatarsophalangeal joint exposed. **D,** lateral release of capsule, ligament, and adductor tendon. Medial capsule is attenuated and redundant. **E,** exostosectomy performed. Resection of metatarsal head **(F)** and proximal phalanx **(G,H). I,** Swanson implant in place within medullary canal of metatarsal and phalanx. **J,** capsular repair of metatarsophalangeal joint.

aligning the sesamoids) and, while holding the hallux in a slightly overcorrected position, suturing it to the metatarsal (Fig 16–22,I and J).

When there is significant metatarsal varus deformity, a basal osteotomy of the hallux metatarsal may be performed. In this case, Cracchiolo[17, 18] prefers an opening wedge osteotomy using a bone graft from the medial eminence of the head to hold the metatarsal in place. More recently, Sculco has performed a capsulotomy of the tarsometatarsal joint (Fig 16–23,A–D) with lateral deviation of the metatarsal. A circumferential capsular release must be performed in order to fully mobilize the first metatarsal. The tarsometatarsal joint is fixed with two 0.62-in. Kirschner wires which are removed at 6 weeks. Maintenance of correction has been achieved in ten patients followed at least 2 years.

Cracchiolo[17, 18] has advocated implant arthro-

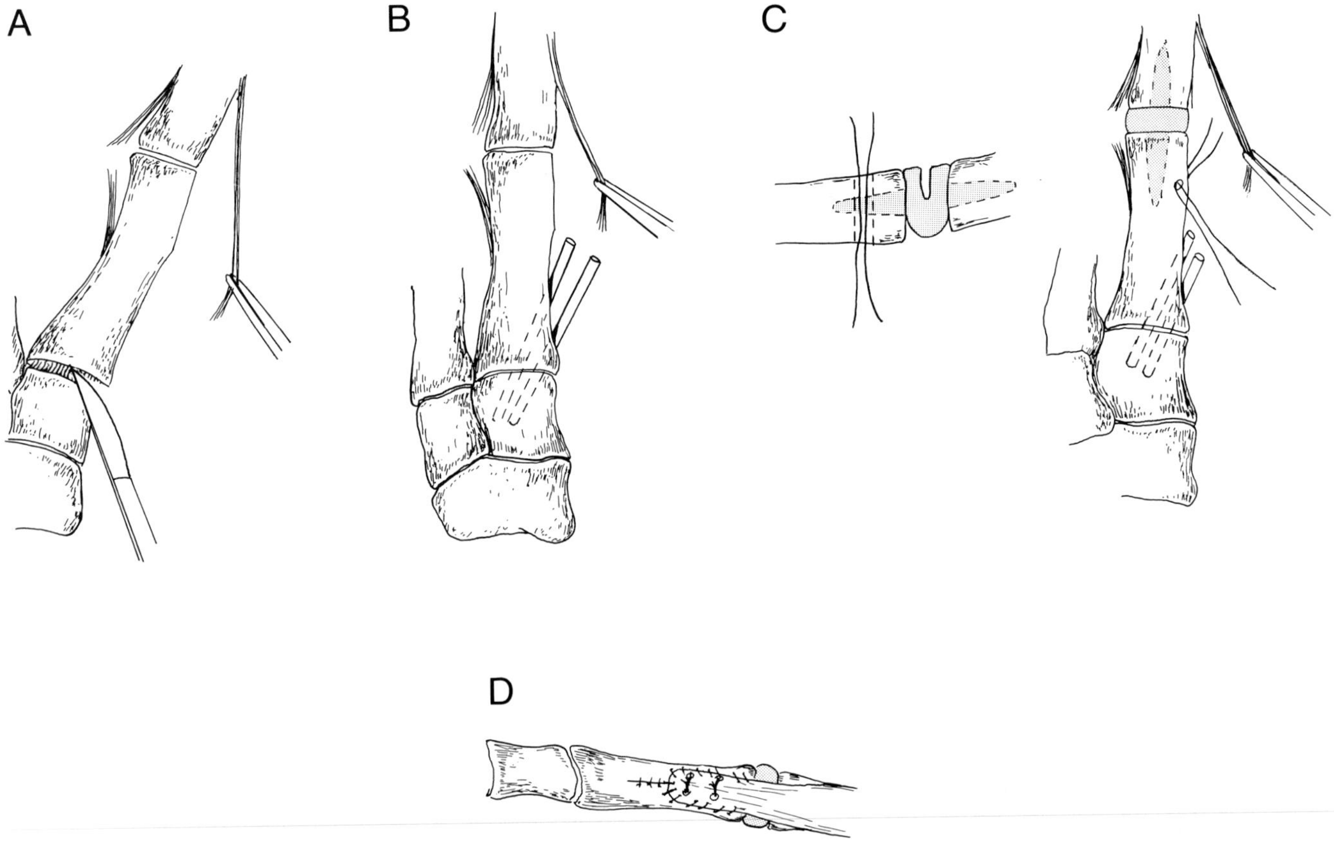

FIG 16–23.
A, total capsulotomy of tarsometatarsal joint. **B,** lateral displacement of first metatarsal at tarsometatarsal joint with internal fixation by two 0.62-mm Kirschner wires. **C,** *(left),* Swanson implant in place after capsulotomy. *(Right)* Medial reefing of capsule through fixation hole in first metatarsal. **D,** repair of goblet capsulorrhaphy.

plasty of the lesser MTP joints which is carried out in a fashion similar to the hallux procedure. Two dorsal longitudinal incisions over the second and fourth web spaces provide exposure to all MTP joints (Fig 16–24,A–F).

Arthrodesis

Arthrodesis of the first MTP joint has been used by Watson,[82] DuVries,[25] Leavitt,[51] and Morrison,[64] and was more recently popularized by Mann and Thompson.[57] Mann and Thompson reported on 18 feet at an average follow-up of 4 years in which fusion of the first MTP joint was used with resection of metatarsal heads 2 through 5. They reported a 94% fusion rate. All patients could wear ordinary shoes postoperatively. There were no cases of recurrent hallux valgus. The authors emphasize that the rationale for this approach is that the great toe length is preserved and the lesser toes are protected from further deformity by the stable medial buttress of the fused hallux. In addition, the plantar fat pad is stabilized.[57] The disadvantages of this approach are: (1) prolonged immobilization, (2) pain beneath the retained first metatarsal head, (3) elongated first toe, (4) the procedure should not be done in the presence of interphalangeal joint disease, (5) nonunion, and (6) malunion.

Watson[82] compared the results of a Keller arthroplasty to a first MTP fusion in conjunction with resection arthroplasty of the lesser four toes, and favored the arthrodesis group. He noted that fusion of the first MTP joint prevented the lateral migration of the hallux that is seen with the Keller arthroplasty and resulted in a high percentage of painless feet following surgery.

Watson also emphasized that the Keller arthroplasty creates a flail great toe which allows the gradual valgus tendency to displace the surgically destabilized lesser toes dorsally and laterally. The end result is increased weightbearing on the remaining metatarsal ends with resultant callus formation.[82]

Henry and Waugh[36] compared the weightbear-

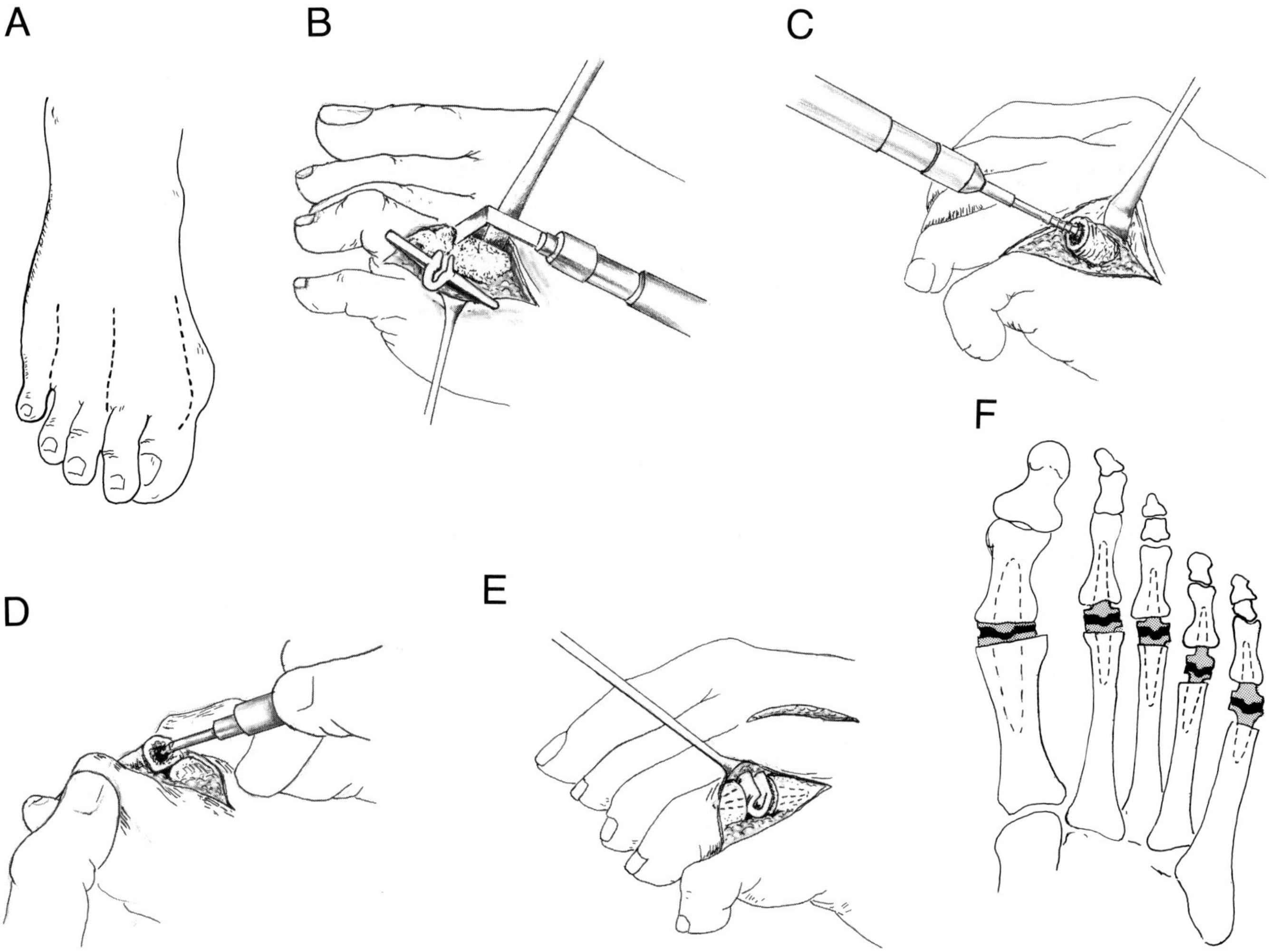

FIG 16–24.
Cracchiolo technique for Silastic replacement of metatarsophalangeal joints of lesser toes. **A,** skin incision. **B,** metatarsal head resection. **C,** intramedullary metatarsal reaming. **D,** phalangeal reaming. **E,** Silastic implant in situ. **F,** replacement of all metatarsophalangeal joints with Silastic implants.

ing patterns of the foot in first MTP joint arthrodesis with Keller arthroplasty and demonstrated a twofold decrease in the amount of first metatarsal weight-bearing and a greater tendency toward development of postoperative metatarsalgia compared with patients undergoing first MTP joint arthrodesis.

More recently, Donegan et al.[23] reviewed 27 rheumatoid feet in which the first MTP joint was fused with staples and the lesser metatarsal heads were resected through a plantar skin incision. At an average follow-up of 20 months, there were 24 good or excellent results and 3 poor results. Fusion was obtained in 100% of patients at an average of 58 days. The authors concluded that first MTP joint arthrodesis with resection arthroplasty of the lesser toes was an excellent method of forefoot reconstruction in the rheumatoid patient.

The type of fusion technique has been debated and good results have been reported with a number of techniques. Mann and Thompson[57] prefer the biplanar osteotomy with either double-threaded fixation with Steinmann's pins or an interfragment compression screw with a dorsal neutralization plate.

Techniques of Mann and Thompson,[57] Mann and Oates,[56] and Coughlin[13, 14] (Fig 16–25).—A longitudinal dorsal incision is made which is centered over the first MTP joint. The extensor tendon is retracted medially or laterally and the capsule is exposed. Next, the capsule and synovial tissue of the first MTP joint are completely excised. The distal aspect of the first metatarsal is resected in a biplanar manner using an oscillating power saw to create a flat surface which is angled slightly dorsally and in a

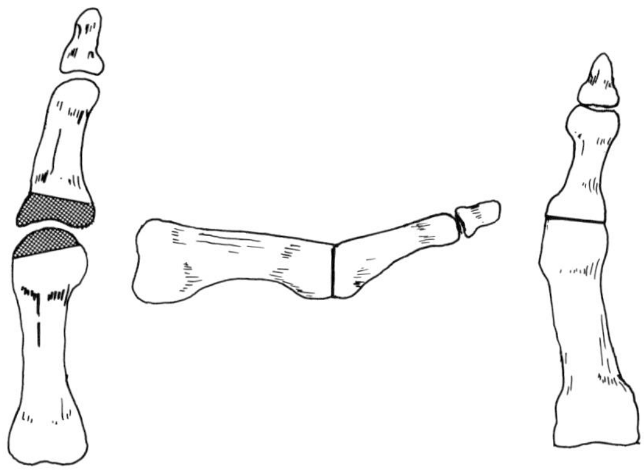

FIG 16–25.
Biplanar osteotomy and arthrodesis of first metatarsophalangeal joint (Mann technique).

few degrees of valgus alignment. The prominent medial eminence of the metatarsal head is resected. Next, the base of the proximal phalanx is resected perpendicular to the axis of the shaft. Care is taken to achieve maximal bone-to-bone contact. The ideal position of the hallux is approximately 15 degrees of valgus angulation and 15 degrees of dorsiflexion (measured from the floor) or 30 degrees of dorsiflexion (measured from the first metatarsal shaft).

Prior to internal fixation of the first MTP joint, the lesser toes are corrected. The overall length of the hallux is assessed and, if necessary, it is shortened at the base of the proximal phalanx so that the hallux does not protrude more than 5 mm beyond the second toe at the completion of the procedure. Internal fixation can be achieved in a variety of ways. Initial reports favored the use of two heavy 9/64-in. (3.6 mm) and 1/8-in. (3.2 mm) double-ended threaded Steinmann's pins. These are inserted using a power instrument from the site of resection of the proximal phalanx out to the tip of the hallux and then driven retrograde across the MTP joint. Care is taken to maintain neutral rotation (avoid pronation) of the hallux before the second pin is inserted. Care is taken to drill slowly so as not to strip the threads in the soft rheumatoid bone.

The distal aspect of each pin is then cut off, leaving 6 mm of each pin protruding from the tip of the hallux. The wound is irrigated and the skin is closed. A well-padded compression dressing is applied for 18 to 24 hours and is then changed to a firm, soft dressing. Fixation is usually rigid enough to permit weightbearing in a wooden shoe on the second postoperative day. The soft, firm dressing is changed every 10 to 14 days for 4 to 6 weeks and is then discontinued. At this point, the patient is permitted to shower and the pins are covered with small adhesive bandages. Ambulation is continued in a wooden-soled shoe until fusion is radiographically apparent (approximately 14 weeks). The pins are then removed.

Alternatively, internal fixation may be accomplished with a compression screw, crossed Kirschner wires, Kirschner wires and pins, staples, wire, sutures, compression plate fixation, Rush nail fixation, compression clamps, and minifragment plate fixation. All have been used successfully with acceptable fusion rates.

Many authors have advocated the use of the flat surface biplanar arthrodesis owing to its relative technical simplicity. The problem with this technique is that if any one of the variables needs to be adjusted, i.e., varus-valgus, dorsiflexion, plantar flexion, or rotation, the first ray must be further shortened to obtain proper alignment of the joint. In addition, in attempting to realign one variable, the others may become malaligned.

The difficulty in achieving acceptable alignment in all planes has led to the development of conical surfaces that allow for adjustment at the fusion site before internal fixation devices are inserted. Accordingly, Lipscomb et al.[53] and Johnson[40] favor the McKeever's[62] "articular surface contouring" technique of fusion for severely destroyed first MTP joints with relative sparing of the interphalangeal joint (Fig 16–26).

Coughlin[14] has developed an advanced form of the Marin[59] reamer for the preparation of bony surfaces. In an excellent review article, he details the history of the first MTP joint arthrodesis, the various methods of fixation, and the surgical approaches.

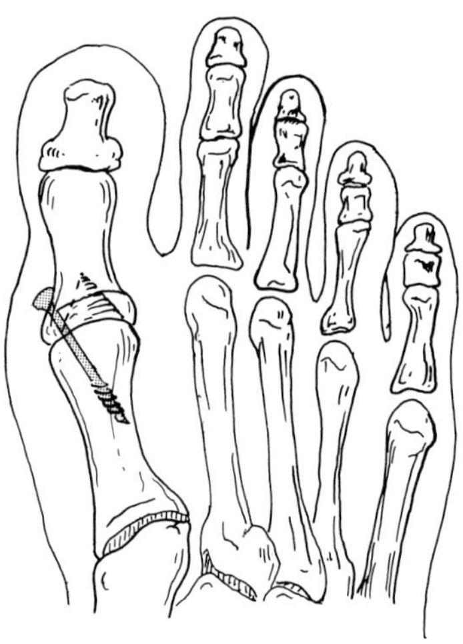

FIG 16–26.
McKeever-type arthrodesis of the first metatarsophalangeal joint (Johnson technique).

The desired position is neutral rotation, 15 to 20 degrees of valgus alignment and 15 to 20 degrees of dorsiflexion. However, the magnitude of dorsiflexion may vary depending on the heel height desired by female patients and upon the length of the hallux.

Lesser Toes—Surgical Treatment

The goals of surgery for the subluxed or dislocated lesser toes include (1) realignment to restore a normal weightbearing pattern to the forefoot and to allow use of more normal shoewear; (2) relocation of the plantar fat pad for comfort in walking; and (3) providing stability to maintain alignment and allow a propulsive gait.

Surgical treatment of the lesser toes has ranged from amputation of all toes[28] to excisional arthroplasty of varying gradations (Fig 16–27). Excision of the metatarsal heads or proximal phalanges or both has been successful in relieving the pain due to clawtoes and dislocated MTP joints with resultant intractable plantar keratoses (Fig 16–28,A–C).

Hoffman, in 1911,[37] wrote the classic paper describing the operation of excision of the metatarsal heads, and, if necessary, parts of the necks of the metatarsal bones of all the affected toes through a transverse curved plantar incision behind the web of the toes. Hoffman wrote:

> . . . the operation is simply to get rid of the metatarsal heads, because they make the patient's life miserable. Every step he takes hurts him so, he is afraid to get up from his chair. Mild grades of contracted toes should not be operated upon in this way.[37]

The Hoffman procedure has been used with success rates averaging 84% by Amuso et al.,[1] Barton,[2] Faithful and Savill,[26] Joplin,[41] Kates et al.,[43] Kuhns,[49] Morrison,[64] and Watson.[82]

Indications for the Hoffman procedure include rheumatoid disease with subluxation in three or more MTP joints. The procedure includes resection of all metatarsal heads, including the first. Consideration is given to a bilateral procedure if the opposite foot has two or more involved MTP joints to avoid the necessity of wearing shoes of different sizes.

In 115 forefoot arthroplasties (removal of five metatarsal heads) in 74 patients, Robson and Taylor[70] reported that cosmetic appearance improved in 89% of patients and that most patients had doubled their walking distance at 4-year follow-up. Amuso et al.[1] reported good or satisfactory results in 88% of patients in 179 operations at an average 28-month follow-up. They noted that the usual cause for an unsatisfactory result was (1) insufficient bone resection or (2) irregular bone resection. These causes for failure have also been recently emphasized by Johnson.[40] Both Clayton[8–12] and Amuso et al.[1] reported that 8% to 10% of patients needed supplemental sur-

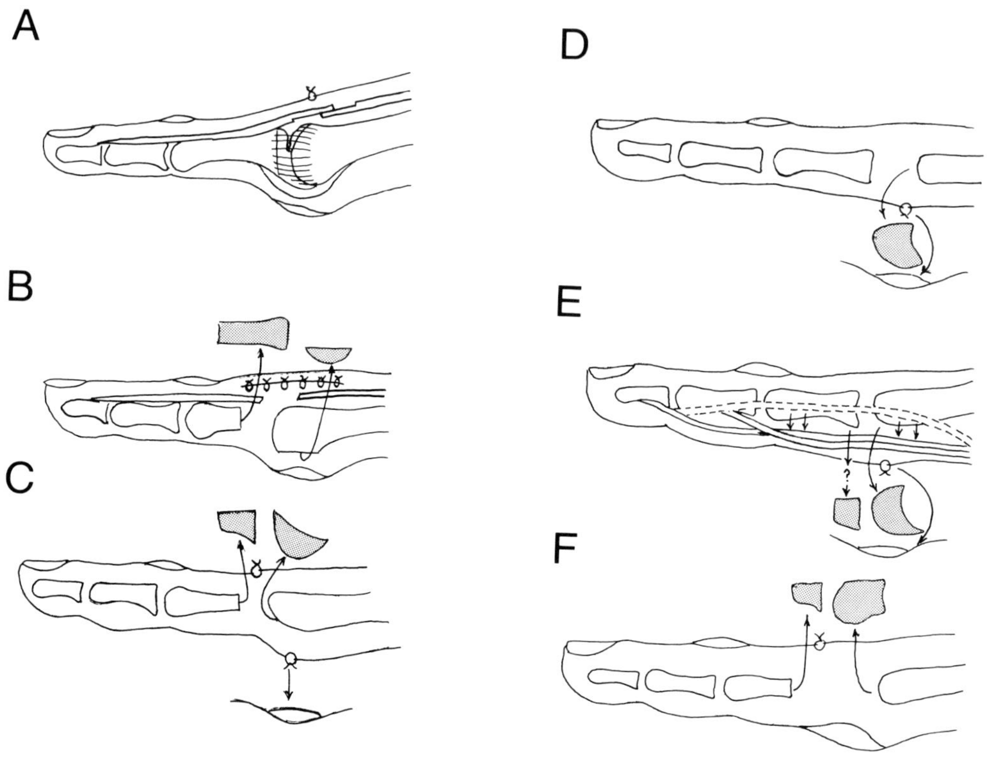

FIG 16–27.
Variations of resection arthroplasty for metatarsophalangeal joints of the lesser toes.

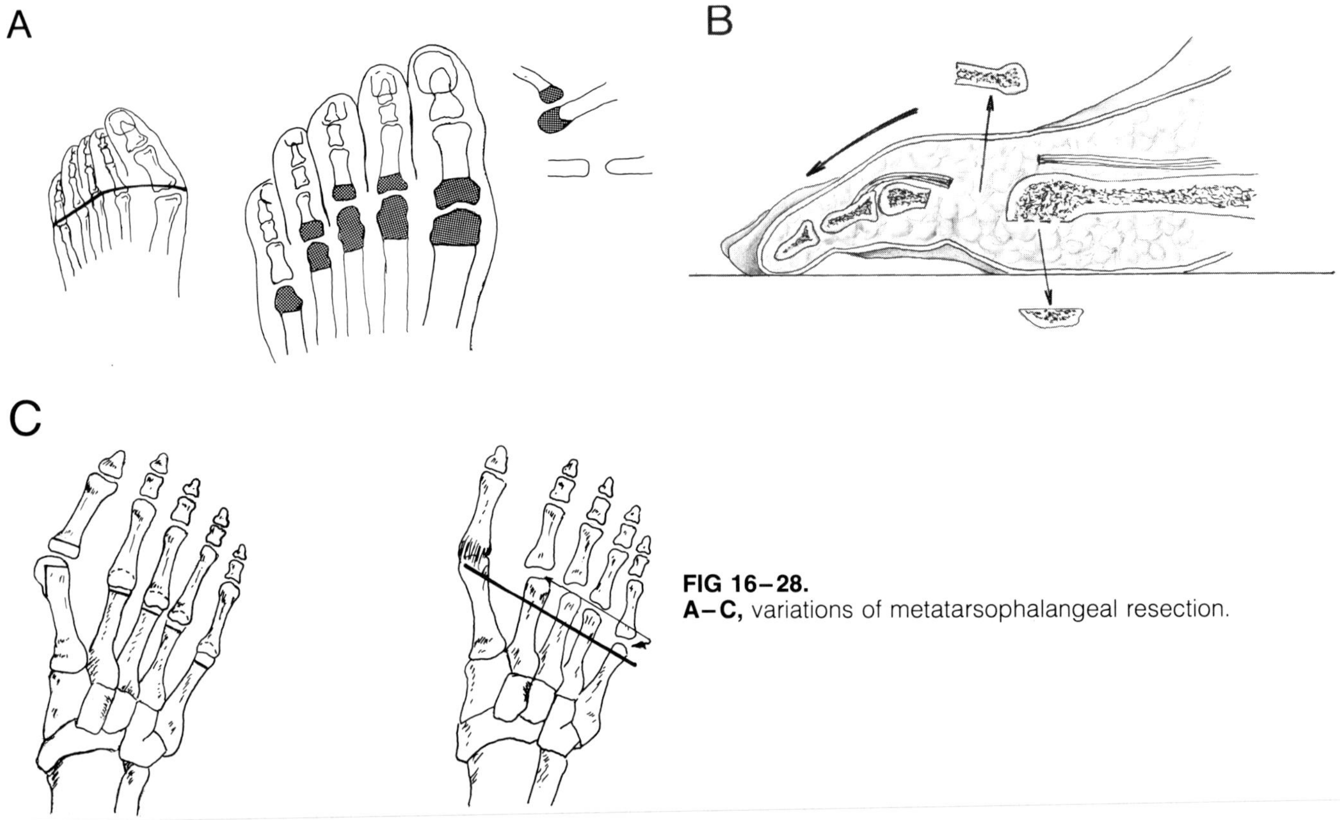

FIG 16–28.
A–C, variations of metatarsophalangeal resection.

gery which usually consisted of resection of one metatarsal. Kates et al.[43] recommended that after generous resection of the metatarsal head the contour of the remaining distal metatarsal shafts be shaped carefully in a flat arc to prevent uneven pressure points across the forefoot. In Schwartzman's[71] review of excisional arthroplasty in the rheumatoid forefoot, he concluded that partial proximal phalangectomies were rarely needed. Barton[2] suggested that retaining the base of the proximal phalanx actually preserved lesser toe function. Johnson[40] emphasizes that the amount of phalangeal resection depends on the degree of deformity. He resects appropriate amounts of the proximal phalanges of the second to fifth toes to allow the toes to return to a more normal position. The disadvantage of phalangeal resection is significant toe shortening with possible dorsal subluxation or lateral drift.

Larmon,[50] in 1951, recommended a Keller procedure on the great toe, excision of the proximal phalanges of the small toes, and osteoplasty of the individual metatarsal heads rather than excision of the heads. With respect to the metatarsal heads, Larmon[50] disagreed with Hoffman. Leavitt[51] and Fowler[29] also criticized the Hoffman procedure as they felt that without the addition of a partial proximal phalangectomy, a large amount of metatarsal bone needed to be excised to correct the dorsal displacement of the toes. Kates et al.,[43] however, emphasized that the Hoffman procedure enabled their patients to walk in a plantigrade manner and justified resection of the metatarsal head.

Fowler,[29] in 1959, described his version of forefoot arthroplasty which included a partial proximal phalangectomy with distal and plantar metatarsal condylectomy. The Fowler procedure[29] has been used successfully by Barton,[2] Benson and Johnson,[3] Larmon,[50] Leavitt,[51] Lipscomb et al.,[53] Peterson,[66] and Watson.[82] Their results parallel those achieved with the Hoffman procedure. Clayton,[9] in 1960, described proximal partial phalangectomy in addition to metatarsal head resection as a means to obtain a "weight tolerant foot." The use of the Clayton procedure by Amuso et al.[1] Brattstrom and Brattstrom,[5, 6] and Marmor[60] in over 400 forefoot reconstructions has resulted in satisfactory results in over 80% of patients. In addition, Barton's review[2] of 65 forefoot arthroplasties in 38 patients found similar postoperative results in patients treated with Fowler, Hoffman, and Clayton procedures. Flint and Sweetnam[28] suggested amputation of all toes. This procedure was found to be unacceptable from a cosmetic point of view. Marmor[60] noted that the plantar prominence of the metatarsal heads was not addressed by Flint and Sweetmann and therefore had no indication in the rheumatoid foot.

Pfeiffer et al.[67] presented their experience with double-stem Silastic implant arthroplasty of the hallux and lateral toe MTP joints in 69 feet. At an average follow-up of 5 years there was improvement of the hallux valgus angle with no loss of correction over time. The lesser toes were improved clinically and radiographically with respect to plantar callus, dorsal corn, malalignment, and hammering. Range-of-motion, pain, and function scores were all improved, but walking scores were not. Complications included implant fracture in six hallux (8%) and seven lateral toe (2%) implants. Three lateral toe implants were removed. There were four toes that developed recurrent deformity, one infection, and one stem dislocation.

Hoffman[37] and Kates[42] have advocated the use of synovectomy of the MTP joints as a way to delay progression of disease. Brattstrom and Brattstrom,[5, 6] Lipscomb et al.,[53] and Peterson[66] advocate the combination of excisional arthroplasty with synovectomy.

Technique of Mann and Johnson

The four lesser MTP joints are approached through two dorsal longitudinal incisions, one between the second and third toes, and one between the fourth and fifth toes. Next, the bases of the proximal phalanges are identified and the soft tissue attachment to the proximal phalanx bases are removed. Approximately one third to one half of the proximal phalanx is then resected depending on the degree of deformity. Next, the contracted dorsal aspect of the MTP joint, i.e., capsule, tendons and collateral ligaments, are released and allowed to slip plantarward to either side of the metatarsal. This soft tissue release allows relocation of the distally displaced plantar fat pad to its more normal proximal location under the metatarsal heads. Next, an assessment is made as to how much metatarsal head or plantar condyle, or both, need to be removed. Usually, the nature of the advanced rigid deformity with significant soft tissue contractures necessitates a generous metatarsal head resection in a smooth arc (Fig 16–29,A and B).

It is important to avoid an insufficient or irregular resection, and care must be taken to avoid any single metatarsal head prominence at the conclusion of the procedure. Variations on this general theme have been advocated by other authors. Johnson[40] prefers to perform the metatarsal head resection prior to assessing the need for proximal phalanx resection. The use of Kirschner wire fixation has also led to differences of opinion. Barton[2] reported improved wound healing, while Watson[82] suggested that Kirschner wire fixation leads to joint stiffness. Tillman[79] avoids Kirschner wire fixation but instead uses a pull-through wire through the tip of the toes that is pulled over a Böhler frame. The frame is attached to a plaster sole which the patient wears for

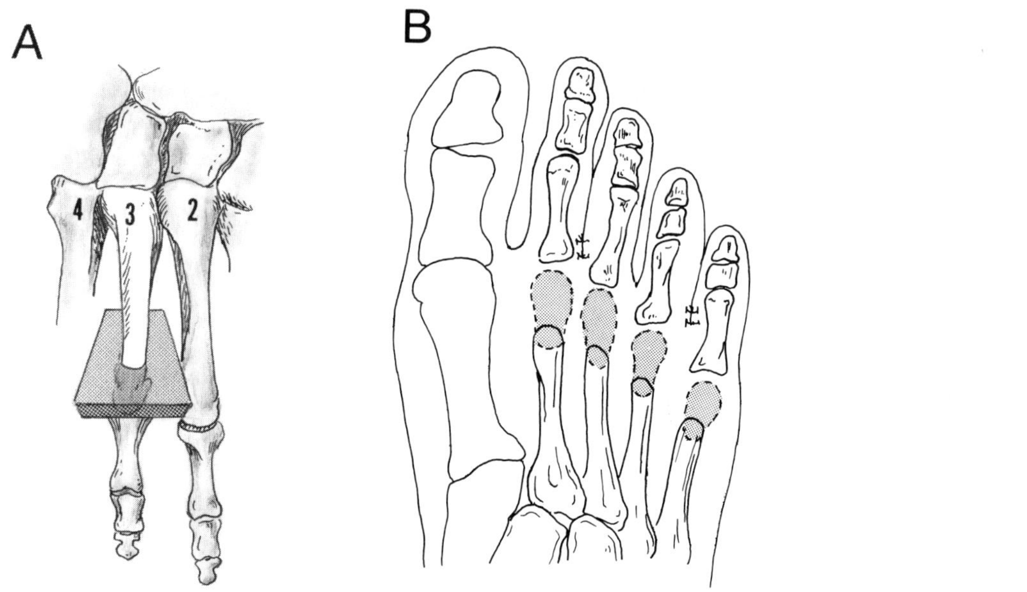

FIG 16–29.
A, Metatarsal resection in Hoffman procedure should be adequate to allow reduction of the metatarsophalangeal joints. **B,** a smooth resection arcade should be present after metatarsal head resection.

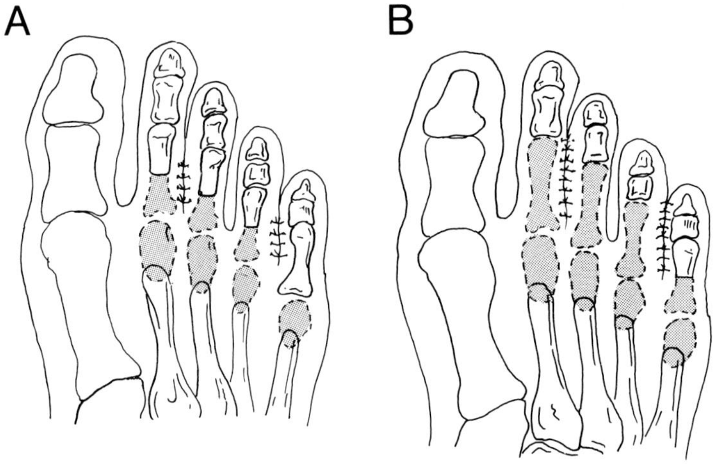

FIG 16–30.
A, B, metatarsophalangeal resection with syndactylization of toes to prevent recurrent subluxation.

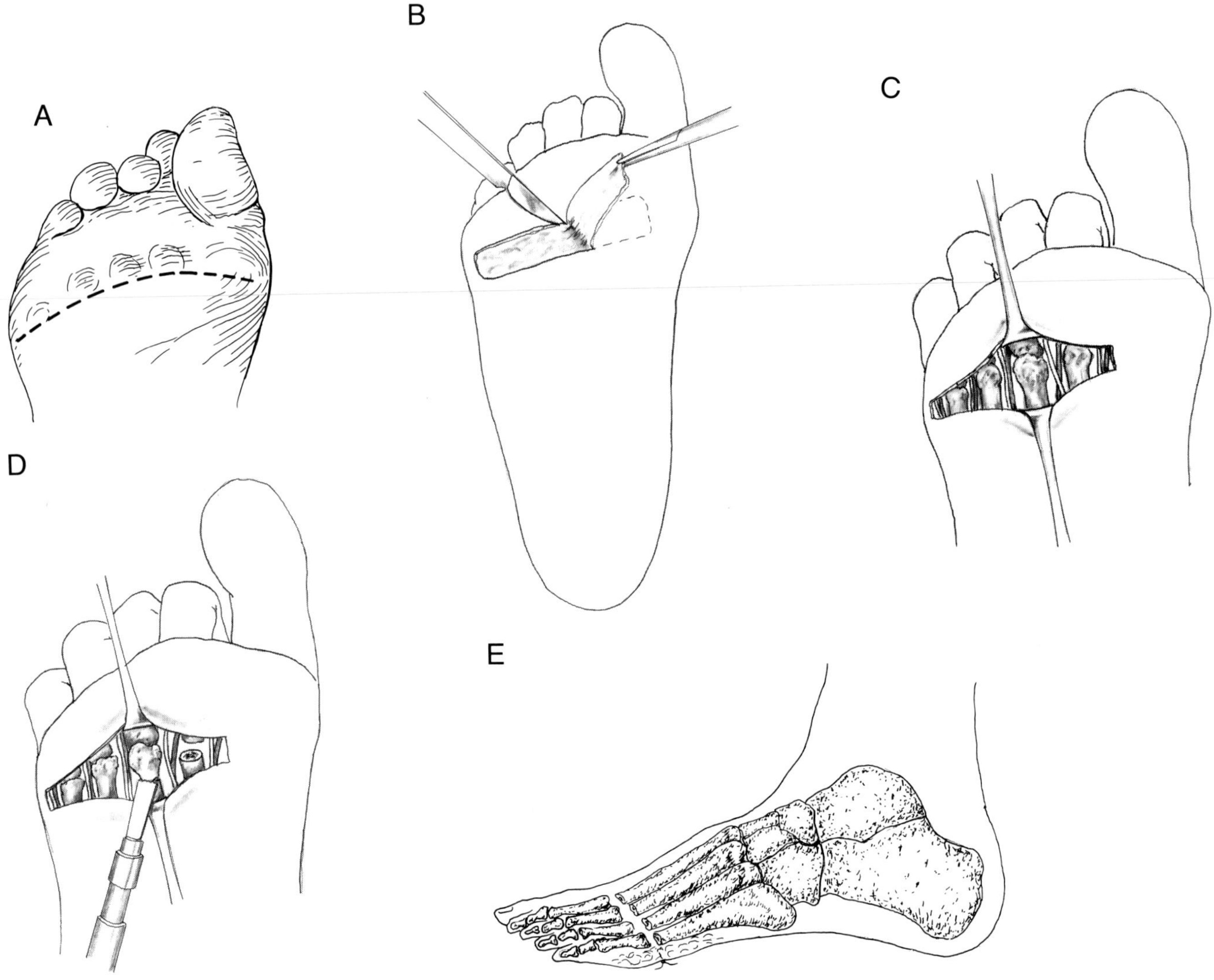

FIG 16–31.
A, plantar incision over dislocated metatarsal heads and proximal to the distally displaced metatarsal fat pad. **B,** excision of an ellipse of skin proximal to the fat pad. **C,** metatarsal head exposed after excision of the metatarsophalangeal joint plantar capsule. **D,** a saw is used to resect the metatarsal heads at the metatarsal neck. **E,** resection must be adequate to allow reduction of toes after dermatoplasty.

the first 14 postoperative days. As an alternative to pin fixation, Johnson[40] has recommended resection arthroplasty with webbing for the subluxed or dislocated lesser MTP joint (Fig 16–30,A and B).

The Plantar Approach (Sculco).—The plantar approach is recommended for metatarsal head resection. This allows easy visualization of the plantarflexed metatarsal head and a plantar dermatoplasty can be performed through the same approach. An elliptic incision is made extending from the base of the distally displaced plantar fat pad (Fig 16–31,A). A 1-cm ellipse of skin is removed (Fig 16–31,B). The metatarsal heads are palpable and are exposed through an excisional plantar capsulotomy (Fig 16–31,C). The flexor tendons are generally dislocated in the intermetatarsal recesses and these are identified and retracted. Resection of the metatarsal head is performed at the metatarsal neck just proximal to the metatarsal head (Fig 16–31,D). Reduction of the digits should then be possible. A gap of 1 cm should be present between the metatarsal shaft and proximal phalanx after reduction of the toes. Complete soft tissue release may be necessary at the base of the phalanx to allow reduction. Rarely, in severe fixed deformities, is there need for proximal phalangeal resection. Internal fixation is not used. Approximation of the plantar dermatoplasty should restore the digits to the reduced position easily (Fig 16–31,E). Bulky compression dressings are used and changed weekly. The patient is able to ambulate on postoperative day 2.

Different surgical approaches to the forefoot have gained popularity and each has its advantages and disadvantages. Hoffman,[37] Key,[47] Faithful and Savill,[26] and Brattstrom and Brattstrom[5, 6] have used the transverse plantar incision. In addition, Fowler[29] and Kates et al.[43] have used the transverse plantar excision to excise the excess plantar skin, and accordingly relocate the plantar fat pad. The observations of Lipscomb et al.[53] suggested that the plantar fat pad eventually relocated after forefoot reconstruction and that elliptic plantar skin excision was unnecessary. A dorsal transverse incision is advocated by Fowler,[29] Clayton,[8–12] Marmor,[60] and Peterson[66] (Fig 16–32). The use of multiple longitudinal incisions has been advocated by Benson and Johnson,[3] Johnson,[40] DuVries,[25] Larmon,[50] and Lipscomb et al.[53] (Fig 16–33). They noted rapid healing and less wound complications with this approach. Clayton[8–12] and Fowler[29] warned against this more limiting approach and emphasized that less optimal exposure could potentiate sloppy metatarsal contouring and accordingly an increased incidence of late plantar callosities.

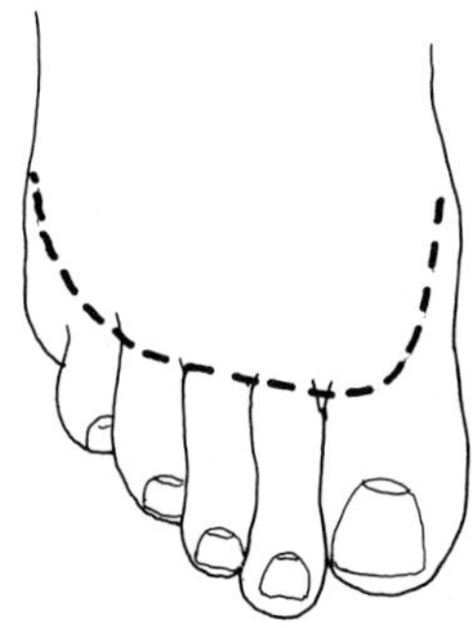

FIG 16–32.
Dorsal transverse incision for metatarsophalangeal resection.

CONCLUSION

The results of resection arthroplasty have generally been very good with satisfactory rates ranging from 70% to 100%.[55] Forefoot surgery in the rheumatoid patient can significantly improve ambulatory capacity by relieving painful weightbearing and achieving forefoot realignment that is more accomodating to shoewear. Recovery is slow but progressive. Swelling may be significant and delay recovery. Wound healing may be problematic and should infection or wound slough occur, aggressive management is mandatory. Frequent dressing changes and careful toe realignment and wound care with the use of dressings can improve the surgical result considerably.

The forefoot is a major component in the complex group of joints of the lower extremity that allow

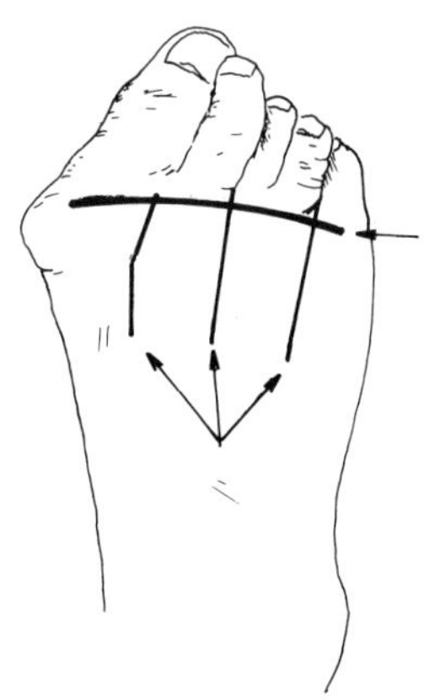

FIG 16–33.
Multiple dorsal incisions for metatarsophalangeal resection.

ambulation in rheumatoid arthritis. Although the joints are the most distal and small, their treatment is complex and demanding. Their weightbearing tolerance is as pivotal to ambulation as the more proximal lower extremity joints. Comprehensive evaluation and treatment is mandatory for successful ambulation in rheumatoid arthritis.

REFERENCES

1. Amuso SJ, Wissinger A, Margolis HM, et al: Metatarsal head resection in the treatment of rheumatoid arthritis. *Clin Orthop* 1971; 74:94–100.
2. Barton NJ: Arthroplasty of the forefoot in rheumatoid arthritis. *J Bone Joint Surg [Br]* 1973; 55:126–133.
3. Benson GM, Johnson EW Jr: Management of the foot in rheumatoid arthritis. *Orthop Clin North Am* 1971; 2:733–744.
4. Bojsen-Moller F: Anatomy of the forefoot, normal and pathologic. *Clin Orthop* 1979; 142:10–18.
5. Brattstrom H, Brattstrom M: Resection of the metatarsophalangeal joints in rheumatoid arthritis. *Acta Orthop Scand* 1970; 41:213–224.
6. Brattstrom M, Brattstrom H: Metatarsophalangeal joints in rheumatoid arthritis. *J Bone Joint Surg [Br]* 1968; 50:221.
7. Calabro JJ: A critical evaluation of the diagnostic features of the feet in rheumatoid arthritis. *Arthritis Rheum* 1962; 5:19–29.
8. Clayton ML: Surgery of the forefoot in rheumatoid arthritis. *Arthritis Rheum* 1959; 2:84–85.
9. Clayton ML: Surgery of the forefoot in rheumatoid arthritis. *Clin Orthop* 1960; 16:136–140.
10. Clayton ML: Surgery of the lower extremity in rheumatoid arthritis. *J Bone Joint Surg [Am]* 1963; 45:1517–1536.
11. Clayton ML: Discussion of paper by Marmor L: Rheumatoid deformity of the foot. *Arthritis Rheum* 1963; 6:754–755.
12. Clayton ML: Surgical treatment of the rheumatoid foot, in Giannestras NJ (ed): *Foot Disorders: Medical and Surgical Management,* ed 2. Philadelphia, Lea & Febiger, 1973, pp 444–466.
13. Coughlin MJ: The rheumatoid foot, in Chapman MW (ed): *Operative Orthopedics,* vol 3, Philadelphia, JB Lippincott Co, 1988, pp 1845–1855.
14. Coughlin MJ: Arthrodesis of the first metarsophalangeal joint. *Orthop Rev* 1990; 12:177–186.
15. Cracchiolo A III: The use of shoes to treat foot disorders. *Orthop Rev* 1979; 8:73–83.
16. Cracchiolo A III: Implant arthroplasty of all metatarsophalangel (MTP) joints of the rheumatoid forefoot. *Orthop Trans* 1981; 5:454.
17. Cracchiolo A III: Management of the arthritic forefoot. *Foot Ankle* 1982; 3:17–23.
18. Cracchiolo A III: Surgery for rheumatoid disease. *Instr Course Lect* 1984; 33:386–411.
19. Cracchiolo A III, Swanson A, Swanson G DeG: The arthritic great toe metatarsophalangeal joint: A review of flexible silicone implant arthroplasty from two medical centers. *Clin Orthop* 1981; 157:64–69.
20. Craxford AD, Stevens J, Park C: Management of the deformed rheumatoid forefoot: A comparison of conservative and surgical methods. *Clin Orthop* 1982; 166:121–126.
21. Dedrick DK, McCune WJ, Smith WS: Rheumatoid arthritis presenting as spreading of the toes. *J Bone Joint Surg [Am]* 1990; 72:463–464.
22. Dixon ASJ: The rheumatoid foot. *Proc R Soc Med* 1970; 63:677–679.
23. Donegan K, DeLee JC, Evans JA: Rheumatoid forefoot reconstruction. Presented at the American Orthopaedic Foot and Ankle Society. 21st Annual Meeting, Anaheim, Calif. March 1991.
24. Duncan H, Frost HM, Villanueva AR, et al: The osteoporosis of rheumatoid arthritis. *Arthritis Rheum* 1965; 8:943–954.
25. DuVries HL: *Surgery of the Foot,* ed 2. St Louis, Mosby–Year Book, Inc, 1965.
26. Faithful DK, Savill DL: Review of the results of excision of the metatarsal heads in patients with rheumatoid arthritis. *Ann Rheum Dis* 1971; 30:201–202.
27. Figgie MP, Ranawat CS, O'Malley MD, et al: Triple arthrodesis in rheumatoid arthritis. Presented at the American Orthopaedic Foot and Ankle Society 56th Annual Meeting, Las Vegas, February 1989.
28. Flint M, Sweetnam R: Amputation of all toes: A review of forty-seven amputations. *J Bone Joint Surg [Br]* 1960; 42:90–96.
29. Fowler AW: A method of forefoot reconstruction. *J Bone Joint Surg [Br]* 1959; 41:507–513.
30. Gold RH, Basset LW: Radiologic evaluation of the arthritic foot. *Foot Ankle* 1982; 2:332–341.
31. Goldberg VM: Early management of the rheumatoid joint. *Instr Course Lect* 1984; 33:404–411.
32. Gordon M, Bullough PG: Synovial and osseous inflammation in failed silicone-rubber prostheses. *J Bone Joint Surg [Am]* 1982; 64:574–580.
33. Gorevic P: Rheumatoid arthritis, in Dee R, Margo E, Hurstic C (eds): *Principles of Orthopaedic Practice.* New York, McGraw-Hill Book Co, 1989, pp 200–210.
34. Gould JS: Conservative management of the hypersensitive foot in rheumatoid arthritis. *Foot Ankle* 1982; 2:224–229.
35. Guerra J, Resnick D: Arthritides affecting the foot: Radiographic-pathological correlation. *Foot Ankle* 1982; 2:325–331.
36. Henry APJ, Waugh W: The use of footprints in assessing the results of operations for hallux valgus: A comparison of Keller's operation and arthrodesis. *J Bone Joint Surg [Br]* 1975; 57:478–482.

37. Hoffman P: An operation for severe grades of contracted or clawed toes. *Am J Orthop Surg* 1912; 9:441–449.
38. Inman VT: *The Joints of the Ankle.* Baltimore, Williams & Wilkins Co, 1976.
39. Jacoby RK, Vidigal E, Kirkup J, et al: The great toe as a clinical problem in rheumatoid arthritis. *Rheum Rehabil* 1976; 15:143–147.
40. Johnson K: *Surgery of the Foot and Ankle.* New York, Raven Press, 1989.
41. Joplin RJ: Surgery of the forefoot in the rheumatoid arthritis patient. *Surg Clin North Am* 1969; 49:847–878.
42. Kates A: Surgery of the rheumatoid foot. *Proc R Soc Med* 1970; 63:679–680.
43. Kates A, Kessel L, Kay A: Arthroplasty of the forefoot. *J Bone Joint Surg [Br]* 1967; 49:552–557.
44. Keenan MAE, Peabody TD, Gronley TK, et al: Valgus deformities of the feet and characteristics of gait in patients who have rheumatoid arthritis. *J Bone Joint Surg [Am]* 1991; 73:237–247.
45. Keller WL: The surgical treatment of bunions and hallux valgus. *N Y State J Med* 1904; 80:741–742.
46. Keller WL: Further observations on the surgical treatment of hallux valgus and bunions. *N Y State J Med* 1912; 95:696–698.
47. Key JA: Surgical revision of arthritic feet. *Am J Surg* 1950; 69:667–672.
48. Kirkup JR, Vidigal E, Jacoby RK: The hallux and rheumatoid arthritis. *Acta Orthop Scand* 1977; 48:527–544.
49. Kuhns JG: The foot in chronic arthritis. *Clin Orthop* 1960; 16:141–151.
50. Larmon, WA: Surgical treatment of deformities of rheumatoid arthritis of the forefoot and toes. *Bull Northwestern Univ Med Sch* 1951; 25:39–42.
51. Leavitt DC: Surgical treatment of arthritic feet. *Northwest Med* 1956; 55:1086–1088.
52. Lian GJ, Cracchiolo A III: Double-stem silicone implant arthroplasty of the hallux metatarsophalangeal joint in the rheumatoid patient. Presented at the American Orthopaedic Foot and Ankle Society. 20th Annual Meeting, New Orleans, February, 1990.
53. Lipscomb PR, Benson GM, Sones DA: Resection of proximal phalanges and metatarsal condyles for deformities of the forefoot due to rheumatoid arthritis. *Clin Orthop* 1972; 82:24–31.
54. Mann RA (ed): *Surgery of the foot,* ed 5. St Louis, Mosby–Year Book, Inc, 1986.
55. Mann RA, Coughlin MJ: The rheumatoid foot: Review of the literature and method of treatment. *Orthop Rev* 1979; 8:105–112.
56. Mann RA, Oates JC: Arthrodesis of the first metatarsophalangeal joint. *Foot Ankle* 1980; 1:159–166.
57. Mann RA, Thompson FM: Arthrodesis of the first metatarsophalangeal joint for hallux valgus in rheumatoid arthritis. *J Bone Joint Surg [Am]* 1984; 66:687–692.
58. Manoli A III: Personal communication, 1991.
59. Marin, GA: Arthrodesis of the metatarsophalangeal joint of the big toe for hallux valgus and hallux rigidis. *Int Surg* 1968; 50:175–180.
60. Marmor L: Resection of the forefoot in rheumatoid arthritis. *Clin Orthop* 1975; 108:223–227.
61. McGarvey, Johnson: Keller arthroplasty and resection of metatarsal heads 2-5. Presented at the Mid-American Orthopedic Society Annual Meeting, April 1986.
62. McKeever DC: Arthrodesis of the first metatarsophalangeal joint for hallux valgus, hallux rigidis, and metatarsus primus varus. *J Bone Joint Surg [Am]* 1952; 34:129–134.
63. Moeckel BH, Sculco TP, Alexiader MM, et al: The management of the rheumatoid forefoot: The long term result of the double-stemmed Silastic implant. 1991, in press.
64. Morrison P: Complication of forefoot operations in rheumatoid arthritis. *Proc R Soc Med* 1974; 67:110–111.
65. Nakano KK: The entrapment neuropathies of rheumatoid arthritis. *Orthop Clin North Am* 1975; 6:837–860.
66. Peterson LFA: Surgery for rheumatoid arthritis—timing and technique: The lower extremity. *J Bone Joint Surg [Am]* 1968; 50:587–604.
67. Pfeiffer WH, Cracchiolo A, Dorey F: Double stem silicone implant arthroplasty of the hallux and lateral toe metatarsophalangeal joints in patients with rheumatoid arthritis. Presented at the American Orthopaedic Foot and Ankle Society Sixth Annual Summer Meeting, Banff, Canada, June 1990.
68. Rana NA: Rheumatoid arthritis, other collagen diseases, and psoriasis of the foot, in Jahss MH (ed): *Disorders of the Foot and Ankle,* ed 2, vol 2. Philadelphia, WB Saunders Co, 1991, pp 1003–1011.
69. Resnick D, Niwayama G: Rheumatoid arthritis, in Resnick D (ed): *Diagnosis of Bone and Joint Disorders,* ed 2, vol 2. Philadelphia, WB Saunders Co, 1988, pp.
70. Robson MJ, Taylor AR: Excision arthroplasty of the forefoot in rheumatoid arthritis. *J Bone Joint Surg [Br]* 1979; 61:519–520.
71. Schwartzman JR: The surgical management of foot deformities in rheumatoid arthritis. *Clin Orthop* 1964; 36:86–95.
72. Shereff MJ, Jahss MH: Complication of Silastic implant arthroplasty in the hallux. *Foot Ankle* 1980; 1:95–101.
73. Short CL, Bauer W, Reynold WE: *Rheumatoid Arthritis.* Cambridge, Harvard University Press, 1957.
74. Spiegel TM, Spiegel JS: Rheumatoid arthritis in the foot and ankle—diagnosis, pathology, and treatment. *Foot Ankle* 1982; 2:318–324.
75. Stockley I, et al: The importance of the valgus hindfoot in forefoot surgery in rheumatoid arthritis. *J Bone Joint Surg [Br]* 1990; 72:705–708.

76. Swanson AB, Lumsden RM, Swanson G DeG: Silicone implant arthroplasty of the great toe. *Clin Orthop* 1979; 142:30.
77. Thomas WH: *Surgery of the foot in rheumatoid arthritis. Orthop Clin North Am* 1975; 6:831–835.
78. Thomas WH: Rheumatoid arthritis of the ankle and foot. *Instr Course Lect* 1979; 28:325–336.
79. Tillman K: *The Rheumatoid Foot—Diagnosis, Pathomechanics and Treatment.* Littleton, Mass, PSG Publishing Co, 1979.
80. Vainio K: The rheumatoid foot: A clinical study with pathologic and rheumatologic comments. *Ann Chir Gynaecol* 1956; 45 (suppl 1) 1–107.
81. Vidigal EC: Forefoot in chronic rheumatoid arthritis. *Orthop Rev* 1978; 7:43–46.
82. Watson MS: A long-term follow-up of forefoot arthroplasty. *J Bone Joint Surg [Br]* 1974; 56:527–533.
83. Weissman BNW, Sosman JL: The radiology of rheumatoid arthritis. *Orthop Clin North Am* 1975; 6:653–672.
84. Wenger RJ, Whalley RC: Total replacement of the first metatarsophalangeal joint. *J Bone Joint Surg [Br]* 1978; 60:88–92.

CHAPTER 17

Lower Extremity Function

Jay D. Mabrey, M.D.

James C. Otis, Ph.D.

INTRODUCTION

Patients with severe rheumatoid arthritis (RA) lose muscle strength over time, prolonging rehabilitation following corrective measures, and their aberrant preoperative gait patterns fail to return to normal following surgery.[1, 2, 4, 5, 8, 13, 17, 19, 22, 24] Those who have walked with a stiff-legged gait for an extended period may have difficulty relearning normal gait patterns.[9] Some joints may display only transient symptoms while others never improve and eventually require surgical correction. For the surgeon, documentation of preoperative and postoperative function in the lower extremities relies on recording the range of motion and stability of each joint as the patient lies on the examination table as well as an observational assessment of the patient's gait in the clinic setting. Gross abnormalities relating to antalgic gait or decreased range of motion are readily apparent, but subtle changes will go unnoticed even by the trained observer.

The accumulated knowledge of lower extremity function in RA has changed the way physicians look at the disease and has improved our understanding of its end effect upon the patient. Details added by a variety of researchers provide a clearer picture of gait pathology in RA and have opened new pathways for investigation. With orthopaedists entering earlier into the treatment process with more aggressive interventions, it is now essential that the surgeon be familiar with the latest findings and the latest techniques.

Normal Human Gait

A normal walk begins with a relatively short *development phase* followed by a much longer period of uniform, cyclic movements known as the *rhythmic phase,* and ends with a short period of controlled stoppage, the *decay phase.*[10] Virtually all published gait studies deal with the uniform rhythmic phase, observing the subject in straight-line motion walking at a comfortable speed over a level surface. The speed and cadence of normal subjects in this phase is close to that required for minimum energy expenditure.[25]

The fundamental unit of gait is the *gait cycle* and refers to the sequence of motions occurring between two consecutive repetitions of a gait event, such as one right heel contact to the next right heel contact. Stride length defines the major displacements of the body during the walking cycle as depicted in Figure 17–1,A. Stride duration defines the time in which those displacements occur and is normalized to a percentage of one complete cycle (Fig 17–1,B). The time and distance of an individual's stride influences the overall pattern of motion during gait.[11] In each stride during rhythmic walking on a level surface, each foot is either on the ground or swinging forward. *Heel contact* and *toe-off* define the beginning and end of the *stance phase* for a given limb and *swing phase* refers to that portion of the gait cycle

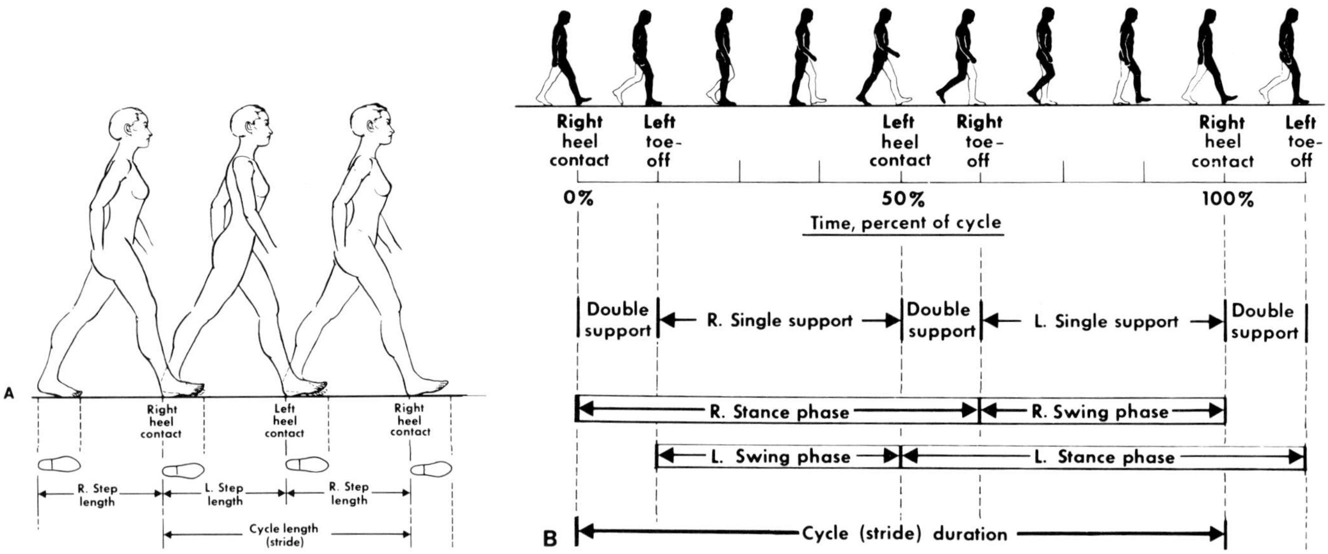

FIG 17–1.
A, distance dimensions of gait cycle. Cycle length equals distance of right heel strike to next right heel strike. **B,** time dimensions of gait cycle. (From Inman VT, Ralston HJ, Todd F: *Human Walking.* Baltimore, Williams & Wilkins Co, 1981. Used by permission.)

when the foot is not in contact with the ground. *Single limb support* is that time during which one extremity is full weightbearing. When both feet are simultaneously in contact with the ground it is referred to as the *double support phase.*

Techniques

Kinematics, the study of motion, has been utilized to determine limb segment motion during gait.[14] Earlier techniques used film and stroboscopic photography to record these displacements and required a technician to manually reduce the data. Many of the earlier studies did not examine true three-dimensional motion, but rather two-dimensional motion in multiple planes. Earlier methods for looking at three-dimensional motion utilized triplanar electrogoniometers to measure changing joint angles. Many laboratories today employ solid-state video cameras to record the images along with sophisticated computer hardware and software to generate the motion in three dimensions. Multiple cameras allow the simultaneous analysis of both sides of the body in three-dimensional space.

Kinetics is the study of how forces effect changes in motion. The subject steps on an instrumented plate embedded in the walking surface and the force is recorded as its components in the *x*-, *y*-, and *z*-axes. This information is combined with the kinematic data to determine the forces and moments at the hip, knee, and ankle joints.

STUDIES OF PATIENTS WITH RHEUMATOID ARTHRITIS

Gait characteristics of patients with RA are important in that they establish a baseline for comparison with operative cases and provide a greater understanding of the overall nature of the disease. The purpose of this chapter is to present the variety of techniques employed. Because of the diverse nature of the various study groups, each investigation is considered separately along with the conclusions of the respective authors.

General Studies in Nonoperative Patients

Marshall et al.[17] evaluated six women with seropositive, erosive RA, ranging in age from 49 to 62 years. Each subject had involvement of the subtalar joint together with associated symmetric involvement of the knees. Two had hip involvement as well and three had symptoms in the ankle joint. Stride analysis was obtained on all six subjects and revealed a decrease in single limb support time (33% vs. 40% for normals) with a concomitant increase in stance (67% vs. 60.5%) and double leg support times (17% vs. 10.5% for normals). Using cine film analysis, linear and angular kinematic data were obtained for three patients, which demonstrated several qualitative differences between the gait patterns of the rheumatoid group and the normals. Early plantar flexion of the ankle during swing phase led the patients to place the entire foot on the ground instead of using plantar flexion after heel strike to absorb impact. Additional flexion of the knee in these patients occurred later in stance phase and was believed to be a compensatory mechanism for the decreased ankle motion. Additionally, heel rise occurred later in stance than normal, accommodating the planovalgus deformity of the foot while prolonging the double support phase.

Isacson and Broström[11] looked at the early changes in the gait of patients with RA in a larger cohort of 17 women with RA and compared their results with 11 healthy female controls. The RA patients had no major deformities and had essentially normal mobility of the lower extremities, and none had undergone any operations with bony involvement. Clinically, only two hips in the group were painful and all had full range of motion; 12 knees were painful and 17 were swollen, but all had flexion exceeding 90 degrees. Minimum dorsiflexion of all ankles was 10 degrees and minimum plantar flexion was 30 degrees. Twelve ankles were painful as were ten subtalar joints; 14 feet were painful with pressure on the footpad and 8 feet had subluxation of the metatarsal heads. Walking speed of the patients with RA was half of that chosen by the healthy controls and was associated with reductions in stride length and gait cycle duration. The gait parameters of the normal subjects approached those of the RA patients when the normals reduced their speed to that of the RA patients. Range of motion during gait was studied using electrogoniometers with the most obvious differences noted in ankle motion. Absolute ankle joint excursion was the same in both patients and normals, but just as Marshall et al.[17] discovered, the pattern of motion was different. Plantar flexion at toe-off was reduced when compared with the normals, as was adduction of the foot. The primary abnormality was the difficulty encountered by the foot and ankle in acting as a support and a stable lever for the leg just prior to toe-off.[11] Adduction of the subtalar joint near the end of stance phase normally locks the foot into a rigid lever and prepares it for push-off[18] but RA patients with involvement of the joints of the foot appear to be less capable of this maneuver.[7]

Lechner et al.[15] used cine film analysis to perform quantitative gait studies on 30 children with juvenile rheumatoid arthritis (JRA), comparing those results with data from 30 healthy children. Criteria for exclusion included any history of orthopaedic or neurologic problems; a requirement for an assistive device; or the concurrent administration of oral steroids. The study included 22 girls and 8 boys ranging in age from 4 to 20 years with an average age of 11 years. This population of patients was therefore weighted toward those with less involvement, although no attempt was made to control for location of joint involvement, stage of arthritis, disease activity, or duration. Only one fourth of the patient population had hips affected by JRA but more than half had involvement of the ankle or the foot. Significant differences between values obtained for the JRA patients and those for the healthy group included slower mean velocity, excessive tilting of the pelvis, lack of full hip extension with contralateral heel contact, and lack of full ankle plantar flexion at toe-off. The decreased hip extension at the end of stance may have resulted from several factors including direct involvement of the hip by the disease, disuse weakness of the gluteus maximus or hip flexor tightness, and decreased knee extension or ankle plantar flexion at the end of single limb support. In contrast to the findings of Marshall et al. in adult patients,[17] this study found that the JRA patients did not increase their percentage of time spent in double limb support even though they demonstrated a slower cadence.

Total Hip Arthroplasty

There are few studies in the literature of lower extremity function after total hip arthroplasty and the number of patients with RA is correspondingly small. Murray et al.[19] were among the first investigators to apply kinesiologic testing to the clinical evaluation of patients following total hip replacement (with a McKee-Farrar prosthesis.) Four women out of the 30 patients in this study had RA. While velocity and stride length improved in virtually all of the patients in the study, the most dramatic improvements were made by the patients with RA. In these 4 patients free walking velocity increased from 18.0 m/min on the average preoperatively to 43.8 m/min 6 months after their total hip arthroplasty, and stride length also improved from an average of 0.44 m in the RA patients to 0.86 m during that period. Additionally, the arc of motion of the hip increased from 15 degrees preoperatively to 33 degrees at 6 months and knee flexion increased from 38 to 62 degrees.

Knee Studies in Patients With Rheumatoid Arthritis

In contrast to the hip, there are more studies in the literature on patients with knee involvement, perhaps because the motion segments of the thigh and shank are more clearly defined than those of the pelvis and thigh. Stauffer et al.[23] conducted a classic study of involved knee joints utilizing dynamic force plates and triplanar electrogoniometers. Ninety-five patients with 162 diseased knee joints were studied. Thirty of those patients had RA and accounted for 54 of the involved knees. Twelve patients were men, 11 with bilateral involvement, and 18 were women, 13 with bilateral disease. The walking velocity of the patients with RA was only 36% of that of the normals. The female patients with bilateral RA involvement walked at 25.2 m/min vs. 56.4 m/min for healthy women. For comparison, patients with osteoarthritis (OA) walked at 55% of normal speed. The authors found no difference in walking velocity between unilaterally and bilaterally involved patients. The significant reduction in walking velocity was related directly to decreased cadence and stride length.

Kettlekamp et al.[13] also using electrogoniometric techniques, reached similar conclusions in their study of 27 patients with RA with a total of 41 involved knees. Cadence averaged 73 steps per minute in these patients[13] compared with 117 to 120 in normals.[12, 20] Stride length averaged 0.81 m in this patient population. Normal stride length averages 1.56 m.[20]

Stance phase time on the involved leg in the unilateral patients of the RA subjects of Stauffer et al.[23] was shorter than normal as they attempted to reduce the load on the painful, affected knee. However, stance phase time in the bilateral patients actually increased as they sought to spend as much time as possible in double limb support to enhance reduction of compressive forces on both knees.[23] The patients with RA also stood with the knee joint in 22 degrees of flexion, while the normal subjects stood within 1 degree of neutral. Osteoarthritis patients stood with their involved knees flexed slightly over 9 degrees. Standing knee flexion in the study of Kettlekamp et al.[13] averaged 17 degrees compared to a normal value for that study of only 5 degrees. These patients had an average of 114 degrees of available flexion yet they used only 25% of that available motion, compared with 46% in the normal population.

Three-dimensional motion analysis during level walking of the diseased knees in the investigation of Stauffer et al.[23] revealed a significant reduction in sagittal plane motion. Patients with RA had 43% of the normal flexion. The 13 women with both RA and bilateral disease had an average of 32 degrees of sagittal motion vs. the 54 degrees seen in the study's normal population. These authors also found that the amount of sagittal motion during stance phase in both the RA and OA groups was markedly reduced and significantly related to the severity of weight-bearing pain.[23] In normals, this value was 19 degrees in women and 17 degrees in men, but in the patients with RA it was less than 4 degrees in women (with bilateral and unilateral involvement) and less than 3 degrees in men (Fig 17–2). Knee motion in the coronal plane was slightly less than normal for both the RA and OA groups and results assumed a bimodal distribution: the patients with "tight" stiff knees clinically had less coronal motion than knees that were "loose" and unstable on examination. Internal and external rotation of the knee in

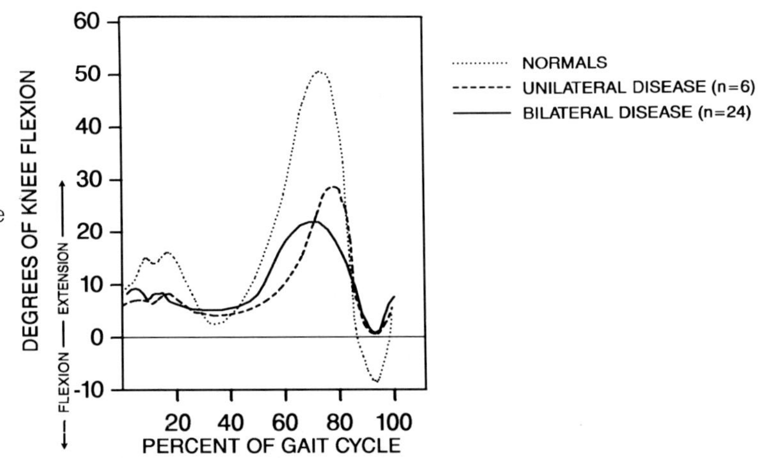

FIG 17–2.
Mean patterns for sagittal plane motion of the knee in patients with RA compared with those of normal subjects. (Adapted from Stauffer RN, Chao EYS, Györy AN: *Clin Orthop* 1977; 126:246–255.)

the transverse plane was also reduced, again in both the RA and OA patients.

Maximal isometric hamstring contraction was reduced in the RA patients to 45% of the normal average of 52 newton-meters. Quadriceps contraction in normals produced 134 newton-meters of torque and was significantly reduced in the RA group to 23% of that value.[23] Isometric torque values for the hamstring and quadriceps were correlated with severity of knee pain in patients with RA but not in those with OA. The pain from the involved joint may have reduced the strength of contraction by reflex inhibition. One must also consider that lower extremity strength in RA patients may be decreased secondary to their prolonged period of diminished activity.

Vertical reaction force in both RA and OA patients demonstrate a slower rate of vertical loading during heel strike as well as decreased peak values.[23] Interestingly, peak values for normal subjects correlate significantly with walking velocity but no such relationship existed in the two patient groups. Vertical floor reaction force in the study by Kettlekamp et al.[13] was evaluated in one patient with severe rheumatoid involvement who had pain with every step. The patient demonstrated a pattern of slow weight acceptance and release as well as a loss of peak loading. Stauffer et al. demonstrated that lateral shear force was also increased in both of their patient groups, more so in those with RA.[23] This suggested an exaggerated displacement of the body's center of gravity and resulted in a waddling type of gait that was felt to be an attempt to even out the more painful vertical compressive forces by substituting a lateral thrust. The gait mechanics of patients with knee joint disease is a compromise between decreasing pain at the expense of energy efficiency.[23]

Total Knee Arthroplasty

Several prospective and retrospective studies of RA patients after total knee arthroplasty are available in the literature[1–3, 5, 25] with many investigators reporting that patients with diseased knees walk significantly slower preoperatively than normal subjects but improve significantly in the postoperative period. An increase in voluntary walking speed was also documented in a mixed group of 9 RA and 15 OA knees studied by Andersson et al.[1] preoperatively and postoperatively, using three different types of prostheses. In general, the walking speed increased up to 1 year after surgery, but the authors did not break down their results by disease group.

Andriacchi et al.[4] were among the first to address the problem of the velocity dependence of gait measurements when attempting to classify gait abnormalities. Five of the 16 patients in their study had RA although the results were not broken down by abnormality. Normal subjects were asked to walk at the same average forward velocity as patients with knee disabilities and their decrease in velocity was accompanied by a linear decrease in stride length. Swing time and support time were inversely proportional to walking speeds. Despite taking this difference in velocity into account, the knee patients were still noted to have a shorter step length and higher cadence than the normals walking at the same speed. In contrast to these findings, Isacson and Broström[11] found that the gait parameters of normals approached those of RA patients without major deformities as the normals decreased their velocities to match those of the RA patients.

Otis et al.[21] documented significant improvements in gait performance after total knee arthroplasty in a study restricted to OA patients. They demonstrated that even in the patients with unilateral disease, preoperatively there was not only a significant reduction in single limb support time for the involved extremity but of the uninvolved side as well. They concluded that those patients were compensating in their gait pattern by increasing their period of double support to minimize the asymmetry of their gait.

Collopy et al.[5] studied seven patients with RA along with nine OA patients both before geometric total knee arthroplasty and postoperatively at 3, 6, and 12 months. The knee flexor and extensor strength of the patients with RA increased progressively in the postoperative period. Standing knee flexion also improved for these same patients from 27 degrees average flexion preoperatively to 13 degrees 1 year postoperatively. The knee flexion-extension patterns of the RA patients demonstrated markedly more flexion during stance phase and less during swing phase than either normals or the OA patients (Fig 17–3). Although the RA patients continued to improve with respect to their knee flexion pattern for up to a year postoperatively, the average pattern remained outside of normal limits. The authors suggested that in many of these patients, the persistence of the abnormal pattern was related to involvement of joints other than the operative knee as well as unsolved problems about the operative knee itself such as flexion contractures and quadriceps weakness.

Andriacchi et al.[3] studied the relationship of gait and prosthetic design in five different designs in a

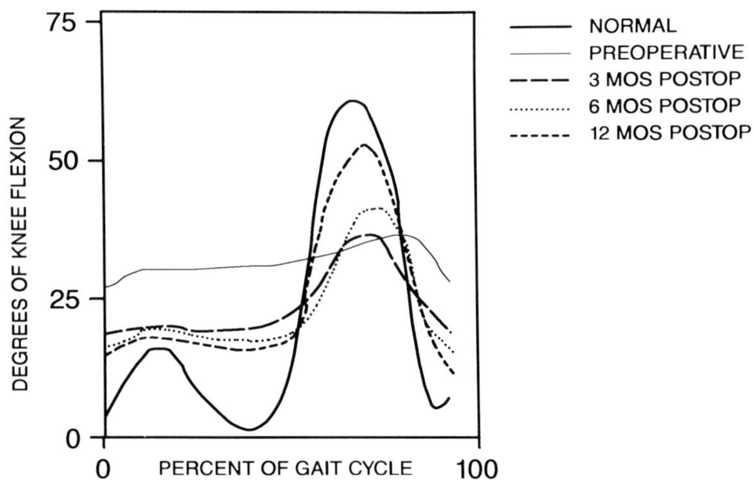

FIG 17–3.
Mean patterns for sagittal plane motion of the knee during free speed walking for seven patients with OA and nine patients with RA before and 3, 6, and 12 months status post total knee arthroplasty and *shaded areas* represent 2 SE above and below the mean patterns for 24 men, 50 to 73 years of age. (Adapted from Collopy MC, Murray MP, Gardner GM, et al: *Clin Orthop* 1977; 126:196–202.)

mixed group of 26 patients. Rheumatoid and OA patients were distributed among all five devices and results were reported based upon the device, not the diagnosis. Interestingly, they found that despite the lack of homogeneity of the study population, there were still common characteristics of gait present, especially during level walking. These included decreased stride length, reduced midstance knee flexion, and abnormal patterns of flexion-extension moments. These differences transcended any prosthetic grouping, suggesting that factors other than component design were at work, including a persistence of learned preoperative gait patterns.

At our laboratory, researchers are using a solid-state video system and force plates to compare two different knee prostheses during level walking and stair ascent and descent (Fig 17–4,A and B) in an otherwise homogeneous patient population. Preliminary results indicate that stair ascent may bring out the greatest differences between prostheses.

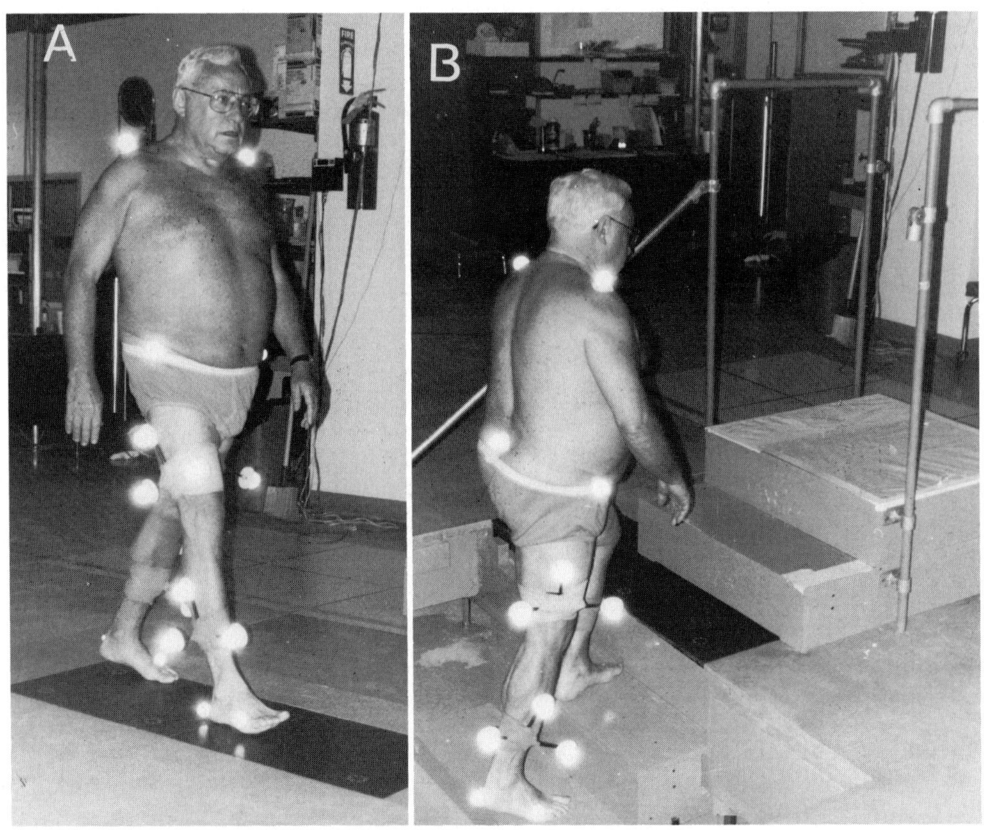

FIG 17–4.
A, experimental setup for gait and kinetic analysis. This subject is 65 years old and 5 years status post total knee arthroplasty on the right side. *Single reflective markers* indicate specific anatomic landmarks such as the acromion, anterior superior iliac spine, and the calcaneus. *Triangular arrays of markers* are used to delineate limb segments of the thigh and shank. Subject is approaching left toe-off from the first black force plate as his right heel contacts the second plate. (Courtesy of The Hospital for Special Surgery, New York.) **B,** same subject in stair ascent. The black step is the force plate. Acromial and sacral markers are necessary to calculate forward trunk lean during ascent. (Courtesy of The Hospital for Special Surgery, New York.)

Ankle Studies in Patients With Rheumatoid Arthritis

Ankle and subtalar involvement of the foot affects a majority of patients with RA at some point in the course of their disease. At the University of California Biomechanics Laboratory (UCBL), Locke et al.[16] studied the motion of these two joints in 25 patients with RA and compared their results with 20 healthy subjects. Ten of the healthy subjects were subclassified as a "young" group ranging in age from 29 to 45 years, and the other 10 as an "old" group with ages from 60 to 84. Fifteen of the patients had used or were using the UCBL orthotic leaving a subset of 10 patients who had not had orthotic intervention. Of these 10, five complained of a painful ankle and hindfoot and 5 were symptom-free. The investigators employed insole foot switches along with ankle and subtalar electrogoniometers. Mean passive dorsiflexion for the 5 RA patients with pain was 8 degrees and for those 5 without pain it was 10 degrees. Young healthy subjects averaged 18 degrees of passive dorsiflexion compared to the 11 degrees registered by the older, healthy group. Active dorsiflexion during walking was virtually the same for the painful and pain-free RA patients at 14 and 13 degrees, respectively. Mean passive plantar flexion for the RA patients was 33 and 34 degrees for the painful and pain-free groups, respectively. Both healthy groups demonstrated more passive plantar flexion at 48 and 40 degrees, respectively, for the young and old healthy subjects. The greatest differences between normal and involved groups, however, occurred in active plantar flexion with the painful and pain-free RA patients demonstrating 1 and 6 degrees, respectively, compared to the 17 to 25 degrees, respectively, of active plantar flexion in the older and younger normals.

Total Ankle Arthroplasty

Demottaz et al.[6] examined 21 total ankle replacements in 19 patients, 14 of whom had RA. Pain was the primary indication for surgery in all 19 patients. Fourteen ankles had a single-axis (Mayo, TPR, Bucholz, or Oregon) and seven had a multiple-axis (Smith or Waugh) prosthesis. Gait measurements were made by cine technique along with electromyographic and force plate data. Average preoperative range of motion was 22 degrees in all patients; 29 degrees postoperatively in the RA patients; and 35 degrees in the OA patients. Subtalar motion remained essentially unchanged after the procedure. The RA patients walked significantly slower than the normals for this study (42 m/min vs. 90.6 m/min). This was a factor in both decreased cadence of the total ankle–RA patients (49 steps/min vs. 113 steps/min in normals) and their shorter stride lengths (0.86 m in RA patients vs. 1.56 m in normals). All of the total ankle patients, RA and OA, spent less of their cycle time in single limb stance than the normal subjects (31.7% vs. 39%).

Anteroposterior and medial-lateral forces were normal for all patients but the vertical forces were reduced at both heel strike and just prior to toe-off.[6] This reduction could have been from either the slower velocity of the patients or as a conscious effort to reduce stress on the ankle. Force vector analysis revealed a significant difference in the coronal plane projection. In the normals this vector was parallel to the tibia but in the total ankle patients, RA and OA, it followed a more medial direction, reaching its maximum just before midstance. In part this could have been explained by the wider-based gait of the patients when compared with the normals. There was also a consistent weakness of the calf and peroneal muscle groups on the operative side in all patients. It is possible that these patients compensated for this weakness by establishing a similar pattern in the contralateral extremity in order to maintain a symmetric gait pattern while increasing activity in the proximal musculature in order to maintain normal patterns of motion in the hips and knees.[6]

CONCLUSIONS

Assessment of lower extremity function in the patient with RA poses a significant challenge to the clinical investigator. Evaluation of function before and after a single procedure represents, at best, a brief interval in the course of a given patient's illness. The condition of other joints can change with respect to range of motion, pain, and functionality over a relatively short period of time, in contrast to the relatively constant nature of the uninvolved joints in OA patients with monarticular disease. Moreover, functional recovery in any patient undergoing lower extremity total joint arthroplasty depends heavily upon the joints distal and proximal to the joint operated on. A total ankle arthroplasty requires relatively uninvolved knees and hips to achieve a good result. Studies of young RA patients without crippling disease are useful in characterizing the disease, but clinically they do not appear to be as useful to the orthopaedic surgeon as postoperative studies in more severely involved patients.

Many of the studies reviewed in this chapter examine both RA and OA patients and while some separate their results by abnormality, others do not. Given the inherent differences between RA and OA, comparisons should be made between normals and patients for a given cohort, but not between RA and OA patients.

Those RA patients with the broadest involvement of joints and the most severe deformities have the most to gain from surgical correction of their abnormalities. These patients, however, are not only the most difficult to treat but also to test. More efforts should be directed toward studies of patients with multiple involvement in an effort to characterize the best combination and sequence of operative intervention. Moreover, many studies of OA and RA patients tend to group bilateral and unilateral cases together and treat each joint as a separate entity during statistical analysis. Future investigations must carefully select their patient populations to avoid the confounding variables introduced by bilateral arthroplasties, or evaluate the bilateral cases separately.

Advances in technology and software have placed sophisticated gait analysis systems within the budget of many laboratories. Accompanying the extended scope of research and clinical laboratories, the orthopaedist should see a greater number of gait studies relating to patients with RA as well as OA. Currently under investigation are the effects of porous-coated hip prostheses upon gait, changes in femoral anteversion after custom hip arthroplasty, and the influence upon gait of posterior cruciate ligament (PCL)–sparing and PCL-substituting total knee arthroplasties.

REFERENCES

1. Andersson GBJ, Andriacchi TP, Galante JO: Correlations between changes in gait and in clinical status after knee arthroplasty. *Acta Orthop Scand* 1981; 52:569–573.
2. Andriacchi TP, Andersson GBJ, Fermier RW, et al: A study of lower limb mechanics during stair climbing. *J Bone Joint Surg [Am]* 1980; 62:749–757.
3. Andriacchi TP, Galante JO, Fermier RW: The influence of total knee replacement design on walking and stair climbing. *J Bone Joint Surg [Am]* 1982; 64:1328–1335.
4. Andriacchi TP, Ogle JA, Galante JO: Walking speed as a basis for normal and abnormal gait measurements. *J Biomech,* 10:261–268, 1977.
5. Collopy MC, Murray MP, Gardner GM, et al: Kinesiologic measurements of functional performance before and after geometric total knee replacement. *Clin Orthop* 1977; 126:196–202.
6. Demottaz JD, Mazur JM, Thomas WH, et al: Clinical study of total ankle replacement with gait analysis. *J Bone Joint Surg [Am]* 1979; 61:976–988.
7. Dimonte P, Light H: Pathomechanics, gait deviations, and treatment of the rheumatoid foot—A clinical report. *Phys Ther* 1982; 62:1148–1156.
8. Dorr LD, Ochsner JL, Gronley J, et al: Functional comparison of posterior cruciate retained *versus* cruciate-sacrificed total knee arthroplasty. *Clin Orthop* 1988; 236:36–43.
9. Hungerford DS, Kenna RV, Haynes DS: Relevant biomechanics of the knee for knee replacements, in Hungerford DS, Krackow KA, Kenna RV (eds): *Total Knee Arthroplasty: A Comprehensive Approach.* Baltimore, Williams & Wilkins Co, 1984, pp 21–34.
10. Inman VT, Ralston HJ, Todd F: *Human Walking.* Baltimore, Williams & Wilkins Co, 1981.
11. Isacson J, Broström L: Gait in rheumatoid arthritis: An electrogoniometric investigation. *J Biomech* 1988; 21:451–457.
12. Johnson RC, Smidt GL: Measurement of hip joint motion during walking—Evaluation of an electrogoniometric method. *J Bone Joint Surg [Am]* 1969; 51:1083–1094.
13. Kettlekamp DB, Leaverton PE, Misol S: Gait characteristics of the rheumatoid knee. *Arch Surg* 1972; 104:30–34.
14. Kroll M: Gait evaluation in total knee arthroplasty—A review of current literature. Unpublished manuscript, 1989.
15. Lechner DE, McCarthy CF, Holden MK: Gait deviations in patients with juvenile rheumatoid arthritis. *Phys Ther* 1987; 67:1335–1341.
16. Locke M, Perry J, Campbell J, et al: Ankle and subtalar motion during gait in arthritic patients. *Phys Ther* 1984; 64:504–509.
17. Marshall RN, Meyers DB, Palmer DG: Disturbance of gait due to rheumatoid disease. *J Rheumatol* 1980; 7:617–623.
18. Morris JM: Biomechanics of the foot and ankle. *Clin Orthop* 1977; 122:10–17.
19. Murray MP, Brewer BJ, Zuege RC: Kinesiologic measurements of functional performance before and after McKee-Farrar total hip replacement. *J Bone Joint Surg [Am]* 1972; 54:237–256.
20. Murray MP, Drought AB, Kory RC: Walking patterns of normal men. *J Bone Joint Surg [Am]* 1964; 46:335–360.
21. Otis JC, Fabian DF, Burstein AH, et al: Evaluation of total knee arthroplasty patients using the VA-Rancho

Gait Analyzer, in Matsui H, Kobayashi K (eds): *Biomechanics VIII-B.* Champaign, Ill, Human Kinetics Publishers, 1983, pp 1075–1080.
22. Rittman N, Kettlekamp DB, Pryor P, et al: Analysis of patterns of knee motion walking for four types of total knee implants. *Clin Orthop* 1981; 155:111–117.
23. Stauffer R, Kettlekamp DB, Thompson C, et al: The MacIntosh prosthesis: Prospective clinical and gait evaluation. *Arch Surg* 1975; 110:717–720.
24. Stauffer RN, Chao EYS, Györy AN: Biomechanical gait analysis of the diseased knee joint. *Clin Orthop* 1977; 126:246–255.
25. Winter DA, Quanbury AO, Reimer GD: Analysis of the instantaneous energy of normal gait. *J Biomech* 1976; 9:253–257.

CHAPTER 18

Soft Tissue

Michael M. Alexiades, M.D.

INTRODUCTION

Rheumatoid arthritis (RA) is a chronic systemic inflammatory disorder characterized mainly by its involvement of synovial joints. However, the extraarticular features of the disease are of significance and include soft tissue involvement, e.g., rheumatoid nodules, vasculitis, neuropathy, lymphadenopathy, pericarditis, pleuritis, and scleritis. It can also involve nonarticular cartilage such as the cricothyroid cartilage, necessitating, on occasion, tracheostomy. These extraarticular manifestations of RA were initially thought to be complications of the disease but currently are recognized as part of the natural history of RA and reinforce its systemic nature. This chapter reviews the extraarticular features of the disease and their surgical treatment. Of note is that these conditions occur more often in patients who are rheumatoid factor–positive and correlate with the severity of the disease but not necessarily with the duration of the disease.

RHEUMATOID NODULES

Rheumatoid nodules are the most common extraarticular feature of RA. They are subcutaneous, localized, and generally not tender or painful (Fig 18–1). They occur in approximately 20% to 25% of patients and are almost always associated with seropositive disease. They are present in the rapidly progressive and most destructive types of rheumatoid arthritis.[10] Rhematoid nodules occur primarily in periarticular areas and on the exterior surface of limbs. Common areas of involvement include the olecranon, extensor surface of the forearms, and along the anterior knee and Achilles tendon. Nodules are also commonly located in the occipital and sacral areas. Pressure from being in the recumbent position can lead to ulceration of these nodules and secondary infection. Rheumatoid nodules can also occur in areas of joint deformity, particularly the metacarpophalangeal joints and the hand. Since nodule recurrence tends to be more common in patients in whom deformity related to nodular disease persists, it is recommended that underlying joint deformity be corrected at the time of the nodule removal. In general, most subcutaneous nodules are asymptomatic and require no treatment. They can persist indefinitely or regress at any time, generally depending on disease activity. Clinically, rheumatoid nodules can be confused with gouty tophi, sebaceous cysts, and carcinoma of the skin. Histologically, the rheumatoid nodule is composed of a central zone of fibrinoid necrosis surrounded by palisading elongated connective tissue cells. There is an outer envelope of chronic inflammatory cells consisting of fibroblasts, lymphocytes, and plasma cells (Fig 18–2,A and B).

Because rheumatoid nodules occur subcutaneously and over bony prominences they can be locally quite sensitive to direct pressure. An attempt should be made to pad over areas where nodules

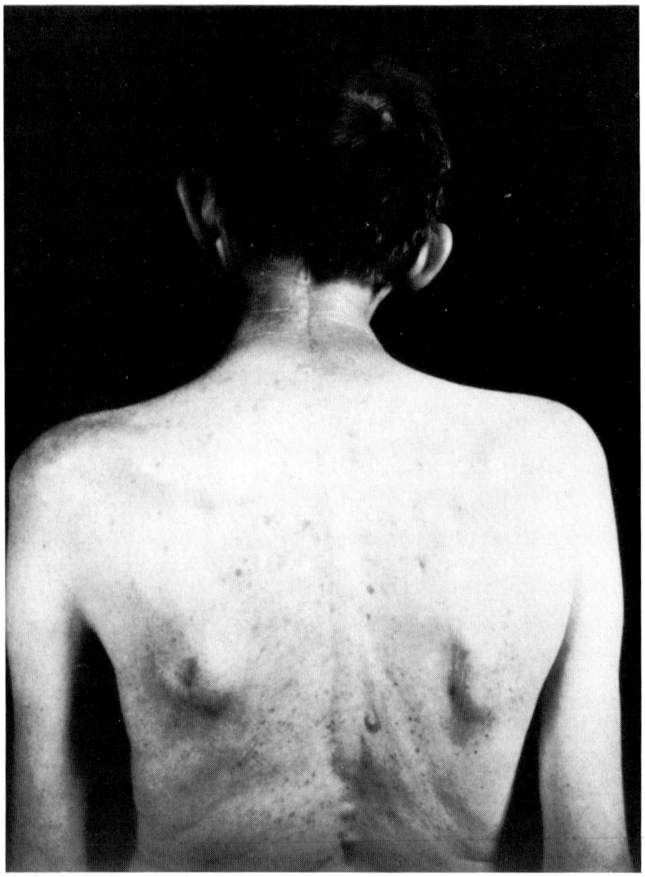

FIG 18–1.
Rheumatoid nodules on the scapula with some skin breakdown *(left).*

can be problematic, particularly about the elbows. Various padded elbow splints and protective supports may be helpful in preventing local areas of skin pressure and breakdown. If rheumatoid nodules are painful and interfere with surrounding joint function, excision is recommended. Recurrence is not uncommon after excision and the patient should be appraised of this tendency. Surgical excision should be considered to differentiate rheumatoid nodules from other skin lesions if the diagnosis is unclear. Excisional biopsy is recommended. In areas of local nodular infection or ulceration, nodular excision should be performed with an effort made to obtain wound closure without excess tension on skin margins. Wound healing may be compromised if there is inadequate soft tissue and skin coverage after nodule excision. Because of the poor healing qualities of RA patients secondary to their disease or medications, excision of nodules should be done only for the above-specified reasons. Excision of nodules over the sacrum and over the olecranon have posed problems with poor healing and drainage which have required a rotation flap or free flap for closure. The nodule should be removed in its entirety with an ellipse of overlying skin so that a primary closure of full-thickness skin can be performed. Planning the incision for the removal of rheumatoid nodules is very important in that later reconstructive surgery may be required. Whenever possible, incisions should be directed toward providing optimal surgical exposure and ample soft tis-

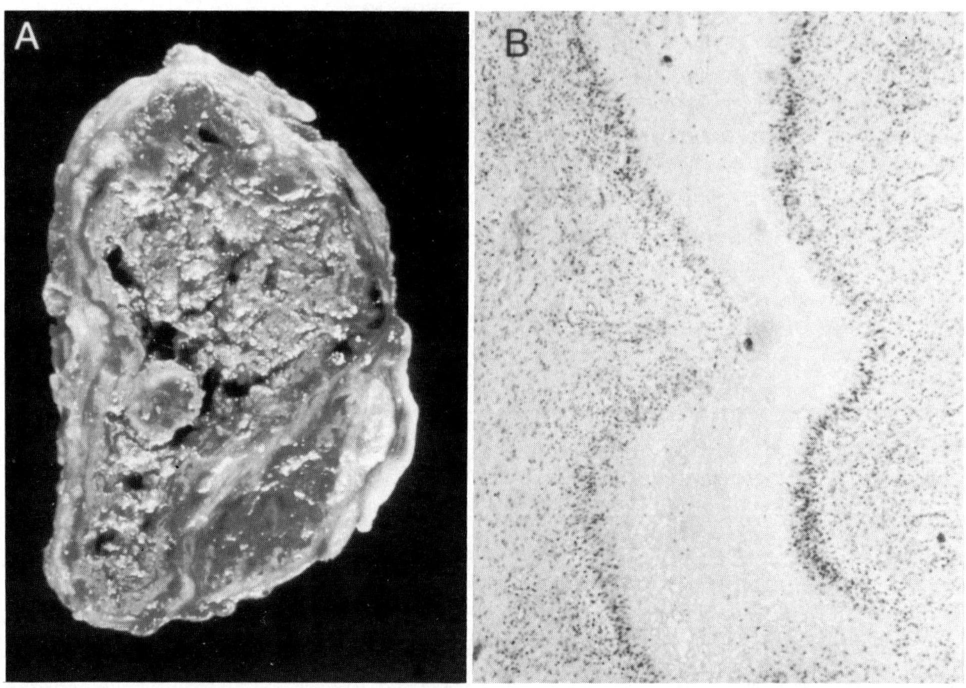

FIG 18–2.
A, gross specimen of a rheumatoid nodule. **B,** histologic appearance of a rheumatoid nodule.

sue coverage in the event they are utilized for further surgery. The incision should never compromise a skin flap between two incisions.

VASCULITIS

Vasculitis is common in RA, and is most often subclinical and found only at postmortem histologic examination of vessels.[10] The vasculitis can affect both small vessels (it may be the cause of the formation of rheumatoid nodules) and major vessels such as mesenteric and extremity vessels. There also exists a more severe type of necrotizing vasculitis that affects small and medium-sized arteries and is indistinguishable from polyarteritis nodosa. The skin lesions can appear in clusters of small brown spots usually affecting nail folds and digital pulp. On occasion purpura may be noted which involves the postcapillary venules (Fig 18–3,A and B). Large areas of ischemic involvement affecting the legs and feet may produce vasculitic ulcerations in the pretibial and malleolar areas. Infarction and necrosis of fingers or toes may also occur secondary to vasculitis.

Rheumatoid vasculitis may be associated with fever and an elevated white blood cell count and sedimentation rate, and other manifestations of severe systemic disease. Neuropathy may also occur secondary to vasculitis.[5] In the most severe type of rheumatoid vasculitis there may be sensory or motor neuropathies, skin necrosis, ulceration, gangrene, and visceral infarction, and death may follow within weeks or months. The prognosis in this rare form of generalized necrosing vasculitis is poor and is usually further complicated by gastrointestinal bleeding, heart failure, and infection secondary to myocarditis or pericarditis.

The pathogenesis of rheumatoid vasculitis is unclear but disposition of immune complexes within vessel walls has been suggested. Most patients have a high serum rheumatoid factor and unlike most rheumatoid patients have a normal or low complement level.[10]

The treatment of vasculitis is primarily systemic. However, the complications related to vasculitis may require surgical intervention. Gangrene of the toes, should it occur, is treated in the same manner as gangrene secondary to diabetic vascular disease (Fig 18–4). If the gangrene is dry, not painful, and without evidence of infection, local nonocclusive dressings to the ischemic toes are permitted and systemic treatment is instituted. The gangrenous digits will often demarcate and eventually autoamputate (see Fig 18–4). The onset of wet gangrene is more problematic and generally requires amputation. Secondary infection is the major complication of this type of ischemia and ascending deep limb infections may develop rapidly. Amputation must be performed at a level that is appropriate for uncomplicated skin healing. If severe cellulitis is present, an open amputation and secondary closure may also be required. Digital, transmetatarsal, or below-knee amputations are not uncommon.

When vasculitic ulcers occur, frequent debridement should be instituted until a clean granulating bed can be obtained. Once this is established a soft cast or Unna boot can be applied which will allow healing of the underlying ulcer by secondary intention. Large ulcers and ulcers more proximal in the leg may benefit from close-fitting skintight casts. These casts must be properly applied and in several

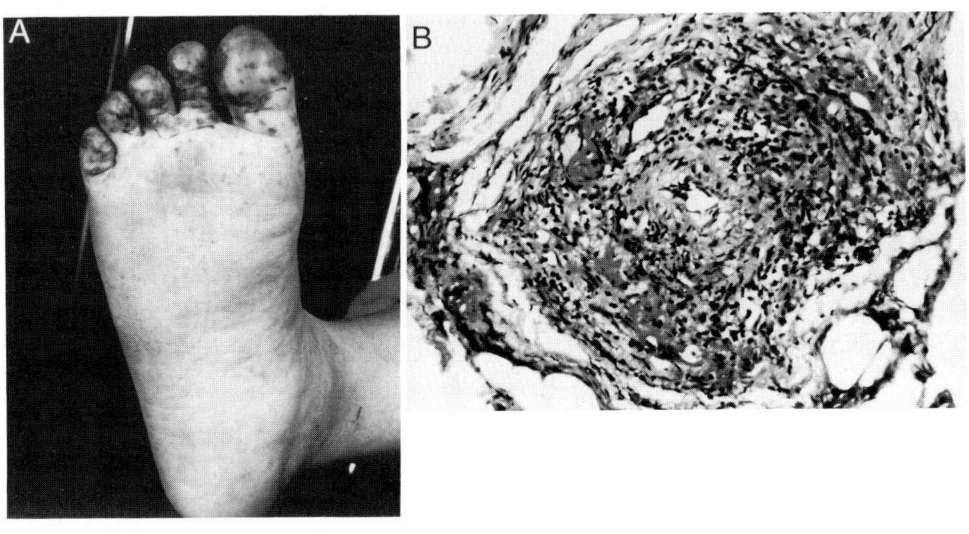

FIG 18–3.
A, vasculitis involving the foot. **B,** histologic appearance of small vessel vasculitis.

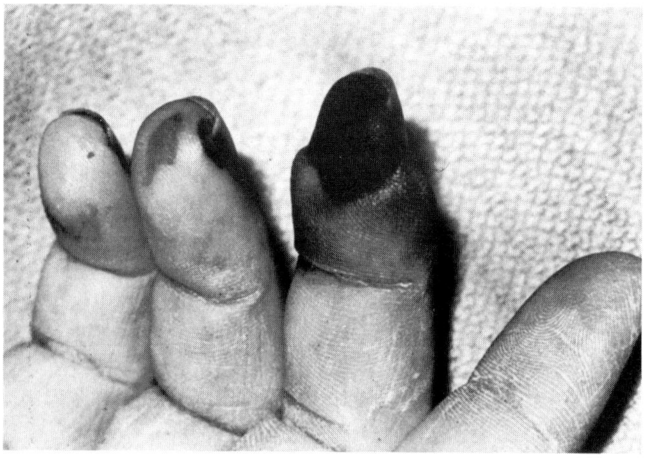

FIG 18–4.
Gangrene with demarcation secondary to vasculitis.

weeks ulcers can significantly reduce in size or heal completely. Repeated casting may be necessary in intractable ulcers. Secondary infections in these ulcers are a severe complication and may be a source of systemic infection and metastatic prosthetic joint infection. It is therefore imperative that healing be effected as quickly as possible with a combined systemic treatment of vasculitis and local treatment of the wound. Healing has been poor or completely absent in soft tissue flap reconstructions, including free flaps and grafts. The active vasculitic process persists both in the bed of the ulcer and in the vessels that are used for anastomosis of the soft tissue flap and this impedes revascularization. Treatment has concentrated on local debridement, immobilization of the limb, appropriate dressings, and systemic treatment of the disease. Occasionally, skin punch biopsies at the ulcer margin are required to differentiate vasculitis from other skin disorders such as carcinoma.

NEUROPATHY

Rheumatoid arthritis usually spares the central nervous system but may affect peripheral nerves. Mononeuritis multiplex is a frequent manifestation of vasculitis and can result in a foot- or wristdrop with patch sensory loss.[5] Elderly patients can also develop a mild symmetric distal sensory neuropathy associated with vasculitis that predominates in the lower extremities, and has a more favorable prognosis. To differentiate a mild sensory neuropathy from a mononeuritis multiplex, a sural nerve biopsy is needed (Fig 18–5). The sural nerve is exposed via a short transverse incision posterior to the lateral malleolus. It is separated bluntly from the lesser saphenous vein which lies just anterior to it. Once identified and isolated the nerve is transected and the distal end of the proximal stump is buried in the underlying fascia to prevent painful neuroma formation. The excised nerve segment is then sent for pathologic examination and evaluation of active perineural vasculitis.

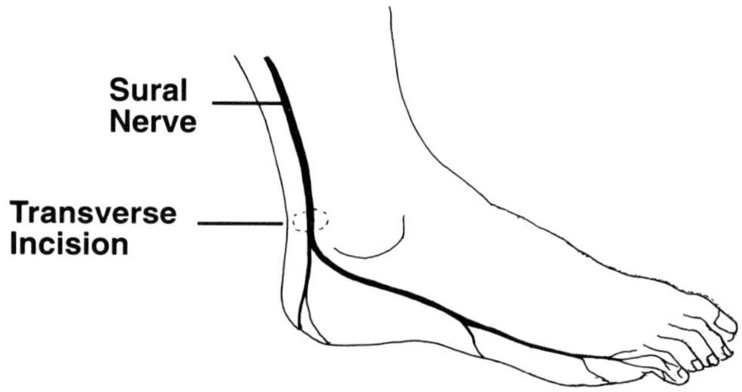

FIG 18–5.
Sural nerve anatomy and transverse incision.

Neurologic complaints in patients with RA are not necessarily secondary to neural intrinsic disease and may be related to nerve compression. Median neuropathy is the most common nerve compression syndrome seen in RA. Tenosynovitis of the wrist (flexor compartment) and flexor tendons results in compression of the median nerve in the carpal canal. In general, the prognosis for return of function and sensation of the median nerve is worse in patients with RA than in the general population.[12] Nonsurgical treatment of the tenosynovitis (e.g., splints, injections) may improve symptoms, but early decompression is advised in refractory patients. Compressive ulnar nerve neuropathy at the elbow or wrist from synovitis of those joints is also common. Release of Guyon's canal or ulnar nerve transposition at the elbow may be necessary. Underlying wrist and elbow synovitis should also be treated. Intraarticular cortisone injections may be used. If synovitis persists, synovectomy or arthroplasty, or both, may be considered. Other peripheral nerve compressive neuropathies can include the anterior tibial nerve resulting in footdrop and tarsal tunnel syndrome.

GIANT CELL ARTERITIS

Giant cell arteritis, also known as cranial arteritis or temporal arteritis, occurs in RA. The vessels most often involved are those originating from the arch of the aorta although vessels traversing the extremities may be affected. The population affected is similar to polymyalgia rheumatica and a relationship between the two has been recognized for over 25 years.[4] Female patients have a twofold increased incidence of this condition, especially those over age 50 years. The incidence has been reported to be as high as 20 per 100,000 people and is more prevalent in the northern United States. Approximately half of the patients with temporal arteritis will have polymyalgia rheumatica.[8] The vessels involved are frequently affected in a discontinuous fashion with some vessels demonstrating sections infiltrated with lymphocytes and other inflammatory cells.[11] There is thickening of the intima which can result in narrowing or occlusion of the vessel lumen. Panarteritis may also be seen which can result in complete disruption of the vessel wall layers. Onset may be insidious or sudden with constitutional symptoms including fever, malaise, and weight loss. Headaches localized to the temporo-occipital region are common. Tenderness or enlargement of the involved arteries of the head and neck is often present. Severe ophthalmic involvement has been reported in 8% to 15% of patients.[2, 4, 7] Patients may have sudden loss of vision due to involvement of ophthalmic vessels. Visual effects can be permanent in these cases. Patients may manifest symptoms of cerebral vascular ischemia such as transient ischemic attacks or strokes.

The laboratory findings reveal an elevated erythrocyte sedimentation rate in almost all patients. Definitive diagnosis is made by temporal artery biopsy. The superficial temporal artery is the small terminal branch of the external carotid and originates in the parotid gland behind the neck as the mandible crosses over the zygomatic process of the temporal bone. Approximately 5 cm above the zygomatic process the artery divides into anterior and posterior branches (Fig 18–6,A). A temporal artery biopsy is performed under local anesthesia that is administered in the region of the branches of the superficial temporal artery (Fig 18–6,B). Epinephrine should not be used with the local anesthetic as it may lead to severe vasoconstriction and increase the difficulty in identifying the temporal artery branches. Since the area to be biopsied is always behind the hairline, local shaving is necessary. Palpation of the pulse can be unreliable in identifying the artery and its branches and therefore a portable Doppler instrument is preferred. With the Doppler and a marking pen, the artery can be traced from the zygoma superiorly and its branches marked out. The two easiest branches to identify and biopsy are (1) the anterior branch or frontal branch which runs cephalad and anterior toward the tuberosity of the frontal bone, and (2) the parietal or posterior branch, which is larger and curves cephalad and posterior on the side of the head lying superficial to the temporal fascia, and which anastomoses with the postero-occipital and opposite parietal branch. As large a segment as possible is obtained for biopsy to insure that an involved portion of the vessel is sent for pathologic evaluation. Both ends of the artery are clamped, and the central portion and the ends of the vessels are li-

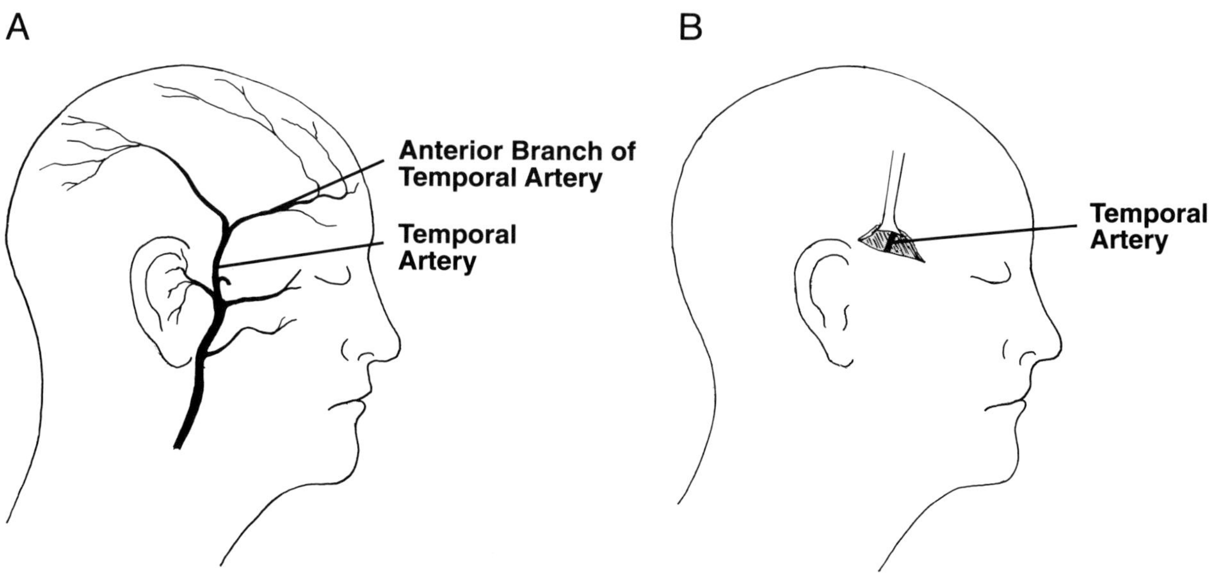

FIG 18–6.
A, temporal artery anatomy. **B,** temporal artery biopsy incision.

gated. Histologic examination of the vessels will often reveal an inflammatory reaction involving primarily the internal elastic membrane and again, occasionally, a panarteritis may be present. Histochemical studies have shown helper T cells involved in the inflammatory reaction. Immunoglobulin deposits have also been found in the walls of inflamed temporal arteries.[1]

MYOPATHY

Inflammatory myopathies such as polymyositis or dermatomyositis are recognized as separate entities in autoimmune disease. They are among the least common of the connective tissue disease.[9] The clinical hallmark of these diseases is proximal limb and neck weakness associated with muscle pain. Almost all of these patients have an elevated creatinine phosphokinase (CPK) level. The inflammatory myopathies can be seen in association with other autoimmune and connective tissue diseases. In RA and systemic lupus erythematosus, myositis is usually mild and often asymptomatic. However, with continued progression of disease in RA, muscle weakness is often a frequent complaint. The differential diagnosis of progressive muscle weakness in the rheumatoid patient includes:

1. Peripheral neuropathy, possibly secondary to vasculitis
2. Brainstem or spinal cord compression secondary to basilar impression or vertebral instability
3. Weakness secondary to muscle atrophy from disuse and malnutrition
4. Proximal muscle myopathy secondary to corticosteroid use
5. Myositis

It is thus very important that all RA patients with muscle weakness undergo a good history and physical examination; cervical spine radiographs, including lateral flexion and extension views; electrodiagnostic studies, including an electromyogram and electrocardiogram; and blood chemistry analysis, including serum enzyme assays which include CPK, aldolase, lactic dehydrogenase, and transaminases. Many of these patients will then require a muscle biopsy for appropriate histochemical studies. Before formal muscle biopsy, consultation with a rheumatologist, neurologist, and a pathologist skilled in muscle tissue evaluation should be obtained to more clearly define the diagnosis.

An electromyogram of normal muscle reveals relative silence when the muscle is at rest and on voluntary contraction the electromyogram shows characteristic frequency duration and amplitude ac-

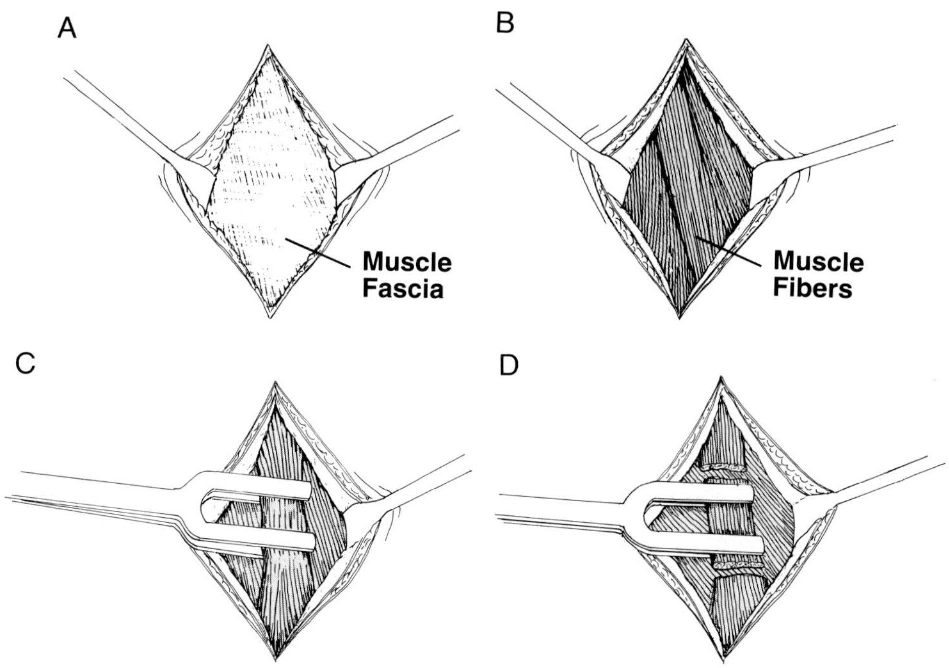

FIG 18–7.
Muscle biopsy: **A,** superficial incision. **B,** deep dissection. **C,** muscle biopsy clamp. **D,** muscle biopsy excision.

tion potentials. The electromyogram can differentiate myopathy from neuropathy. The electromyogram reveals increased frequency, amplitude, and duration of the action potential, whereas neuropathy reveals the exact opposite.

TECHNIQUE FOR MUSCLE BIOPSY

In general, a regional or local anesthetic in the overlying skin and subcutaneous tissue is performed. The fascia overlying muscle is then split to expose the underlying muscle bundles (Fig 18–7,A). The most reliable technique for obtaining muscle specimens while maintaining muscle length is use of a holding clamp (Fig 18–7,B–D). This device grasps the muscle in the direction of its fibers, after which the muscle is sectioned around the outside of the arms of the clamps. If small biopsy specimens are obtained using the clamp, bleeding is usually not a problem. Three muscle specimens from the same site are obtained since different histologic staining techniques and special fixative techniques are required. The pathologist must be alerted prior to the biopsy to insure that the specimens in the clamps are processed rapidly without preservatives and without dessication of the tissues. Once hemostasis is achieved the fascia and wound can be closed in layers in the usual fashion. Histologic examination (Fig 18–8) will usually reveal inflammatory infiltrates consisting primarily of chronic inflammatory cells. Examination of the muscle will reveal variation of fiber size with most atrophied fibers being peripheral. Areas of fibrinoid necrosis are seen and in long-standing cases, interstitial fibrosis. The biopsy of a severely involved muscle may reveal severe fibrosis and fibrofatty degeneration which makes the biopsy less useful. Sometimes biopsies will be normal histologically because pathologic changes can be focal within the muscle. Proper biopsy site selection is integral to making a pathologic diagnosis.

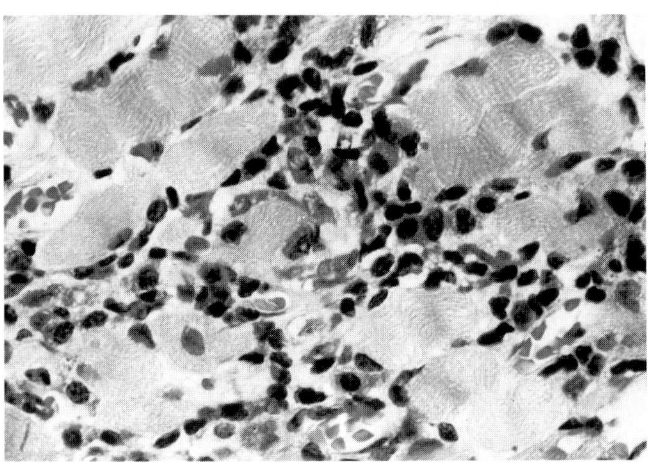

FIG 18–8.
Histologic appearance of myositis.

CONCLUSION

The use of these simple techniques in soft tissue management and biopsy are helpful in the management of the rheumatoid patient with extraarticular manifestations. Skin punch biopsy, sural nerve biopsy, temporal artery biopsy, and muscle biopsy techniques are essential in establishing the diagnosis for the various types of vasculitis, neuropathies, and myopathies that involve the rheumatoid patient. Knowledge of treatment modalities for skin ulceration and necrosis can help shorten the period of disability and pain for the rheumatoid patient and promote a rapid return to a maximal level of functioning. One must be aware, particularly in patients with evidence of neuromuscular disease, that spinal cord compression may actually be the cause, and simple radiographic techniques can establish this diagnosis before extensive invasive biopsy techniques are performed.

REFERENCES

1. Banks PM, Cohen MD, Ginsburg WW, et al: Immunohistologic and cytochemical Studies of temporal arteritis. *Arthritis Rheum* 1983; 26:1201–1207.
2. Bednar M, Alexiades MM, Inglis AE: Carpal tunnel syndrome in rheumatoid arthritis. Presented to the American Society for Surgery of the Hand, Seattle, September, 1989.
3. Bengtsson BA, Malmvall BE: The epidemiology of giant cell arteritis including temporal arteritis. *Arthritis Rheum* 1981; 24:899–904.
4. Berman AT, Garbarino JL, Rosenberg H, et al: Muscle biopsy: Proper surgical technique. *CORR* 1985; 198:240–243.
5. Calamia KT, Hunder GG: Clinical manifestations of giant cell arteritis. *Clin Rheum Dis* 1980; 6:389–403.
6. Cohen RD, Coun DL, Illstrup DM: Clinical features, prognosis and response to treatment in polyarteritis. *Mayo Clin Proc* 1980; 55:146–155.
7. Dubowitz V, Brooke MH: *Muscle Biopsy: A Modern Approach. Major Problems in Neurology,* vol 2. Philadelphia, WB Saunders Co, 1973, pp 5–20.

8. Healy LA, Wilske UR: Manifestations of giant cell arteritis. *Med Clin North Am* 1977; 61:261–270.
9. Huston KA, Hunder GG, Lie JT, et al: Temporal arteritis: A 25 year epidemiologic, clinical and pathological study. *Ann Intern Med* 1978; 88:162–167.
10. Medsger TA, Dawson NN, Masi AT: The epidemiology of polymyositis. *Am J Med* 1970; 48:715–723.
11. Schumacher HR Jr (ed): *Primer on the Rheumatic Diseases.* Atlanta, Arthritis Foundation, 1988.
12. Wilkinson IM, Russell RW: Arteries of the head and neck in giant cell arteritis: A patholic study to show the pattern of arterial involvement. *Arch Neurol* 1972; 27:378–391.

CHAPTER 19

Surgery in Juvenile Rheumatoid Arthritis

Norman A. Johanson, M.D.

INTRODUCTION

Juvenile rheumatoid arthritis (JRA) presents a challenge to the orthopaedic surgeon, both in the planning of surgery and its timing.[2] To meet this challenge, the surgeon must see his or her contribution as but one part of a team process that has as its goal the optimal physical and emotional development of the pediatric patient. This chapter focuses first on the patient and the context in which care should be given, and then on the surgical principles and procedures that may be useful in the treatment of JRA. At the outset it should be stated that JRA has such a wide variety of clinical presentations that each patient must be individually planned and treated. Moreover, severe chronic musculoskeletal involvement in JRA is rare.

The orthopaedic surgeon most commonly addresses pain and functional disability. These two parameters are usually intimately connected in adult reconstructive surgery, but it is usually pain which precipitates surgical treatment. In JRA, however, functional problems are more prevalent, and the prevention or treatment of functional impairment is more likely to be the goal of surgery. The surgical management of JRA requires careful consideration of the patient's psychosocial status, the pattern of the disease, and the goals that can realistically be achieved. This comprehensive understanding of a patient's condition is most reliably developed in an interdisciplinary setting.

It is not unusual for a patient with polyarticular disease to have both upper and lower extremity involvement, and therefore a surgeon caring for JRA patients should be well acquainted with both upper and lower extremity surgery, and be able to prioritize the sequence of procedures for the patient. A surgeon should become acquainted with patients early in the disease process, as it is undesirable to perform multiple major reconstructive procedures in the upper and lower extremities within a short period of time. Even though this latter approach is feasible and sometimes gratifying, it can place the patient in a precarious physical and emotional state that is preventable if the patient is cared for appropriately from the onset of the disease.

Even under the best of circumstances a patient may move from the "preventive" soft tissue procedures to the reconstructive bony procedures with the disease relentless in its course of joint destruction. Here is where the clinical team approach is necessary, and where the orthopaedic surgeon is reminded that he or she cannot function alone. A pediatric rheumatologist, physical therapist, occupational therapist, nurse, and social worker, all are needed for the success of surgical intervention. If one procedure fails, another may be needed. The confidence of the patient and family may be shaken, and contact with another team member may be needed to restore confidence that everything that can be done is being done. Education regarding the disease itself or physical therapy to compensate for the recent loss of function may be all that is needed. In any case, care of the patient with JRA is a long-term commitment. A surgical outcome that is less than perfect is successful if it has prevented more severe loss of function.

THE PATIENT

In the best of circumstances, the orthopaedic surgeon will be consulted on a newly diagnosed case of JRA and be apprised regularly throughout the course of the illness, particularly in problematic patients. This may not always be possible because of late referrals of patients who have not responded to medical therapy elsewhere. In those cases, careful attention should be given to the history. In the patient under 6 years of age with systemic-onset JRA, medical problems such as fever, rash, lymphadenopathy, hepatosplenomegaly, and pericarditis may be of primary concern. The orthopaedic surgeon must observe the patient for musculoskeletal problems that may arise during the systemic illness and persist or progress after constitutional symptoms have subsided. It is important to have an accurate record of the joints affected and the objective findings at each visit. This is especially true early in the course of systemic or pauciarticular disease, when there is risk for evolution toward polyarticular involvement. Attention to only one or a few actively inflamed joints with a fixed treatment plan may lead to failure to identify more ominous problems developing in other joints. Care of the JRA patient should be comprehensive rather than anatomic in its orientation.

The very young patient with JRA cannot be expected to understand the nature of his or her disease and the treatment alternatives being considered. As the patient's communication skills improve, interaction with the pediatric, nursing, and other staff should help reduce the anxiety associated with this disabling illness. Fortunately, most young patients are successfully treated with medication and conservative measures such as splinting and physical therapy. But should more aggressive treatment be required the orthopaedic surgeon should be mindful of the relatively helpless feeling a child has in the midst of the process. This may also apply to family members, who may have a limited understanding of JRA and its course. The incidence of significant family events such as divorce, separation, death, or adoption has been associated with a predisposition for important psychosocial problems that can confound treatment plans.[5] The relationship of the patient to his or her family is of utmost importance from the standpoint of providing informed consent for surgery and assuring an optimal environment for recovery.

There is a great difference between a 10-year-old girl who has been intermittently sick for 5 years and has progressed to polyarticular destructive arthritis, and a 15-year-old girl who has a swollen right knee with patellofemoral pain. From a physical standpoint, the first patient may be unusually small, having experienced little in the way of vigorous activity, and be poorly motivated to undergo any treatment to enable her to do so. The second patient may have participated in competitive athletics, may view her knee as an obstacle to enjoying sports, and be highly motivated to undergo any procedure recommended. These extreme examples illustrate the need to consider the marked disparity in disease manifestation and patient motivation before recommending surgery. Intellectual development is also important to assess because of its potential interaction with physical development. A sick or disabled patient with JRA may be negatively affected intellectually and socially by limited school participation. In general, surgery will be much more successful if it results in improved school attendance.

Functional assessment in a child with JRA is difficult because it involves both the functions that the patient has lost and those functions that would have otherwise developed were it not for the illness. The child may never have been able to perform a certain function prior to the onset of JRA. Moreover, if the disease progresses to a chronic state, that function may never be expected of the child, even though the potential for learning it may exist. The child's emotional state, degree of dependence on family or caregiver, and true physical limitations constantly interact. They must be assessed by the most qualified person in each discipline and articulated such that the other team members can integrate the information. The orthopaedic surgeon needs to hear these evaluations before planning surgery.

The patient's resources for making a full recovery should be thoroughly considered prior to initiating surgical treatment. Emotional, physical, and intellectual resources are important, but availability of financial and human resources necessary to carry a treatment plan through to completion are equally crucial. Hospitalization, transportation, home or outpatient physical and occupational therapy, and mechanical equipment are expensive, and their availability must be resolved prior to surgery. In many cases the surgical result is ultimately determined by these and other nonsurgical factors.

THE CONTEXT OF TREATMENT

Facilities

With few exceptions the comprehensive care of JRA should take place within an academic medical center that offers a full range of professional expertise to deal with the complexities of the disease. The patient should be seen in an ambulatory setting on a particular day when all members of the health team will be present. This facilitates the rapid interchange of information among the staff, and is most convenient for the patient and family. A large referral network is necessary so that an adequate number of newly diagnosed patients are encountered. From a surgical standpoint this is important because of the level of expertise necessary to appropriately treat these patients. Surgery in JRA is not common, and a centralized clinical facility enables the orthopaedic surgeon to maintain his or her skills and judgment. It is also desirable from the standpoint of clinical research.

The institution in which surgery for JRA is performed should have a full capacity for arthroscopic surgery and joint arthroplasty utilizing modern techniques. Financial support from the hospital may be necessary to support a JRA clinic. Promotion of the clinic in the community and helping to fund the care of financially needy patients is often necessary. It is clear that the type of care required may be very expensive in terms of human and financial resources. For a JRA clinical service to succeed it must be given a relatively high institutional priority.

The Team

The clinical director of a JRA service should be a pediatric rheumatologist or the service can be jointly directed by a rheumatologist and a pediatrician. Since there is overlap care by a pediatrician and rheumatologist, there may be some variation in the leadership of the clinic according to location. The clinic must have an orthopaedic consultant with skills in pediatric orthopaedics, arthroscopy, and total joint replacement. It is desirable to have one surgeon managing the patient in all of these areas because the severely affected patient may in fact require the full spectrum of orthopaedic procedures within a relatively short period of time. Multiple orthopaedic surgeons may lead to fragmented care and to patient and family anxiety. Ultimately, this could compromise the surgical results.

The clinical service should be managed by an administrative coordinator with organizational and communication skills. The importance of this position cannot be overemphasized. The coordinator of a JRA service provides the important functions of the service organization, including schedules, conferences, parental and patient education, and medical and surgical consultation.

A nurse-clinician is an important link between the patient and the JRA clinic, often providing the necessary sensitivity and care on a day-to-day basis that is needed to maintain the trust of existing patients and to encourage new patient enrollment. The nurse is also essential for the research effort that should be a high priority in a JRA service. The nurse-clinician should manage all data collection instruments for clinical research. This will give the highest probability that reliable medical information is being collected in a comprehensive fashion. This interaction provides an excellent opportunity for feedback of information to the patient for educational purposes.

A social worker should be assigned to a JRA service to help the patient and family obtain the necessary resources to facilitate ambulatory visits, hospitalizations, surgical aftercare, and social needs that may arise during the course of the illness. An experienced social worker is a fundamental source of information on the many resources that the patient may require and that might otherwise be overlooked during discussions of medical details and surgical planning.

Physical and occupational therapists play an essential role in the pre- and postoperative care of the patient with JRA. It is necessary to include the therapist's evaluation in any decision regarding surgical treatment. Just as the social worker provides information regarding the social realities facing the patient, the physical therapist is best qualified to assess the patient's interaction with his or her physical environment. This type of observation often offers the best description of the patient's true functional disability and his or her motivation to overcome it.

The place of resident house staff in the milieu of a JRA comprehensive care service is problematic from several standpoints. The usual structure of residency training programs provides for relatively short (6 weeks to 3 months) rotations. A resident, especially at the junior level, enters a situation where he or she is expected to be an authority on a complex clinical area. The natural inclination is either to assert authority inappropriately, or to sit back apathetically. The appropriate experience for a house officer on a comprehensive care JRA service is to develop competence in the area of clinical evaluation, patient presentation to the clinical conference, the summary and formulation of treatment plans with the team, and surgical experience appropriate for the level of training. Residents should not be asked to make crucial day-to-day decisions on patient management issues with long-term implications. This is the responsibility of either the fellow or the attending orthopaedic surgeon. A JRA service should seek an orthopaedic fellow who has completed an orthopaedic residency. A clinical research fellow is an important bridge between the educational and service functions of the service and he or she should have ample time for research endeavors. Continuity of patient care is greatly enhanced by the presence of a fellow on the team.

PRINCIPLES FOR EVALUATING SURGICAL INDICATIONS AND OUTCOMES

1. *Avoid surgery during periods of crisis.* In general it is unlikely that performing musculoskeletal surgery in a JRA patient during a period of metabolic instability will be any more beneficial than waiting for the patient's medical condition to stabilize. Surgery should be deferred until systemic manifestations of the arthritis have reached a relatively quiescent baseline. The patient's emotional state should be considered an important indicator of the appropriateness of surgery, especially when multiple operations are planned. If possible, a psychosocial crisis must be identified and managed prior to surgery. Unfortunately, many JRA patients have chronically disrupted lives and are emotionally distraught.[5] Such adverse conditions must often be regarded as the patient's functional normal status, and surgical planning should proceed in order to prevent other, potentially more severe problems. The quality of the patient's family life should have an influence on surgical planning. Whenever possible, important family members should be present when the plans are discussed. It is helpful for the clinical team to listen in a conference setting to the family's observations on the patient's pain and functional status prior to making a final recommendation.

2. *Perform surgery prior to sharp functional decline.* The patient's level of disability, especially in polyarticular JRA, should be monitored closely in order to detect subtle changes that may presage a more rapid functional decline. It is desirable to regularly take inventory of the patient's functional capabilities in light of his or her physical and intellectual development. A very important variable is the patient's ambulatory status. An ominous change in the time spent walking, use of assistive devices, gait pattern, and range of joint motion will frequently precede by several months the need for a wheelchair. The lack of ambulatory capacity is a catastrophe, and bilateral joint involvement can amplify and accelerate this process. Surgery that is performed prior to rapid deterioration in function is likely to be less complex, with less associated morbidity, and a significantly better chance of an improved outcome.

3. *Consider pain and function separately.* Although pain and function are intimately related, it is helpful for the surgeon to ferret out the distinctive features of each area. The difference between what a patient can do and what he or she will do is often determined by pain. Variability in age of onset, duration, disease activity, and number of joints affected tends to confound the direct relationship between pain and function. For example, early in the course of the disease a painful swollen joint may not cause significant dysfunction because it is still mobile and the patient is motivated to essentially continue his or her activities. At the other extreme, a patient with polyarticular disease may have ankylosed joints, be completely disabled and with markedly limited range of motion, but without significant pain. Both patients are severely affected by either pain or dysfunction, but they cannot be considered equal from the standpoint of overall health status or appropriateness for surgery.

4. *Discuss surgical treatment in an open forum.* One of the benefits of the team approach is the wealth of information that can be brought to bear on treatment issues. With an experienced staff, knowledgeable about how each surgical treatment has affected previous patients, important feedback is available for discussion. Short-circuiting this process invites ill-informed decisions, and ultimately undermines the process of the clinic.

5. *Maintain records of objective outcome evaluation.* Important clinical information on patients should be maintained as part of a computerized database to facilitate prospective research. The data variables

should be carefully chosen to suit the particular research interests of the JRA service. Health assessment questionnaires are a convenient way to regularly evaluate patients. Several validated instruments are currently available, but there is a need for further development of joint-specific instruments that are useful in surgical outcome assessment.[16]

6. *Learn from mistakes.* Every suboptimal surgical result offers an opportunity for improvement in the future. In a disease like JRA, error is often very hard to define when a less-than-perfect surgical result is compared to nonsurgical alternatives. Analysis of failures should be an important part of the JRA service. A surgeon should be able to discuss the operative results with knowledgeable colleagues and accept the observations of others on the service so that future error may be avoided.

SURGICAL PROCEDURES

Surgery in JRA is contemplated only after conservative measures have.[24] Besides medical therapy, physical and occupational therapy are the cornerstones of conservative management. Manipulation and serial casting, particularly of the knee, is often an important adjunct to conservative or surgical therapy. Traction for the treatment of acute hip or knee arthritis may be helpful, but has limited use in long-term management.

JRA surgery may be divided into (1) soft tissue procedures and (2) bone and joint procedures. Soft tissue procedures are most often thought of as preventive in that their success is contingent on having essentially intact articular cartilage and major supporting ligaments that will allow physiologic motion and stability after the joint has been mobilized. As a rule, the recovery period following soft tissue procedures is shorter, and morbidity is less perioperative. Consequently, soft tissue surgery is performed earlier in the course of the disease. However, defining the ideal surgical timing and evaluating the outcome of these procedures may be difficult.

With few exceptions, the bone and joint procedures are performed at the end stage of joint disease and involve more extensive postoperative therapy and longer recovery times. These procedures are demanding in terms of patient motivation for recovery and therefore the risks of surgery must be weighed against the expected benefits.

Soft Tissue Procedures

Tenotomy and Capsulotomy

Tendon and capsular releases may be performed for incipient contractures, most commonly in the hip and knee, that do not respond to physical therapy.[4, 25] The timing of release is largely subjective, and underscores the necessity for the surgeon to carefully follow the progress of the patient in physical therapy. When contractures are fixed and interfere with function, surgical release should be considered.

In the operating room prior to surgery an examination under anesthesia is helpful to rule out the presence of fibrous ankylosis. If a hip or knee cannot be moved at least through a partial range of motion under anesthesia, soft tissue release will be unsuccessful.

The hip joint is best approached medially for optimal exposure during release of the iliopsoas and adductor tendons, and the hip capsule.[25] Postoperatively the patient should receive immediate physical therapy, and be encouraged to lie prone as much as possible to bring the hip into extension. Swann performed 89 releases in the hips of 52 children with a mean age of 11 years using this regimen.[25] He found good relief of pain, improved range of motion, and in some cases radiographically demonstrable improvement. This phenomenon was attributed to the effect of mechanically decompressing the joint. Tendon and capsular release around the hip is low risk and may help to defer more complicated surgical procedures until growth is completed.

The knee in JRA presents a more complex deformity in that there are usually three components: flexion, angulation, and rotation. As the deformity progresses, the growth disturbance in the distal femoral and proximal tibial epiphyses, and the tightening of the cruciate ligaments, posterior capsule, and soft tissues render the joint unable to be fully extended, even in the absence of actual joint space narrowing. Growth disturbances are common in JRA, particularly at the knee. The bizarre knee deformities seen in JRA exemplify the important contribution of epiphyseal growth to the ultimate shape and mechanical behavior of the joint. (Fig 19–1,A and B).

Soft tissue procedures for correcting knee deformities in JRA should be performed before cartilage degeneration and before significant fixed valgus (>15 degrees), flexion, or rotational deformity has occurred.[4] Two incisions, medial and lateral, should be used. Medial and lateral hamstring tenotomies are performed in conjunction with a posterior capsu-

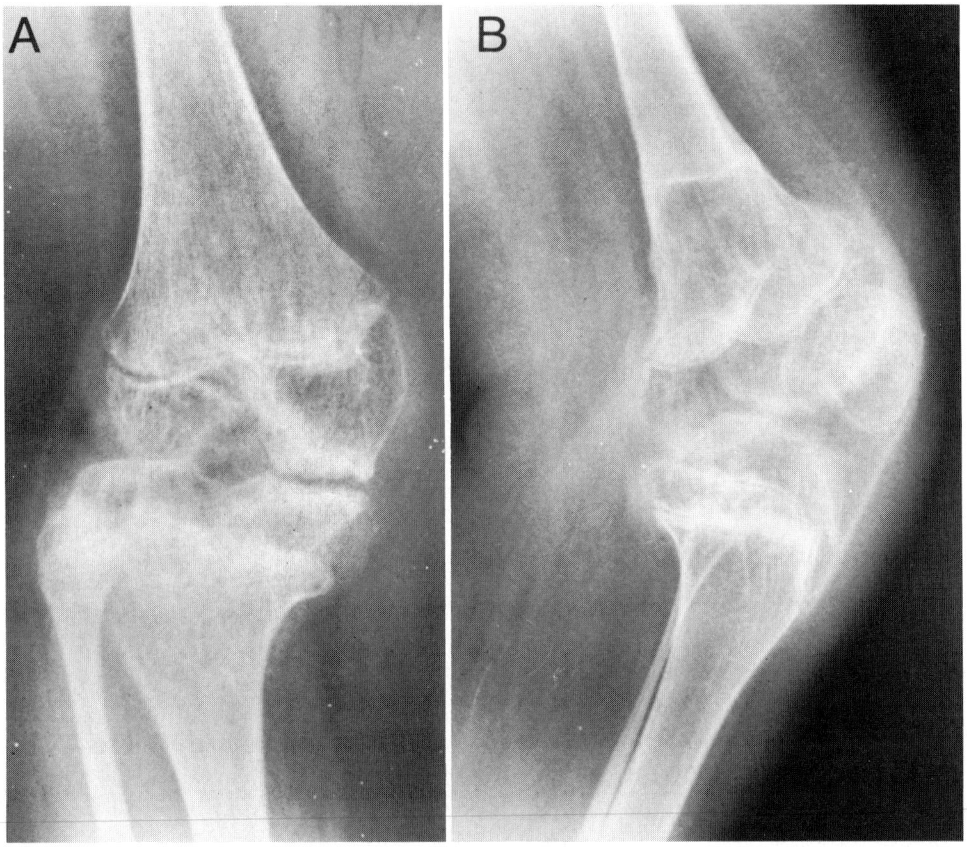

FIG 19–1.
A,B, marked deformity of the knee joint with severe osteopenia in a 12-year-old girl with JRA.

lotomy. Postoperative serial casting is utilized until the contracture is fully corrected, and night splinting with a posterior molded splint for at least 1 year helps to maintain the correction. Clark et al. reported on 23 tenotomyocapsulotomy procedures in the knees of 15 patients with a mean age of 13 years.[4] This procedure was modestly successful in improving pain, mobility, and function over the short term.

Tenosynovectomy

Tenosynovitis in the hand, wrist, and foot may cause significant pain and disability in the JRA patient, and ultimately result in spontaneous rupture of the wrist and finger extensors, and the tibialis posterior tendon at the ankle. The first sign of a wrist abnormality is loss of complete wrist extension and ulnar deviation.[7] Later, loss of metacarpophalangeal and proximal interphalangeal joint motion is seen. Aggressive occupational therapy is the optimal treatment for the vast majority of JRA patients. In severe cases of tenosynovitis, tenosynovectomy of the extensor tendons of the wrist may be indicated to prevent tendon rupture. This may be combined with a formal wrist synovectomy and resection of the distal ulna. Often the severely affected wrist progresses to carpal fusion and ankylosis (Fig 19–2,A and B). It has not been proved that synovectomy can prevent this from occurring. The goal of all therapy should be to maintain optimal functional position for the hand and wrist. Dynamic splinting, resting splints, and occupational therapy are important adjuncts to tenosynovectomy about the hand and wrist.

Tenosynovitis of the foot and ankle, although not as frequently reported, can be a problem in the active patient with a mobile ankle and subtalar joint. A chronically inflamed posterior tibial tendon is at risk for spontaneous rupture. Tenosynovectomy at an early symptomatic stage may prevent rupture. Repair of a ruptured posterior tibial tendon in JRA may be unsuccessful because of the stress of weight-bearing and the poor healing properties of a tendon that is already affected by attrition. Transfer of the flexor hallucis longus may be more effective in restoring medial support to the midfoot. If the subtalar and/or talonavicular is destroyed, a subtalar or triple arthrodesis is the treatment of choice.

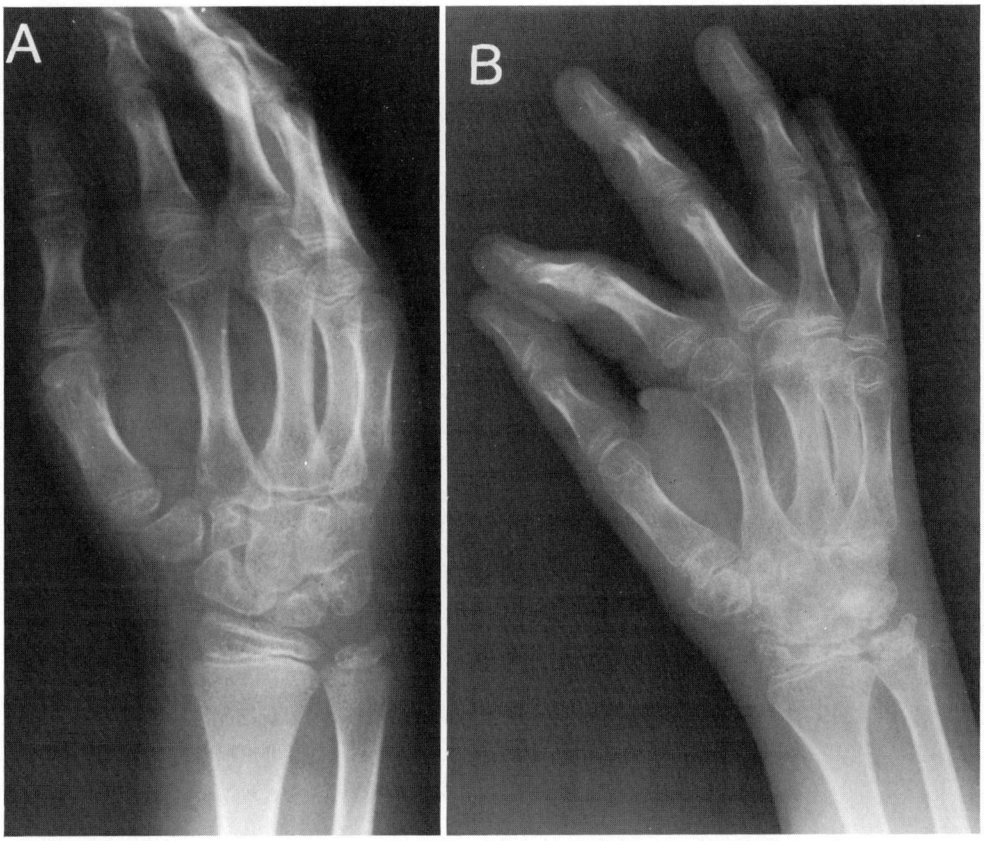

FIG 19–2.
A, hand and wrist of a 10-year-old girl with polyarticular JRA shortly after the onset of wrist swelling and pain. **B,** 2 years later, the patient had wrist stiffness and radiographic evidence of carpal coalescence and radiocarpal degeneration.

Synovectomy

Removal of the inflamed synovium from an arthritic joint is a rational and theoretically preventive measure that has been performed most commonly in the knee. Other less commonly synovectomized joints are the wrist, elbow, ankle, metacarpophalangeal joint, proximal interphalangeal joint, and hip. With the evolution of arthroscopic techniques and instrumentation, both large and small joints may be approached in a relatively atraumatic fashion, and substantial amounts of synovial tissue may be removed.[11, 17] Arthroscopic synovectomy now appears to be preferable to open synovectomy, but long-term follow-up studies, particularly in JRA, are not available.

There are several long-term studies of open synovectomy in JRA.[6, 12, 13, 18, 19] Unfortunately, the results are difficult to interpret because of the lack of standardized reporting and the inclusion of procedures on multiple joints in these reports. In general, most studies indicate favorable early results provided that there is not excessive joint destruction, joint range of motion is normal or nearly normal, and that adequate (>75%) synovium is removed. Patients with pauciarticular arthritis were found to have more favorable results. With follow-up longer than 2 years, the results of synovectomy tend to deteriorate, with recurrent swelling and stiffness being the major problems. Although the stiffness that often complicated open synovectomy was used as an argument against the procedure, it has been reported that patients were generally satisfied with the results. It is likely that with arthroscopic techniques, the procedure may be performed earlier in the course of the disease and repeated as necessary with low risk to the patient and with minimal residual stiffness.

Bone Procedures

Osteotomy

Osteotomy for the correction of deformity in JRA is rarely indicated.[24] In general, it is a poor choice because of the limited fixation alternatives in the osteopenic bone that is often encountered, and because of the extended time that a joint must be immobilized postoperatively. This is particularly true in pelvic or proximal femoral osteotomy. The treatment of valgus knee deformities with supracondylar femoral osteotomy is similarly fraught with problems in that knee stiffness may result if the joint is immobilized. In the case of severe deformity in an ankylosed knee, osteotomy to improve position and facilitate ambulation may be performed, provided that the patient is motivated to walk and is willing to tolerate the inconvenience of sitting with the knee extended (Fig 19–3,A–C).

Resection Arthroplasty

Resection arthroplasty of the femoral head, a salvage procedure, may provide pain relief in patients with severe hip arthritis who are not candidates for total joint arthroplasty. History of hip sepsis, nonambulatory status, and severe osteopenia are indications for considering resection arthroplasty. The advantages of this procedure over arthrodesis are the relatively uncomplicated postoperative care, without the need for immobilization, and the mobility that is preserved for sitting. Hip motion is especially important in the patient with lumbar spine ankylosis.

In severe planovalgus foot deformities that cannot be corrected with bracing or appropriate footwear, surgery may be required to allow the fitting of shoes and to prevent breakdown of the skin overlying the medial malleolus or head of the talus. The treatment of choice is a triple arthrodesis, but in severe cases the talus may actually need to be excised in order to bring the calcaneus back under the mechanical axis of the tibia and to swing the mid- and forefoot medially. It is expected that surgery of this magnitude can be prevented by proper conservative foot care.

Arthritis of the first metatarsophalangeal joint with either hallux valgus or hallux varus is a common foot deformity in JRA. In most patients the deformity is rigid, and may lead to a severely painful interphalangeal joint. Resection arthroplasty of 25% to 50% of the proximal phalanx, and if necessary, the metatarsal head, corrects the deformity and restores partial mobility that relieves the stress on the interphalangeal joint. Nonthreaded wire fixation is useful in holding the correction while adequate fibrous tissue forms at the pseudarthrosis.

Symptomatic clawtoe deformities leading to pain underneath the metatarsal heads may occur in JRA, although owing to the better soft tissue turgor in the plantar fat pad of young patients, pain is not as frequent as in older rheumatoid patients. Resection arthroplasty of the second to fifth metatarsal heads is useful in refractory cases that do not respond to footwear modification. The procedure can be used in conjunction with treatment of deformity of the great toe.

The distal radioulnar joint may become arthritic and cause significant pain on pronation and supination of the forearm. This may be complicated by dorsal subluxation of the distal ulna. If functional impairment results, resection of the distal ulna may lead to dramatic improvement of motion. This pro-

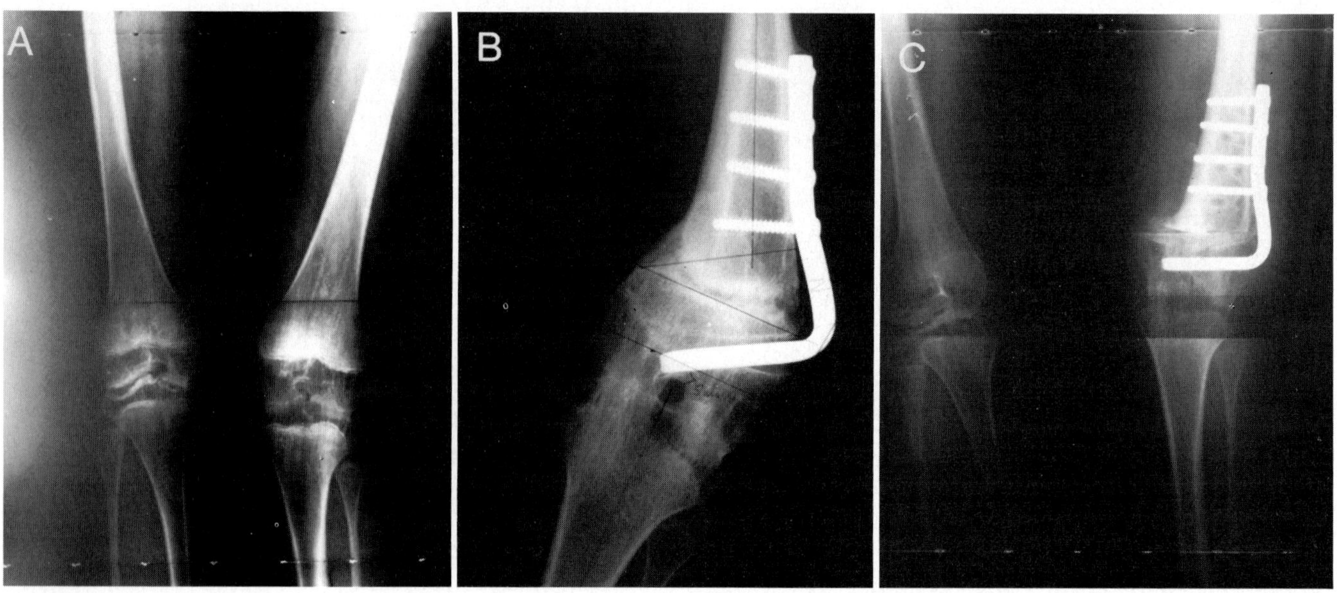

FIG 19–3.
A, a 14-year-old girl treated with supracondylar femoral osteotomy for valgus deformity and ankylosed knee. **B,** nonunion at the osteotomy site with loss of position and varus deformity. **C,** the position of the limb shows improvement after revision osteotomy.

cedure is frequently performed in conjunction with a dorsal tenosynovectomy.

Arthrodesis

Arthrodesis is performed when joint motion produces severe pain, or a joint is ankylosed in a position that compromises function. In JRA the joints most commonly considered for arthrodesis are the ankle, hindfoot, wrist, metacarpophalangeal joint, and proximal interphalangeal joints of the hand.

The ankle is frequently involved in polyarticular JRA, and synovitis of this joint can result in severe pain and disability. Ankylosis in neutral or mild equinus can usually be managed with shoe modifications. Significant equinus deformity can lead to exacerbation of forefoot or midfoot pain. This may be complicated by a flexion contracture of the hip and knee. Ankle arthrodesis that corrects the equinus deformity to neutral is the treatment of choice for this problem. Crossed cancellous bone screws from the medial and lateral tibia help to compress the bone surfaces, and provide rigid internal fixation (Fig 19–4,A and B).

Arthrodesis of the ankle results in increased stress across the hindfoot and midfoot joints. These joints may also be affected by arthritis and be adversely affected by ankle arthrodesis. It is therefore important to assess the whole foot preoperatively, particularly the subtalar joint, to make certain that the pain is in fact arising from the ankle. A helpful diagnostic method is sequential joint injection with local anesthetic. After the painful joint is localized, a short period of cast immobilization may help to predict the effectiveness of arthrodesis. If the ankle and the joints of the hindfoot all appear to be painful, a pantalar arthrodesis is the treatment of choice.

The wrist, when severely affected, tends to become ankylosed in flexion and ulnar deviation as the carpal bones fuse. Conservative measures are usually successful in preventing severe deformity. When the deformity causes significant functional disturbance, surgical correction with arthrodesis should be performed. This may be combined with a dorsal tenosynovectomy if refractory tenosynovitis is present, and distal ulnar resection arthroplasty if there is limitation of pronation or supination of the forearm.

The proximal and distal interphalangeal joints of the hand are common sites of JRA involvement. When deformity or pain cause significant functional impairment, arthrodesis in a functional position is indicated. Crossed smooth wires or small screws provide acceptable fixation alternatives.

Total Joint Replacement

During the past 20 years the art and science of total joint replacement have progressed to the point where even the young patient with JRA can be offered these procedures with increasing confidence. In most cases joint replacement is deferred until growth is completed, but in severely affected patients with polyarticular arthritis, i.e., those threatened with a wheelchair, there may be a justification

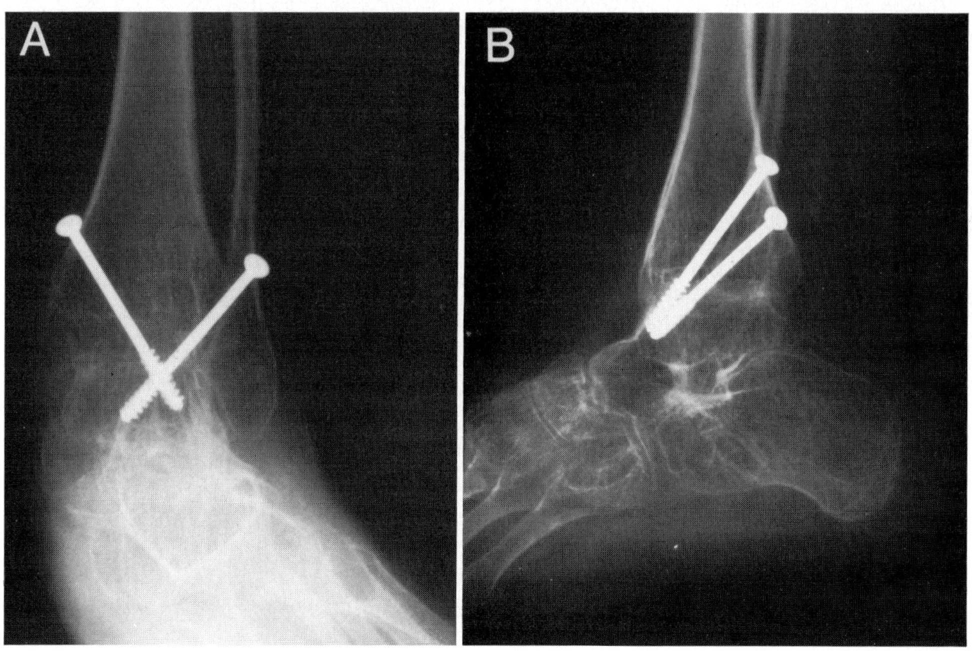

FIG 19–4.
A, a 13-year-old girl with polyarticular JRA who complained of severe ankle pain while walking and at rest. She had previously undergone bilateral total hip and total knee replacement. This anteroposterior (AP) radiograph demonstrates an ankle arthrodesis with crossed cancellous bone screw fixation. **B,** lateral projection of the ankle in the same patient.

for aggressive early treatment with multiple bilateral procedures. This type of treatment has been performed in patients under 10 years old, but it remains extremely rare and should not be undertaken without serious consideration by the surgeon, patient, family, and clinic staff. The most commonly replaced joints in JRA are the hip and knee, and they receive most of the consideration in this chapter. Shoulder and elbow replacement have an increasingly important role in the relief of pain and restoration of function in selected patients, but the long-term results are less certain.

Principles.— Joint contracture is more frequently a problem with JRA than with other forms of arthritis. This often presents a challenge to the surgeon, who should attempt to obtain correction of the contracture intraoperatively at the time of joint replacement. Successful correction of contracture is achieved by releasing soft tissues and resecting bone. In the hip and shoulder most of the correction can be obtained by extensive soft tissue release. Knee replacement requires a judicious mix of both soft tissue and bone resection, with extreme care for the posterior neurovascular structures. The management of joint contracture in the JRA patient is a primary determinant of the surgical outcome in total joint replacement.

The quality of bone in the JRA patient is frequently poor, especially in polyarticular disease. This may be caused by poor nutrition, inactivity, corticosteroid therapy, or a combination of all three. Bone quality should be considered when deciding the mode of fixation and prosthetic design. The fragility of the bone must be kept in mind intraoperatively when placing retractors or performing trial reductions. During maneuvers that apply relatively little stress during joint replacement, ligamentous attachments are more vulnerable to avulsion. Even the utilization of routine pulsatile lavage, in certain severe cases, may unnecessarily destroy metaphyseal cancellous bone around the knee.

The diminutive size of the bone necessitates careful preoperative planning to either assure an adequate inventory of small prosthetic components, or initiate the manufacture of a patient-matched custom implant. A computed tomography (CT) scan is helpful in defining the size and shape of the bone, and is used for computer-assisted implant design and manufacture.

Methylmethacrylate acrylic cement remains important in total joint replacement in JRA because of several features mentioned above. Cement should be used when bone quality is poor. Also, a more equitable initial load transfer to bone can be achieved using cement, with stable immediate fixation that will facilitate early weightbearing. This is particularly applicable in noncustom hip implants that may not precisely fit and fill the femoral canal. The cancellous bone structure of the proximal tibia is often deficient and not amenable to the fixation screws used in most uncemented tibial components. Moreover, residual contracture following joint replacement may result in unphysiologic loading, and accelerate loosening of an uncemented prosthesis. Therefore cement should be considered in any case where prosthetic fit is suboptimal, bone quality is poor, or the initial deformity cannot be completely corrected intraoperatively.

When several surgical procedures on a single extremity are contemplated, it is useful to have a systematic approach to the sequence in which the procedures should be performed. Severe pain usually commands top priority over other functional considerations. If a painful joint is not addressed, the results of all other procedures may be compromised. In general, bilateral or simultaneous procedures are desirable so that the number of anesthetics can be minimized. Anesthesia in these patients is frequently complicated by difficult airway access requiring fiberoptic intubation. Physical therapy progresses more rapidly when painful, disabling joints are replaced at one operative setting than in a staged manner.

In the upper extremity, procedures should proceed from distal to proximal. Adequate function of the hand and wrist is a prerequisite to undertaking reconstructive procedures on the elbow and shoulder, unless a severely painful condition is present proximally. In the lower extremity, reconstruction of the hips should precede knee replacement.[22, 23] Rehabilitation of a hip in the presence of a stiff knee is easier that mobilizing a knee when the hip is stiff. It is also technically easier to perform a hip replacement with a stiff ipsilateral knee than it is to perform a knee replacement with ankylosis of the ipsilateral hip. Other less important reasons to perform hip surgery first include ruling out referred pain to the knee, proceeding with conservative casting or manipulation of the knee during the same anesthesia, and building the confidence of the young patient by doing the less painful hip surgery first.

Total Hip Replacement.— Total hip replacement (THR) is a well-accepted procedure for use in end-stage arthritis. About 90% of all THRs in JRA are performed for systemic-onset or polyarticular disease, and 10% for pauciarticular involvement.[15, 23] Therefore, most patients undergoing this procedure have significant functional impairment, particularly with regard to ambulation. Pain, however, appears to be less of a problem. In one reported series, only 13% of the patients complained of severe pain at the time of surgery.[23]

THR in JRA is a technical challenge because of severe joint contracture, and the distorted bony anatomy. Capsular release and psoas tenotomy are frequently required, and occasionally transection of the iliotibial band and fascia lata is necessary to fully correct the flexion deformity. Acetabular deficiencies are frequently encountered which may be anterior, superior, or central (Figs 19–5,A–D and 19–6,A and B). Anterior deficiency is associated with excessive femoral neck antetorsion, and superior deficiency with chronic subluxation of the femoral head, similar radiographically to congenital hip dysplasia. Central deficiency, or protrusio deformity, results from chronic synovitis and medial bone remodeling. All of these acetabular deficiencies present problems with cup positioning and fixation, and should be corrected so as to optimize hip stability, range of motion, and leg length.

Anterior acetabular deficiencies are usually superior, and if medial reaming is possible, enough of the anterior column can be recovered to provide cup stability. Increasing the socket anteversion will also aid in coverage, but great care must be taken to avoid anterior instability with hip extension. This problem is exacerbated by associated excessive femoral neck antetorsion. Superior bone grafting of defects is rarely necessary in JRA because medial reaming usually provides adequate coverage.

Mild protrusio deformities may be best addressed by reaming the acetabulum to accommodate a larger uncemented socket, while taking extreme care not to destroy the anterior or posterior columns. This procedure redistributes load to the acetabular margin, and moves the center of rotation of the joint laterally. Severe protrusio deformities should be bone-grafted using a bulk femoral head autograft or allograft. Uncemented acetabular com-

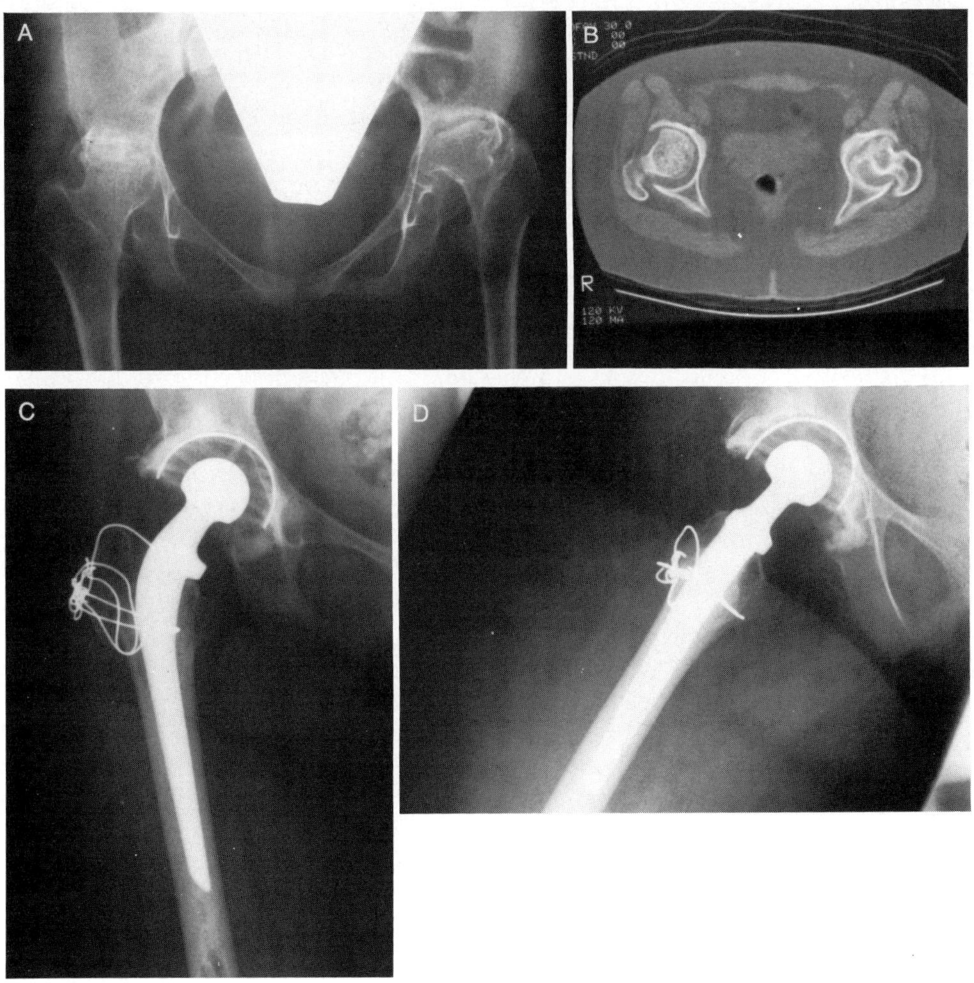

FIG 19–5.
A, AP pelvis radiograph of a 16-year-old girl with polyarticular JRA and involvement of both hips. There is a mild protusio deformity on the left, marked head deformity, and relative sparing of the joint space. The right hip demonstrates marked concentric joint space obliteration. **B,** CT scan of both hips showing the destructive changes in the femoral heads and the relative acetabular enlargement secondary to inflammatory arthritis. Note the thinning of both medial acetabular walls, and the intrapelvic new bone formation in response to the bone resorption inside the acetabulum. **C,** 2-year follow-up radiograph of a cemented right total hip replacement performed with a trochanteric osteotomy. Fixation is stable. **D,** lateral radiograph of a well-fixed total hip replacement.

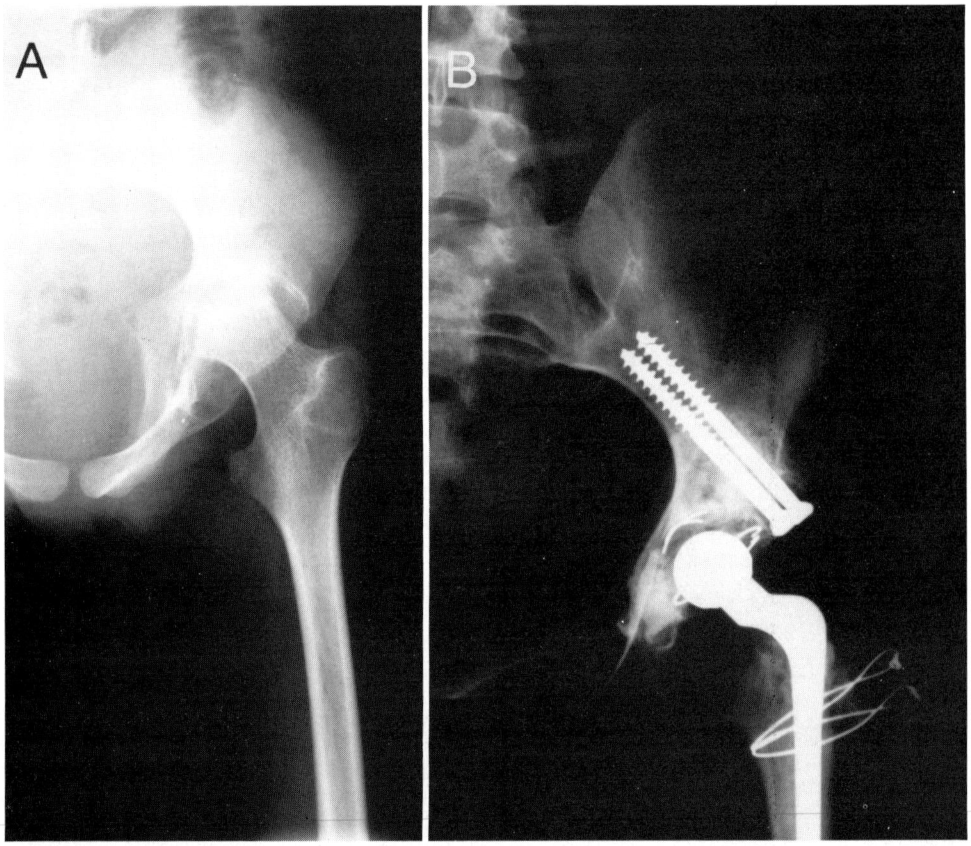

FIG 19–6.
A, a 14-year-old with supermedial migration of the femoral head. **B,** postoperative radiograph at 3-year follow-up. A custom femoral component has been used with bone grafting.

ponents are desirable in JRA, unless adequate initial implant stability is unobtainable (Fig 19–7,A and B).

The distorted anatomy of the proximal femur in JRA often necessitates the use of a custom femoral component. Excessive femoral neck antetorsion, a relatively small femoral neck compared to the medullary canal, and disproportionate growth of the greater trochanter pose technical problems during surgery. Trochanteric osteotomy is frequently necessary to obtain adequate exposure, and minimize the risk of periprosthetic fracture, particularly in the osteopenic patient. If a patient-matched custom implant is not available, a modular system that allows for independent fitting of the metaphysis and diaphysis is desirable.[3] This system also allows for adjustment of neck version to enhance stability and range

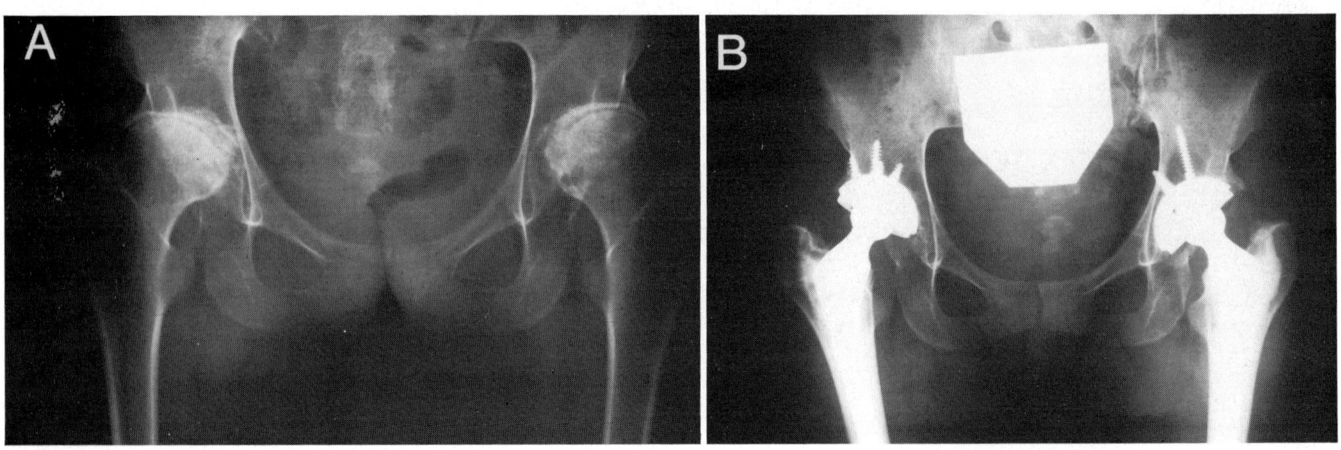

FIG 19–7.
A, AP pelvis radiograph of a 21-year-old woman with polyarticular JRA and bilateral destructive arthritis of the hips. **B,** 2-year follow-up radiograph of bilateral hybrid total hip replacement.

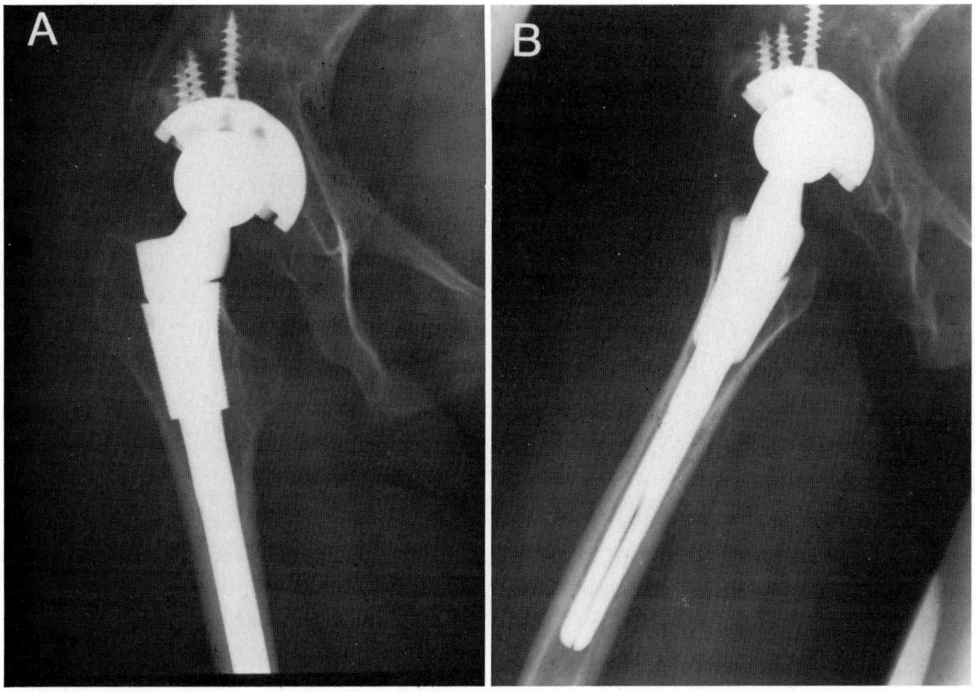

FIG 19–8.
A, uncemented modular femoral component that allows for precise fitting of the metaphysis and diaphysis, and adjustment of the femoral neck version. **B,** lateral radiograph showing excellent metaphyseal and diaphyseal fit.

of motion (Fig 19–8,A and B). Uncemented fixation is indicated in the young patient with adequate bone stock and a good prosthetic fit (Fig 19–9,A and B). Otherwise, cement should be used. In most cases a 22-mm femoral head component is indicated for the purpose of maximizing the amount of polyethylene in the acetabular component.

The results of THR in JRA have been generally good, although they must be interpreted in the light of other lower extremity problems. In one series reporting on hip and knee replacement, 20% of the patients had both procedures.[23] However, pain and function are both improved by THR, even in those patients operated on during the first decade of THR in this country (the 1970s). Loosening of cemented acetabular components is the most commonly en-

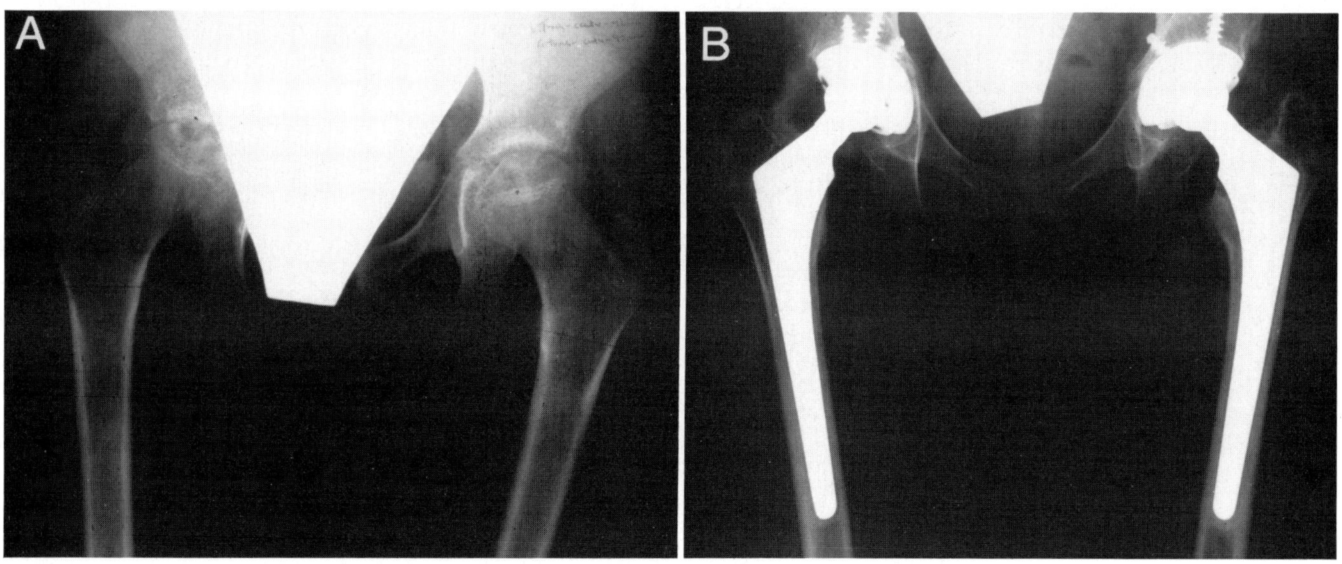

FIG 19–9.
A, a 12-year-old girl with JRA and bilateral osteonecrosis. **B,** the patient was treated with bilateral noncemented total hip replacements.

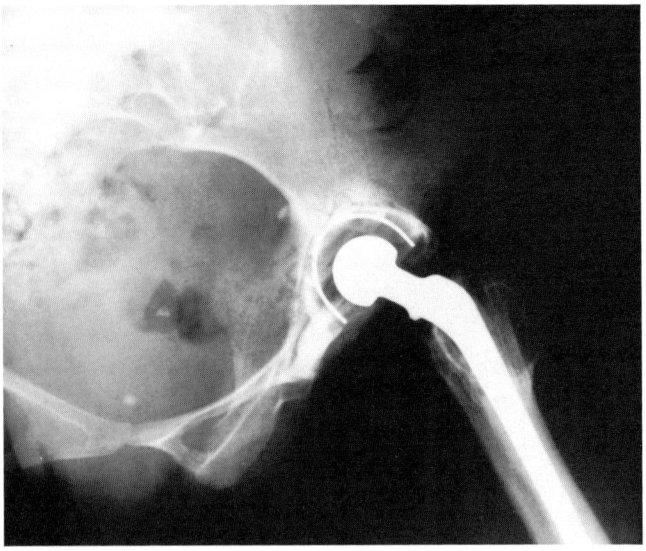

FIG 19–10.
Loose acetabular component 6 years after replacement in 24-year-old woman.

countered late complication.[20] (Fig 19–10). This result is similar to that seen in the adult rheumatoid population. Modern cement techniques and improved design of uncemented implants should help to further improve the long-term results.

Total Knee Replacement.— Total knee replacement (TKR) has been useful in providing improved ambulation and relief of pain in JRA if the deformity is adequately corrected and stability is maintained.[21] Contracture is the most important factor that influences the outcome of this procedure. Often a complete posterior capsular release with a greater distal femoral resection than usual is necessary to correct a fixed flexion deformity. Extensive lateral release may also be necessary to address valgus and rotational problems and optimize patellar tracking. A posterior stabilized prosthesis should be used (Fig 19–11,A and B).

The extensive distal femoral resection and soft tissue release required to fully correct a deformity may lead to unacceptable instability, in which case a constrained prosthesis is required. Resecting a disproportionately large amount of distal femur also raises the joint line and lowers the relative position of the patella on the femoral component. This relationship compromises quadriceps function and may exacerbate the flexion deformity.

There is controversy as to how much postoperative flexion contracture can be accepted. One report on TKR in 17 JRA patients advocates accepting up to 20 degrees, and utilizing serial casting for correction.[21] If stability can be preserved, it is probably beneficial to correct the contracture to less than 15 degrees intraoperatively and avoid postoperative casting. Intermittent dynamic splinting may be of benefit in the postoperative knee contracture.

Total Shoulder Replacement.— Even in the presence of an ankylosed glenohumeral joint, most patients with JRA have scapulothoracic motion that provides acceptable function. When there is severe pain or bilateral ankylosis, total shoulder replacement should be considered.[8, 10] Shoulder replacement has characteristically been more reliable in its relief of pain than in restoration of motion, especially in rheumatoid patients with severe rotator cuff

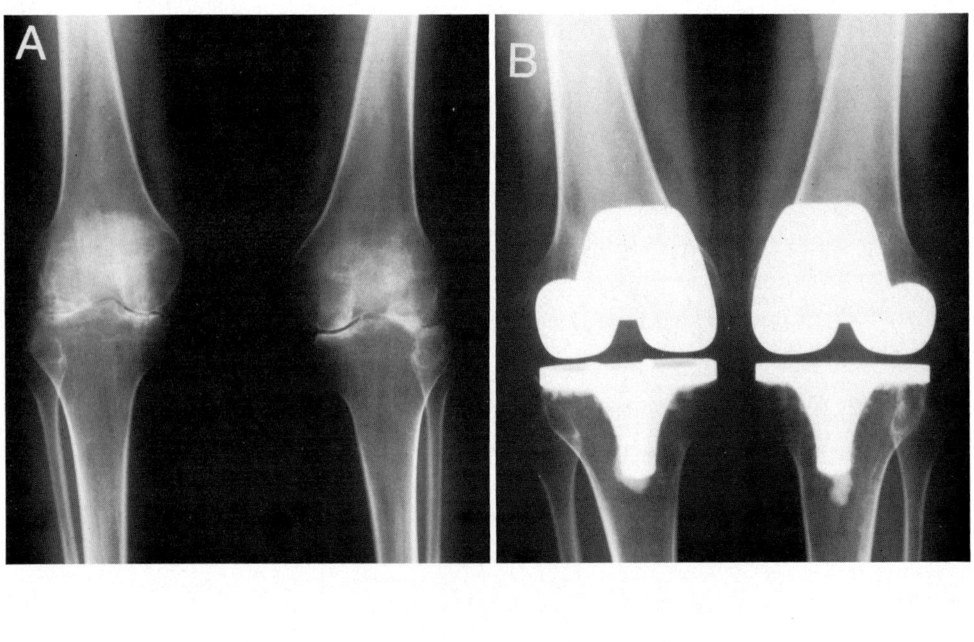

FIG 19–11.
A, AP radiograph of a 21-year-old woman (same patient as in Figure 18–7) who had 30-degree knee flexion contractures. **B,** 2-year follow-up radiograph of bilateral posterior stabilized total knee replacement. The patient underwent bilateral knee replacement 10 days after total hip replacement.

impairment. It is important to clearly define the goals and the range of potential outcomes for the patient and family prior to proceeding with surgery.

The surgical exposure is often difficult, and extensive soft tissue release is required. Retraction should be monitored carefully to avoid stretch injuries to the brachial plexus. A custom prosthesis may be required in very small patients. Short-stemmed humeral components should be used to allow for the option of elbow replacement (Fig 19–12,A and B). Cementless fixation of the glenoid component with screws may be done if bone stock is acceptable and prosthetic fit is good. Otherwise, cemented fixation is indicated. The humeral component should be cemented. Even with extensive soft tissue release and early motion, prolonged aggressive postoperative therapy is required to improve glenohumeral motion.

Total Elbow Replacement.— Elbow involvement in JRA often results in partial or complete ankylosis. Bilateral disease is frequently associated with significant functional impairment. It is remarkable, however, to observe how well these patients adapt to and compensate for the disability. In severe cases total elbow replacement may be considered with the caveat that this procedure can lead to unacceptably high complication rates, wound problems and infection being the most important. Elbow replacement is a rapidly evolving procedure, and there is hope that with more durable implants matched to the patient's anatomy, reliably good results will be seen.[9] Currently an unacceptably high rate of long-term wear and loosening does not allow routine use of this procedure in young patients.

Total Ankle Replacement.— Total ankle replacement is almost exclusively used in rheumatoid arthritis, where patients tend to be smaller, lighter, and less active.[1, 14] It may be useful in the severely affected foot that has an ankylosed subtalar joint and midfoot. Materials and design features still pose grave limitations to its utility. Uncemented arthroplasties are now becoming available as an answer to the problems caused by using cement in this small and heavily loaded joint. Until this procedure evolves to a more sophisticated level, it should not be considered in the JRA patient.

CONCLUSIONS

JRA patients must be cared for in a comprehensive service concept with a clinical team composed of surgeon, rheumatologist, physical therapist, social worker, and, most important, patient and family. The disease is traumatic, both physically and psychologically, and planned surgical treatment must carefully take this into consideration. Surgical treat-

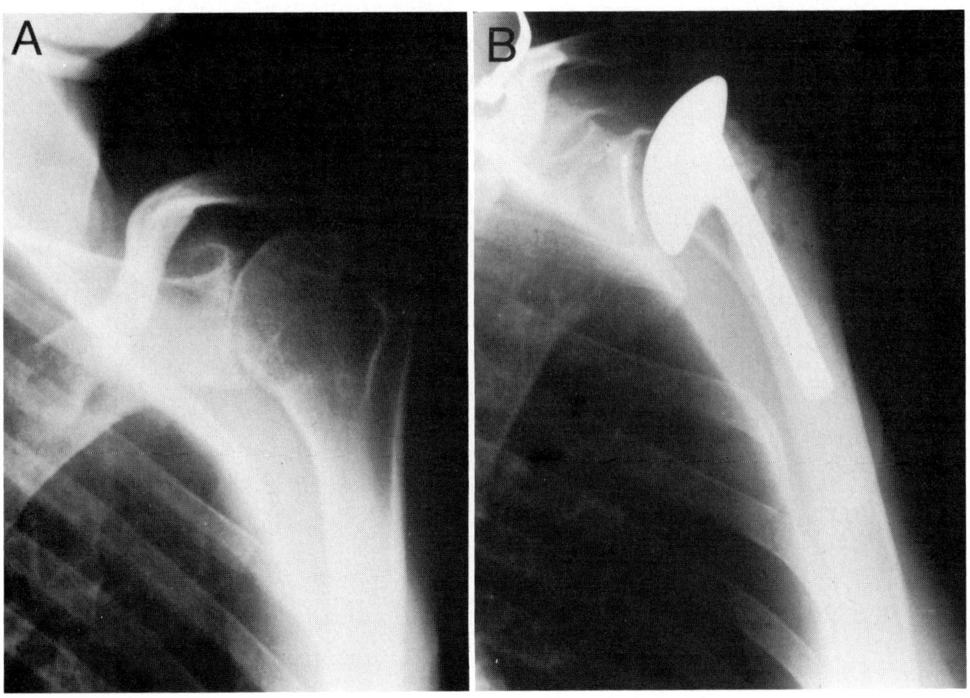

FIG 19–12.
A, AP radiograph of the shoulder of a 22-year-old woman with polyarticular JRA. Marked joint space narrowing, pain, and loss of glenohumeral motion was noted. **B,** AP radiograph in the same patient 1 year following cemented left total shoulder replacement.

ment is complex and complications are devastating when they occur. The need for careful preoperative planning is paramount to avoid intraoperative problems. Implant sizing is often inadequate and custom implants must be fabricated frequently. The comprehensive and carefully planned surgical treatment in the JRA patient will provide marked improvement in pain relief and function in these disabled patients.

REFERENCES

1. Alvine FG: Total ankle arthroplasty: New concepts and approach. *Contemp Orthop* 1991; 22:397.
2. Ansell BM, Swann M: The management of chronic arthritis of children. *J Bone Joint Surg [Br]* 1983; 65B:536.
3. Cameron HU, Bhimji S: Early clinical trials with a proximally-fixed uncemented hip stem. *Contemp Orthop* 1988; 17:31.
4. Clark DW, Ansell BM, Swann M: Soft tissue release of the knee in children with juvenile chronic arthritis. *J Bone Joint Surg [Br]* 1988; 70B:224.
5. Cleveland SE, Reitman EE, Brewer EJ Jr.: Psychological factors in juvenile rheumatoid arthritis. *Arthritis Rheum* 1965; 8:1152.
6. Eyring EJ, Longent A, Bass, JC: Synovectomy in juvenile rheumatoid arthritis: Indications and short-term results. *J Bone Joint Surg [Am]* 1971; 53A:638.
7. Flatt AE: *Care of the Arthritic Hand,* ed 4. St Louis, Mosby–Year Book, Inc, 1983.
8. Friedman RJ, Thornhill TS, Thomas WH, et al: Nonconstrained total shoulder replacement in patients who have rheumatoid arthritis and class-IV function. *J Bone Joint Surg [Am]* 1989; 71A:494.
9. Goldberg VM, Figgie HE, Inglis AE, et al: Current concepts review: Total elbow arthroplasty. *J Bone Joint Surg [Am]* 1988; 70A:778.
10. Hawkins RJ, Bell RH, Jallay B: Total shoulder arthroplasty. *Clin Orthop* 1989; 242:188.
11. Highgenboten CL: Arthroscopic synovectomy. *Orthop Clin North Am* 1982; 13:399.
12. Jacobsen ST, Levinson JE, Crawford AH: Late results of synovectomy in juvenile rheumatoid arthritis. *J Bone Joint Surg [Am]* 1985; 67A:8.
13. Kampner SL, Ferguson AB: Efficacy of synovectomy in juvenile rheumatoid arthritis. *Clin Orthop* 1972; 88:94.
14. Lachiewicz PF, Inglis AE, Ranawat CS: Total ankle replacement in rheumatoid arthritis. *J Bone Joint Surg [Am]* 1984; 68A:340.
15. Lachiewicz PF, McCaskill B, Inglis AE, et al: Total hip arthroplasty in juvenile rheumatoid arthritis: Two to eleven year results. *J Bone Joint Surg [Am]* 1986; 68:502.
16. Liang MH, Larson MG, Cullen KE, et al: Comparative measurement efficiency and sensitivity of five health status instruments for arthritis research. *Arthritis Rheum* 1985; 28:542.
17. Matsui N: Arthroscopic versus open synovectomy in the rheumatoid knee. *Int Orthop* 1989; 13:17.
18. McMaster M: Synovectomy of the knee in juvenile rheumatoid arthritis. *J Bone Joint Surg [Br]* 1972; 54B:263.
19. Ovregard T, Hoyeraal HM, Pahle JA, et al: A three-year retrospective study of synovectomies in children. *Clin Orthop* 1990; 259:76.
20. Ruddlesdin C, Ansell BM, Arden GP, et al: Total hip replacement in juvenile chronic arthritis. *J Bone Joint Surg [Br]* 1984; 66B:141.
21. Sarokhan A, Scott RD, Thomas WH, et al: Total knee replacement in juvenile rheumatoid arthritis. *J Bone Joint Surg [Am]* 1983; 65A:1071.
22. Scott RD: Total hip and knee arthroplasty in juvenile rheumatoid arthritis. *Clin Orthop* 1990; 259:83.
23. Scott RD, Sarokhan AJ, Dalziel R: Total hip and knee arthroplasty in juvenile rheumatoid arthritis. *Clin Orthop* 1984; 182:90.
24. Swann M: The surgery of juvenile chronic arthritis: An overview. *Clin Orthop* 1990; 259:70.
25. Swann M, Ansell BM: Soft tissue release of the hips in children with juvenile chronic arthritis. *J Bone Joint Surg [Br]* 1986; 68B:404.

PART III

Rehabilitation

CHAPTER 20

Rehabilitation in Rheumatoid Arthritis

Sandy B. Ganz, M.S.P.T.

Louis L. Harris, M.S.P.T.

Toni I. Golin, O.T.R.

Nancy Nichols, O.T.R.

CHAPTER 20A

Physical Therapy

Sandy B. Ganz, M.S.P.T.

Louis L. Harris, M.S.P.T.

INTRODUCTION

Rheumatoid arthritis (RA) is a chronic systemic disease with severe musculoskeletal involvement that is characterized by acute and disabling exacerbations. Since the disease is of a chronic nature, surgical treatment of affected joints represents focal acute care in a continuum of the disease. Providers of care to the polyarticular rheumatoid patient will be required in varying intensities depending on the course of the disease. Continuing care of these patients by physical and occupational therapists is necessary during the acute, chronic, and quiescent phases of their disease. During the perisurgical period, physical therapy provides preoperative instruction to the patient in such diverse areas as pulmonary toilet, gait training, dealing with functional deficits in the postoperative period, and plan of rehabilitation after surgery. Preoperative physical therapy provides an opportunity to identify the potential problems that may increase the risk of postoperative complications and enables the clinical team to plan for appropriate home care assistance. In so doing patients have the opportunity to communicate their concerns in these areas, and by the teaching provided by the therapist, many of their fears and anxieties can be allayed. For continuity of patient care, an attempt should be made to have the same therapist see the patient during the pre- and postoperative period.

In the more chronic periods of the disease the therapist is invaluable in instructing the patient on various techniques to improve function. Assistive devices and advice as to methods to facilitate activities of daily living (ADLs), and maintain strength and joint range of motion are given to the patient and the therapist can modify programs according to individual needs and disease activity. Rest is also essential in management of active inflammatory disease and the amount of rest vs. activity is the subject of extensive debate. The proper balance between rest and exercise is the key to successful treatment.[13, 18] The problem-oriented approach to modalities employed by physical and occupational therapists is outlined in Table 20A–1.

PHYSICAL THERAPY MANAGEMENT IN THE RHEUMATOID PATIENT UNDERGOING SURGERY

Preoperative Management

A preoperative physical therapy evaluation should be performed on patients with RA prior to reconstructive musculoskeletal surgery, in order to identify and address potential problems that may occur in the postoperative period. Clinically, the patient's gait is first evaluated for abnormal loading on the affected limb and weightbearing ability with and without assistive devices. Patients with a painful limb will have a decreased stance phase of gait. Obvious limp patterns are documented, e.g., antalgic, coxalgic, and so forth. The patient's gait may then be evaluated more objectively using a stride analysis

TABLE 20A–1.
Physical Therapy Management of Rheumatoid Arthritis

Problem	Physical Therapy Treatment
Acute inflammatory disease	Rest
	Systemic (body) rest
	Articular (joint) rest
	Emotional rest
	Joint protection
	Assistive devices
	Ambulatory aids
	Splinting
	Relaxation, stress reduction
	Patient education
Pain	Physical modalities
	Superficial heat: moist hot pack, therapeutic pool
	Cryotherapy
	Transcutaneous electrical nerve stimulation
Decreased range of motion	Passive range-of-motion exercises
	Active assisted range of motion exercises
	Stretching
Weakness	Muscle strengthening
	Isometric
	Isotonic
	Isokinetic
Ambulation	Ambulatory aids
	Orthotics
	Gait training
Decreased endurance	Energy conservation techniques
	Aerobic exercise program
Difficulty with activities of daily living	Adaptive equipment
	Assistive devices

with a foot switch stride analyzer. Cadence, velocity, and single limb support time are recorded by a waistpack recorder. The state of the art in gait analysis is an automated three-dimensional system that utilizes six video cameras suspended by fine wire from the ceiling. The cameras enable the therapist to view the patient while walking and instantaneously analyze the angles and positions of the joints and overall motion patterns (Fig 20A–1).

The primary role of the cameras is to record special reflective markers that are placed at selected sites on the patient's body to quantify specific elements of the walking cycle. Instrumented stairs are an added feature of this system. Force plates are mounted in the floor and act as a sophisticated bathroom scale. As the patient steps on the force plate a voltage is generated to the computer indicating the direction as well as the magnitude of the forces on the lower extremities during different phases of stair climbing (Fig 20A–2).

The data collected during the testing period emerge on a computer as an animated stick figure that reproduces the patient's movement. The stick figure can be viewed from the front, back, and side. Gait analysis can also be performed at various intervals postoperatively (Fig 20A–3). There have been many studies using biomechanical and quantitative gait analysis on pre- and postoperative functional changes in total knee patients.[1, 2, 23]

Range-of-motion measurements of all joints,

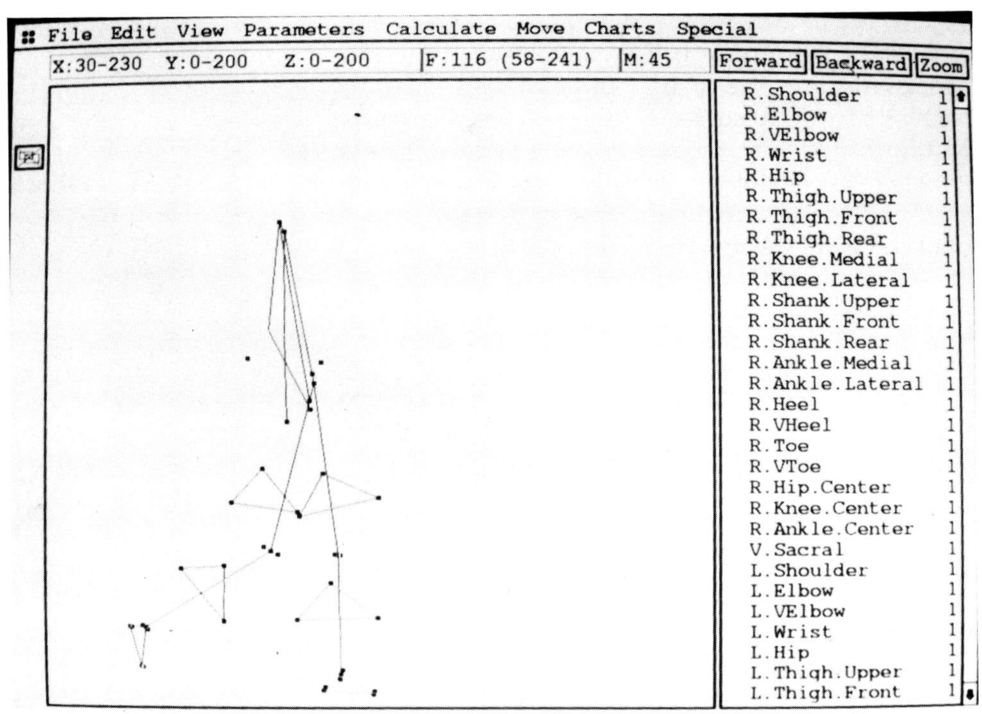

FIG 20A–1.
Three-dimensional gait analysis of ambulation on level surfaces.

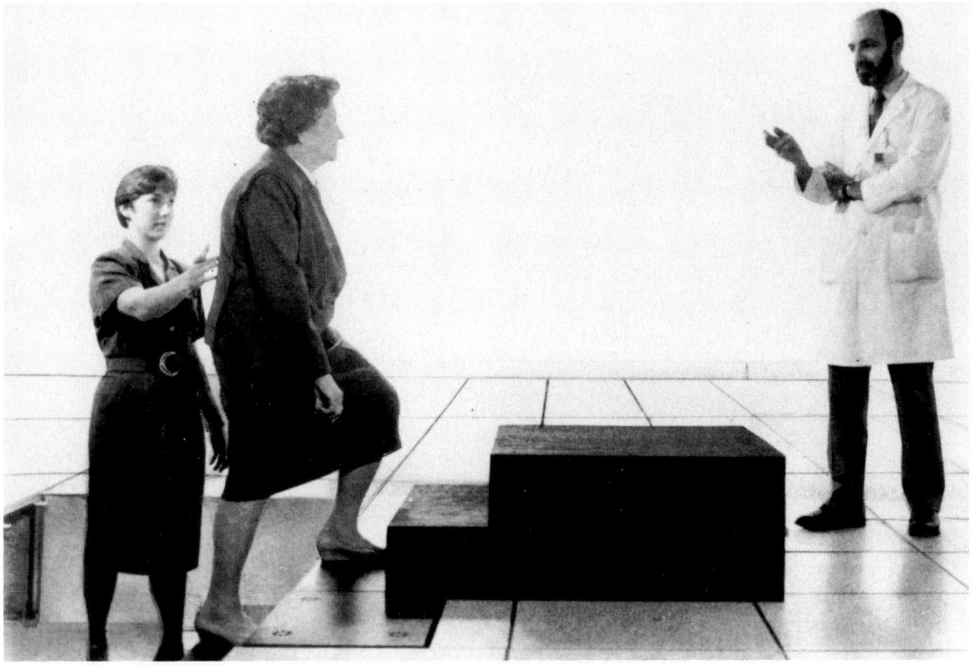

FIG 20A–2.
Three-dimensional gait analysis: ambulation on instrumented stairs.

and gross manual muscle testing of the upper extremities and the uninvolved lower extremity are performed to assess weightbearing ability and to determine the ambulatory aids that will be needed postoperatively. Strength is also assessed biomechanically using an isokinetic system. Cybex,* Lido,† and Kin-Com,‡ are the most common isokinetic systems used today.

The patient's respiratory status is evaluated through ascultation. Assessment of inspiration and expiration is performed using an incentive inspirometer. Following the preoperative assessment patients are then instructed in chest physical therapy, precautions, ambulation, and exercises that they will be performing postoperatively.

In patients with RA who have multiple joint involvement and might need modifications and adaptations, a preoperative assessment is essential in order to avoid a prolonged hospital stay. The following case study demonstrates these concepts involving preoperative modifications of an assistive device.

E.P., a 60-year-old woman with RA and severe bilateral hand deformities (Fig 20A–4), underwent bilateral total knee replacement with subsequent removal of the right knee secondary to an infection. She also had severe genu recurvatum of the left knee and had previously had bilateral total hip replacement and bilateral ankle fusion. She is currently maintained in a Philadelphia collar because of cervical spine instability. The patient became wheelchair-bound because of severe left hip pain from mechanical loosening of her total hip replacement. A revision total hip replacement was necessary, but there was concern as to whether the patient could ambulate with her upper extremity deformities. Custom hand grips were constructed out of dental material and molded to her hands (Figs 20A–5 and 20A–6). These allowed her to use an assistive device to ambulate and she underwent a successful total hip revision. Because this patient was nonambulatory for an extended period of time, and had severe hand deformities with multiple joint involvement, there was considerable debate as to whether to perform surgery. This patient, despite many poor prognostic indicators, was highly motivated, compliant with physical therapy in the past, and therefore an excellent candidate for rehabilitation. Postoperatively E.P. is able to ambulate unassisted on level surfaces (Fig 20A–7).

Total hip and total knee replacement surgery have become common procedures in patients with RA. A more detailed review of the physical therapy rehabilitation program for these patients follows.

*Cybex Corp., Lake Ronkonkoma, N.Y.
†Lido Systems (Loredan Biomedical, Davis, Calif.).
‡Kin-Com (Chatteck Corp., Chattanooga, Tenn.).

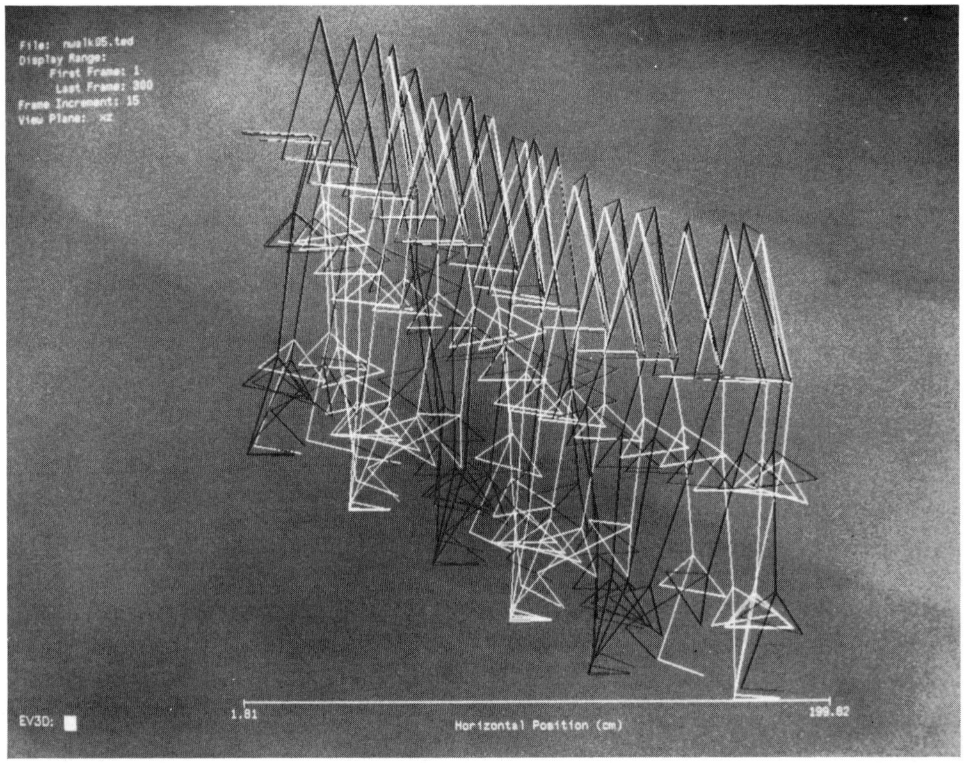

FIG 20A–3.
Three-dimensional animated stick figures descending stairs.

PHYSICAL AGENTS USED IN THE TREATMENT OF RHEUMATOID ARTHRITIS

Various modalities are employed by the physical therapist in the treatment of patients with RA, including the application of heat, cold, electrical stimulation, mechanical traction, and mobilization and massage. These are generally provided to control pain and enhance the patient's physiologic responses, as an adjunct to a comprehensive rehabilitative program. A complete treatment strategy should also include therapeutic exercise, and postural awareness, body mechanics training, and patient education programs.[36] An in-depth literature review explaining the principles and applications of all the physical modalities used is beyond the scope and intent of this section. Instead, the most common agents have been selected and are described.

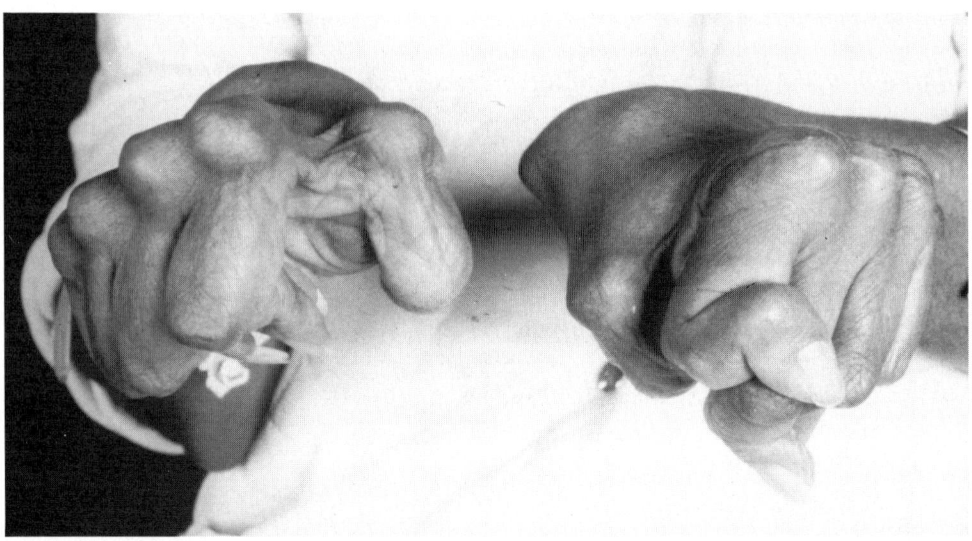

FIG 20A–4.
Severe bilateral hand deformities secondary to rheumatoid arthritis.

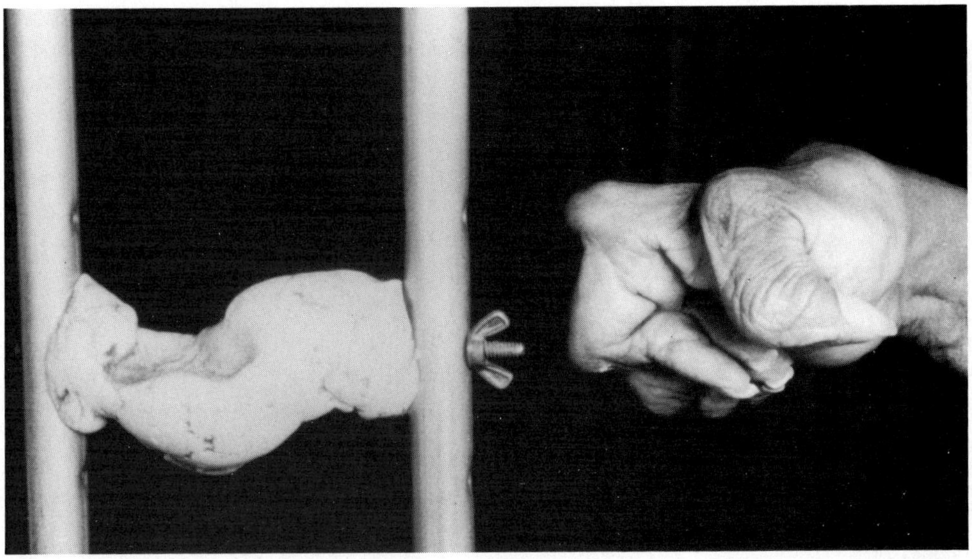

FIG 20A–5.
Molded hand grips.

Heat

It is widely accepted that the therapeutic application of heat produces the following physiologic effects:[3, 24–26]

- Increases collagen tissue elasticity
- Decreases joint stiffness
- Provides pain relief
- Decreases muscle spasm
- Increases blood flow

Superficial Heating

Hot Packs.— Hot packs contain a silica gel which absorbs water. The packs are kept in thermostatically controlled water at 70 to 80°C and are then wrapped in towels for application. They are effective at a depth of 1 cm and increase skin temperature by 10°C. This increase achieves its peak temperature approximately 8 minutes after application.[24, 36, 37] Hot packs, therefore, offer superficial muscle relaxation and may be used to prepare the skin for other forms of treatment (e.g., exercise, ultrasound).

1. *Indications:* pain relief, muscle spasm, decreased range of motion
2. *Contraindications:* local sensory loss, open lesions, malignancy

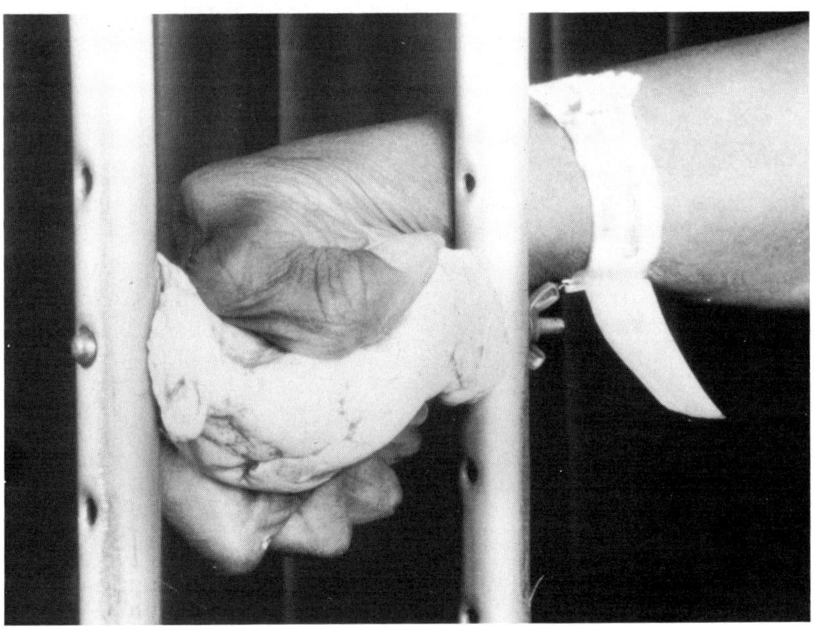

FIG 20A–6.
Molded hand grips attached to axillary crutches.

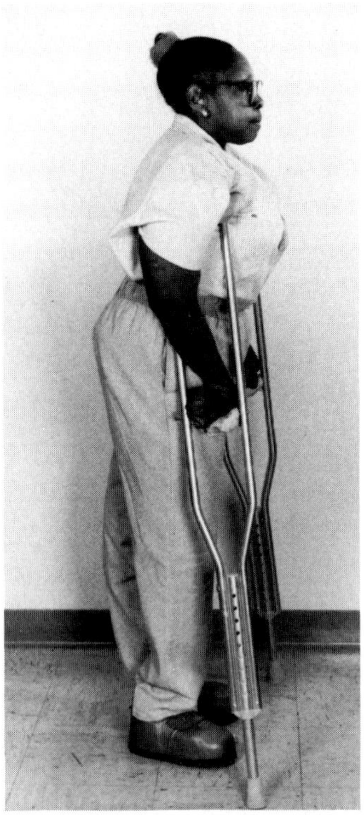

FIG 20A–7.
Patient ambulating independently with modifed crutches.

Paraffin Bath.— Paraffin wax is mixed with mineral oil and maintained at a melting point of 51.7°C. It is most useful in the treatment of arthritic involvement of the hands. The wax mold conforms to the hand and provides heat to all joint surfaces. The heating benefits are similar to those obtained with hot packs.[5]

1. *Indications:* pain relief, muscle spasm, decreased range of motion
2. *Contraindications:* local sensory loss, open lesions

Hydrotherapy (therapeutic pool, whirlpool).— Water is maintained at 34 to 36°C and by eliminating the effect of gravity (buoyancy) excellent moist heat limb contact and exercise are provided simultaneously. Whirlpools for individual limbs (37.7°C) also promote wound cleaning and healing.

1. *Indications:* muscle spasms, pain relief, decreased range of motion, open lesions
2. *Contraindications:* patients with decreased heat tolerance; therapeutic pool: open lesions, urinary tract infections, diarrhea, incontinence

Fluidotherapy.— This is dry application of heat. A bed of finely ground solids (e.g., glass beads, average diameter 0.0165 in.) is blown with thermostatically controlled warm air (47.7°C). This produces a warm semifluid mixture for treatment of the hand or foot. Studies comparing the effective heating therapy of fluidotherapy to that of a paraffin bath and whirlpool found them to be similar.[5, 24]

1. *Indications:* pain relief, muscle spasms, decreased range of motion
2. *Contraindications:* local sensory loss, open lesions

Deep Heating

Ultrasound.—The application of ultrasonic radiation to the musculoskeletal system causes a deep heating response. Energy levels of 50% are observed at 5 cm of tissue depth.[36] Ultrasound has also been demonstrated to raise the intraarticular temperature of the hip joint by 1.43°C after a properly applied dose.[24] Additional evidence indicates that it is safe to use with metal and synthetic implants. Very little increase in temperature has been noted either by the implant or at the tissue-implant interface.[6, 24, 36] Typical patient exposure is 1 to 2 W/cm^2 for 5 to 10 minutes. Ultrasound can also be combined with electrical stimulation.

1. *Indications:* pain relief in a joint or limb, muscle spasm, decreased range of motion
2. *Contraindications:* local malignancy, unstable vertebrae (post laminectomy), pregnancy, spinal cord disease; should not be applied directly over the eyes, brain, or spinal cord.

Cold

Cryotherapy is very effective in the treatment of mechanical trauma by promoting vascoconstriction which reduces the acute inflammatory response. Range of motion and function are improved. It also contributes to pain relief by elevating the pain threshold as a direct result of the temperature reduction at the neural receptors.[27] Cold modalities include ice packs, frozen gel packs (cold packs), and ice massage. Recently, several types of mechanical cryotherapy units have been developed; however, experimental data are not conclusive as to their effectiveness at this time.

1. *Indications:* acute and chronic swelling and inflammatory reactions, muscle spasms, con-

tusions, active arthritis, musculoskeletal trauma
2. *Contraindications:* decreased sensation, sensitivity to cold, Raynaud's phenomenon

Electrical Stimulation

Electrical stimulation is one of the oldest and most effective physical agents. Its purpose is to contract or reeducate muscle, relax muscle spasms, stimulate nerves to promote motion and pain relief, and to generally improve circulation.[21, 34] The use of electrical stimulation to stimulate nerve and contract muscle is well documented; but its general application as an effective musculoskeletal pain-relieving modality has not been conclusively established.[21, 37]

The most widely studied form of electrical stimulation has been transcutaneous electrical nerve stimulation (TENS). Although TENS is not always effective, its effectiveness in acute and chronic pain, sports injuries, and in immediate postoperative management is documented.[12, 30, 33] There are currently available a wide range of types (e.g., AC or DC) and variety of electrical generators (e.g., low-volt, high-volt, biofeedback, and interferential current (IFC) TENS). No one system or model is ideal for all clinical situations and the therapist's choice is dependent on the desired therapeutic response.[21, 36]

1. *Indications:* muscle reeducation, stimulation of denervated muscles, pain relief, increase in general circulation, maintenance of muscle strength during immobilization, maintenance or increase in range of motion
2. *Contraindications:* phlebitis, demand pacemakers, hemorrhage, recent fractures

Mechanical Traction

Mechanical traction is used in the treatment of spinal disorders. It has demonstrated its effectiveness in promoting relaxation through muscle stretching, in relieving nerve root compression, and in promoting pain relief; however, researchers cannot agree on the amount of force necessary to provide a therapeutic effect. For the lumbar spine, a weight range of 60 to 120 lb is recommended.[10, 15, 20]

In the case of cervical intermittent traction, the supine position has been determined to be more beneficial than sitting, with a force vector direction of approximately 25 to 30 degrees in an anterior plane. This allows for a maximum posterior structure separation when applied with a weight of 10 to 30 lb.[8, 11] In RA where there is associated cervical instability, it should not be used.

1. *Indications:* muscle spasm, mild nerve compression, vertebral osteoarthritis
2. *Contraindications:* unstable vertebrae, local malignancy, spinal cord disease, osteoporosis, pregnancy

Mobilization and Massage

Mobilization generally means moving joints, including spinal joints,[29] through a range of motion that is designed to stretch the joint capsule and, in some instances, to move the joint beyond the plane of its associated muscles. The technique is used primarily in patients with musculoskeletal pain.[29] The goal of treatment is to attempt to normalize the joint movement by delivering a thrust with minimum force in the direction of the limitation.[39]

1. *Indications:* joint hypomobility, decreased proprioception, restriction of accessory joint motion, ligamentous tightness, adhesions, joint dysfunction
2. *Contraindications:* ligamentous laxity, unstable joints, osteoporosis

Massage is a widely practiced modality. It is intended to relieve pain, soft tissue tightness, and muscle spasm. It is often used in conjunction with heat or cold. Other forms of massage include acupressure, connective tissue massage, postural integration (rolling), and deep friction massage. By stimulating the skin and local soft tissues, including tendon, ligament, and muscle, local blood is increased and an anti-inflammatory effect is achieved.

1. *Indications:* muscle spasm, decreased extensibility of soft tissues, musculoskeletal pain
2. *Contraindications:* cellulitis, malignancy, phlebitis

POSTOPERATIVE MANAGEMENT FOLLOWING TOTAL HIP ARTHROPLASTY

In the two decades of treating total joint replacement patients, methods and philosophies of rehabilitation have changed but the goals of physical therapy remain the same. The principal goals in the management of any joint replacement patient are threefold:

(1) prevention of disability, (2) restoration of function, and (3) pain relief.[7]

Rehabilitation following cemented and porous total hip arthroplasty (THA) is influenced by the surgical technique and approach used. In our institution the most common approach is posterolateral. Precautions following this approach are to avoid extremes of hip flexion, adduction, and internal rotation. Dislocation may occur in any one or a combination of these positions. When a trochanteric osteotomy is performed, in addition to dislocation precautions, weightbearing is protected for 6 to 12 weeks and active abduction is avoided until the osteotomy site is well healed. The above precautions may be altered by varying component placement. The most common maneuvers in which dislocations have occurred following a posterolateral approach are: twisting in a low chair, where the feet are planted on the floor and the hip is in increased internal rotation and flexion (Fig 20A–8); bending down from a seated position; and twisting toward the side operated on from a supine position. In our institution over 2000 total joint arthroplasty replacements were performed last year, and, 60% of these were THAs. Ninety-five percent were performed under epidural anesthesia.

Patients are brought to the recovery room and placed in balanced suspension slings with 10 lb of weight, or whatever is needed to suspend the limb. Some institutions use abduction pillows and splints which are effective in preventing dislocation, but they are uncomfortable and the patient cannot move about easily in bed. The slings maintain the hip in a supported and stable position as well as balance the pelvic femoral relationship. It is not uncommon for patients using the bed controls to place the bed in an improper position, with the head and foot of the bed in a flexed position. We advocate keeping the bed as flat as possible and locking it in that position. This is recommended for two reasons: Firstly, patients that undergo a THA often have tight hip flexors preoperatively which is not always recognized at surgery and because of postoperative pain the hip is placed in a flexed position. A flat position helps to stretch the hip flexors. Secondly, patients performing bedside exercises with the head of the bed elevated could place the hip in an unstable position and cause a dislocation. In an effort to prevent thrombophlebitis antiembolism stockings are applied within the first 24 hours postoperatively and the patient is instructed on their proper use if limb swelling occurs. After postoperative drains are removed, usually within 24 hours postoperatively, the patient begins performing quadriceps and gluteal setting exercises, supine hip flexion to 45 degrees, supine hip internal rotation to neutral, and ankle pumps. Postoperative exercise programs vary with the surgical procedure used. Depending on the patient's ability and motivation he or she then progresses to an advanced exercise program, which consists of hip flexion in the seated position, straight leg raising, prone hip extension, and hip abduction in standing and lying on the side. If straight leg raising elicits groin pain, it is delayed. Active hip abduction in lying on the side is delayed 4 to 6 weeks postoperatively by some surgeons.

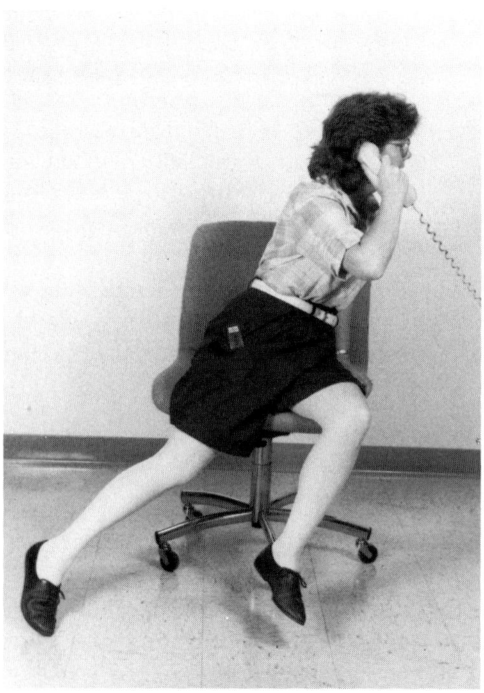

FIG 20A–8.
A hip-dislocating position: twisting to answer the telephone (hip flexion, adduction, internal rotation).

Transfer activities are initiated on postoperative day 1 or 2. Patients are taught to get in and out of bed on the side operated on and if they exhibit good control of the limb on that side they are taught prior to discharge to get in and out of bed on both sides. We strongly discourage the use of the overhead trapeze for transfers, unless absolutely necessary. In our experience the overhead trapeze often leads to pectoral strain, which may mimic the symptoms of cardiac ischemia or pulmonary embolism. Transfer training should simulate what the patient has available at home.

Ambulation is initiated on postoperative day 1 or 2 following a routine cemented or uncemented

THA. There exists controversy over the degree of weightbearing. In our institution, weightbearing can vary from partial weightbearing with crutches to full weightbearing with a cane, with both cemented and uncemented THA. In hybrid THAs, where the stem is cemented and the cup is uncemented, partial to full weightbearing is used for 4 to 6 weeks (see Table 20A–2 for THA protocols). Some believe that loading the bone with full weightbearing is harmful to the bone-cement interface and have their patients maintain partial weightbearing for 6 to 8 weeks.[31] Others believe that loading the bone with full weightbearing is harmful to bone ingrowth in noncemented hip systems and maintain protected weightbearing for 6 to 8 weeks. However, it is uniformly agreed that a cemented or uncemented THA with a trochanteric osteotomy is placed on protected weightbearing with crutches for 6 to 12 weeks. This decreases the load across the hip joint and osteotomy site by minimizing abductor muscle activity.[7, 31]

It is not uncommon for patients to have the sensation in the early postoperative period that the limb operated on is longer, as temporary abduction contractures may result from enforced abduction in bed or from distal advancement of the trochanter. We usually refrain from measuring and ordering a shoe lift for 4 to 6 weeks unless there is a true leg length discrepancy on radiograph.

There is controversy regarding whether patients who have undergone THA should return to recreational activities. Some surgeons allow their patients to return to nonimpact sports like bicycle riding, swimming, dancing, tennis (doubles), and golf. Because of the clinical evidence that impact loading of the prosthesis during certain activities places high stress on the cement-bone interface and can lead to loss of fixation, we discourage our patients from participating in sports that involve running, jumping, and singles tennis.[31]

Prior to discharge from the hospital patients are instructed on proper transfers on an off the toilet, and are provided with an elevated toilet seat. In addition, patients are also seen for a joint physical and occupational therapy session for ADLs and are given a set of long-handled devices consisting of a reacher, sock aid, sponge, and shoehorn.

The two most commonly asked questions prior to discharge are: When can I drive? and When can I resume sexual activity. Macdonald and Owen studied the effect of THA on right foot braking reaction time and found that most patients who underwent unilateral THA had recovered sufficiently by the eighth postoperative week to return to driving.[28] Our patients are told that they may resume driving at 6 or 8 weeks. We advise resuming sexual activity 4 to 6 weeks postoperatively in the supine position to avoid dislocation. Patients are provided with a sexual activity pamphlet and advised to continue to adhere to total hip replacement precautions when engaging in sexual activity.[38]

Once the patient is discharged from the hospital the long-term goals are to develop and maintain gait without abductor weakness or lurch. Prolonged weakness in the hip abductors causes abnormal stress on the hip joint, and these abnormal forces can, over a period of time, lead to implant loosening. As Blount emphasized in an article entitled "Don't Throw Away the Cane," the cane should be used until abductor weakness is resolved.[4] The patient must be conscious of the fact that although the artificial joint causes little or no pain and functions extremely well, it is in fact an *artificial* joint and not a normal joint.

TABLE 20A–2.
Total Hip Arthroplasty Protocols*

Surgeon	Initiate Ambulation (Postoperative Day)	Prosthesis	Weightbearing
Sculco	2	C,H	FWB (cane)
		U	TTWB
Ranawat	2	C,H	PWB (crutches)
		U	TTWB
Galante	2	C	FWB (crutches)
		U	PWB
Ritter	1	U	TTWB
Harris	2	H	One-third weightbearing
Borden	2	C,U	PWB
Welch	4	C,H	FWB (crutches)

*C = cemented; H = hybrid; U = uncemented; FWB = full weightbearing; TTWB = toe-touch weightbearing; PWB = partial weightbearing.

POSTOPERATIVE MANAGEMENT FOLLOWING TOTAL KNEE ARTHROPLASTY

The art and science of total knee arthroplasty (TKA) has evolved considerably over the past 10 years. More than a decade ago TKA patients were immobilized in cylinder casts, flexion was not initiated for at least a week, and the average length of stay was 3 weeks. Flexion is now initiated in the recovery room or on the first postoperative day with continuous passive motion (CPM) machines and the average length of stay has decreased to 8 days.

In 1990 over 800 total knee replacements were performed at The Hospital for Special Surgery in New York City. All were cemented, and the most common were the posterior stabilizer and total condylar types, both of which are cruciate ligament–sacrificing prostheses. CPM is routinely utilized by all surgeons at our institution. Studies indicate that CPM may be beneficial in counteracting the effect of joint immobilization, by improving postoperative venous flow, and in maintenance of articular cartilage.[9, 14, 35] Coutts et al., in a multi-institutional study,[9] found a more rapid gain in knee motion and a shorter hospital stay in patients who had CPM compared with a control group that did not have CPM. Ritter et al.[32] did a similar study but had significantly different results. They found that there was no significant increase in range of motion with CPM compared to conventional physical therapy. The authors concluded that knees that were in CPM felt weaker, noting more extensor lags. In addition, patients appeared to exhibit less endurance because of the confinement to bed to allow use of CPM.[32]

Contraindications to use of CPM are: sensory deficits excluding epidural anesthesia, excessive drainage, and postoperative confusion.[9, 14, 32] Some physical therapists believe that patients with knee flexion contractures should not be placed in CPM. For patients who have difficulty bending in addition to a knee flexion contracture, the time in the CPM should be reduced and a knee immobilizer used at night. For those patients who have knee flexion contractures and are not having difficulty with flexion, CPM should not be used and emphasis should be on extension during physical therapy sessions. A night splint is also recommended in these patients.

It is not uncommon for CPM to be initiated in the recovery room while the patient is still under epidural anesthesia, although some surgeons prefer to begin CPM on postoperative day 1. They argue that the combination of CPM and freshly cut bone combine to produce excessive blood loss within the first 24 hours. If CPM is applied immediately postoperatively it is set at a range from 0 to 45 degrees as the compression dressings tend to kink and create pressure areas on the posterior surface of the knee. After the dressing is removed, which is usually postoperative day 1, CPM is increased to the patient's tolerance. It is imperative that the aides, orderlies, and nursing staff have a thorough understanding of the mechanics of CPM and the proper placement of the limb. We routinely instruct the inpatient nursing staff and recovery room staff on CPM to avoid potential problems. In addition, the patient must be fully aware of the rationale for use of CPM and how to control it.

In an effort to decrease the incidence of deep-vein thrombosis, pneumatic sequential-compression boots are applied to many patients in the recovery room. Haas et al.[16] compared the effectiveness of pneumatic sequential-compression boots with that of aspirin in preventing deep vein thrombosis. The results showed that the incidence of deep vein thrombosis was significantly lower in patients who used the boots. The boots are applied to both limbs in the recovery room. The limb operated on is then placed securely in CPM. The boots are removed only for hygiene, ambulation, and therapeutic exercise.

Many of our rheumatoid patients, particularly those undergoing bilateral procedures, are placed on warfarin. The prothrombin time (PT) is monitored daily by the physical therapist. Normal PT is 11 to 14 seconds. If the PT is greater than 20 seconds, the patient is placed on bed rest, and the knee is removed from CPM and placed in a knee immobilizer. Physical therapy is stopped to prevent bleeding into the joint. Following a routine cemented TKA, three important factors that influence postoperative range of motion are (1) type of prosthesis, (2) preoperative deformity, and (3) intraoperative bone resection.[19, 31] Ambulation, weightbearing as tolerated, and therapeutic exercises are initiated to enhance the redevelopment of the quadriceps. Active range of motion and ambulation are initiated on the second postoperative day. Our exercise program consists of: active, active assisted, and passive range-of motion exercises, quadriceps and hamstring isometrics, straight leg raising, short-arc quadriceps strengthening exercises, patellar mobilization, and stationary bicycle riding. Cryotherapy is usually used in conjunction with daily exercise sessions. Insall[19] believes that quadriceps strengthening exercises are contraindicated during the acute stage of treatment (1–2 weeks) because of the risk of damaging the capsular closure.[19] While bracing is not commonly used, individual cases may dictate the use of an orthosis. For patients who have varus or valgus instability postoperatively, a polycentric hinged knee brace is used (Fig 20A–9).

In patients who have undergone bilateral total knee replacements and have profound quadriceps weakness, knee immobilizers are used. In difficult patients, when flexion is problematic, many therapeutic exercise techniques may be utilized. With the patient in a seated position a 5- to 10-lb ankle weight is applied, or an elastic exercise band is used, in an effort to gain flexion. The patient does not try to extend the knee with the weight or exercise band in place. The intention is to fatigue the quadriceps allowing the hamstrings to contract. Stair stretching exercises are commonly used, and having the patient descend the stairs with the leg not operated on usually succeeds in gaining knee flexion.

During rehabilitation of patients following TKA, extension lags and inability to actively extend the knee to zero degrees are commonly seen. Functional electrical stimulation of the knee extensors can be used to increase quadriceps strength and decrease extensor lag. Haug and Wood at the Mayo Clinic looked at the efficacy of neuromuscular stimulation of the quadriceps during CPM after TKA.[17] They concluded that CPM combined with electrical stimulation in the treatment of TKA patients is a worthwhile adjunctive therapy when muscle reeducation is necessary. For patients who complain of severe pain, and who are unable to achieve optimal flexion, TENS is used in conjunction with heat or cold modalities.

Patients are usually discharged with 90 degrees of knee flexion, and ability to ambulate weightbearing as tolerated with a cane independently on level surfaces and stairs. We allow our patients to return to the following recreational activities: swimming, golf, bicycling, gardening, and walking (see Table 20A–3 for TKA protocols).

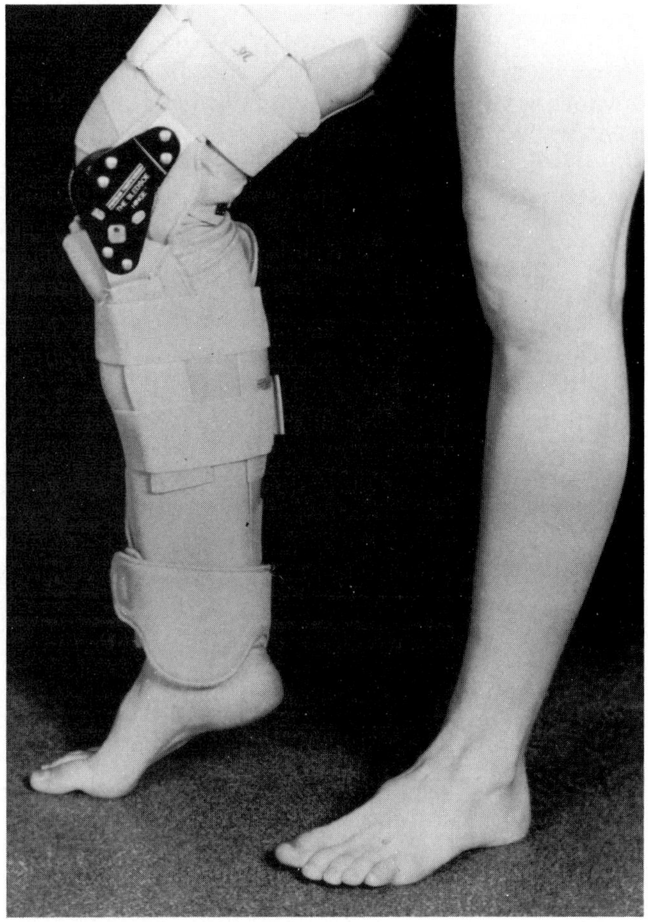

FIG 20A–9.
Polycentric hinge brace (Bledsoe brace).

A very important aspect of rehabilitation during

TABLE 20A–3.
Total Knee Arthroplasty Protocols*

	Initiate (Postoperative Day)				
Surgeon	CPM	ROM	AMB	Prosthesis	Weightbearing
Insall	RR (0–45)	2	2	C	FWB (cane
Sculco	1 (0–45)	2	2	C	FWB (cane)
Ranawat	1 (0–45)	2	2	C	FWB (cane)
Krackow	1 (0–30)	3	3	C	PWB
				U	TTWB
Sledge	1 (0–30)	2	2	C	PWB
Galante	Not used	2	2	C	FWB (crutches)
		5		U	TTWB-PWB
Ritter	Not used	1	1	H	FWB

*CPM = continuous passive motion; ROM = range of motion; AMB = ambulation; C = cemented; H = hybrid; U = uncemented; FWB = full weightbearing; PWB = partial weightbearing; TTWB = toe-touch weightbearing hospitalization is measuring functional outcomes. After total joint replacement, patients rapidly increase their level of function prior to discharge. This improvement in function must be carried out in the face of chronic shortages in physical therapy staff and the fiscal constraints of new hospital reimbursement policies. In our institution it was necessary to carefully measure functional progress to assure that patients achieved the desired level of function in a timely fashion. By consensual agreement of our inpatient staff, functional progress of THA and TKA patients was defined by the attainment of specific

TOTAL HIP ARTHROPLASTY - FUNCTIONAL MILESTONES

DEPARTMENT OF REHABILITATION SERVICES
PHYSICAL THERAPY

DIAGNOSIS__________ PT ______

RIGHT/LEFT/BILAT EPI/SPIN/GEN ♀ ♂

HT(in.)______ WT(lbs.)______

COMPLICATIONS/CO-MORBIDITY/COMMENTS __________

DISCHARGE																					
STAIRS UNASSISTED*																					
STAIRS ASSISTED																					
CANE UNASSISTED*																					
CANE ASSISTED																					
CRUTCHES UNASSISTED*																					
CRUTCHES ASSISTED																					
WALKER UNASSISTED*																					
WALKER ASSISTED																					
TRANSFER UNASSISTED*																					
TRANSFER ASSISTED																					
DATE																					
DATE OF SUGERY: ______ P.O.D.	PRE	1	2	3	4	5	6	7	8	9	10	11	12	13	14	15	16	17	18	19	20

COMMENTS: __________

*UNASSISTED = Not requiring the presence of another person to perform the activity

FIG 20A–10.
A, total hip arthroplasty: functional milestone form. **B,** total knee arthroplasty: functional milestone form.

functional milestones that patients were required to achieve prior to discharge. A reliable functional milestone form (Fig 20A–10,A and B) was used to determine the mean postoperative day of achievement of each milestone.[22]

The milestones that we addressed were transfers in and out of bed; walker, crutch, and cane ambulation; stair ambulation; and postoperative day of discharge. Function was characterized by two levels of achievement: assisted and unassisted. *Assisted* was defined as that requiring assistance from another person to perform the task. This consisted of contact guarding, supervision, and verbal cuing. We did not consider the use of an ambulatory aid as

TOTAL KNEE ARTHROPLASTY - FUNCTIONAL MILESTONES

DEPARTMENT OF REHABILITATION SERVICES
PHYSICAL THERAPY

DIAGNOSIS__________ PT_____

RIGHT/LEFT/BILAT EPI/SPIN/GEN ♀ ♂

HT(in.)_______ WT(lbs.)_______

MANIP/R/L COMPRESSION BOOTS Y/N

VENOGRAM L +/- R +/-

COMPLICATIONS/CO-MORBIDITY/COMMENTS __________

DISCHARGE																					
STAIRS UNASSISTED*																					
STAIRS ASSISTED																					
CANE UNASSISTED*																					
CANE ASSISTED																					
WALKER UNASSISTED*																					
WALKER ASSISTED																					
TRANSFER UNASSISTED*																					
TRANSFER ASSISTED																					
DANGLE UNSUPPORTED																					
DANGLE SUPPORTED																					
CPM (R/L)																					
ACTIVE EXT R																					
ACTIVE FLEX R																					
ACTIVE EXT L																					
ACTIVE FLEX L																					
DATE OF SURGERY:______ P.O.D.	RR	1	2	3	4	5	6	7	8	9	10	11	12	13	14	15	16	17	18	19	20

COMMENTS:__________

*UNASSISTED = Not requiring the presence of another person to perform the activity

FIG 20A–10 (cont'd.).

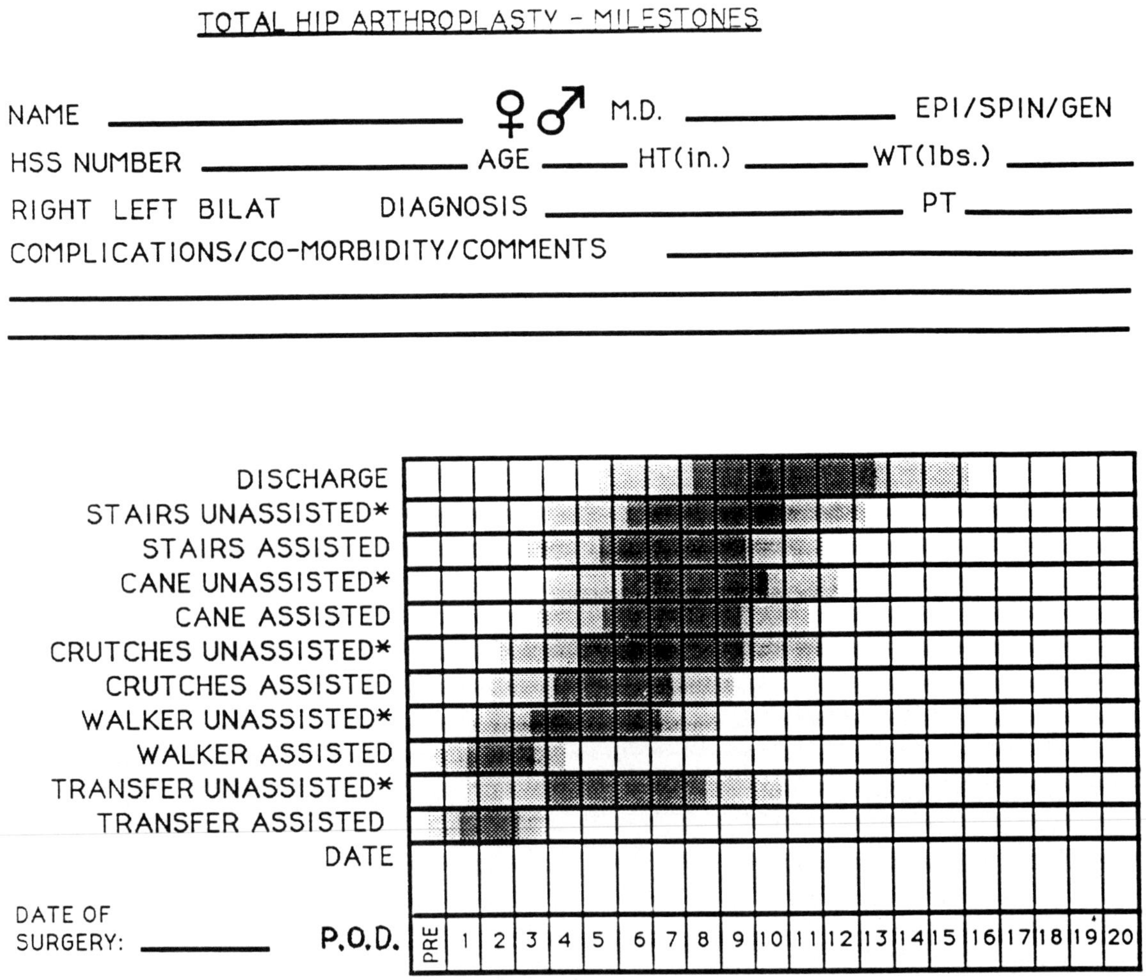

FIG 20A–11.
Total hip arthroplasty: functional milestone form depicting the mean postoperative day of 300 unilateral uncomplicated total hip arthroplasty patients. *Darker-shaded areas* = 1SD; *lighter-shaded* areas = 2 SD from the mean.

"assisted," because every patient was discharged from the hospital with an assistive device. Figure 20A–11 illustrates the functional course of 300 patients who underwent unilateral THA without complication.

CONCLUSIONS

The treatment of patients with RA can be a challenging and rewarding experience, necessitating a multidisciplinary team approach. Treatment programs and goals must be individualized to the needs of the patient with chronic dysfunction.

REFERENCES

1. Andersson G, Andriacchi TP, Galante JO: Correlations between changes in gait and in clinical status after knee arthroplasty. *Acta Orthop Scand* 1981; 52:569.
2. Andriacchi TP, Galante JO, Fermier RW: The influence of total knee replacement design in walking and stairclimbing. *J Bone Joint Surg [Am]* 1982; 64:1235.
3. Bishop B: Pain. Parts 1, 2, and 3. *Phys Ther* 1980; 60:21.
4. Blount WP: Don't Throw Away the Cane. *J Bone Joint Surg [Am]* 1956; 38:695–708.
5. Borrell RM, Parker R, Henley EJ, et al: Comparison of in vivo temperatures produced by hydrotherapy, paraffin wax treatment, and fluidotherapy. *Phys Ther* 1980; 60:1273–1276.
6. Brunner GD: Can ultrasound be used in the presence of surgical metal implants? *Phys Ther* 1958; 38:823.

7. Chandler HP: Postoperative rehabilitation of the total hip patient, in Stillwell W (ed): *The Art of Total Hip Arthroplasty.* New York, Grune & Stratton, Inc, 1987, pp 371–401.
8. Colachis S, Stohm M: Cervical traction. *Arch Phys Med* 1965; 46:815.
9. Coutts RD, Kaita J, Barr R, et al: The role of continuous passive motion in the postoperative rehabilitation of the total knee patient. *Orthop Trans* 1982; 6:277.
10. Cyriax J: The treatment of lumbar disc lesions. *Br Med J* 1950; 2:1434.
11. Deets D, Hands K, Hopp S: Cervical traction: A comparison of sitting and supine positions. *Phys Ther* 1977; 57:253.
12. Ersek RA: Low back pain: Prompt relief with transcutaneous neurostimulation. *Orthop Rev* 1976; 5:12.
13. Ganz SB: Physical therapy, in Spiera H, Oreskes I (eds): *Rheumatology for the Health Care Professional.* St Louis, Warren H Green, Inc, 1991, pp 210–217.
14. Gose JC: CPM in the postoperative treatment of patients with total knee replacement: A retrospective study. *Phys Ther* 1987; 67:39.
15. Gupta R, Ramarood S: Epidurography in reduction of lumbar disc prolapse by traction. *Arch Phys Med Rehabil* 1978; 59:322.
16. Haas SB, Insall JN, Scuderi GR, et al: Pneumatic sequential-compression boots compared with aspirin prophylaxis of deep-vein thrombosis after total knee arthroplasty. *J Bone Joint Surg [Am]* 1990; 72:27.
17. Haug J, Wood LT: Efficacy of neuromuscular stimulation of the quadriceps femoris during continuous passive motion following total knee arthroplasty. *Arch Phys Med Rehabil* 1988; 69:423.
18. Hicks JE, Nicholas JJ, Sweezey RL (eds): *Handbook of Rehabilitative Rheumatology.* Atlanta, American Rheumatism Association, 1988.
19. Insall JN (ed): *Surgery of the Knee.* New York, Churchill Livingstone Inc, 1982, pp 587–695.
20. Judovich B: Lumbar traction therapy. *JAMA* 1955; 159:549.
21. Kahn J: Electrical stimulation, in *Principles and Practices of Electrotherapy.* New York, Churchill Livingstone Inc, 1987.
22. Kroll MA, Ganz SB, Backus SI, et al: A scale for measuring functional outcomes following total joint arthroplasty, in *Proceedings of the 25th Scientific Meeting of Arthritis Health Profession Association,* (abstract), 1988.
23. Kroll MA, Otis JC, Sculco TP, et al: The relationship of stride characteristics to pain before and after total knee arthroplasty. *Clin Orthop* 1989; 239:191–195.
24. Lehman JF: Effects of therapeutic temperature on tendon extensibility. *Arch Phys Med Rehabil* 1970; 51:481.
25. Lehman JF (ed): *Therapeutic Heat and Cold,* ed 3. Baltimore, Williams & Wilkins Co, 1982.
26. Lehman JF, DeLateur BS: Therapeutic heat, in Lehman JF (ed): *Therapeutic Heat and Cold,* ed 3. Baltimore, Williams & Wilkins Co, 1982, pp
27. Lehman JF, DeLateur BS: Cryotherapy, in Lehman JF (ed): *Therapeutic Heat and Cold,* ed 3. Baltimore, Williams & Wilkins Co, 1982, pp 563–602.
28. Macdonald W, Owen JW: The effect of total hip replacement on driving time. *J Bone Joint Surg [Br]* 1988; 70:202–205.
29. Paris SV: Mobilization of the spine. *Phys Ther* 1979; 49:988–995.
30. Pike PMH: Transcutaneous electrical nerve stimulations: Its uses in the management of postoperative pain. *Anaesthesia* 1978; 33:165.
31. Ranawat CS, Figgie HE, Paget SA, et al: What to expect from joint replacement. *Patient Care.* 1990; 24:105.
32. Ritter MA, Gandolf VS, Holston KS: Continuous passive motion versus physical therapy in total knee replacements *Clin Orthop* 1989; 244:239.
33. Roeser WM, Meeks LW, Venis R, et al: The use of transcutaneous nerve stimulation for pain control in athletic medicine: A preliminary report. *Am J Sports Med* 1976; 4:5:210.
34. Rose S, Rothstein J: Muscle mutability, 1 and 2. *Phys Ther* 1982; 62:12.
35. Salter RB, Clements ND, Ogilvie-Harris D, et al: The healing of articular tissues through continuous passive motion. Essence of the first 10 years of experimental investigations. *J Bone Joint Surg* 1982; 64B:640.
36. Santiesteban AT: Physical agents and musculoskeletal pain, in Gould T (ed): *Orthopaedic and Sports Physical Therapy,* ed 2. St. Louis, Mosby–Year Book, 1990.
37. Shriber WJ: *A Manual of Electrotherapy.* Philadelphia, Lea & Febiger, 1975.
38. Stern SH, Ganz SB, Sculco TP, et al: Sexual function following total hip arthroplasty. *Clin Orthop* (submitted for publication).
39. Stoddard A: *Manual of Osteopathic Technique.* London, Hutchinson, 1974.

CHAPTER 20B

Occupational Therapy

Toni I. Golin, O.T.R.

Nancy Nichols, O.T.R.

INTRODUCTION

Occupational therapy provides assistance to persons whose functional level of performance has been altered by physical, psychological, or developmental disabilities. The role of the occupational therapist in the treatment of rheumatoid arthritis (RA) is to improve or maintain the patient's maximum level of functioning. The basic goals of treatment include:

1. Maintenance of, or increase in upper extremity range of motion, strength, and endurance.
2. Correction and prevention of development or progression of upper extremity deformities.
3. Improvement of functional abilities in activities of daily living (ADLs).
4. Patient education, primarily in the areas of joint protection and energy conservation.
5. In the postoperative upper extremity patient, increase range of motion, function, and strength.

The first approach in the rheumatoid patient is the evaluation. Careful observation of the extremity for heat, redness, edema, deformity, pain, and stage of disease process helps determine treatment plans and goals. Active and passive upper extremity range of motion and muscle strength are determined using goniometry, and individual and functional muscle testing. Objective strength measurements can be performed using a dynamometer, sphygomometer, and pinch gauge or computer-assisted equipment. Based on these findings, an exercise program can be designed specifically for the patient. A thorough hand evaluation is performed assessing grasp, prehension, strength, deformity, and pain. Joint stability, crepitus, and muscle imbalance should be noted. This information is necessary also when determining a patient's splinting needs. An ADL evaluation is performed to assess the patient's level of independence. Repeated ADL evaluations over a period of time can help define progression of the rheumatoid disease and alterations in function. ADLs include feeding, writing, dressing, grooming, and personal hygiene, homemaking, and the ability to perform work-related skills. The evaluation measures the ease with which the task is accomplished, and the potentially deforming stresses to the involved joints.

EXERCISE

The goals of exercise in the rheumatoid patient are to strengthen muscles, improve range of motion, and increase endurance, all of which contribute to an improved overall level of functioning. Heat, cryotherapy, paraffin baths, and fluidotherapy are often used to augment exercise programs.

Active, active assistive, and passive range-of-motion exercises, along with resistive exercises, are used with the rheumatoid patient depending on the disease activity. In the acute stage, when the joints are inflamed, rest accompanied by splinting is generally indicated. Active and gentle passive range-of-motion exercises are performed to maintain joint mobility. Isometric exercises can also be performed. Stretching or resistive exercises are often too painful and are not performed at this stage.

In the subacute stage, gentle passive stretch and active isotonic exercises with minimal joint stress can be added to the regimen. Their purpose is to regain lost active joint range of motion and improve endurance. In the chronic stage, stretch at the end of the range-of-motion, active range-of-motion, and isometric exercises are employed. Patients are encouraged to maintain general conditioning and function by performing ADLs routinely.

Hand exercises are done to counteract potentially deforming forces. An adequate grip strength necessary to perform most ADLs is approximately 20 lb, as measured by a Jamar goniometer. With less grip strength patients have difficulty lifting a coffee cup and brushing their hair. Pinch strength of 5 to 7 lb is adequate in the performance of such tasks as writing and holding a feeding utensil.

SPLINTING

Splinting is frequently used by the occupational therapist in treatment of the rheumatoid patient. Indications for splinting include:

1. Immobilization of painful, inflamed joints.
2. Prevention of contractures by maintaining proper joint alignment.
3. Prevention of repetitive stress in a joint during activities.
4. Improvement of function by increasing support and stability.
5. Maintenance of surgical correction.

Static splints maintain the affected limb in an appropriate position. Dynamic splints assist movement in specific planes of motion by applying constant force. Hinges, springs, or outriggers with elastic tension are all used. It is important to fabricate a splint that is both functional and acceptable to the patient. A functional splint that the patient can easily apply is a better choice than a more complicated splint that attempts to accomplish too many goals at once, and is uncomfortable and awkward to use. Also, a splint may immobilize one joint and alter the biomechanical forces on adjacent joints, causing increased stress, and inflammation and pain.

Common problems that may require splinting, the types of splints used, and the rationale for their use are listed in Table 20B–1.

ACTIVITIES OF DAILY LIVING

At any stage of the disease the patient can experience functional limitations in his ADLs due to pain, decreased joint range of motion, decreased muscle power, joint deformity, or fatigue. The occupational therapist assists the rheumatoid patient in ADLs by teaching alternative ways to perform a task and providing assistive devices to maintain independent function.

Feeding

Limited upper extremity function may make bringing food to the mouth difficult. Hand weakness and finger deformity may make it difficult to manipulate utensils and cut food. Utensils with enlarged or extended handles can facilitate the process of eating. Swiveled or curved forks and spoons can compensate for lack of supination and radial deviation of the wrist. When weakness or poor pinch is present, an insulated mug which does not transfer heat permits a patient to bring the cup to the mouth by using both hands. A long straw eliminates the need to raise a glass from the table. A universal cuff can hold utensils when hand use is markedly impaired.

Dressing

Painful and limited range of motion in both upper and lower extremity joints may make it difficult to get clothing over the head or onto the lower limbs. Impaired grasp and pinch loss of fine prehension ability can greatly complicate zippers, buttoning clothing, and pulling on pants. A dressing stick will facilitate putting on and removing shirts when there is shoulder involvement and decreased range of motion. A sock aid and a long-handled shoehorn can assist with lower extremity dressing. A zipper pull and Velcro fasteners to replace buttons (or the top button at the neck of the shirt) are useful.

Bathing

Lower extremity arthritic involvement and limited transfer skills can make getting in and out of the bath or shower extremely difficult. Loss of upper extremity strength and range of motion can make it difficult to reach body parts, adjust faucets, and wash hair. Grab bars and tub or shower seats are

TABLE 20B–1.
Splinting*

Problem	Splint	Rationale
Acute wrist synovitis	Volar wrist cockup (Fig 20B–1)	Provides wrist support while allowing digital movement
Wrist and hand synovitis	Resting hand splint (Fig 20B–2)	Provides support for wrist, MCP and IP joints, and thumb by resting hand in a functional position—for nighttime use, or in acute flare
Carpal tunnel syndrome	Volar or dorsal wrist cockup (see Fig 20B–1)	Holds wrist in neutral position; relieves pressure on median nerve; usually worn at night
MCP-ulnar drift	Volar splint with finger separators; splint can incorporate wrist or be hand based (Fig 20B–3,A,B)	Allows use of hand while preventing ulnar deviation at MCP joints
de Quervain's tenosynovitis	Thumb spica splint (Fig 20B–4)	Splint restricts wrist deviation and thumb CMC flexion, but allows IP flexion and some wrist flexion and extension.
Thumb CMC-MCP synovitis	CMC-MCP–stabilizing splint ("shorty" thumb spica) (Fig 20B–5)	Restricts motion at CMC and MCP joints, but allows motion at wrist and thumb IP joints.
Swan-neck deformity, boutonnière deformity	Figure-of-8 or silver ring splint. (Fig 20B–6)	Applies three-point pressure to restrict PIP hyperextension, and permit, or prevent, PIP flexion

*MCP = metacarpophalangeal; IP = interphalangeal; CMC = carpometacarpal; PIP = proximal interphalangeal.

strongly recommended for safety. Lever-type faucet handles can replace traditional faucets, or tap-turning devices can be placed on existing faucets when hand strength and range of motion are limited. A hand-held showerhead can be placed on the side of the tub for easy access, and can aid in reaching body parts and washing hair.

Homemaking

The common homemaking activities of reaching into cabinets, holding and opening containers, lifting pots and pans, and chopping food are complex for the person with rheumatoid arthritis. Many labor-saving appliances, such as a food processor, are use-

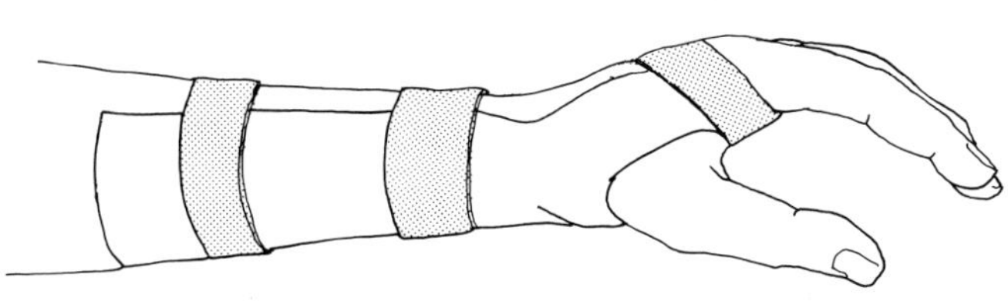

FIG 20B–1.
Volar wrist cockup.

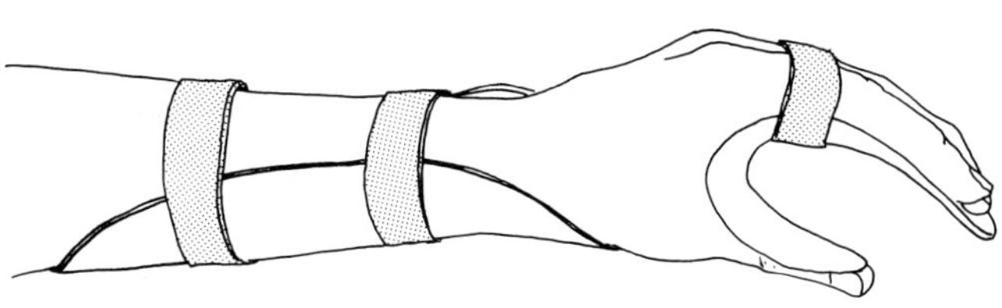

FIG 20B–2.
Resting hand splint.

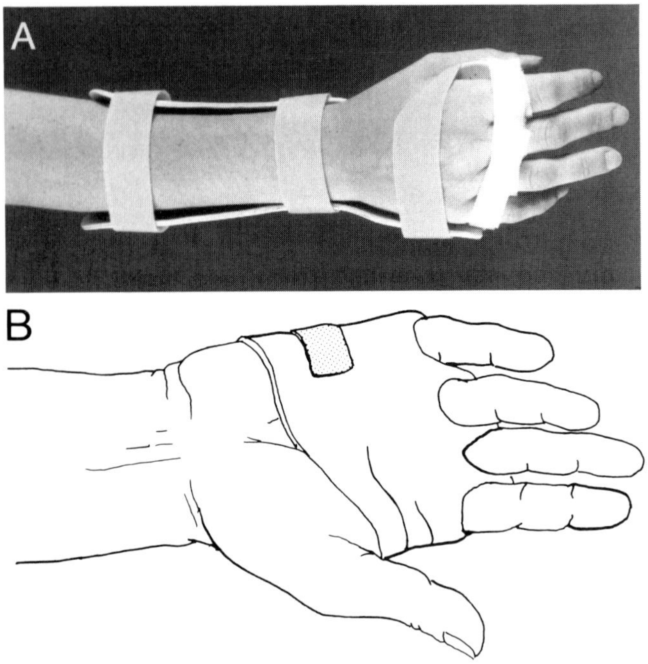

FIG 20B–3.
A, forearm-based ulnar drift splint. **B,** hand-based ulnar drift splint.

ful when lightweight and easy to operate. The use of roller knives and pizza cutters to cut food places less stress on joints. Many devices are currently available to improve ADLs for people with a disability. Many homemaking devices can often be fabricated or adapted by the occupational therapist to meet the patient's specific problems and needs.

PATIENT EDUCATION

Protection of Joints and Energy Conservation

The occupational therapist can instruct the rheumatoid patient in techniques to protect joints. These methods enable the patient to perform his or her daily tasks with a minimum amount of stress on the joints. To preserve the integrity of the joint structures, and reduce pain and inflammation, the patient must be educated in how particular joints work and how forces used during activities can alter their function. Some principles are:

1. Avoid deforming positions.
2. Avoid ulnar-deviating pressures in the fingers.
3. Avoid holding a joint in one position for an extended length of time.
4. Use the strongest joint available for any activity.
5. Let pain be the limiting factor during activity.
6. Design a range-of-motion program to prevent development or progression of a fixed deformity.

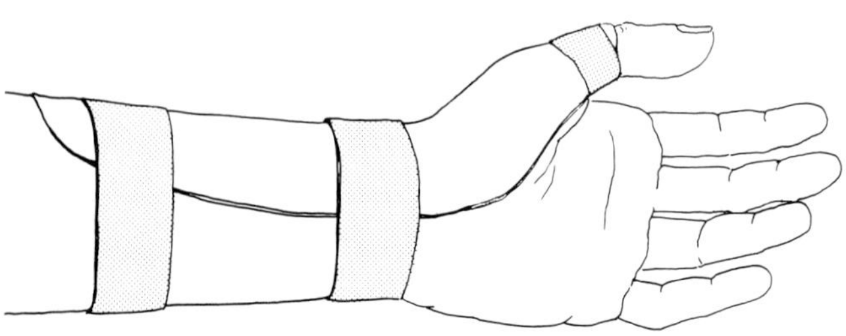

FIG 20B–4.
Thumb spica splint.

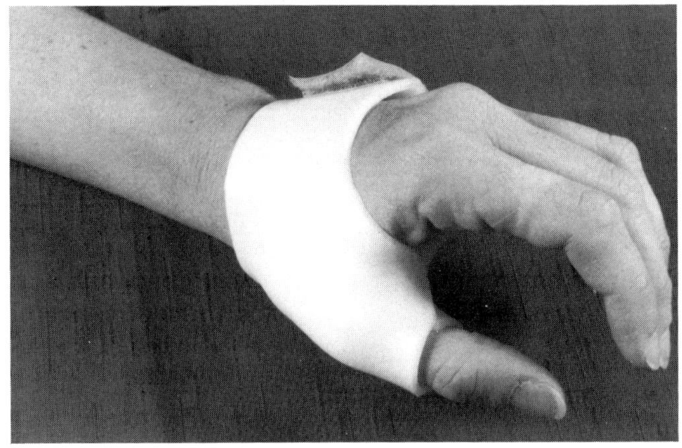

FIG 20B–5.
"Shorty" thumb spica.

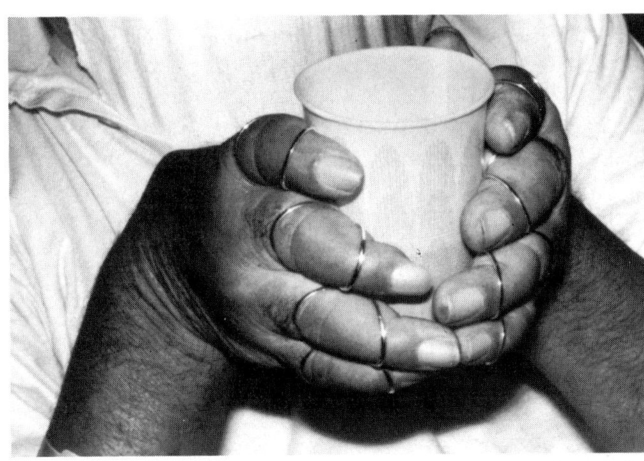

FIG 20B–6.
Silver ring splints.

Energy Conservation

The rheumatoid patient must be instructed in techniques that encourage accomplishment of tasks with a minimal amount of energy expenditure. An appropriate balance of work and rest should be determined for the patient. There is a tendency for patients to try to get everything accomplished quickly on days when their arthritic symptoms are quiescent. Short rest breaks of 5 to 10 minutes during daily activities can be helpful in increasing overall endurance.

Since the purpose of total joint replacement surgery is to relieve pain, correct the deformity, and improve or maintain function in ADLs, occupational therapy plays an important role in the treatment of patients undergoing this surgery. Preoperative evaluation of the patient's range of motion, strength, sensation, and function is invaluable to determine postoperative treatment goals. Since patients with rheumatoid arthritis frequently have multiple joint involvement, deficiencies in other joints may be noted, so that necessary alterations in the treatment procedures can be planned. The postoperative rehabilitation program is reviewed at this time, and therapy appointments scheduled. Information regarding immobilization following surgery can be given so that appropriate plans for transportation, housework, and self-care can be made. If assistive devices are needed, they can be issued at this time to maximize the patient's level of functioning during the rehabilitation phase. A clear understanding of postoperative procedures and realistic planning will reduce many of the patient's fears and concerns.

OCCUPATIONAL THERAPY FOLLOWING TOTAL JOINT REPLACEMENT SURGERY

Treatment guidelines and considerations in the management of patients following total shoulder replacement, total elbow replacement, and metacarpophalangeal (MCP) joint replacement are outlined below. Treatments may vary depending on the surgical approach and modifications.

Total Shoulder Replacements

Treatment goals following total shoulder replacement are pain relief and improved functional use of the extremity. During the initial week following surgery, the extremity is maintained in an immobilizer. Pendulum exercises are initiated with the immobilizer removed, the elbow bent, and the arm supported by the therapist, if necessary. In a supine position, with a pillow wedge placed under the elbow to avoid shoulder hyperextension, gentle passive forward flexion is performed to the patient's tolerance and externally rotated to neutral with the arm at zero degrees abduction. Care should be taken at this phase to encourage normal motion, as well as to avoid compensatory movement patterns. This can only be achieved if the extremity is moved within a pain-free arc. Range-of-motion exercises are performed to distal joints to prevent stiffness from disuse. Massage and other edema-reducing methods may be administered to control postoperative swelling. Overhead pulleys can be installed at bedside and performed three or four times daily for 5- to 10-minute sessions. The incision is monitored on a daily basis for drainage.

Patients are discharged from the hospital approximately 1 week following surgery. Outpatient therapy continues two to three times weekly. The patient is instructed in a home exercise program including pendulum exercise with the elbow extended, active assisted forward flexion, and external rotation to neutral in the supine position, and assisted extension using a dowel stick (wand exercises) is performed three or four times daily (Figs 20B–7,A and B). The use of a sling is decreased at this time and gradually discontinued.

Dowel exercises continue into the second week with assisted horizontal abduction and abduction, external rotation beyond neutral as tolerated with the arm held at zero degrees abduction, and assisted internal rotation. Isometric strengthening of the deltoids and internal and external rotators is initiated. After week 2, exercise continues as above with additions as follows:

1. Active forward flexion in the supine position with the elbow flexed.
2. Active forward flexion raising the arm from the table top.
3. Gradual increase of activities progressing from the supine to the vertical position, with care taken to avoid compensatory movements.
4. The main emphasis is on flexion and external rotation.

By week 3 strengthening exercises using the Theraband and light resistive exercises can be initiated

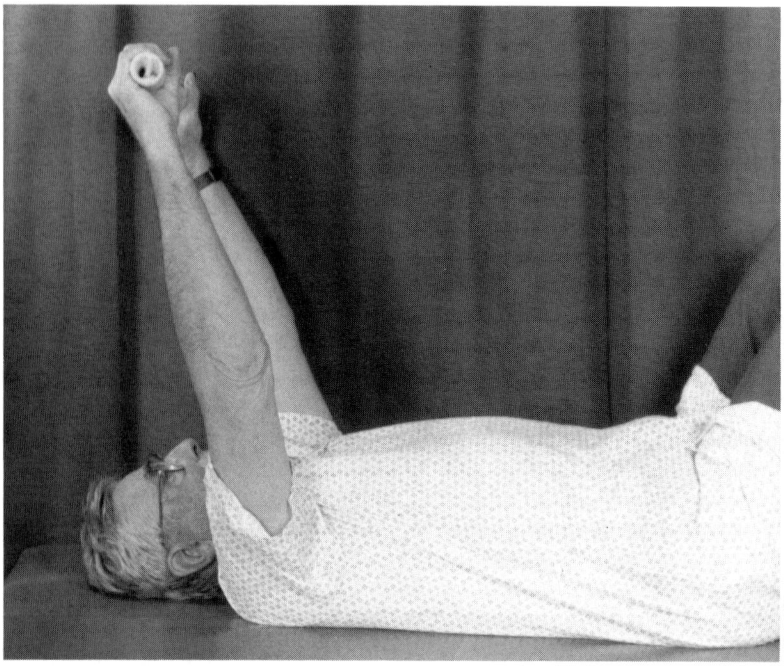

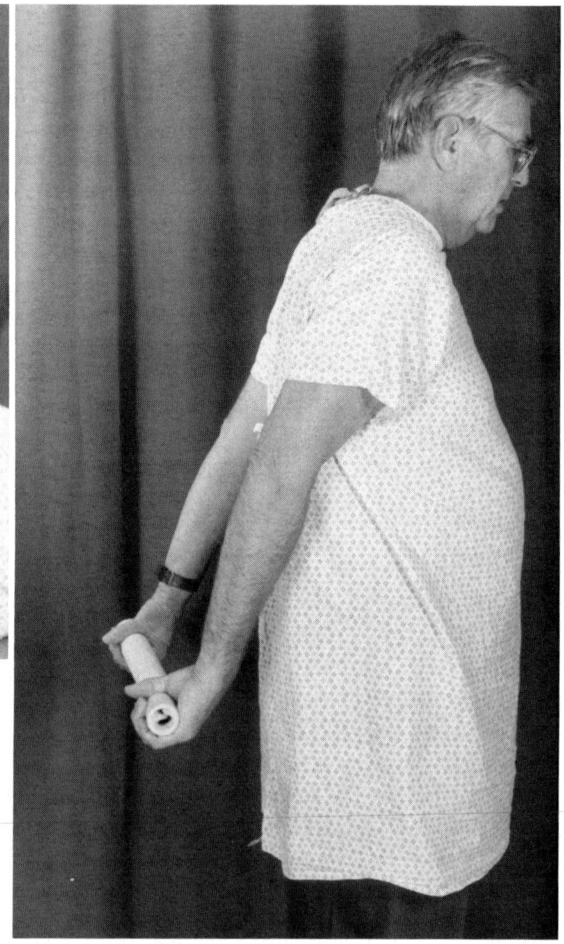

FIG 20B–7.
Wand exercises for assisted forward flexion **(A)** and assisted extension **(B).**

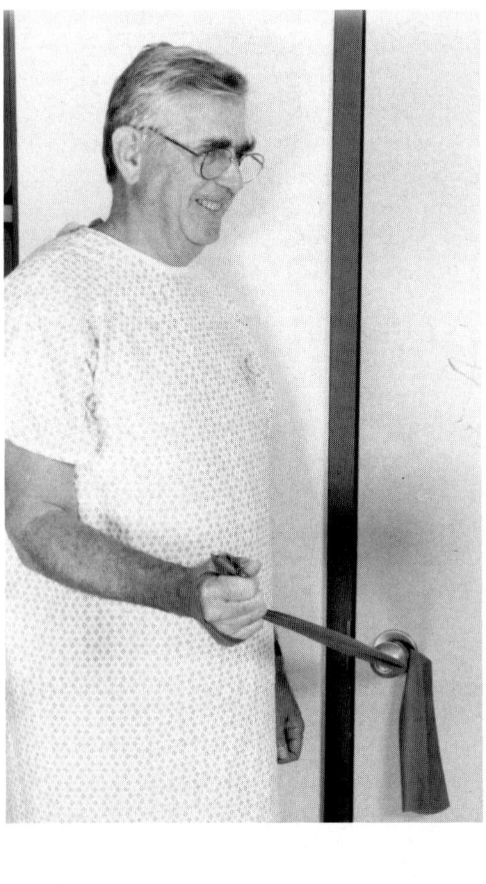

FIG 20B–8.
Theraband exercise for external rotators.

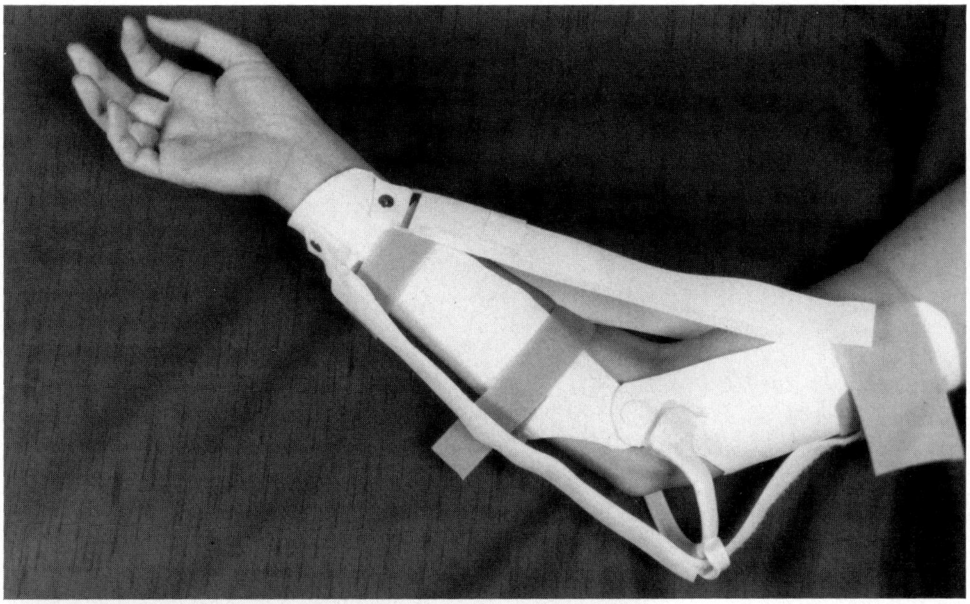

FIG 20B–9.
Flexible hinge splint for total elbow replacement.

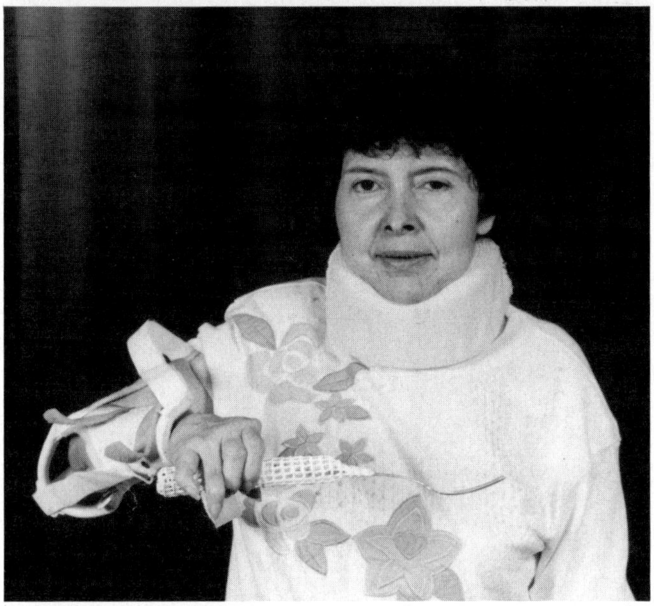

FIG 20B–10.
A long-handled fork used for self-feeding following total elbow replacement.

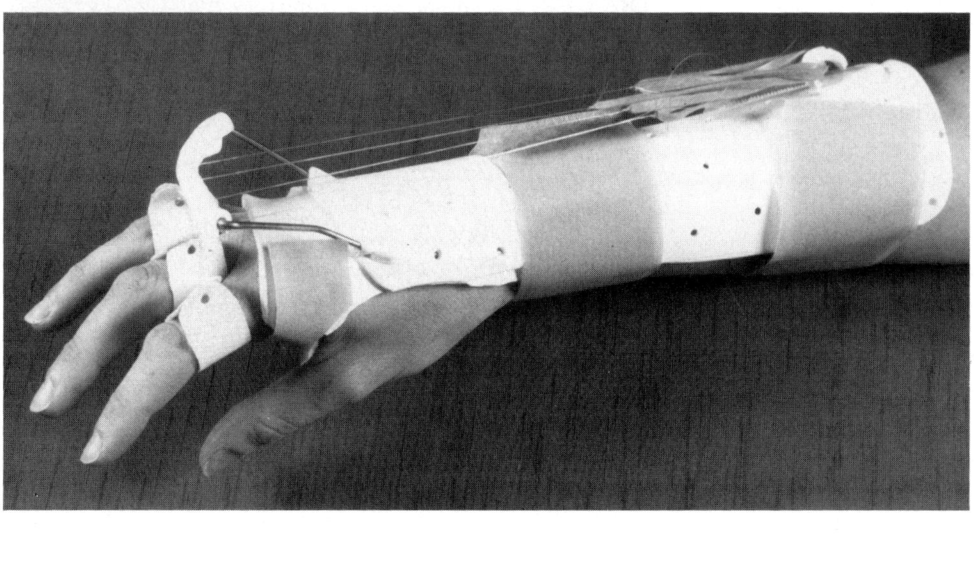

FIG 20B–11.
Dynamic metacarpophalangeal extension splint used following arthroplasty.

(Fig 20B–8). The outpatient therapy program continues for approximately 3 months and the patient is encouraged to continue with a modified program of daily exercises for 6 months to gain muscle strength and endurance for normal activities.

Total Elbow Replacement

Following total elbow replacement, patients are seen on postoperative day 3 or 4 depending on the amount of swelling and the status of the incision. Treatment goals are decreased pain and increased range of motion. A flexible hinge splint is fabricated that allows flexion and extension in a fixed neutral plane (Fig 20B–9), and exercises are initiated. The initial emphasis is on active flexion and assisted extension, thus protecting the triceps muscle which was partially detached and repaired. Active assisted exercises are started to promote forearm rotation. Active elbow extension is gradually encouraged, as tolerated by the patient, usually 2 or 3 days after therapy begins.

Within the first week on a therapy program, patients are encouraged to perform light ADLs within the dynamic splint. Adapted devices may be fabricated to assist with ADLs when initial range of motion is limited. For example, long-handled feeding utensils may be necessary to aid in self-feeding (Fig 20B–10). These may be altered as range of motion improves. By week 4 therapy has progressed to light resistive elbow flexion and isometric extension, as tolerated. The dynamic splint is worn at all times,

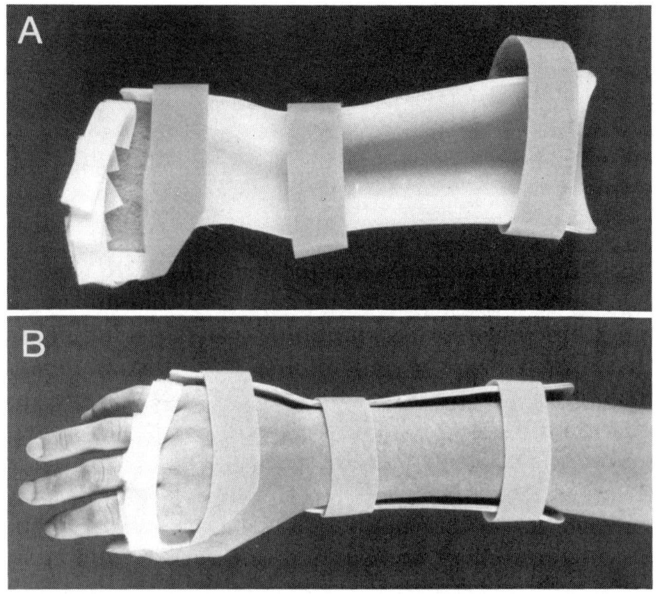

FIG 20B–13.
A, resting splint with finger separators. **B,** resting splint being worn by a patient.

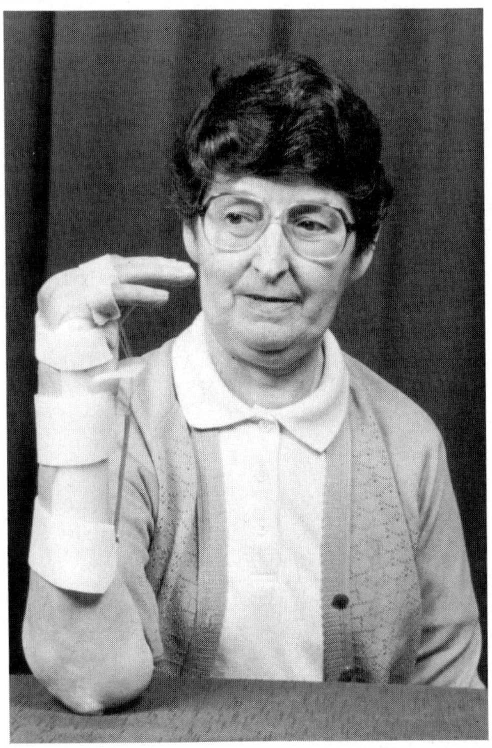

FIG 20B–12.
Dynamic metacarpophalangeal flexion splint used following arthroplasty.

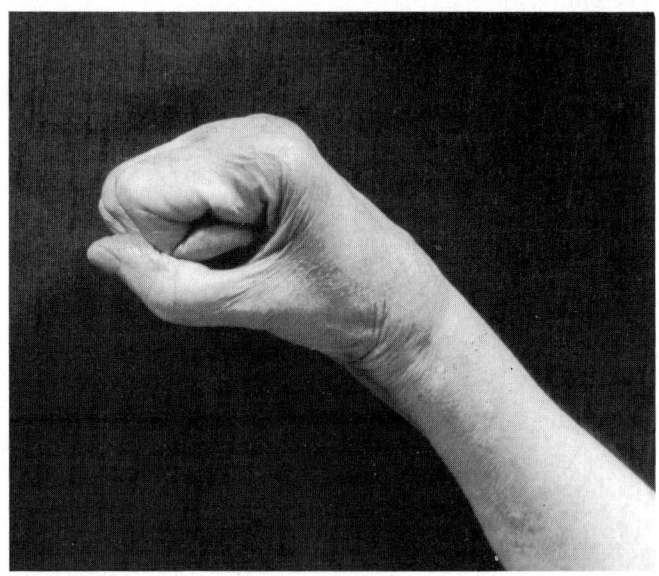

FIG 20B–14.
Significantly improved range of motion following metacarpophalangeal arthroplasty.

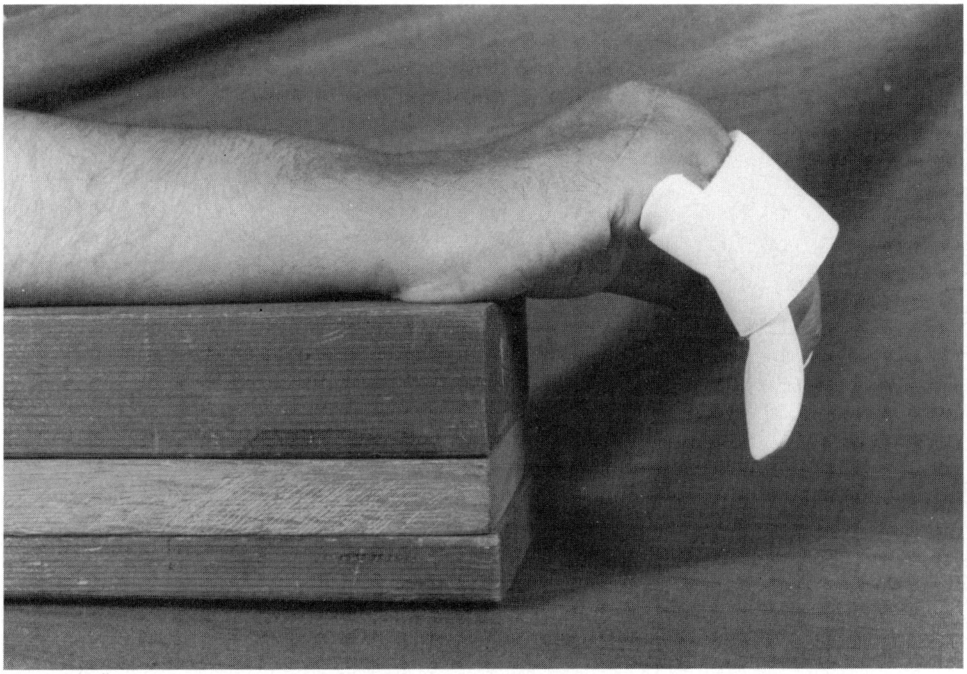

FIG 20B–15.
Proximal interphalangeal block splint to assist in methcarpophalangeal flexion exercise.

except for exercise and personal hygiene. The adjustable straps allow the splint to be set at varying degrees of elbow flexion or extension and is maintained during the night in the position most lacking in range of motion.

In our experience patients achieve good functional range of motion following this procedure, but overzealous exercises can compromise triceps repair and healing of the incision and should be avoided.

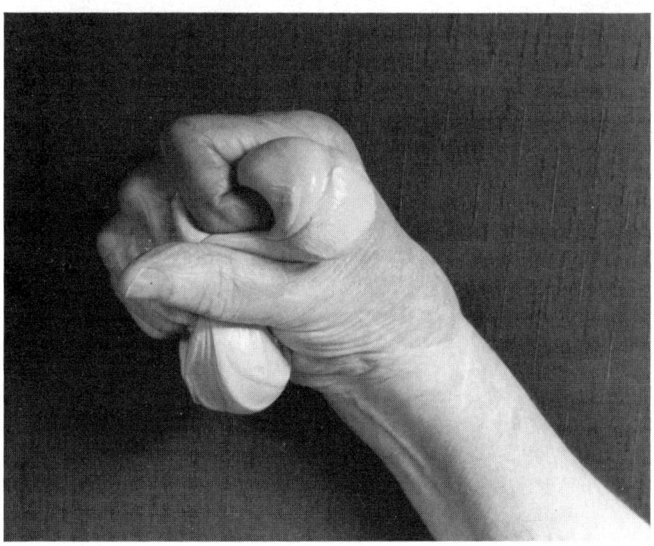

FIG 20B–16.
Exercise to increase hand strength.

Metacarpophalangeal Arthroplasty

Treatment goals following MCP arthroplasty are relief of pain, improved cosmesis, improved digital alignment, and stability. Therapy begins when the bulky dressing is removed 4 days following surgery if postoperative swelling has decreased. Patients are fitted with thermoplastic splints to position and control joint movement during the encapsulation process and instructed to elevate the extremity for control of edema. A dorsal dynamic MCP extension splint is fabricated to hold the MCP joint in zero degrees extension and radial deviation (Fig 20B–11). The splint's pulley system is constructed of a nylon cord attached to finger slings, within rubber bands at the proximal hook attachment. Attempts should be made to maintain the joint in extension with the least amount of force necessary, so that the patient is able to flex the joint with the splint. The exterior of the sling is made of plastic and the interior is lined with moleskin. Moleskin is comfortable and is easily replaced when soiled. The splint should be worn continuously throughout the day except for periods of exercise and personal hygiene. The patient should be able to remove the finger slings while keeping the dorsal splint intact to perform exercises, then to reapply the slings following exercise. A dynamic flexion splint is fabricated to hold the MCP joints in a flexed position during nighttime (Fig 20B–12). The splint is constructed with moleskin

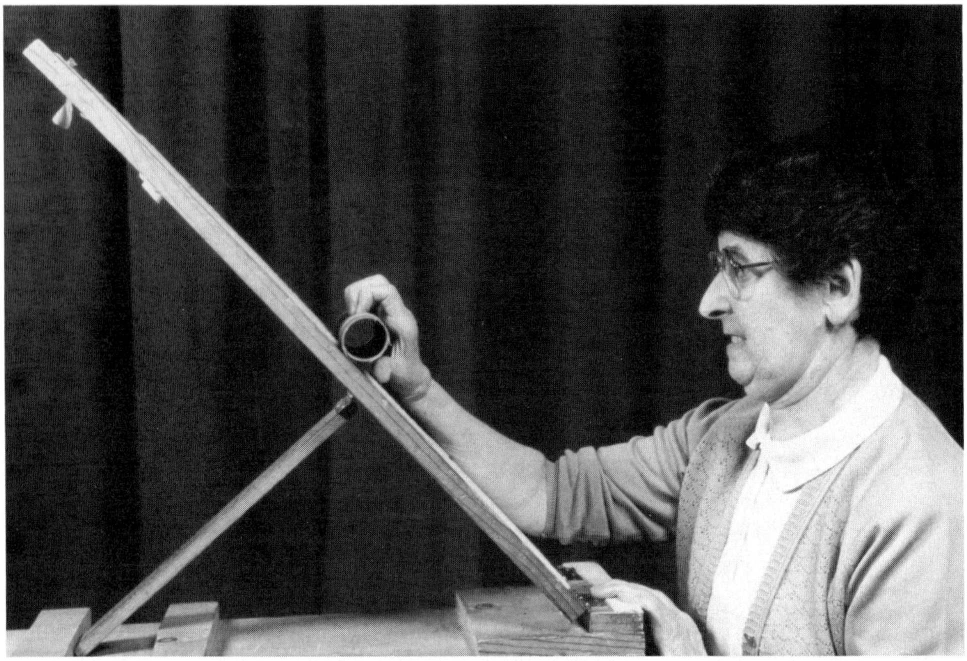

FIG 20B–17.
Rolling a cylinder against Velcro resistance to stretch the intrinsic muscles.

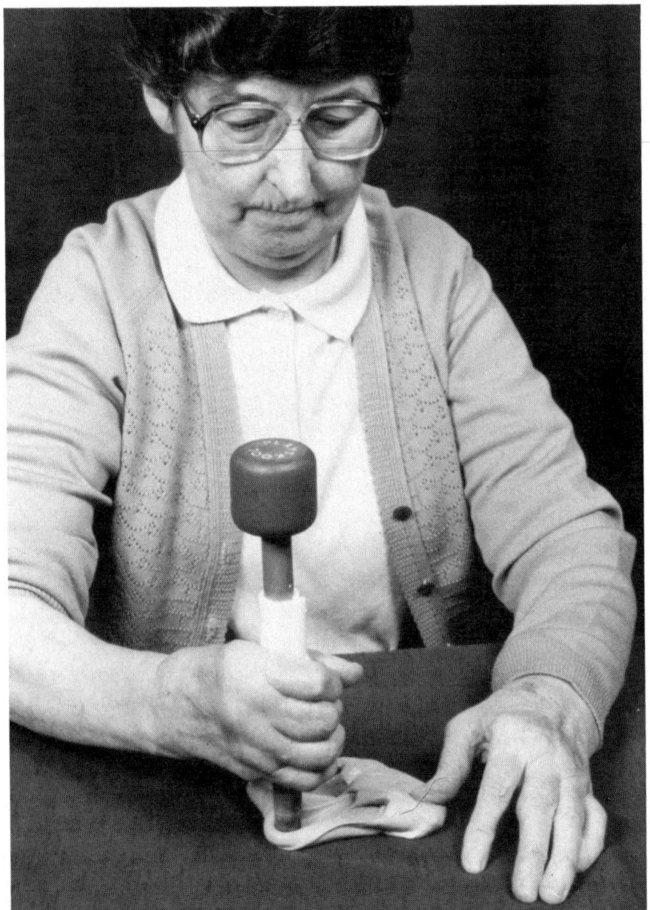

FIG 20B–18.
Putty-pull exercise to stretch extrinsic muscles.

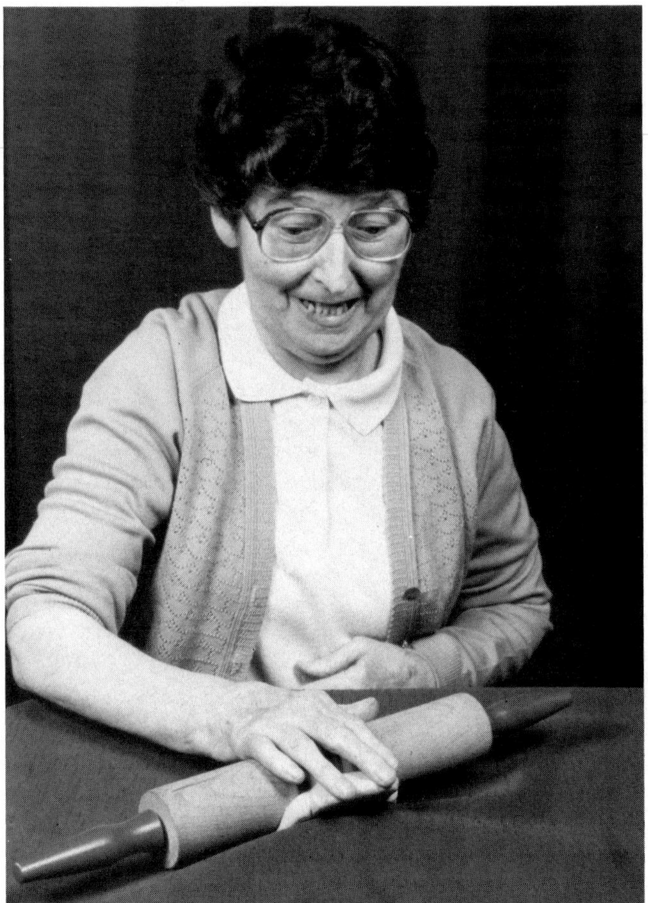

FIG 20B–19.
Rolling pin exercise to increase metacarpophalangeal extension.

finger slings, and rubber bands, attached to the proximal hook attachment. The splint should be comfortable and not too forcible. Care should be taken to ensure adequate circulation to the fingers is maintained. Patients should be able to tolerate the usage of the splints for extended periods of time.

The splints are worn for 6 weeks postoperation. Night splinting in either flexion or extension or alternating between both continues if necessary. If good motion is obtained, a resting splint with finger separators to maintain radial deviation can be worn at nighttime (Fig 20B–13).

Exercise begins the day after the splint is made. Range-of-motion goals are zero to 65 or 75 degrees of MCP flexion (Fig 20B–14). Active and assisted MCP flexion and extension, and exercises to correct ulnar drift (radial walking) are performed initially with the therapist, then independently by the patient on an hourly basis.

Gentle massage can be performed over the incisional area (Fig 20B–15). Patients are instructed to progress to 15-minute exercise sessions three to four times daily. A proximal interphalangeal joint (PIP) block splint can be fabricated out of Orthoplast to prevent PIP flexion and isolate MCP flexion. Patients are usually discharged from the hospital within the first week and are seen three times weekly as outpatients. After 10 days, light functional hand activities are started to encourage opposition and basic grasp patterns.

The patient is encouraged to use the hand during ADLs while still in the splint. Light resistive and isometric exercises for flexion, extension, and intrinsic muscles are initiated and progressed as tolerated (Figs 20B–16 to 20B–19). Outpatient treatment generally continues for 3 months. After 3 months the patient can use the hand for normal ADLs. Instruction in the principles of joint protection are emphasized to prevent recurrence of the deformity and to maintain the surgical correction. Excessive weight-bearing or lifting with the affected hand should be avoided.

CONCLUSIONS

The role of therapy following total joint replacement extends beyond guiding the patient through range-of-motion exercises. Objective measurements taken frequently throughout the course of treatment encourage the patient and help the therapist gauge the efficacy of treatment. A positive relationship between patient and therapist provides reassurance and motivation to achieve therapeutic goals.

SUGGESTED READINGS

Hicks JE, Nicholas JJ, Sweezey RL (eds): *Handbook of Rehabilitative Rheumatology.* Atlanta, American Rheumatism Association, 1988.

Hunter JM, Schneider LH, Mackin EQ (eds): *Rehabilitation of the Hand: Surgery and Therapy,* ed 3. St Louis, Mosby–Year Book, 1990.

Kottke FJ, Lehmann JF: *Krusen's Handbook of Physical Medicine and Rehabilitation,* ed 4. Philadelphia, WB Saunders Co, 1990.

Melvin JL: *Rheumatic Disease in the Adult and Child,* ed 3. Philadelphia, FA Davis Co, 1989.

Pedretti LW: *Occupational Therapy Practice Skills for Physical Dysfunction.* St Louis, Mosby–Year Book, Inc, 1990.

Index

A

Acetabulum
  deformities, 371, 372
  dysplasia, 62
  locating position of, 219
  loosening of cemented components, 233, 373–374
  reconstruction, 219, 220, 223–225
Acetylsalicylic acid, for JRA, 18, 19
Acromegaly, hip destruction from, 213
Activities of daily living (ADLs), 397, 398–400
Admininistrative coordinator, of JRA service, 363
Adrenocortical steroids (*see* Corticosteroids)
Adult-onset rheumatoid arthritis (*see* Rheumatoid arthritis, adult)
Airway abnormalities, anesthesia and, 74, 75–79
Ambulation (*see also* Lower extremity function)
  in bilateral hip and knee replacement, 265, 266, 267
  with modified crutches, 386
  as surgical and rehabilitative goal, 62–63
  wheelchair dependency and, 20
American College of Rheumatology, RA classification criteria, 6–7
Ancillary therapies, 19–20
Anemia of chronic disease, anesthesia and, 70
Anesthesia, 69–81
  airway abnormalities and, 74, 75–79
  cervical spine and, 74, 75–76
  choice of, 72–74
  epidural, potential benefits of, 73–74
  general, 74
  perioperative monitoring, 72, 73
  preoperative evaluation
    anemia of chronic disease, 70
    cardiovascular disease associated with RA, 70–71
    effects of steroids, 69
    increased risk of infection, 70
    metabolic rate, 69
    personality disorders associated with RA, 72
    pulmonary disease associated with RA, 71–72
  regional, 60, 73–74
  temporomandibular joint and, 76–79
Ankle
  arthrography, oblique view showing capsulitis, 29
  biomechanics, 273–274
  MRI showing subchondral cysts in talus, 278
  physical examination, 276–277
  radiographic findings, 60, 277–280
  tenosynovitis, 366
Ankle studies, in RA patients, 349
Ankle surgery
  arthrodesis, 282–283, 369
    biomechanics, 283
    complications, 291
    fixation screws, 290–291
    indications and contraindications, 283
    optimal position, 282–283
    problems with external fixation, 282
    results, 287–291
    surgical approaches, 284–287
  arthroplasty (*see* Total ankle arthroplasty)
  synovectomy, 282
Ankylosing spondylitis, 17, 212
Ankylosis
  apophyseal joint, radiography, 39, 40
  radiographic detection of, 25–26
Appendicular skeleton imaging
  arthrography, 27, 28–29, 30
  plain film analysis, 23–27, 28
  scintigraphy, 29, 31
  ultrasound, 27, 29
Arteritis, giant cell, 356–358
Arthritis
  osteoarthritis, lower extremity function in RA vs., 346–348, 349–350
  psoriasiform, 18
  rheumatoid (*see* Rheumatoid arthritis)
  tuberculous, 13
Arthrodesis, 369
Arthrography, of appendicular skeleton, 27, 28–29, 30
Articular cartilage, pathology, 49–51
Atlantoaxial impaction, 105–106, 108
  imaging, 110, 111–112
  measurement, 110
  surgical treatment, 116–119
Atlantoaxial subluxation, 103–105, 106, 107
  imaging, 110, 111, 112, 113
  surgical treatment, 114–116
Auranofin
  for adult RA, 8
  for JRA, 18
Aurothioglucose
  for adult RA, 8
  for JRA, 18, 19
Azathioprine
  for adult RA, 8
  for JRA, 18, 19

B

Basilar invagination, imaging, 36, 37
Bathing, in occupational therapy, 398–399
Bicipital tenosynovitis, 130
Bilateral hip and knee replacement (*see* Hip and knee replacement, bilateral)
Biopsy
  muscle, 358, 359
  temporal artery, 357–358
Bledsoe brace, 391
Blood replacement, perioperative, 61
Bone deficit management (*see also* Osteopenia)
  in revision knee procedures, 66, 259, 260
  in total knee arthroplasty, 246–249
    bone grafting for tibial deficiency, 246, 249, 250
    patellofemoral joint, 249, 251
Bone grafting, 60, 61
  from fibula, for ankle arthrodesis, 283, 284

Bone grafting *(cont.)*
  in hip, 219, 220, 223
  from iliac crest
    for compression arthrodesis in ankle, 300
    in subaxial subluxation surgery, 119, 120
  radiography, 66
  of subtalar joint, 308
  in talonavicular arthrodesis, 303
  from tibia, for ankle arthrodesis, 285–287
  for tibial deficiency, 246, 249, 250
  in triple arthrodesis, 304
Bone pathology, 51
Bone quality, joint replacement and, 370
Bone scintigraphy, 29, 31
  joint replacement and, 40, 41
Boutonnière deformity, of hand, 202, 203–204, 206
Brainstem compression, 111, 112
Bursitis
  rotator cuff disease and impingement syndrome, 128–129
  subdeltoid, 129–130

C

Calcaneus
  radiography, lateral view showing erosion, 28
  stress fracture, 279
Callus formation, on forefoot, 316, 317, 321, 322
Capsular contracture, 142, 143
Capsulotomy, 365–366
Cardiovascular disease, RA-associated, 70–71
Carpal fusion, 366, 367
Carpal measurements, 167–168
Carpal tunnel syndrome, 167
Carpometacarpal joint destruction, with ankylosis of carpal bones, 193, 194
Cartilage, articular, pathology of, 49–51
Casting, for rheumatoid hindfoot, 280
Cement fixation, in total hip arthroplasty, 223–225, 228
Cervical collars, 112
Cervical myelopathy, rehabiltation and, 64–65
Cervical spine, 103–125
  anesthesia and, 74, 75–76
  imaging
    apophyseal joint ankylosis, 39
    cord compression, 35, 64
    modalities, 31–32, 34–37
    normal relationships, 36
    radiographic features, 109–112, 113
    subluxation, 34, 35
    thecal sac constriction, 35
  ligamentous complex at atlantoaxial level, 104
  manifestations of involvement, 103
    atlantoaxial impaction, 105–106, 108
    atlantoaxial subluxation, 103–105, 106, 107
    subaxial subluxation, 106–107, 108
  methylmethacrylate-augmented cervical fusions, 122–123
  myelopathy, 64
  nonsurgical management, 112–113
  postoperative rehabilitation, 113–114
  preoperative examination, 64
  sagittal section through cervico-occipital junction, 104
  subluxation below cervical arthrodesis site, 123
  surgical treatment
    for atlantoaxial impaction, 116–119
    for atlantoaxial subluxation, 114–116
    evaluation for, 113–114
    indications for, 114
    for subaxial subluxation, 119–122
Charnley compression arthrodesis, of ankle, 288, 289
Charnley low friction arthroplasties, 211, 232
Chin implants, 98, 99, 100
Chisel toe, 320
Chlorambucil, for JRA, 18, 19
Clawtoe deformity, 320
Clayton resection arthroplasty, 328
Cold therapy, 386–387
Complications, of RA surgery, 65–67
Comprehensive Arthritis Program (CAP), at The Hospital for Special Surgery (NYC), 58–59
Computed tomography, 29–30, 31
  in cervical spine evaluation, 111
Conaxial ankle prosthesis, 294
Condylar revision surgery, modular constrained, 260–262
Connective tissue disease, hip involvement with, 213
Conoidal ankle prosthesis, 294
Constant/continuous passive motion (CPM), in knee replacement rehabilitation, 251, 394–395
Coonrad implant, 154
Coronary artery disease, RA-associated, 71
Cortical index of femoral shaft, 220, 221
Corticosteroids
  for adult RA, 9
  anesthesia and, 69–70
  for elbow, 149, 150
  for forefoot, 325
  for JRA, 19
    pauciarticular-onset, 14
    polyarticular, 15
  for metacarpophalangeal joints, 197
  for proximal interphalangeal joint, 205
  systemic lupus erythematosus and, 131
Costochondral grafts, for mandibular deformities, 93–94, 96
Coughlin MTP joint arthrodesis, 334–335
Coxarthrosis etiologies, 211
CPM, in knee replacement rehabilitation, 251, 390–391
Cracchiolo implant arthroplasty, 329–332, 333
Cranial arteritis, 356–358
Cranial settling, 105–106, 108
Craniomandibular myalgia, 88, 89
Cricoarytenoid joints, anesthesia and, 79
Cryotherapy, 386–387
Cyclophosphamide, for adult RA, 8
Cyclosporine, for JRA, 18, 19

D

Darrach procedure, 173
Deep vein thrombosis
  after total hip arthroplasty, 212
  after total knee arthroplasty, 256, 390
Dens (*see* Odontoid process of axis)
Dental treatment, for RA-TMJ patient, 88–90
Diarthrodial joint pathology, 49
  articular cartilage, 49–51
  bone, 51
Digital synovitis, 207–209
Disease-modifying antirheumatic drugs, for adult RA, 8–9

Distal interphalangeal joint, flexion deformity at, 320, 321
Distal ulnar resection, 368–369
  complications, 175
  goals, 172
  indications and contraindications, 172–174
  modifications, 174–175
  technique, 174
DMARDs, for adult RA, 8–9
Dorsal stabilization, 175, 176
Dorsal tenosynovectomy
  goals, 175–176
  indications, 176
  results, 177
  technique, 176
Dressing, in occupational therapy, 398
Drug therapy
  for adult RA, 7–9
  for JRA, 18–19
  surgery and, 57–58

E

E. coli infection, in bilateral hip and knee replacement, 268, 269, 270
Eating, in occupational therapy, 398
Eaton implant, 192, 193
Elbow, 147–159
  conservative treatment, 149–150
  evaluation, 149
  flexion and extension, 147, 148
  medial side, 148
  movements, 147
  postoperative rehabilitation, 158
  splint, 404–405
  stability, 146
  surgical considerations, 150–153
  synovectomy, 151
    postoperative radiograph, 151
    technique, 151–153
  synovial mass on, 150
  total elbow arthroplasty (*see* Total elbow arthroplasty)
Electrical stimulation therapy, 387
Electromyogram, 358–359
Emotional disorders, RA-associated, 72
Energy conservation, patient education for, 401
Epidemiology, 11
Escherichia coli infection, in bilateral hip and knee replacement, 268, 269, 270
Etiology
  of JRA, 12
  of severe coxarthrosis, 211
Exercise, in occupational therapy, 397–398
  after metacarpophalangeal arthroplasty, 405, 406, 407
  after total knee arthroplasty, 390–391
  after total shoulder replacement, 401–402, 404
Extensor digitorum communis tendon
  in metacarpophalangeal joint surgery, 199–200, 201
  rupture, 164–165
    surgery for, 177
Extensor retinaculum, 162–163
Extremities (*see* Lower extremity(ies); Upper extremity)

F

Feeding, in occupational therapy, 398, 403
Feet (*see* Foot)
Femoral head
  migration, 214, 372
  prosthesis
    complications, after total hip arthroplasty, 230–231, 233
  resection arthroplasty, 368
Femur
  bone deficiency, in revision knee replacement, 259
  dysplasia, 62
  medullary canal, 226, 227–228
  reconstruction, 225–229
  shaft, cortical index of, 220, 221
Fibrin, in synovium pathology, 46
Fibula, stress fractures, 276
Fibular strut graft, 283, 284
Fingers
  lesser, metacarpophalangeal joints, 196–203
  synovitis of, 207–209
  thumb (*see* Thumb)
Flexor pollicis longus, rupture of, 191
Fluidotherapy, 386
Foot (*see also* Forefoot disorders; Hindfoot)
  biomechanics, 273–274
  resection arthroplasty, 368
  tenosynovitis, 366
  vasculitis, 281, 355
Forefoot disorders, 315–340
  clinical presentation and physical examination, 317–318
    great toe, 319–320
    lesser toes, 320
    neurovascular, 320–321
  conservative treatment, 324–326
  nodules, 277
  pathophysiology, 315–317
  radiographic evaluation, 322–324
  skin and soft tissues, 321–322
  surgical treatment, 326–327
    great toe, 327–335
Fracture, stress, of hindfoot, 276, 279, 299

G

Gait analysis, three-dimensional, 382, 383, 384
Gait cycle, 343–344
Gangrene, 355, 356
Genetics, 12
Genioplasty, sliding, 100
Germinal centers, in RA pathology, 49, 52
Giant cell arteritis, 356–358
Girdlestone resection, 216
Glenohumeral joint
  motion loss, 375
  normal motion, 127, 128
  resurfacing, by total shoulder arthroplasty, 132–139
  synovectomy, 131–132
Glenoid component loosening, after total shoulder arthroplasty, 143–144
Gold compounds, for adult RA, 8
Gold salts, for JRA, 19
Gold sodium thiomalate
  for adult RA, 8
  for JRA, 18, 19
Gout, hip arthritis from, 213
GUEPAR replacement, 243

H

Hallux rigidus, 320
Hallux tortus, 320
Hallux valgus deformity, 316, 317, 319
  contributing factors, 319
  radiograph, 323
  surgery, 327–335
Hand, 189–209
  deformities, 189, 384
    advanced, 190
    boutonnière, 202, 203–204, 206
  functions, 189
  grips, 385
  interphalangeal joints, 203–207
  metacarpophalangeal joint of thumb, 194–196
  metacarpophalangeal joints of lesser fingers, 196–203
  neural damage, 189
  radiography
    Norgaard view in normal patient, 24
    oblique view showing erosions at MCP joints, 25
    oblique view showing erosions with resultant ulnar subluxation, 25

Hand *(cont.)*
PA and oblique views showing premature epiphyseal fusion, 38
in patient with joint replacement, 42
PA view in older patient with erosive arthritis, 28
PA view showing cystic changes in carpus and erosions of MCP joints, 27
PA view showing DIP joint involvement and ankylosis of fifth ray, 26
PA view showing osteoporosis, 24
rheumatoid thumb involvement, 190–194
rheumatoid vasculitis, 190
splints, 399, 400
strength exercise, 405
surgical caveats, 209
tendon damage, 189, 191
volar and digital synovitis, 207–209
Heart disease, RA-associated, 70–71
Heat therapy, 385–386
Hematoma, after total knee arthroplasty, 253
Hemochromatosis, hip destruction from, 213
Heterotopic ossification, after total hip arthroplasty, 231
Hindfoot
biomechanics, 273–274
conservative treatment, 280
evaluation, 318–319
MRI showing subchondral cysts in talus, 278
pathophysiology, 274–275
pes planovalgus deformity, 275, 279
physical examination, 276–277
radiographic findings, 277–280
talonavicular joint dislocation, 301
valgus deformity, 301, 307
Hindfoot surgery, 280–310
ankle joint
arthrodesis, 282–291
synovectomy, 282
total ankle arthroplasty (*see* Total ankle arthroplasty)
arthrodesis, 301–310
complications, 310
indications and contraindications, 301–302
isolated talonavicular arthrodesis, 302–303
lower extremity involvement and, 281
pantalar arthrodesis, 309–310
triple arthrodesis, 303–309
closing wedge osteotomies after, 306
complications, 306, 307
dowel technique, 304, 305, 308
incisions for, 305
metaphyseal stapling, 308
results, 307–309
screw fixation, 309
Hip, 211–212
arthroplasty, 216–217 (*see also* Total hip arthroplasty)
clinical and radiographic features, 26, 213–214
flexion contracture, 266
fusion, 215
girdlestone resection, 216
joint destruction, 62
joint space narrowing, 26
medical considerations, 217
osteonecrosis, 215
osteotomy, 215
in other arthritides, 212–213
protrusion deformity, 26, 214, 218
soft tissue procedures, 214–215, 365
surgical considerations, 217–218
surgical indications, 214–217
synovectomy, 214
total hip arthroplasty (*see* Total hip arthroplasty)
Hip and knee replacement, bilateral, 265–271
clinical results, 267–270
surgical approach, 266–267
Hip-dislocating maneuvers, 388
Hip surgery, physical therapy and, 383, 384, 385, 386
Histiocytes, in RA pathology, 52
HLA-B27 testing, 17
Hoffman excisional arthroplasty, 335, 337
Homemaking, in occupational therapy, 399–400
Hospital for Special Surgery, The (NYC)
bicondylar implant, 295
Comprehensive Arthritis Program (CAP), 58–59
triaxial implant, 154, 156
Hot packs, 385
Humeral head, avascular necrosis of, 131
Humerus
component loosening, after total shoulder arthroplasty, 142, 143–144
fracture
infection after, 159
in shoulder arthroplasty, 141–142
osteotomy, 135–137
Hydrotherapy, 386
Hydroxychloroquine sulfate, for adult RA, 8
Hydroxychloroquinine, for JRA, 19
Hyperextension deformity, of proximal interphalangeal joint, 202, 204, 205, 206–207

I

Ibuprofen, for JRA, 18, 19
ICLH ankle prosthesis, 294, 298
Iliac crest bone graft
for compression arthrodesis in ankle, 300
in subaxial subluxation surgery, 119, 120
Imaging
of appendicular skeleton
arthrography, 27, 28–29, 30
plain film analysis, 23–27, 28
scintigraphy, 29, 31
ultrasound, 27, 29
of juvenile rheumatoid patient, 38–40
of postoperative patient, 40–41
of spine, 31–32, 34–37
Impingement syndrome, 128–129
Implants (*see* Prostheses)
Indomethacin, for JRA, 18
Infection
after elbow arthroplasty, 158, 159
after shoulder arthroplasty, 141
after total ankle arthroplasty, 298–299
after total hip arthroplasty, 230
after total knee arthroplasty
deep, 254–256
superficial, 253–254
anesthesia and, 70
in bilateral hip and knee replacement, 268, 269, 270
postoperative, 61, 67
Interphalangeal joint(s), 203–207
of thumb, 195–196
Ischium, cement fixation holes in, 224

J

Jaw (*see also* Temporomandibular joint)
  dislocated disc, 84, 86
  opening of, biomechanics, 83, 85
Johnson resection arthroplasty, 328, 329
Joint(s)
  multiple involvement, surgical planning considerations, 217–218
  protection, patient education for, 400
  replacement, radiography and, 40, 41, 42
  surface pathology, 49, 50
Joint space narrowing, radiographic detection, 26
Jugular vein, internal, location of, 73
Juncturae tendinum, 200
Juvenile rheumatoid arthritis
  ancillary therapies, 19–20
  anesthetic management, 69–81
  definitions and terminology, 11
  drug therapy, 18–19
  epidemiology, 11
  etiology and genetics, 12
  medical concepts and treatment, 11–20
  multidisciplinary approach, 58–59, 60, 363–364
  natural history, 12
  occupational therapy, 397–407
  pathology, 45–53
  pauciarticular-onset, 12–13
    exclusions, 13–14
    medical treatment, 14
  physical therapy, 381–395
  polyarticular, 14–15
    exclusions, 15
    medical therapy, 15–16
  postoperative rehabilitation, 62–65
  radiographic evaluation, 23–43
  subtypes, 12
  surgery, 361–376
    introduction to rheumatoid patient, 57–68
  systemic-onset, 16
    exclusions, 15, 16
    medical therapy, 17

K

Keller procedure, of resection arthroplasty, arthrodesis vs., 332–333
Keller resection arthroplasty, 327–328
Kinematics/kinetics, 344, 348
Knee, 237–261
  arthrodesis, 256
  arthroscopic synovectomy, 240–241
  biplane and triplane deformity, 245–246, 247
  brace, 391
  conservative treatment, 239
  flexion contracture, 63, 266, 374
  imaging
    arthrography of popliteal cyst, 30
    flexion-valgus deformity, 238
    joint deformity with bone loss, 61
    lateral view for Still's disease, 38
    MRI of erosions, joint effusion and fluid, and popliteal cyst, 33
    150-degree fixed flexion deformity, 243
    osteopenia and tibial cyst, 238
    scintigraphy of stress fracture, 31
    total knee replacement with bone grafting, 61
  patient presentation, 237–239
  prostheses, 245–250, 257, 258, 374
    cemented prostheses and porous implants, 251–252
    implantation technique, 260–262
    removal, 258–259
    selection for knee revision surgery, 260
    wound infection and, 254, 255, 256
  radiation synovectomy, 239
  soft tissue procedures, 365
  stability, implants and, 246, 247
  surgical treatment, 239–240
  total knee arthroplasty (*see* Total knee arthroplasty)
  valgus deformity, 281
Knee and hip replacement, bilateral (*see* Hip and knee replacement, bilateral)
Knee joint, 242, 243
Knee studies, in RA patients, 346–348
Knowles pin, 192

L

Larynx, anesthesia and, 80
LCS ankle prosthesis, 293, 297
Le Fort I ostectomy, 99, 100
Leg(s) (*see* Lower extremity(ies))
Ligaments, in atlantoaxial subluxation, 103–104
Lower extremity function, 343–351
  motion analysis, 344
  normal human gait, 343–344
  studies of RA patients, 344
    ankle studies, 349
    general studies in nonoperative patients, 344–345
    knee studies, 346–347
    total ankle arthroplasty, 349
    total hip arthroplasty, 345
    total knee arthroplasty, 347–348
Lower extremity(ies)
  contrast venography showing venous thrombosis, 40
  length discrepancy, after total hip arthroplasty, 231
  multiple joint involvement, 218
  postoperative rehabilitation, 62–63
Lung disease
  chest radiograph and CT image, 32
  RA-associated, 71–72
Lyme disease, 13
Lymph node pathology, 52, 53
Lymphocytes, in synovium pathology, 47

M

Magnetic resonance imaging, 30–31, 33–34
  in cervical spine evaluation, 111
Malleolus fracture, 299
Mandible
  anterior horizontal osteotomy, 100
  erosive changes of condyle, 87, 88
  ligaments limiting movement of, 85
  limited opening of, anesthesia and, 76, 77
  orthopaedic repositioning appliance, 89–90
  retrognathia, 98, 99, 100
  surgery, 98–100
Mandibular disorders
  in adult RA, 91, 93
    imaging, 95–96, 97
  costochondral grafts for, 93–94, 96
  in JRA, 91, 92
Mann and Johnson excisional arthroplasty, 337–339
Mann and Thompson/Mann and Oates MTP joint arthrodesis, 333–334

Mann resection arthroplasty, 327–328
Massage therapy, 387
Maxillary surgery, 98–100
Mayo ankle prosthesis, 294, 298
Mayo-type resection arthroplasty, 328, 329
McIntosh prosthesis, 245
McKeever-type arthrodesis of MTP joint, 334
Mechanical traction, 387
Medications
  for adult RA, 7–9
  for JRA, 18–19
  surgery and, 57–58
Medullary canal of femur, 226, 227–228
Metabolic rate, anesthesia and, 69
Metacarpophalangeal joint(s)
  arthrodesis, 369
  of lesser fingers, 196–203
    conservative treatment, 196
    deformities, 196, 197
    implant arthroplasty, 200–203
    realignment of extensor mechanism without synovectomy, 199–200, 201
    resting splints for ulnar drift, 196–197
    steroid instillation into, 196, 197
    synovectomy, 198–199
  occupational therapy after arthroplasty, 403, 404, 405–407
  radiography, 25, 26
  of thumb, 194–196
    arthrodesis, 195
    implant arthroplasty, 195
    radiography, 196
    synovectomy, 194–195
Metal toxicity, after total hip arthroplasty, 231–232
Metatarsal head, bursa over, 317
Metatarsophalangeal joint
  dislocation, 316, 323
  dorsal subluxation, 320
  hallux valgus deformity (*see* Hallux valgus deformity)
  infected implant, 330
  surgery, 327–339
Methotrexate
  for adult RA, 8
  for JRA, 18–19
Methylmethacrylate
  in atlantoaxial impaction surgery, 116, 118
  benefits, 370
  for bone deficiency, 247, 248
  for cervical fusions, clinical experience, 122–123
  in subaxial subluxation surgery, 119, 120, 121, 122
Meuli prosthesis, 182
Mobilization therapy, 387
Multidisciplinary team, 58–59, 60, 363–364
Muscle biopsy, 358, 359
Myelopathy, cervical, 105, 106, 107
  MRI of, 111–112
  rehabilitation and, 64–65
Myocardial disease, RA-associated, 71
Myopathy, 358–359
Myositis, histologic appearance, 359

N

Naproxen, for JRA, 18, 19
Neer prosthesis, 135, 140
Neuropathy, 356
  in forefoot disorders, 320–321
  in hand, 189, 190
  after shoulder arthroplasty, 141
Neuroses, RA-associated, 72
Newton ankle prosthesis, 293, 297
Nightguard appliance, 89–90
Nodules (*see* Rheumatoid nodules)
Nonsteroidal anti-inflammatory drugs (NSAIDs)
  for adult RA, 7–8
  for JRA, 18
    pauciarticular-onset, 14
    polyarticular, 15
Nursing staff, in clinical team, 58, 59, 363

O

Occipitocervical fusion, surgery for, 116–118
Occupational therapist, in clinical team, 58, 59, 363
Occupational therapy, 397–407
  activities of daily living, 397, 398–400
  evaluation for, 397
  exercise, 397–398
  for JRA, 19–20
  patient education, 400–401
  splinting, 398, 399
  after total joint replacement, 401
    of elbow, 403, 404–405
    metacarpophalangeal arthroplasty, 403, 404, 405–407
    of shoulder, 401, 402, 404
  treatment goals, 397
  for upper extremity rehabilitation, 64, 65
Ochronosis, hip destruction from, 213
Odontoid process of axis
  in atlantoaxial subluxation, 103–104
  erosion, 104, 105, 109–110, 111
  imaging, 36, 37, 109–110, 111
  transverse axial ligament and, 74, 75, 104
  vertical migration, 105–106, 108
Olecranon process, rheumatoid nodules over, 150
Oregon I and II ankle prostheses, 294, 298
Orthognathic surgery, 98–100
Orthopaedic surgeon, in clinical team, 58, 59, 363
Orthotic shoe devices, 324–325
Osteoarthritis, RA vs., lower extremity function in, 346–348, 349–350
Osteopenia, 60, 67 (*see also* Bone deficit management)
  in bilateral hip and knee replacement, 265, 266
  in knee, 238
  in knee joint, 366
  radiography, 60, 66
  in shoulder, 131
Osteoporosis
  pathology, 51
  radiographic detection, 23, 24, 27
Osteotomy, 367–368

P

Palmar shelf arthroplasty, 180
Palmar synovectomy, 207–209
Pannus
  MRI, 31, 37
  in RA pathology, 49, 50, 51
Pantalar arthrodesis, 309–310
Paraffin bath, 385
Patellofemoral joint, in total knee arthroplasty, 249, 251
Pathology, 45–53
  of diarthrodial joints, 49
    articular cartilage, 49–51
    bone, 51
  of soft tissue, 51
    lymph nodes, 52, 53
    rheumatoid nodules, 51–53
  of synovium, 45–49
Patient, surgery and, 57–68, 362–363
Patient education, for occupational therapy, 400–401
Pauciarticular-onset JRA, 12–13
  exclusions, 13–14
  medical treatment, 14

Pediatrician, in clinical team, 363
Penicillamine, for adult RA, 8
Pericarditis, RA-associated, 70–71
Personality disorders, RA-associated, 72
Pes planovalgus deformity, 275, 279
Physical therapist, in clinical team, 58, 59, 363
Physical therapy, 381–395
  for adult RA, 7
  for JRA, 19–20
  modalities, 384–385
    cold, 386–387
    electrical stimulation, 387
    heat, 385–386
    mechanical traction, 387
    mobilization and massage, 387
    problem-oriented approach, 382
  preoperative, 381–384, 385, 386
    case study, 383, 384, 385, 386
    three-dimensional gait analysis, 382, 383, 384
  after total hip arthroplasty, 387–389
    functional milestone form, 392, 394
    protocols, 389
  after total knee arthroplasty, 390–394
    functional milestone form, 393
    protocols, 391
Plantar callosity, 316, 317
Plant thorn synovitis, 250
Plasma cells
  in lymph node pathology, 53
  in synovium pathology, 45–46, 47, 48
Plastazote, 324, 325
Pleural effusion, RA-associated, 71
Polyarticular JRA, 14–15
  exclusions, 15
  medical therapy, 15–16
Polycentric hinge brace, 391
Prostheses *(see also specific types)*
  for elbow, 153–154, 155, 156, 157
  in forefoot arthroplasty, 329–332, 333, 337
  knee (*see* Knee prostheses)
  for metacarpophalangeal joints, 202
  planning, 61
  radiography and, 40, 41
  resorption of femoral neck under, 269
  for TMJ, 93, 95, 96–98
  in total ankle arthroplasty, 293–295
    results, 296–300
  in total hip arthroplasty, 219–220, 225, 232–234
  in total hip replacement, 371–374
  in total knee replacement, 374
  in total shoulder arthroplasty, 134, 135, 137–138, 141
    complications, 142, 143–144
  for total wrist arthroplasty, 180–182, 183, 184
Proximal interphalangeal joint(s), 203–207
  arthrodesis, 205–206, 369
  block splint, 405
  flexion deformity, 320, 321
  swan-neck deformity, 202, 204, 205, 206–207
Pseudobasilar invagination, 105–106, 108
Psoriaform arthritis, 18
Psoriasis, hip involvement with, 213
Pubis, cement fixation holes in, 224
Pulmonary disease, RA-associated, 71–72

Q

Quadricepsplasty, 242–243, 244

R

Radiation synovectomy, of knee, 239
Radiocapitellar joint narrowing, 149
Radiocarpal collapse, 163–164
Radiographic evaluation
  appendicular skeleton
    arthrography, 27, 28–29, 30
    plain film analysis, 23–27, 28
    scintigraphy, 29, 31
    ultrasound, 27, 29
  computed tomography, 29–30, 31
  of JRA, 23–43
  of JRA patient, 38–40
  magnetic resonance imaging, 30–31, 33–34
  of postoperative patient, 40–41
  spine, 31–32, 34–37, 109–112, 113
Radiolunate and radioscapholunate arthrodesis, 177–178, 179
Radioulnar joint, distal, 162
Ramusotomy, bilateral sagittal, 98, 99, 100
Ranawat index, for atlantoaxial impaction, 110
Rehabilitation
  occupational therapy (*see* Occupational therapy)
  physical therapy (*see* Physical therapy)
  postoperative, 62–65
Resection arthroplasty, 368–369
Residents, in JRA service, 363–364
Respiratory disease, RA-associated, 71–72
Revision knee replacement, 258
  bone deficits, 259, 260
  implant removal, 258–259
Rheumatoid arthritis
  adult
    adrenocortical steroid therapy, 9
    clinical course and natural history, 7
    diagnosis, 6–7
    disease-modifying drugs, 8–9
    etiology, 6
    experimental models of chronic synovitis, 6
    mandibular condyles in, 91, 93
    medical concepts and treatment, 5–9
    NSAIDs, 7–8
    pathology, 5–6
    physical therapy, 7
    subset variations, 6
    surgical rehabilitation, 9
  juvenile (*see* Juvenile rheumatoid arthritis)
  types, 317–318
Rheumatoid factor, 315
Rheumatoid nodules, 353–355
  excision, 354–355
  of forefoot, 277, 321, 322
  of hand, 190–191, 207
  histologic appearance, 353, 354
  pathology, 51–53
Rheumatologist
  in clinical team, 58, 59, 363
  surgeon communicating with, 57–58
Rice bodies, in synovium pathology, 46
Rotator cuff
  disease, 128–129
  in total shoulder arthroplasty, 133, 134, 140, 143

S

Scallop sign, 168
Scapula, nodules on, 354
Scintigraphy
  of appendicular skeleton, 29, 31
  joint replacement and, 40, 41
Scoliosis, 39
Sculco implant arthroplasty, 329–332
SEA syndrome, 17
Seroma, after total knee arthroplasty, 253
Seronegative enthesopathy arthropathy, 17

Shoewear
for forefoot disorders, 324–325, 326
for rheumatoid hindfoot, 280
Shoulder, 127–144
arthrography, 28, 29
bicipital tenosynovitis, 130
biomechanics and function, 127–128
computed tomography, 31
rheumatoid arthropathy, 130–131
rotator cuff disease and impingement syndrome, 128–129
subdeltoid bursitis, 129–130
surgical treatment, 131–139
arthrodesis and resection arthroplasty, 132
glenohumeral synovectomy, 131–132
hemiarthroplasty, 132
total shoulder arthroplasty (*see* Total shoulder arthroplasty)
Silcone/Silastic implant arthroplasty, 329–332, 337
Silicone synovitis, 181–182
Skin flaps, 60
Sliding genioplasty, 100
Smith ankle prosthesis, 293, 296–297, 299
Social work, 20
Social worker, in clinical team, 58, 59, 363
Soft tissue, 353–359
giant cell arteritis, 356–358
lymph nodes, 52, 53
myopathy, 358–359
neuropathy, 356
pathology, 51–53
rheumatoid nodules (*see* Rheumatoid nodules)
vasculitis, 317, 355–356
Spherical triaxial total wrist arthroplasty, 182–186
Spinal cord compression
in atlantoaxial impaction, 105, 108
in atlantoaxial subluxation, 104, 106
imaging, 35, 64, 111, 112, 113
in subaxial subluxation, 106
surgical treatment, 115, 116, 120
Spine
cervical (*see* Cervical spine)
imaging, 31–32, 34–37
Splinting, 398
elbow, 149–150, 404, 405
metacarpophalangeal, 403, 404, 405, 407
problems, splint types, and rationale, 399
for ulnar drift involving MP joints, 196–197
upper extremity, 64
wrist, 170
Splints, illustrations, 399, 400
Spondylitis, ankylosing, 17, 212
Spondyloarthropathies, 17
Steroids (*see* Corticosteroids)
Still's disease, radiography, 38
Stress fracture, of hindfoot, 276, 279, 299
Subacromial impingement, after shoulder arthroplasty, 142
Subaxial subluxation, 106–107, 108
MRI, 111, 112, 113
surgical treatment, 119–122
Subluxation
atlantoaxial, 103–105, 106, 107
imaging, 110, 111, 112, 113
surgical treatment, 114–116
below cervical arthrodesis site, 123
imaging, 34, 35, 36
subaxial, 64, 106–107, 108
MRI, 111, 112, 113
surgical treatment, 119–122
Subtalar joint, 274
bone grafting, 308
radiography, 278
Sulfasalazine
for adult RA, 8
for JRA, 19
Sural nerve anatomy, 356
Surgeon, rheumatologist communicating with, 57–58
Surgery, 361–376 (*see also specific types*)
bone procedures
arthrodesis, 369
osteotomy, 367–368
resection arthroplasty, 368–369
total joint replacement, 369–375
facilities, 363
intraoperative planning, 60–62
planning for multiple joint involvement, 217–218
postoperative complications, 65–67
postoperative rehabilitation, 62–65
preoperative evaluation, 57–60
principles for evaluating surgical indications and outcomes, 364–365
procedures, 365
in rheumatoid patient, 57–68, 362–363
soft tissue procedures
synovectomy, 367
tenosynovectomy, 366–367
tenotomy and capsulotomy, 365–366
team, 363–364
Swan-neck deformity, of proximal interphalangeal joint, 202, 204, 205, 206–207
Swanson prosthesis, 181–182, 192, 193, 194, 330
Synovectomy, 367
of ankle, 282
of elbow, 151–153
of hip, 214
of knee
arthroscopic, 240–241
open, 239–240
radiation, 239
of metacarpophalangeal joint, 198–199
of shoulder, 131–132
volar, 207–208
Synoviocytes, 47
Synovitis
chronic, experimental models, 6
plant thorn, 13–14
silicone, 181–182
Synovium pathology, 45–49
Systemic lupus erythematosus, 131, 213
Systemic-onset JRA, 16
exclusions, 15, 16
medical therapy, 17

T

Talonavicular joint, 275
arthrodesis, 301, 302
surgical technique, 302–303, 304
dislocation, 301
pseudarthrosis after triple arthrodesis, 306
Talus, subchondral cysts in, MRI of, 278
Tarsal tunnel syndrome, 275–276, 321
Team, clinical, 58–59, 60, 363–364
Temporal arteritis, 356–358
Temporal artery biopsy, 357–358
Temporomandibular joint, 83–102
anatomy, 83, 84, 85
anesthesia and, 76–79
larynx, 80
limitation of mandibular opening, 76, 77
preanesthesia examination, 76–77, 79
upper airway obstruction, 76, 78
biomechanics, 83–84, 85–86
dental treatment, 88
nightguard appliance, 89–90
occlusal force distribution, 89

- physical therapy, 88–89, 90
  - in JRA patients, 90–91
  - nonsurgical and presurgical treatment, 88
  - prostheses, 95, 96–98
  - radiography, 77
  - RA of
    - anterior open bite, 84, 87
    - differential diagnosis, 87–88
    - pathology, 84, 86, 87
    - radiographic evaluation, 87, 88
  - surgical indications, 91, 92, 93
  - surgical management, 91–100
  - surgical procedures
    - arthroplasty, 91–92
    - arthroscopy, 92–93
    - costochondral grafts, 93–94, 96
    - orthognathic surgery, 98–100
    - total joint replacement, 93, 95, 96–98
- Tendon damage, in hand, 189, 191
- Tenosynovectomy, 366–367
  - dorsal (*see* Dorsal tenosynovectomy)
  - volar, 170–172
- Tenosynovitis
  - bicipital, 130
  - of forefoot, 322
  - of hindfoot, 275
  - of wrist, 356, 366
- Tenotomy, 365–366
- Thoracic spine, scoliosis of, 39
- Thumb, 190–194
  - advanced deformities, 193
  - implant arthroplasty, 192–193
  - interphalangeal joint, 195–196
  - metacarpophalangeal joint, 194–196
  - resection arthroplasty, 192
- Tibial cyst, imaging, 238
- Tibial deficiency, 246–249
  - bone grafting for, 61, 246, 249, 250
  - in revision knee replacement, 259, 260
- Tibial graft, for ankle arthrodesis, 285–287
- Titanium
  - in atlantoaxial impaction surgery, 116, 118
  - in subaxial subluxation surgery, 119, 120, 121
- TMJ (*see* Temporomandibular joint)
- Toe(s)
  - great
    - clinical presentation and physical examination, 319–320
    - surgical treatment, 327–335
  - interdigital splaying, 322
  - lesser
    - clinical presentation and physical examination, 320
    - surgical treatment, 335–339
- Tolmetin sodium, for JRA, 18, 19
- Total ankle arthroplasty, 291–310, 375
  - complications, 298–300
  - implant design, 293–295
  - indications and contraindications, 291–292
  - lower extremity function after, 349
  - postoperative care, 296
  - preoperative assessment, 292
  - results
    - nonconstrained implants, 296–298
    - semiconstrained implants, 298–300
  - revision procedures, 300
  - surgical technique, 295
    - anterior approach, 295–296
    - posterior approach, 296, 297
  - technical considerations, 292–293
- Total condylar III prosthesis, 245, 247, 250, 260
- Total elbow arthroplasty, 153–158, 375
  - complications, 158–159
  - indications, 153
  - occupational therapy after, 403, 404–405
  - prostheses, 153–154, 155, 156, 157
  - rehabilitation, 158
- Total hip arthroplasty, 211–234, 370–374
  - cemented vs. noncemented fixation, 219–220, 232–234
  - complications
    - deep vein thrombosis, 230
    - dislocation, 66, 230–231
    - heterotopic ossification, 231
    - infection, 230
    - intraoperative, 229–230
    - leg length discrepancy, 231
    - metal toxicity, 231–232
    - trochanteric nonunion, 231
  - hospital course, 229
  - imaging, 371, 372, 373, 374
  - indications and contraindications, 216
  - long-term results, 232–234
  - lower extremity function after, 345
  - medical considerations, 217
  - osteopenia and, 66, 67
  - physical therapy after, 387–389
    - functional milestone form, 392, 394
    - protocols, 389
  - rehabilitation, 229
  - surgical considerations, 217–218
  - surgical procedure
    - acetabular reconstruction, 219, 220, 223–225
    - course of posterior capsulotomy, 222
    - femoral reconstruction, 225–229
    - immediate preoperative preparation, 220–221
    - line of incision, 221
    - long-range preparation, 218–220
    - position for femoral neck osteotomy, 222
    - surgical approach, 221–222
- Total joint replacement, 370–371
  - occupational therapy after, 401–407
- Total knee arthroplasty, 241, 374
  - biplane and triplane deformity, 245–246, 247
  - bone deficit, 66, 67, 246–249
    - bone grafting for tibial deficiency, 61, 246, 249, 250
    - patellofemoral joint, 249, 251
  - complications
    - deep infection, 254–256
    - deep vein thrombosis, 256
    - delayed wound healing, 252
    - local, 252–254
    - superficial wound infection, 253–254
    - wound hematoma, 253
    - wound slough, 252–253
  - failure due to component loosening, 246
  - knee joint and, 242, 243
  - lower extremity function after, 347–348
  - operative technique
    - exposure, 242–243, 244
    - soft tissue balancing, 243–245
  - orthopaedic evaluation for, 242
  - physical therapy after, 390–394
    - functional milestone form, 393
    - protocols, 391
  - postoperative rehabilitation, 251

Total knee arthroplasty (*cont.*)
 results, 256–258
 revision replacement, 258
  bone deficits, 259–260
  implant removal, 258–259
Total shoulder arthroplasty, 132–133, 374–375
 complications, 141–144
 elbow replacement and, 133
 indications and contraindications, 133
 occupational therapy after, 401, 402, 404
 postoperative rehabilitation, 139–140
 preoperative considerations, 133–134
 prostheses, 134, 135, 137–138, 141
 results, 140–141
 surgical technique, 134–139
Total wrist arthroplasty, 180–182
 complications, 186
 goals, 182
 indications and contraindications, 182, 184
 prostheses, 180–182, 183, 184
 results, 185, 186–187
 technique, 184, 186
Traction, mechanical, 387
Trapezium, removal of, 192
Triple arthrodesis, for rheumatoid hindfoot, 303–309
Trochanteric nonunion, after total hip arthroplasty, 231
Tuberculous arthritis, 13

U

Ulcers, vasculitic, 355–356
Ulna, distal, resection arthroplasty of (*see* Distal ulnar resection)
Ulnar drift, 196, 197–198
Ultrasonography, of appendicular skeleton, 27, 29
Ultrasound therapy, 386
Upper extremity
 multiple joint involvement, 65
 postoperative rehabilitation, 63, 64–65

V

Valvular disease, RA-associated, 71
Vasculitis, 355–356
 types, 317, 355
Venous thrombosis, contrast venography of, 40
Vocal cords, in RA with laryngeal involvement, 79
Volar subluxation, 197–198
Volar synovectomy, 207–209
Volar synovitis, 207–209
Volar tenosynovectomy
 goals, 170
 indications and contraindications, 171
 results, 172
 technique, 171–172
Volz prosthesis, 182

W

Waugh ankle prosthesis, 296
Weichselbaum lacunae, 50
Wheelchair dependency, 20
Whirlpool, 386
Wound closure, 60
Wound considerations, after total knee arthroplasty
 healing, 252
 hematoma, 253
 infection
  deep, 254–256
  superficial, 253–254
 slough, 252–253
Wound problems, in hindfoot surgery, 298–299, 310
Wrist, 161–187
 anatomy, 161–163
 biomechanics, 163
 carpal fusion, 366, 367
 carpal measurements, 167–168
 carpal tunnel syndrome, 167
 carpometacarpal joint destruction, with ankylosis of carpal bones, 193, 194
 clinical presentation, 165–167
 computed tomography, 169
 conservative treatment, 170
 distal radioulnar joint, 162, 164
 dorsal compartments, 162–163
 dorsal synovitis, 166
 injections, 170
 ligaments, 161–162
 magnetic resonance imaging, 33, 169
 pathophysiology, 163–165
 radiocarpal collapse, 163–164
 radiographic findings
  ankylosis of radioscaphoid and radioulnate joints, 26
  arthrography, 169, 170
  normal anatomy, 167–168
  pathologic changes, 168–170
 splints, 170
 tendon rupture, 164–165
 tenosynovitis, 356, 366
 volar synovitis, 166–167
Wrist surgery, 170–186
 algorithm, 186
 arthrodesis, 177, 178, 369
  pan-, 178–180
  radiolunate and radioscapholunate, 177–178, 179
 arthroplasty
  palmar shelf, 180
  total (*see* Total wrist arthroplasty)
 distal ulnar resection, 172–175, 368–369
 dorsal stabilization, 175, 176
 dorsal tenosynovectomy, 175–177
 tendon ruptures, 177
 treatment goals, 170
 volar tenosynovectomy, 170–172